PDR® -for all of your drug information needs.

W9-CKH-712

Physicians' Desk Reference®

Physicians have turned to the PDR for the latest word on prescription drugs for 57 years. Today, PDR is still considered the standard prescription drug reference and can be found in virtually every physician's office, hospital and pharmacy in the United States. You can search the more than 4,000 drugs by using one of many indices and look at more than 2,100 full-color photos of drugs cross-referenced to the label information. More than 3,000 pages!

PDR® Companion Guide™

This unique 1,900-page all-in-one clinical companion to the PDR ensures safe, appropriate drug selection with nine critical checkpoint indices including *Indications, Side Effects, Interactions, Off-Label Treatment* and much more.

PDR® Pharmacopoeia™ Pocket Dosing Guide – Third Edition 2003

This pocket dosing guide brings important dispensing information to the practitioner's fingertips. Organized in tabular format, this small, 300-page quick reference is easy to navigate and gives important FDA-approved dosing information, black box warning summaries and much more, whenever it is needed. At the point of care, rely on PDR Pharmacopoeia for quick dosing information.

PDR® for Nutritional Supplements™ – 1st Edition

The definitive information source for more than 200 nutritional supplements. This first, comprehensive, unbiased source of solid, evidence-based information about nutritional supplements provides practitioners with more than 700 pages of the most current and reliable information available.

PDR for Nonprescription Drugs and Dietary Supplements™

This acknowledged authority offers full FDA-approved descriptions of the most commonly used OTC medicines. Plus, it includes a section on supplements, vitamins and herbal remedies.

PDR® for Herbal Medicines™ – 2nd Edition

This guide, the most comprehensive reference on herbal remedies, is based upon the work of Germany's Commission E and Jöerg Gruenwald, Ph.D., a renowned expert on herbal medicines. This detailed guide provides more than 1,100 pages of thorough descriptions on over 600 botanical remedies.

PDR for Ophthalmic Medicines™

The definitive reference for the eye-care professional offers 230 pages of detailed information on drugs and equipment used in the fields of ophthalmology and optometry. With five full indices and information on specialized instruments, lenses and much more, this guide is the most comprehensive of its kind.

PDR® Medical Dictionary™ – 2nd Edition

This fully updated edition, with more than 2,100 pages, includes extensive images and tables, an innovative Genus Finder to help you find the genus of organisms, and much more!

Complete Your 2003 PDR® Library NOW! Enclose payment and save shipping costs.

Code			Price	$
104901	___ copies **2003 Physicians' Desk Reference®**		$89.95 ea.	$ _____
104919	___ copies **2003 PDR® Companion Guide™**		$66.95 ea.	$ _____
104992	___ copies **PDR Pharmacopoeia™ Pocket Dosing Guide***		$9.95 ea.	$ _____
104968	___ copies **PDR® for Nutritional Supplements™, 1st EDITION!**		$59.95 ea.	$ _____
104935	___ copies **2003 PDR for Nonprescription Drugs and Dietary Supplements™**		$58.95 ea.	$ _____
104950	___ copies **PDR® for Herbal Medicines™, 2nd EDITION!**		$59.95 ea.	$ _____
104927	___ copies **2003 PDR for Ophthalmic Medicines™**		$63.95 ea.	$ _____
104943	___ copies **PDR® Medical Dictionary™, 2nd EDITION!**		$49.95 ea.	$ _____

Shipping & Handling (Add $9.95 S&H per book if paying later*) $ _____
Sales Tax (FL, GA, IA, & NJ) $ _____
Total Amount of Order $ _____

(*Shipping and handling is $1.95 for PDR Pharmacopoeia)

Mail this order form to: **PDR**, P.O. Box 10689, Des Moines, IA 50336-0689
e-mail: customer.service@medec.com

For Faster Service—FAX YOUR ORDER (515) 284-6714 or CALL TOLL-FREE (888) 859-8053
Do not mail a confirmation order in addition to this fax.

Valid for 2003 editions only, prices and shipping & handling higher outside U.S.

SAVE TIME AND MONEY EVERY YEAR AS A STANDING ORDER SUBSCRIBER

☐ Check here to enter your standing order for future editions of publications ordered. They will be shipped to you automatically, after advance notice. As a standing order subscriber, you are **guaranteed** our lowest price offer, earliest delivery and FREE shipping and handling.

PLEASE INDICATE METHOD OF PAYMENT:
Payment Enclosed (shipping & handling FREE)
☐ Check payable to PDR
☐ VISA   ☐ MasterCard
☐ Discover   ☐ American Express

Account No. _____

Exp. Date _____

Telephone No. _____

Signature _____

Name _____

Address _____

City _____

State/Zip _____

☐ **Bill me later** (Add $9.95 per book for shipping and handling*)

KEY 766501

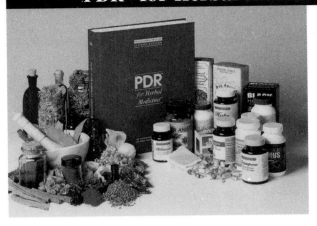
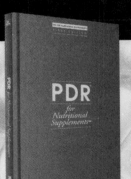

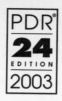

PDR®
24
EDITION
2003

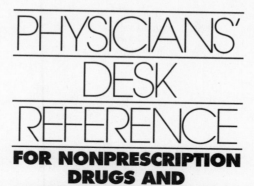

PHYSICIANS' DESK REFERENCE

FOR NONPRESCRIPTION DRUGS AND DIETARY SUPPLEMENTS™

Executive Vice President, Physicians' Desk Reference: Paul Walsh

Vice President, Sales and Marketing:
Dikran N. Barsamian

Director, Pharmaceutical Sales: Anthony Sorce

Senior Account Manager: Frank Karkowsky

Account Managers: Eileen Sullivan,
Suzanne E. Yarrow, RN

Director, Trade Sales: Bill Gaffney

Director of Product Management: Valerie E. Berger

Senior Product Manager: Jeffrey D. Dubin

Director of Financial Planning and Analysis:
Mark S. Ritchin

Senior Director, Publishing Sales and Marketing:
Michael Bennett

Direct Mail Managers: Jennifer M. Fronzaglia,
Lorraine M. Loening

Senior Marketing Analyst: Dina A. Maeder

Promotion Manager: Linda Levine

Vice President, Regulatory Affairs and Labeling:
Mukesh Mehta, RPh

Manager, Professional Data Services:
Thomas Fleming, PharmD

Manager, Concise Data Content:
Christine Wyble, PharmD

Drug Information Specialists: Maria Deutsch, MS,
PharmD; Greg Tallis, RPh

Editor, Directory Services: Bette LaGow

Senior Editor: Lori Murray

Production Editor: Gwynned L. Kelly

Senior Director, Production Services: Brian Holland

Director, PDR Operations: Jeffrey D. Schaefer

PDR Production Manager: Joseph Rizzo

Manager, Production Operations: Thomas Westburgh

Senior Production Coordinator: Christina Klinger

Production Coordinators: Gianna Caradonna,
Yasmin Hernandez

Index Editors: Noel Deloughery, Shannon Reilly

Format Editor: Michelle Guzman

Art Associate: Joan K. Akerlind

Digital Imaging Coordinator: Michael Labruyere

Production Design Supervisor: Adeline Rich

Electronic Publishing Designers: Bryan Dix,
Rosalia Sberna, Livio Udina

Fulfillment Managers: Louis J. Bolcik,
Stephanie Struble

Officers of Thomson Healthcare, Inc.: *President and Chief Executive Officer:* Richard Noble; *Chief Financial Officer:* Paul Hilger; *Executive Vice President, Clinical Trials:* Tom Kelly; *Executive Vice President, Medical Education:* Jeff MacDonald; *Executive Vice President, Clinical Solutions:* Jeff Reihl; *Executive Vice President, Medical Education & Communications:* Terry Meacock; *Executive Vice President, Physicians' Desk Reference:* Paul Walsh; *Senior Vice President, Business Development:* William Gole; *Vice President, Human Resources:* Pamela M. Bilash; *President, Physician's World:* Marty Cearnal

ISBN: 1-56363-451-1

FOREWORD

Physicians' Desk Reference has been providing unparalled drug information to doctors and other allied professionals for more than 50 years. In 2002, mental health professionals welcomed the debut of a PDR reference developed just for them—*The PDR Drug Guide for Mental Health Professionals™*. Now psychologists, social workers, school nurses, and family therapists have a resource to help them understand the effects of certain psychotropic drugs, herbs, and supplements that their clients may be taking. Mental health professionals today need to be as knowledgeable as possible about psychotropic drugs, and this addition to the PDR reference library addresses this need.

For complicated cases and special patient problems, there is of course no substitute for the in-depth data contained in *Physicians' Desk Reference*. But on other occasions, you may find that the new *PDR® Monthly Prescribing Guide™* provides a practical alternative. Distilled from the pages of *PDR*, this 360-page digest-sized reference presents the key facts on more than 1,000 drugs, including the form, strength, and route; therapeutic class; approved indications; dosage; contraindications; warnings; precautions; pregnancy rating; drug interactions; and adverse reactions. Each entry alerts you to the significant precautions you need to take, spells out the most common or dangerous adverse effects, summarizes the recommended adult and pediatric dosages, and supplies you with the *PDR* page number to turn to for further information.

Issued monthly, the guide is continuously updated with the latest FDA-approved revisions to existing product information, augmented with detailed descriptions of recently approved medications. In addition, you'll receive bulletins about major new pharmaceutical developments, an overview of important new agents nearing approval, an update on the latest news on herbal and nutritional supplements, and a handy reminder of upcoming medical meetings. In fact, in one neat package you'll find just about everything you need to make a routine prescribing decision—secure in the knowledge that you're acting on the latest FDA-approved data. To order your personal subscription to this important new monthly publication, simply call 800-232-7379.

If you prefer to keep information such as this on a handheld device like a Palm® or Pocket PC, another of our other reference guides may be just what you're looking for. Called **mobilePDR™**, this easy-to-use software allows you to instantly retrieve the basic facts you need on any drug, lets you run automatic interaction checks on multidrug regimens, and even alerts you to significant events such as product recalls, new product introductions, and new dosing and indication approvals. Covering a total of 1,600 drugs, this portable electronic reference is updated daily based on the latest FDA-approved package inserts. mobilePDR is available for downloading at www.PDR.net. It works with both the Palm and Pocket PC operating systems, and it's free to U.S.–based MDs, DOs, NPs, and PAs in full-time patient practice as well as to medical students and residents. Check it out today.

Other Prescribing Aids from PDR

For those times when all you need is quick confirmation of a particular dosage, you may also want to order a copy of the **PDR Pharmacopoeia™ Pocket Dosing Guide**. This handy little book can accompany you around the office or on rounds. Only slightly larger than an index card and half an inch thick, it fits easily into any pocket, while providing you with FDA-approved dosing recommendations for more than 1,500 drugs. Unlike other condensed drug references, it's drawn almost exclusively from the FDA-approved drug labeling published in *Physicians' Desk Reference*. And its tabular presentation makes lookups a breeze. At $9.95 a copy, it's a tool you really can't afford to be without.

Recently, the use of OTC nutritional supplements has skyrocketed, and PDR has responded with a medical reference covering this unfamiliar—even exotic—set of agents. **PDR® for Nutritional Supplements™** offers the latest scientific consensus on hundreds of popular supplement products, including an array of amino acids, co-factors, fatty acids, probiotics, phytoestrogens, phytosterols, OTC hormones, hormonal precursors, and much more. Focused on the scientific evidence for each supplement's claims, this unique new reference offers you today's most detailed, informed, and objective overview of a burgeoning new area in the field of self-treatment. To protect your patients from bogus remedies and steer them toward truly beneficial products, this book is a must.

For counseling patients who favor herbal remedies, another *PDR* reference may prove equally valuable. Now in its second edition, **PDR® for Herbal Medicines™** provides you with the latest science-based assessment of some 700 botanicals. Indexed by scientific, common, and brand names (as well as Western, Asian, and homeopathic indications) this volume also includes a Side Effects Index, a Drug/Herb Interactions Guide, an Herb Identification Guide with nearly 400 color photos, and a Safety Guide that lists herbs to be avoided during pregnancy and herbs to be used only under professional supervision. Although botanical products are not officially regulated or monitored in the United States, *PDR for Herbal Medicines* provides you with the closest analog to FDA-approved labeling—the findings of the German Regulatory Authority's herbal watchdog agency, Commission E.

To maximize the value of *PDR* itself, you'll also need a copy of the 2003 edition of the **PDR Companion Guide™,** an 1,800-page reference that augments PDR with a total of nine unique decision-making tools, including: an Interactions Index; a Food Interactions Cross-Reference; a Side Effects Index; an Indications Index; an Off-Label Treatment Guide; a Contra-indications Index; an International Drug Name Index; a Generic Availability Guide; and an Imprint Identification Guide. The *PDR Companion Guide* includes all drugs described in *PDR, PDR for Nonprescription Drugs and Dietary Supplements™,* and *PDR for Ophthalmic Medicines™.*

PDR and its major companion volumes are also found in the **PDR® Electronic Library™** on CD-ROM, now used in over 100,000 practices. This Windows compatible disc provides users with a complete database of *PDR* prescribing information, electronically searchable for instant retrieval. A standard subscription includes *PDR*'s sophisticated search software and an extensive file of chemical structures, illustrations, and full-color product photographs. Optional enhancements include the complete contents of *The Merck Manual Seventeenth Edition, Stedman's Medical Dictionary,* and *Stedman's Spellchecker.* For anyone who wants to run a fast double check on a proposed prescription, there's also the *PDR® Drug Interactions and Side Effects System™* — sophisticated software capable of automatically screening a 20-drug regimen for conflicts, then proposing alternatives for any problematic medication. This unique decision-making tool now comes free with the PDR Electronic Library.

For more information on these or any other members of the growing family of PDR products, please call, toll-free, 800-232-7379 or fax 201-722-2680.

How to Use This Book
Physicians' Desk Reference for Nonprescription Drugs and Dietary Supplements is comprised of five color-coded indices and a full-color Product Identification Guide followed by two distinct sections of product information. The first of these, entitled *Nonprescription Drug Information,* presents descriptions of conventional remedies marketed in compliance with the Code of Federal Regulations labeling requirements for over-the-counter drugs. The second section, entitled *Dietary Supplement Information,* contains information on herbal remedies and nutritional supplements marketed under the Dietary Supplement Health and Education Act of 1994. For your convenience, products in both sections are listed in the consolidated indices at the front of the book.

Physicians' Desk Reference for Nonprescription Drugs and Dietary Supplements is published annually by Thomson PDR in cooperation with participating manufacturers. The function of the publisher is the compilation, organization, and distribution of product information obtained from manufacturers. Each product description has been prepared by the manufacturer, and edited and approved by the manufacturer's medical department, medical director, and/or medical consultant. During compilation of this information, the publisher has emphasized the necessity of describing products comprehensively in order to provide all the facts necessary for sound and intelligent decision-making. Descriptions seen here include all information made available by the manufacturer. Please note that descriptions of OTC products marketed under the Dietary Supplement Health and Education Act of 1994 have not been evaluated by the Food and Drug Administration, and that such products are not intended to diagnose, treat, cure, or prevent any disease.

In organizing and presenting the material in *Physicians' Desk Reference for Nonprescription Drugs and Dietary Supplements,* the publisher does not warrant or guarantee any of the products described, or perform any independent analysis in connection with any of the product information contained herein. *Physicians' Desk Reference* does not assume, and expressly disclaims, any obligation to obtain and include any information other than that provided to it by the manufacturer. It should be understood that by making this material available, the publisher is not advocating the use of any product described herein, nor is the publisher responsible for misuse of a product due to typographical error. Additional information on any product may be obtained from the manufacturer.

CONTENTS

MANUFACTURERS' INDEX

This index lists manufacturers that have supplied information for this edition. Each company's entry includes the address, phone, and fax number of its headquarters and regional offices, as well as company contacts for inquiries, orders, and emergency information.

Products with entries in the Nonprescription Drug Information section are listed with their page numbers under the heading "OTC Products Described." Products with entries in the Dietary Supplement Information section are listed with their page numbers under the heading "Dietary Supplements Described." Other OTC products and dietary supplements available from the manufacturer follow these two sections.

If an entry in the index lists multiple page numbers, the first one shown refers to the photograph of the product, the last one to its prescribing information.

- The ◆ symbol marks drugs shown in the Product Identification Guide.

- *Italic page numbers* signify partial information.

A & Z PHARMACEUTICAL INC.   **503, 796**

180 Oser Avenue, Suite 300
Hauppauge, NY 11788
Direct Inquiries to:
Customer Service
(631) 952-3800
FAX: (631) 952-3900

Dietary Supplements Described:
◆ D-Cal Chewable Caplets **503, 796**

A. C. GRACE COMPANY   **602**

1100 Quitman Rd.
P.O. Box 570
Big Sandy, TX 75755
Direct Inquiries to:
(903) 636-4368
Orders Only:
(800) 833-4368

OTC Products Described:
Unique E Vitamin E Capsules **602**

ADAMS LABORATORIES, INC.   **602**

14801 Sovereign Road
Fort Worth, TX 76155
Direct Inquiries to:
Medical Affairs
(817) 786-1200

OTC Products Described:
Mucinex 600mg
    Extended-Release Tablets **602**
Mucinex 1200mg
    Extended-Release Tablets **602**

AK PHARMA INC.   **503, 796**

P.O. Box 111
Pleasantville, NJ 08232-0111
Direct Inquiries to:
Elizabeth Klein
(609) 645-5100
FAX: (609) 645-0767
For Medical Emergencies Contact:
Alan E. Kligerman
(609) 645-5100

Dietary Supplements Described:
◆ Prelief Tablets and Granulate **503, 796**

ALPHARMA   **602**

U.S. Pharmaceuticals Division
7205 Windsor Boulevard
Baltimore, MD 21244
Direct Inquiries to:
Customer Service
(800) 432-8534

OTC Products Described:
Permethrin Lotion. **602**

AMERICAN LONGEVITY   **797**

2400 Boswell Road
Chula Vista, CA 91914
Direct Inquiries to:
Customer Service
(800) 982-3189
FAX: (619) 934-3205
www.americanlongevity.net

Dietary Supplements Described:
Majestic Earth Ultimate Osteo-FX *797*
Plant Derived Minerals Liquid *797*

AMERIFIT NUTRITION, INC.   **503, 797**

166 Highland Park Drive
Bloomfield, CT 06002
Direct Inquiries to:
Consumer Affairs
(800) 722-3476
FAX: (860) 243-9400
www.amerifit.com

Dietary Supplements Described:
◆ Estroven Caplets **503, 797**
◆ Estroven Gelcaps **503, 797**
◆ Vitaball Vitamin Gumballs *503, 797*

AWARENESS CORPORATION/dba AWARENESSLIFE   **503, 798**

25 South Arizona Place, Suite 500
Chandler, AZ 85225
Direct Inquiries to:
(800) 69AWARE
www.awarecorp.com
www.awarenesslife.com

Dietary Supplements Described:
Awareness Clear Capsules **798**
◆ Awareness Female Balance
    Capsules **503, 798**
◆ Daily Complete Liquid. **503, 798**
◆ Experience Capsules **503, 798**
◆ Pure Garden Cream. **503, 799**

BAYER HEALTHCARE LLC CONSUMER CARE DIVISION   **503, 603**

36 Columbia Road
P.O. Box 1910
Morristown, NJ 07962-1910

GLAXOSMITHKLINE CONSUMER HEALTHCARE, L.P.—cont.

GREEN PHARMACEUTICALS INC.,   508, 661

1459 E. Thousand Oaks Blvd., #3
Thousand Oaks, CA 91362
Direct Inquiries and Medical Emergencies to:
(800) 337-4835
E-mail: mail@snorestop.com

OTC Products Described:

HYLAND'S, INC.

(See STANDARD HOMEOPATHIC COMPANY)

JOHNSON & JOHNSON •   508, 662
MERCK CONSUMER PHARMACEUTICALS CO.

7050 Camp Hill Road
Fort Washington, PA 19034
Direct Inquiries to:
Consumer Relationship Center
Fort Washington, PA 19034
(215) 273-7000

OTC Products Described:

KYOWA   509, 809
ENGINEERING-SUNDORY

5-964 Nakamozu-Cho, Sakai-City
Osaka, Japan
Direct Inquiries to:
Consumer Relations
82-722-57-8568
Osaka
FAX: 81-722-57-8655
www.sundory.co.jp

Dietary Supplements Described:

LEDERLE CONSUMER HEALTHCARE

(See WYETH CONSUMER HEALTHCARE)

LEGACY FOR LIFE, LLC   811

P.O. Box 410376
Melbourne, FL 32941-0376
Direct Inquiries to:
(800) 557-8477
(321) 951-8815
www.legacyforlife.net

Dietary Supplements Described:

Other Products Available:
BioChoice FLEX Capsules
BioChoice SLIM Capsules

MAITAKE PRODUCTS, INC.   811

P.O. Box 1534
Paramus, NJ 07653
Direct Inquiries to:
(800) 747-7418
www.maitake.com

Dietary Supplements Described:

MANNATECH, INC.   509, 811

600 S. Royal Lane
Suite 200
Coppell, TX 75019
Direct Inquiries to:
Customer Service
(972) 471-8111
For Medical Information Contact:
Kia Gary, RN LNCC
(972) 471-8189
E-mail: Kgary@mannatech.com
www.mannatech.com
(for product information)
www.glycoscience.com
(for ingredient information)

Dietary Supplements Described:

Other Products Available:
AmbroDerm Lotion
AmbroStart Beverage Mix
CardioBALANCE Heart Support Formula Capsules
EM-PACT Sports Drink
Emprizone Hydrogel
FIRM with Ambrotose Lotion
Glycentials Vitamin, Ambroglycin Mineral and Antioxidant Formula Tablets
Glyco-Bears Children's Chewable Vitamins and Minerals
GlycoLEAN Accelerator 2 Capsules
GlycoLEAN Catalyst with Ambroglycin Caplets
GlycoLEAN Fiber Full Capsules
GlycoSLIM GlycoLEAN Drinks
ImmunoSTART Chewables
Manna-C Capsules
Manna-Cleanse Caplets
Mannatonin Tablets
Phyto-Bear Supplements
Protein MannaBAR Supplement Bar
Sport Capsules
Vanilla Yogurt-Coated Apple Crunch MannaBar Supplement Bar

MATOL BOTANICAL   509, 813
INTERNATIONAL LTD.

290 Labrosse Avenue
Pointe-Claire, Quebec
Canada, H9R 6R6
Direct Inquiries to:
(800) 363-1890
www.matol.com

Dietary Supplements Described:

MAYOR PHARMACEUTICAL   813
LABORATORIES

2401 South 24th Street
Phoenix, AZ 85034
Direct Inquiries to:
Medical Director
(602) 244-8899
www.vitamist.com

Dietary Supplements Described:

(◆) **Shown in Product Identification Guide**   *Italic Page Number* **Indicates Brief Listing**

For Medical Emergencies Contact:
Professional Services
(763) 475-3023
(800) 654-2299
FAX: (763) 475-3410
Branch Offices:
13700 1st Avenue N.
Plymouth, MN 55441
(763) 475-3023
FAX: (763) 475-3410
OTC Products Described:

WARNER-LAMBERT COMPANY
(See PFIZER CONSUMER GROUP, PFIZER INC.)

WARNER-LAMBERT CONSUMER HEALTHCARE
(See PFIZER CONSUMER HEALTHCARE, PFIZER INC.)

WELLNESS INTERNATIONAL NETWORK, LTD.   772
5800 Democracy Drive
Plano, TX 75024
Direct Inquiries to:
Product Coordinator
(972) 312-1100
FAX: (972) 943-5250

OTC Products Described:

WHITEHALL-ROBINS HEALTHCARE
(See WYETH CONSUMER HEALTHCARE)

WYETH CONSUMER HEALTHCARE   774
Wyeth
Five Giralda Farms
Madison, NJ 07940-0871
Direct Inquiries to:
Wyeth Consumer Healthcare
(800) 322-3129 (9-5 E.S.T.)

OTC Products Described:

Other Products Available:

WYETH CONSUMER HEALTHCARE—
cont.
Robitussin Honey Flu Nighttime Mix-In
Robitussin Honey Flu Non-Drowsy Mix-In
Robitussin Night Relief Liquid
Robitussin Pediatric Night Relief Drops

YOUNGEVITY INC., THE   **834**
ANTI-AGING COMPANY
3100 East Plano Parkway
Plano, TX 75074
Direct Inquiries to:
(972) 239-6864, Ext. 108

FAX: (972) 404-3067
E-mail: asd@youngevity.com
www.youngevity.com

Dietary Supplements Described:

SECTION 2

PRODUCT NAME INDEX

This index includes all entries in the Product Information sections. Products are listed alphabetically by brand name.

If an entry in the index lists multiple page numbers, the first one shown refers to the photograph of the product, the last one to its prescribing information.

- **Bold page numbers** indicate that the entry contains full product information.

- *Italic page numbers* signify partial information.

Italic Page Number **Indicates Brief Listing**

Italic Page Number **Indicates Brief Listing**

SECTION 3

PRODUCT CATEGORY INDEX

This index cross-references each brand by pharmaceutical category. All fully described products in the Product Information sections are included.

If an entry in the index lists multiple page numbers, the first one shown refers to the photograph of the product,

the last one to its prescribing information.

The classification of each product is determined by the publisher in cooperation with the product's manufacturer or, when necessary, by the publisher alone.

E

EAR WAX REMOVAL
(*see under:*
OTIC PREPARATIONS
CERUMENOLYTICS)

ELECTROLYTES
(*see under:*
DIETARY SUPPLEMENTS
MINERALS & ELECTROLYTES)

EXPECTORANTS
(*see under:*
RESPIRATORY AGENTS
DECONGESTANTS, EXPECTORANTS & COMBINATIONS
EXPECTORANTS & COMBINATIONS)

F

FEVER PREPARATIONS
(*see under:*
ANALGESICS
ACETAMINOPHEN & COMBINATIONS
NONSTEROIDAL ANTI-INFLAMMATORY DRUGS (NSAIDS)
SALICYLATES)

FOOT CARE PRODUCTS
(*see under:*
SKIN & MUCOUS MEMBRANE AGENTS
FOOT CARE PRODUCTS)

FUNGAL MEDICATIONS
(*see under:*
SKIN & MUCOUS MEMBRANE AGENTS
ANTI-INFECTIVES
ANTIFUNGALS & COMBINATIONS)

G

GASTROINTESTINAL AGENTS

ANTACIDS

SECTION 4

ACTIVE INGREDIENTS INDEX

This index cross-references each brand by its generic ingredients. All entries in the Product Information sections are included. Under each generic heading, all fully described products are listed first, followed by those with only partial descriptions.

If an entry in the index lists multiple page numbers, the first one shown refers to the photograph of the

product, the last one to its prescribing information.

- **Bold page numbers** indicate full product information.
- *Italic page numbers* signify partial information.

Classification of products under these headings has been determined in cooperation with the products' manufacturers or, if necessary, by the publisher alone.

Italic Page Number **Indicates Brief Listing**

DOXYLAMINE SUCCINATE
Alka-Seltzer Plus Night-Time
Cold Medicine Liqui-Gels
(Bayer Healthcare) **503, 608**
Alka-Seltzer Plus Night-Time Cold
Medicine Effervescent Tablets
(Bayer Healthcare) **607**
Maximum Strength Tylenol Flu
NightTime Liquid (McNeil
Consumer) **513, 682**
Maximum Strength Tylenol
Sinus NightTime Caplets
(McNeil Consumer) **513, 684**
Unisom SleepTabs (Pfizer
Consumer Healthcare) **522, 742**
Vicks NyQuil Cough Liquid
(Procter & Gamble) **523, 758**
Vicks NyQuil LiquiCaps/Liquid
Multi-Symptom Cold/Flu
Relief (Procter & Gamble)..... **523, 758**

E
ECHINACEA
Halls Defense Multiblend
Supplement Drops (Pfizer
Consumer Group) **516, 712**
ECHINACEA ANGUSTIFOLIA
VitaMist Intra-Oral Spray (Mayor) **813**
Echinacea + G (Mayor)................ *813*
EGG PRODUCT
Transfer Factor Cardio Capsules
(4Life) **805**
EGG PRODUCT, HYPERIMMUNE
immune[26] Powder and Capsules
(Legacy for Life) **811**
immune Support Powder (Legacy for
Life)................................. **811**
ELECTROLYTE REPLACEMENT
B-Fit Drink Mix (Mayor).................. *813*
EPHEDRA
BioLean Tablets (Wellness
International)......................... **821**
EPHEDRINE HYDROCHLORIDE
Primatene Tablets (Wyeth).............. **785**
EPINEPHRINE
Primatene Mist (Wyeth).................. **785**
ETHYL AMINOBENZOATE
(*see under:* **BENZOCAINE**)
ETHYLHEXYL METHOXYCINNAMATE
Bio-Complex 5000 Revitalizing
Conditioner (Wellness
International)......................... **772**
Bio-Complex 5000 Revitalizing
Shampoo (Wellness
International)......................... **772**
StePHan Bio-Nutritional Nightime
Moisture Creme (Wellness
International)......................... **773**
EUCALYPTOL
Listerine Mouthrinse (Pfizer
Consumer Healthcare)........ **519, 729**
Cool Mint Listerine Mouthrinse
(Pfizer Consumer
Healthcare)................... **519, 729**
FreshBurst Listerine
Mouthrinse (Pfizer
Consumer Healthcare) **519, 729**
Tartar Control Listerine
Mouthwash (Pfizer
Consumer Healthcare)........ **519, 729**
EUCALYPTUS, OIL OF
Vicks VapoRub Cream (Procter &
Gamble) **761**
Vicks VapoRub Ointment (Procter &
Gamble) **761**

F
FAMOTIDINE
Pepcid AC Tablets, Chewable
Tablets, and Gelcaps
(J&J • Merck)............... **509, 665**
Pepcid Complete Chewable
Tablets (J&J • Merck)........ **509, 665**
FATTY ACIDS
Anti-Aging Daily Premium Pak
(Youngevity) **834**
VitaMist Intra-Oral Spray (Mayor) **813**
Blue-Green Sea Spray (Mayor)........ *813*
Premium Hawaiian Noni Juice
(Youngevity) *835*
FERROUS FUMARATE
Ferretts Tablets (Pharmics, Inc.) **818**
FERROUS GLUCONATE
Fergon Iron Tablets (Bayer
Healthcare).................... **504, 799**
FERROUS SULFATE
Feosol Tablets
(GlaxoSmithKline)............ **506, 807**
Slow Fe Tablets (Novartis
Consumer)................... **515, 816**
Slow Fe with Folic Acid Tablets
(Novartis Consumer)......... **515, 817**
FIBER, DIETARY
Benefiber Supplement
(Novartis Consumer).......... **513, 816**
FOLIC ACID
Slow Fe with Folic Acid Tablets
(Novartis Consumer)......... **515, 817**

G
GARLIC
(*see under:* **ALLIUM SATIVUM**)
GARLIC EXTRACT
VitaMist Intra-Oral Spray (Mayor) **813**
Echinacea + G (Mayor)................ *813*
GINKGO BILOBA
Anti-Aging Daily Premium Pak
(Youngevity) **834**
BioLean Free Tablets (Wellness
International)......................... **822**
Centrum Performance Complete
Multivitamin-Multimineral Tablets
(Wyeth)............................. **833**
DHEA Plus Capsules (Wellness
International)......................... **823**
One-A-Day Memory & Concentration
Tablets (Bayer Healthcare).......... **802**
Phyto-Vite Tablets (Wellness
International)......................... **828**
Satiete Tablets (Wellness
International)......................... **825**
StePHan Clarity Capsules (Wellness
International)......................... **826**
StePHan Elixir Capsules (Wellness
International)......................... **827**
VitaMist Intra-Oral Spray (Mayor) **813**
GinkgoMist (Mayor) *813*
St. John's Wort (Mayor)............... *813*
VitaSight (Mayor) *813*
Power Circulation Tablets
(Sunpower) *820*
Premium Hawaiian Noni Juice
(Youngevity) *835*
Sun Cardio Tablets (Sunpower)......... *820*
GINSENG
BioLean Free Tablets (Wellness
International)......................... **822**
Centrum Performance Complete
Multivitamin-Multimineral Tablets
(Wyeth) **833**
Dexatrim Results Caplets (Chattem) ... **631**

One-A-Day Active Tablets (Bayer
Healthcare).......................... **800**
One-A-Day Energy Formula Tablets
(Bayer Healthcare) **800**
5 Seng Tea (Sunpower)................. *820*
Power Refresh (Sunpower) *820*
GLUCOSAMINE
Sun Joint Tablets (Sunpower)........... *820*
GLUCOSAMINE HYDROCHLORIDE
Ambrotose Powder
(Mannatech).................. **509, 811**
Osteo Bi-Flex Plus Calcium
Caplets (Rexall Sundown) **523, 819**
Osteo Bi-Flex Triple Strength
Caplets (Rexall Sundown) **523, 819**
Sure2Endure Tablets (Wellness
International)......................... **830**
GLUCOSAMINE SULFATE
Dona Crystalline Glucosamine
Sulfate Caplets (Rotta) **819**
Dona Crystalline Glucosamine
Sulfate Powder for Oral
Suspension (Rotta) **819**
VitaMist Intra-Oral Spray (Mayor) **813**
ArthriFlex (Mayor) *813*
Majestic Earth Ultimate Osteo-FX
(American Longevity)................ *797*
GLYCERIN
Preparation H Cream (Wyeth).......... **783**
Visine Tears Eye Drops (Pfizer
Consumer Healthcare)........ **522, 744**
Visine Tears Preservative Free
Eye Drops (Pfizer
Consumer Healthcare)........ **522, 744**
GLYCERYL GUAIACOLATE
(*see under:* **GUAIFENESIN**)
GUAIFENESIN
Benylin Cough Suppressant/
Expectorant Liquid (Pfizer
Consumer Healthcare)........ **518, 723**
Mucinex 600mg Extended-Release
Tablets (Adams)..................... **602**
Mucinex 1200mg Extended-Release
Tablets (Adams)..................... **602**
Primatene Tablets (Wyeth)............. **785**
Robitussin Expectorant (Wyeth) **785**
Robitussin-CF Liquid (Wyeth) **792**
Robitussin Cold & Congestion
Caplets (Wyeth) **786**
Robitussin Cold & Congestion
Softgels (Wyeth) **786**
Robitussin Cold Severe Congestion
Softgels (Wyeth) **787**
Robitussin Cold Multi-Symptom Cold
& Flu Caplets (Wyeth)............... **786**
Robitussin Cold Multi-Symptom Cold
& Flu Softgels (Wyeth) **786**
Robitussin-DM Infant Drops (Wyeth) ... **791**
Robitussin-DM Liquid (Wyeth) **791**
Robitussin Cough & Cold Infant
Drops (Wyeth) **792**
Robitussin-PE Liquid (Wyeth) **790**
Robitussin Sinus & Congestion
Caplets (Wyeth) **790**
Robitussin Sugar Free Cough Liquid
(Wyeth) **791**
Sinutab Non-Drying Liquid
Caps (Pfizer Consumer
Healthcare).................. **520, 734**
Sudafed Non-Drowsy Cold &
Cough Liquid Caps (Pfizer
Consumer Healthcare)........ **520, 736**
Sudafed Non-Drying Sinus
Liquid Caps (Pfizer
Consumer Healthcare)........ **521, 737**

Italic Page Number **Indicates Brief Listing**

COMPANION DRUG INDEX

This index is a quick-reference guide to OTC products that may be used in conjunction with prescription drug therapy to reverse drug-induced side effects, relieve symptoms of the illness itself, or treat sequelae of the initial disease. All entries are derived from the FDA-approved prescribing information published by *PDR*.

The products listed are generally considered effective for temporary symptomatic relief. They may not, however, be appropriate for sustained therapy, and each case must be approached on an individual basis. Certain common side effects may be harbingers of more serious reactions. When making a recommendation, be sure to adjust for the patient's age, concurrent medical conditions, and complete drug regimen.

Consider timing as well, since simultaneous ingestion may not be recommended in all instances.

Please note that only products fully described in *Physicians' Desk Reference* and its companion volumes are included in this index. The publisher therefore cannot guarantee that all entries are totally accurate or complete. Keep in mind, too, that although a given OTC product is usually an appropriate companion for an entire class of prescription medications, certain drugs within the class may be exceptions. If you have any doubt about the suitability of a particular OTC product in a given situation, be sure to check the underlying *PDR* prescribing information and the relevant medical literature.

ALCOHOLISM, VITAMINS AND MINERALS DEFICIENCY SECONDARY TO

Alcoholism may be treated with disulfiram or naltrexone hydrochloride. The following products may be recommended for relief of vitamins and minerals deficiency:

ANCYLOSTOMIASIS, IRON-DEFICIENCY ANEMIA SECONDARY TO

Ancylostomiasis may be treated with mebendazole or thiabendazole. The following products may be recommended for relief of iron-deficiency anemia:

ANEMIA, IRON-DEFICIENCY

May result from the use of chronic salicylate therapy or nonsteroidal anti-inflammatory drugs. The following products may be recommended:

ANGINA, UNSTABLE

May be treated with beta blockers, calcium channel blockers or nitrates. The following products may be recommended for relief of symptoms:

ARTHRITIS

May be treated with corticosteroids or nonsteroidal anti-inflammatory drugs. The following products may be recommended for relief of symptoms:

BRONCHITIS, CHRONIC, ACUTE EXACERBATION OF

May be treated with quinolones, sulfamethoxazole-trimethoprim, cefixime, cefpodoxime proxetil, cefprozil, ceftibuten dihydrate, cefuroxime axetil, cilastatin, clarithromycin, imipenem or loracarbef. The following products may be recommended for relief of symptoms:

BURN INFECTIONS, SEVERE, NUTRIENTS DEFICIENCY SECONDARY TO

Severe burn infections may be treated with anti-infectives. The following products may be recommended for relief of nutrients deficiency:

CANCER, NUTRIENTS DEFICIENCY SECONDARY TO

Cancer may be treated with chemotherapeutic agents. The following products may be recommended for relief of nutrients deficiency:

CANDIDIASIS, VAGINAL

May be treated with antifungal agents. The following products may be recommended for relief of symptoms:

FLATULENCE

May result from the use of nonsteroidal anti-inflammatory drugs, potassium supplements, acarbose, cisapride, guanadrel sulfate, mesalamine, metformin hydrochloride, methyldopa, octreotide acetate or ursodiol. The following products may be recommended:

FLU-LIKE SYNDROME

May result from the use of gemcitabine hydrochloride, interferon alfa-2b, recombinant, interferon alfa-n3 (human leukocyte derived), interferon beta-1b, interferon gamma-1b or succimer. The following products may be recommended:

FLU-LIKE SYNDROME —cont.

Vicks DayQuil LiquiCaps/Liquid
Multi-Symptom Cold/Flu Relief..........**757**
Children's Vicks NyQuil
Cold/Cough Relief **756**
Vicks NyQuil LiquiCaps/Liquid
Multi-Symptom Cold/Flu Relief..........**758**

FLUSHING EPISODES
May result from the use of lipid lowering doses of niacin. The following products may be recommended:

Advil Caplets....................................**774**
Advil Gel Caplets..............................**774**
Advil Liqui-Gels...............................**774**
Advil Tablets....................................**774**
Ecotrin Enteric Coated Aspirin
Low Strength Tablets.......................**638**
Ecotrin Enteric Coated Aspirin
Maximum Strength Tablets **638**
Ecotrin Enteric Coated Aspirin
Regular Strength Tablets **638**
Motrin IB Tablets, Caplets,
and Gelcaps **668**

GASTRITIS, IRON-DEFICIENCY SECONDARY TO
Gastritis may be treated with histamine h2 receptor antagonists, proton pump inhibitors or sucralfate. The following products may be recommended for relief of iron deficiency:

Feosol Caplets..................................**806**
Feosol Tablets...................................**807**
Fergon Iron Tablets...........................**799**
Ferretts Tablets.................................**818**
Slow Fe Tablets.................................**816**
Slow Fe with Folic Acid Tablets **817**

GASTROESOPHAGEAL REFLUX DISEASE
May be treated with histamine h2 receptor antagonists, proton pump inhibitors or sucralfate. The following products may be recommended for relief of symptoms:

Alka-Seltzer Original Antacid
and Pain Reliever Effervescent
Tablets...**605**
Alka-Seltzer Cherry Antacid
and Pain Reliever Effervescent
Tablets...**605**
Alka-Seltzer Lemon Lime
Antacid and Pain Reliever
Effervescent Tablets **605**
Alka-Seltzer Extra Strength
Antacid and Pain Reliever
Effervescent Tablets **605**
Alka-Seltzer Heartburn
Relief Tablets **606**
Ex-Lax Milk of Magnesia
Liquid **695**
Gas-X with Maalox Extra
Strength Chewable Tablets **696**
Gaviscon Regular Strength
Liquid **641**
Gaviscon Extra Strength
Liquid **641**
Gaviscon Extra Strength
Tablets...**641**
Gas-X with Maalox Extra
Strength Softgels **696**
Maalox Regular Strength
Antacid/Anti-Gas Liquid **698**
Maalox Max Maximum Strength
Antacid/Anti-Gas Liquid **697**
Maalox Quick Dissolve
Regular Strength Antacid
Chewable Tablets **699**
Maalox Max Quick Dissolve
Maximum Strength
Chewable Tablets **699**
Children's Mylanta Upset
Stomach Relief Tablets **663**
Regular Strength Mylanta
Gelcaps..**664**
Extra Strength Mylanta
Liquid **663**
Regular Strength Mylanta
Liquid **663**
Mylanta Ultra Tabs............................**664**
Pepto-Bismol Original Liquid,
Original and Cherry
Chewable Tablets & Caplets............**753**
Pepto-Bismol Maximum Strength
Liquid **753**
Phillips' Chewable Tablets **621**
Phillips' Milk of Magnesia Liquid
(Original, Cherry, & Mint)................**622**
Rolaids Tablets..................................**734**
Extra Strength Rolaids
Tablets...**734**
Tums E-X Antacid/
Calcium Tablets **660**
Tums E-X Sugar Free
Antacid/Calcium Tablets..................**660**
Tums Regular Antacid/
Calcium Tablets **660**
Tums ULTRA Antacid/
Calcium Tablets **660**

GINGIVAL HYPERPLASIA
May result from the use of calcium channel blockers, cyclosporine, fosphenytoin sodium or phenytoin. The following products may be recommended:

Listerine Mouthrinse..........................**729**
Cool Mint Listerine
Mouthrinse **729**
FreshBurst Listerine
Mouthrinse **729**
Tartar Control Listerine
Mouthwash **729**
Sensodyne Original Flavor **657**
Sensodyne Cool Gel **657**
Sensodyne Extra Whitening **657**
Sensodyne Fresh Mint **657**
Sensodyne Tartar Control....................**657**
Sensodyne Tartar Control
Plus Whitening................................**657**
Sensodyne with Baking Soda **657**

HUMAN IMMUNODEFICIENCY VIRUS (HIV) INFECTIONS, NUTRIENTS DEFICIENCY SECONDARY TO
HIV infections may be treated with non-nucleoside reverse transcriptase inhibitors, nucleoside reverse transcriptase inhibitors or protease inhibitors. The following products may be recommended for relief of nutrients deficiency:

Anti-Aging Daily Premium Pak **834**
Centrum Tablets.................................**832**
Centrum Kids Complete
Children's Chewables.......................**832**
Centrum Performance Complete
Multivitamin-Multimineral
Tablets...**833**
Centrum Silver Tablets........................**833**
Daily Complete Liquid **798**
Flintstones Complete Children's
Mutivitamin/Multimineral
Chewable Tablets **799**
My First Flintstones
Multivitamin Tablets **799**
One-A-Day Kids Complete
Scooby Doo Multivitamin/
Multimineral Tablets **801**
One-A-Day Kids Bugs Bunny and
Friends Complete Sugar Free
Tablets...**801**
One-A-Day Kids Scooby Doo
Plus Calcium Multivitamin
Tablets...**802**

One-A-Day Men's Health
Formula Tablets...............................**802**
One-A-Day Today for
Active Women Tablets **803**
One-A-Day Women's Tablets **804**

HUMAN IMMUNODEFICIENCY VIRUS (HIV) INFECTIONS, SEBORRHEIC DERMATITIS SECONDARY TO
HIV infections may be treated with non-nucleoside reverse transcriptase inhibitors, nucleoside reverse transcriptase inhibitors or protease inhibitors. The following products may be recommended for relief of seborrheic dermatitis:

Nizoral A-D Shampoo **671**
Tegrin Dandruff Shampoo -
Extra Conditioning............................**659**
Tegrin Dandruff Shampoo -
Fresh Herbal....................................**660**
Tegrin Skin Cream **660**

HUMAN IMMUNODEFICIENCY VIRUS (HIV) INFECTIONS, XERODERMA SECONDARY TO
HIV infections may be treated with non-nucleoside reverse transcriptase inhibitors, nucleoside reverse transcriptase inhibitors or protease inhibitors. The following products may be recommended for relief of xeroderma:

Lubriderm Advanced Therapy
Creamy Lotion **730**
Lubriderm Seriously
Sensitive Lotion...............................**730**
Lubriderm Skin Firming Lotion **730**
Lubriderm Skin Therapy
Moisturizing Lotion **731**
StePHan Bio-Nutritional
Daytime Hydrating Creme **772**
StePHan Bio-Nutritional
Nightime Moisture Creme **773**
StePHan Bio-Nutritional
Ultra Hydrating Fluid........................**773**

HYPERTHYROIDISM, NUTRIENTS DEFICIENCY SECONDARY TO
Hyperthyroidism may be treated with methimazole. The following products may be recommended for relief of nutrients deficiency:

Anti-Aging Daily
Premium Pak....................................**834**
Centrum Tablets.................................**832**
Centrum Kids Complete
Children's Chewables.......................**832**
Centrum Performance Complete
Multivitamin-Multimineral
Tablets...**833**
Centrum Silver Tablets........................**833**
Daily Complete Liquid **798**
Flintstones Complete Children's
Mutivitamin/Multimineral
Chewable Tablets **799**
My First Flintstones
Multivitamin Tablets **799**
One-A-Day Kids Complete
Scooby Doo Multivitamin/
Multimineral Tablets **801**
One-A-Day Kids Bugs Bunny and
Friends Complete Sugar Free
Tablets...**801**
One-A-Day Kids Scooby Doo
Plus Calcium Multivitamin
Tablets...**802**
One-A-Day Men's Health
Formula Tablets...............................**802**
One-A-Day Today for
Active Women Tablets **803**
One-A-Day Women's Tablets **804**

HYPOKALEMIA

May result from the use of thiazides, thiazides, corticosteroids, diuretics, diuretics, aldesleukin, amphotericin b, carboplatin, etretinate, foscarnet sodium, mycophenolate mofetil, pamidronate disodium or tacrolimus. The following products may be recommended:

Chlor-3 Shaker **632**

HYPOMAGNESEMIA

May result from the use of aldesleukin, aminoglycosides, amphotericin b, caroboplatin, cisplatin, cyclosporine, diuretics, foscarnet, pamidronate, sargramostim or tacrolimus. The following products may be recommended:

Beelith Tablets **804**
Chlor-3 Shaker **632**
Magonate Liquid **804**
Magonate Natal Liquid **804**
Magonate Tablets **804**

HYPOPARATHYROIDISM

May be treated with vitamin d sterols. The following products may be recommended for relief of symptoms:

Caltrate 600 PLUS Tablets **831**
Caltrate 600 + D Tablets **831**
Caltrate 600 + Soy Tablets **831**
Citracal Liquitab
  Effervescent Tablets **816**
Citracal Tablets **815**
Citracal Caplets + D **816**
D-Cal Chewable Caplets...................**796**
Os-Cal Chewable Tablets **807**
Os-Cal 250 + D Tablets....................**807**
Os-Cal 500 Tablets **808**
Os-Cal 500 + D Tablets....................**808**
Tums E-X Antacid/Calcium
  Tablets.....................................**660**
Tums E-X Sugar Free
  Antacid/Calcium Tablets..................**660**
Tums Regular Antacid/Calcium
  Tablets.....................................**660**
Tums ULTRA Antacid/Calcium
  Tablets.....................................**660**

HYPOTHYROIDISM, CONSTIPATION SECONDARY TO

Hypothyroidism may be treated with thyroid hormones. The following products may be recommended for relief of constipation:

Ceo-Two Evacuant
  Suppository................................**625**
Citrucel Caplets...........................**635**
Citrucel Orange Flavor
  Powder......................................**634**
Citrucel Sugar Free
  Orange Flavor Powder......................**635**
Dulcolax Stool Softener **627**
Dulcolax Suppositories **626**
Ex-Lax Regular Strength
  Pills......................................**695**
Ex-Lax Regular Strength
  Chocolated Pieces **694**
Ex-Lax Maximum Strength
  Pills......................................**695**
Ex-Lax Ultra Pills........................**696**
FiberCon Caplets **782**
Freelax Caplets **783**
Gentlax Tablets **763**
Metamucil Capsules **751**
Metamucil Powder, Original
  Texture Orange Flavor.....................**751**
Metamucil Powder, Original
  Texture Regular Flavor....................**751**
Metamucil Smooth Texture
  Powder, Orange Flavor.....................**751**
Metamucil Smooth Texture
  Powder, Sugar-Free,
   Orange Flavor **751**

Metamucil Smooth Texture
  Powder, Sugar-Free,
   Regular Flavor **751**
Metamucil Wafers,
  Apple Crisp & Cinnamon
   Spice Flavors **751**
Nature's Remedy Tablets **644**
Perdiem Fiber Therapy Caplets **699**
Perdiem Overnight Relief Pills...............**700**
Phillips' Liqui-Gels **622**
Phillips' Milk of Magnesia Liquid
  (Original, Cherry, & Mint)..................**622**
Phillips' M-O Original Formula..............**622**
Phillips' M-O Refreshing
  Mint Formula **622**
Purge Liquid **632**
Senokot Children's Syrup **764**
Senokot Granules **764**
Senokot Syrup **764**
Senokot Tablets **764**
Senokot-S Tablets..........................**764**
SenokotXTRA Tablets **764**

HYPOTHYROIDISM, XERODERMA SECONDARY TO

Hypothyroidism may be treated with thyroid hormones. The following products may be recommended for relief of xeroderma:

Lubriderm Advanced Therapy
  Creamy Lotion **730**
Lubriderm Seriously
  Sensitive Lotion...........................**730**
Lubriderm Skin
  Firming Lotion.............................**730**
Lubriderm Skin Therapy
  Moisturizing Lotion........................**731**
StePHan Bio-Nutritional
  Daytime Hydrating Creme **772**
StePHan Bio-Nutritional
  Nightime Moisture Creme **773**
StePHan Bio-Nutritional
  Ultra Hydrating Fluid.......................**773**

INFECTIONS, BACTERIAL, UPPER RESPIRATORY TRACT

May be treated with amoxicillin-clavulanate, cephalosporins, doxycycline, erythromycin, macrolide antibiotics, penicillins or minocycline hydrochloride. The following products may be recommended for relief of symptoms:

Actifed Cold & Allergy Tablets...............**713**
Actifed Cold & Sinus
  Maximum Strength
   Caplets and Tablets.....................**713**
Advil Caplets **774**
Advil Gel Caplets **774**
Advil Liqui-Gels **774**
Advil Tablets **774**
Advil Allergy Sinus Caplets **774**
Children's Advil Suspension **778**
Children's Advil Chewable
  Tablets.....................................**777**
Advil Cold & Sinus Caplets...................**775**
Advil Cold & Sinus Liqui-Gels...............**775**
Advil Cold & Sinus Tablets..................**775**
Advil Flu & Body Ache Caplets **775**
Children's Advil Cold
  Suspension................................**778**
Infants' Advil Drops **779**
Junior Strength Advil Tablets **777**
Junior Strength Advil
  Chewable Tablets..........................**776**
Aleve Tablets, Caplets and
  Gelcaps **603**
Aleve Cold & Sinus Caplets.................**604**
Aleve Sinus & Headache
  Caplets **604**
Alka-Seltzer Original Antacid and
  Pain Reliever Effervescent
   Tablets.................................**605**

Alka-Seltzer Cherry Antacid and
  Pain Reliever Effervescent
   Tablets.................................**605**
Alka-Seltzer Lemon Lime
  Antacid and Pain Reliever
   Effervescent Tablets....................**605**
Alka-Seltzer Extra Strength
  Antacid and Pain Reliever
   Effervescent Tablets....................**605**
Alka-Seltzer Plus Cold
  Medicine Liqui-Gels.......................**608**
Alka-Seltzer Plus Cold &
  Cough Medicine Effervescent
   Tablets.................................**607**
Alka-Seltzer Plus Cold &
  Sinus Medicine
   Effervescent Tablets....................**607**
Alka-Seltzer Plus Night-Time
  Cold Medicine Liqui-Gels **608**
Alka-Seltzer Plus Cold &
  Cough Medicine Liqui-Gels................**608**
Alka-Seltzer Plus Cold & Sinus
  Medicine Liqui-Gels.......................**608**
Alka-Seltzer Plus Cold Medicine
  Effervescent Tablets
   (Original, Orange & Cherry) **607**
Alka-Seltzer Plus Flu
  Medicine Liqui-Gels.......................**608**
Alka-Seltzer Plus Flu
  Medicine Effervescent
   Tablets.................................**607**
Alka-Seltzer Plus Night-Time
  Cold Medicine Effervescent
   Tablets.................................**607**
Alka-Seltzer Plus PM Tablets...............**609**
Alka-Seltzer Plus Nose &
  Throat Cold Medicine
   Effervescent Tablets....................**607**
Genuine Bayer Tablets,
  Caplets and Gelcaps **611**
Extra Strength Bayer Caplets
  and Gelcaps **616**
Aspirin Regimen Bayer
  Children's Chewable Tablets
   (Orange or Cherry Flavored)...........**613**
Genuine Bayer Professional
  Labeling (Aspirin Regimen
   Bayer)..................................**614**
Extra Strength Bayer Plus
  Caplets **616**
Extra Strength Bayer PM
  Caplets **617**
Bayer Women's Aspirin
  Plus Calcium Caplets **617**
BC Powder..................................**633**
BC Allergy Sinus Cold
  Powder......................................**633**
Arthritis Strength BC
  Powder......................................**633**
BC Sinus Cold Powder **633**
Children's Benadryl
  Allergy Chewables.........................**719**
Benadryl Allergy Kapseal
  Capsules...................................**715**
Children's Benadryl Allergy
  Liquid **718**
Benadryl Allergy Ultratab
  Tablets.....................................**715**
Benadryl Allergy & Cold
  Caplets **716**
Benadryl Allergy & Sinus
  Tablets.....................................**716**
Children's Benadryl Allergy &
  Sinus Liquid **719**
Benadryl Allergy & Sinus
  Fastmelt Tablets **718**
Benadryl Allergy & Sinus
  Headache Caplets & Gelcaps **717**

INFECTIONS, SKIN AND SKIN STRUCTURE

May be treated with aminoglycosides, amoxicillin, amoxicillin-clavulanate, cephalosporins, doxycycline, erythromycin, macrolide antibiotics, penicillins or quinolones. The following products may be recommended for relief of symptoms:

IRRITABLE BOWEL SYNDROME

May be treated with anticholinergic combinations, dicyclomine hydrochloride or hyoscyamine sulfate. The following products may be recommended for relief of symptoms:

ISCHEMIC HEART DISEASE

May be treated with beta blockers, calcium channel blockers, isosorbide dinitrate, isosorbide mononitrate or nitroglycerin. The following products may be recommended for relief of symptoms:

KERATOCONJUNCTIVITIS, VERNAL

May be treated with ophthalmic mast cell stabilizers. The following products may be recommended for relief of symptoms:

MYOCARDIAL INFARCTION, ACUTE

May be treated with ace inhibitors, anticoagulants, beta blockers, thrombolytic agents or nitroglycerin. The following products may be recommended for relief of symptoms:

PANCREATIC INSUFFICIENCY, NUTRIENTS DEFICIENCY SECONDARY TO

Pancreatic insufficiency may be treated with pancrelipase. The following products may be recommended for relief of nutrients deficiency:

PARKINSON'S DISEASE, CONSTIPATION SECONDARY TO

Parkinson's disease may be treated with centrally active anticholinergents, dopaminergic agents or selective inhibitor of mao type b. The following products may be recommended for relief of constipation:

PARKINSON'S DISEASE, SEBORRHEIC DERMATITIS SECONDARY TO

Parkinson's disease may be treated with centrally active anticholinergic agents, dopaminergic agents or selective inhibitor of mao type b. The following products may be recommended for relief of seborrheic dermatitis:

PEPTIC ULCER DISEASE

May be treated with histamine h2 receptor antagonists, proton pump inhibitors or sucralfate. The following products may be recommended for relief of symptoms:

PEPTIC ULCER DISEASE —cont.

PEPTIC ULCER DISEASE, IRON DEFICIENCY SECONDARY TO

Peptic ulcer disease may be treated with histamine h2 receptor antagonists, proton pump inhibitors or sucralfate. The following products may be recommended for relief of iron deficiency:

PHARYNGITIS

May be treated with cephalosporins, macrolide antibiotics or penicillins. The following products may be recommended for relief of symptoms:

PHOTOSENSITIVITY REACTIONS

May result from the use of thiazides, antidepressants, antihistamines, estrogens, nonsteroidal anti-inflammatory drugs, phenothiazines, quinolones, sulfonamides, sulfonylurea
hypoglycemic agents, tetracyclines, topical
retinoids, captopril, diltiazem hydrochloride,
enalapril maleate, fluorouracil, griseofulvin,
labetalol hydrochloride, lisinopril, methoxsalen,
methyldopa, minoxidil, nalidixic acid or nifedipine. The following products may be recommended:

PRURITUS, PERIANAL

May result from the use of broad-spectrum
antibiotics. The following products may be recommended:

PSORALEN WITH UV-A LIGHT (PUVA) THERAPY

May be treated with methoxsalen. The following
products may be recommended for relief of
symptoms:

RENAL OSTEODYSTROPHY, HYPOCALCEMIA SECONDARY TO

Renal osteodystrophy may be treated with vitamin d sterols. The following products may be
recommended for relief of hypocalcemia:

RESPIRATORY TRACT ILLNESS, INFLUENZA A VIRUS-INDUCED

May be treated with amantadine hydrochloride
or rimantadine hydrochloride. The following
products may be recommended for relief of
symptoms:

RHINITIS, NONALLERGIC

May be treated with nasal steroids or ipratropium bromide. The following products may be recommended for relief of symptoms:

SERUM-SICKNESSLIKE REACTIONS

May result from the use of amoxicillin, amoxicillin-clavulanate, penicillins, sulfamethoxazole-trimethoprim, antivenin (crotalidae) polyvalent, antivenin (micrurus fulvius), metronidazole, ofloxacin, streptomycin sulfate, sulfadoxine, sulfamethoxazole or sulfasalazine. The following products may be recommended:

SINUSITIS

May be treated with amoxicillin, amoxicillin-clavulanate, cefprozil, cefuroxime axetil, clarithromycin or loracarbef. The following products may be recommended for relief of symptoms:

SINUSITIS, HALITOSIS SECONDARY TO

Sinusitis may be treated with amoxicillin, amoxicillin-clavulanate, cefprozil, cefuroxime axetil, clarithromycin or loracarbef. The following products may be recommended for relief of halitosis:

SKIN IRRITATION

May result from the use of transdermal drug delivery systems. The following products may be recommended:

STOMATITIS, APHTHOUS

May result from the use of selective serotonin reuptake inhibitors, aldesleukin, clomipramine hydrochloride, didanosine, foscarnet sodium, indinavir sulfate, indomethacin, interferon alfa-2b, recombinant, methotrexate sodium, naproxen, naproxen sodium, nicotine polacrilex or stavudine. The following products may be recommended:

TASTE DISTURBANCES

May result from the use of biguanides, acetazolamide, butorphanol tartrate, captopril, cefuroxime axetil, clarithromycin, etidronate disodium, felbamate, flunisolide, gemfibrozil, griseofulvin, interferon alfa-2b, recombinant, lithium carbonate, lithium citrate, mesna, metronidazole, nedocromil sodium, penicillamine, rifampin or succimer. The following products may be recommended:

TONSILITIS, HALITOSIS SECONDARY TO

Tonsilitis may be treated with erythromycin, macrolide antibiotics, cefaclor, cefadroxil, cefixime, cefpodoxime proxetil, cefprozil, ceftibuten dihydrate or cefuroxime axetil. The following products may be recommended for relief of halitosis:

TUBERCULOSIS, NUTRIENTS DEFICIENCY SECONDARY TO

Tuberculosis may be treated with capreomycin sulfate, ethambutol hydrochloride, ethionamide, isoniazid, pyrazinamide, rifampin or streptomycin sulfate. The following products may be recommended for relief of nutrients deficiency:

VAGINOSIS, BACTERIAL

May be treated with sulfabenzamide/sulfacetamide/sulfathiozole or metronidazole. The following products may be recommended for relief of symptoms:

XERODERMA

May result from the use of aldesleukin, protease inhibitors, retinoids, topical acne preparations, topical corticosteroids, topical retinoids, benzoyl peroxide, clofazimine, interferon alfa-2a, recombinant, interferon alfa-2b, recombinant or pentostatin. The following products may be recommended:

XEROMYCTERIA

May result from the use of anticholinergics, antihistamines, retinoids, apraclonidine hydrochloride, clonidine, etretinate, ipratropium bromide, isotretinoin or Iodoxamide tromethamine. The following products may be recommended:

XEROSTOMIA

May result from the use of anticholinergics, antidepressants, diuretics, phenothiazines, alprazolam, bromocriptine mesylate, buspirone hydrochloride, butorphanol tartrate, clomipramine hydrochloride, clonidine, clozapine, dexfenfluramine hydrochloride, didanosine, disopyramide phosphate, etretinate, flumazenil, fluvoxamine maleate, guanfacine hydrochloride, isotretinoin, leuprolide acetate, pergolide mesylate, selegiline hydrochloride, tramadol hydrochloride or zolpidem tartrate. The following products may be recommended:

VERIFIED HERBAL INDICATIONS

Claims made for herbs in the popular press often outdistance their actual benefits. Which indications should be taken seriously and which dismissed? The most authoritative answers come from Germany, where the efficacy of medicinal herbs undergoes official scrutiny by the German Regulatory Authority's "Commission E." This agency has conducted an intensive analysis of the peer-reviewed literature on some 300 common botanicals, weighing the quality of the clinical evidence and identifying the uses for which the herb can reasonably be considered effective. The results of this effort are summarized in the table below.

Herb	Indications	Herb	Indications
Adonis (Adonis vernalis)	Arrhythmias Anxiety disorders, management of	**Asparagus** (Asparagus officinalis)	Infections, urinary tract Renal calculi
Agrimony (Agrimonia eupatoria)	Diarrhea, symptomatic relief of Skin, inflammatory conditions Stomatitis	**Bean Pod** (Phaseolus vulgaris)	Infections, urinary tract Renal calculi
Aloe Vera (Aloe barbadensis)	Constipation	**Belladonna** (Atropa belladonna)	Liver and gallbladder complaints
Angelica (Angelica archangelica)	Appetite, stimulation of Digestive disorders, symptomatic relief of Cold, common, symptomatic relief of Fever associated with common cold Infections, urinary tract	**Bilberry** (Vaccinium myrtillus)	Diarrhea, symptomatic relief of Stomatitis
		Birch (Betula species)	Infections, urinary tract Renal calculi Rheumatic disorders, unspecified
		Bitter Orange (Citrus aurantium)	Appetite, stimulation of Digestive disorders, symptomatic relief of
Anise (Pimpinella anisum)	Appetite, stimulation of Bronchitis, acute Cold, common, symptomatic relief of Cough, symptomatic relief of Digestive disorders, symptomatic relief of Fever associated with common cold Stomatitis	**Bittersweet Nightshade** (Solanum dulcamara)	Acne, unspecified Furunculosis Dermatitis, eczematoid Warts
		Black Cohosh (Cimicifuga racemosa)	Menopause, climacteric complaints Premenstrual syndrome, management of
Arnica (Arnica montana)	Bronchitis, acute Cold, common, symptomatic relief of Cough, symptomatic relief of Fever associated with common cold Infection, tendency to Rheumatic disorders, unspecified Skin, inflammatory conditions Stomatitis Trauma, blunt	**Blackberry** (Rubus fruticosus)	Diarrhea, symptomatic relief of Stomatitis
		Blessed Thistle (Cnicus benedictus)	Appetite, stimulation of Digestive disorders, symptomatic relief of
		Bog Bean (Menyanthes trifoliata)	Appetite, stimulation of Digestive disorders, symptomatic relief of
Artichoke (Cynara scolymus)	Appetite, stimulation of Liver and gallbladder complaints	**Boldo** (Peumus boldus)	Digestive disorders, symptomatic relief of

Herb	Indications	Herb	Indications
Brewer's Yeast (*Saccharomyces cerevisiae*)	Acne vulgaris Appetite, stimulation of Digestive disorders, symptomatic relief of Furunculosis Skin, inflammatory conditions	**Chaste Tree** (*Vitex agnus-castus*)	Premenstrual syndrome, management of Menopause, climacteric complaints
Buckthorn (*Rhamnus catharticus*)	Constipation	**Chicory** (*Cichorium intybus*)	Appetite, stimulation of Digestive disorders, symptomatic relief of
Bugleweed (*Lycopus virginicus*)	Anxiety disorders, management of Premenstrual syndrome, management of Sleep, induction of	**Chinese Cinnamon** (*Cinnamomum aromaticum*)	Appetite, stimulation of Digestive disorders, symptomatic relief of
Butcher's Broom (*Ruscus aculeatus*)	Hemorrhoids, symptomatic relief of Venous conditions	**Chinese Rhubarb** (*Rheum palmatum*)	Constipation
Cajuput (*Melaleuca leucadendra*)	Rheumatic disorders, unspecified Infection, tendency to Pain, muscular, temporary relief of Pain, neurogenic Wound care, adjunctive therapy in	**Cinnamon** (*Cinnamomum verum*)	Appetite, stimulation of Digestive disorders, symptomatic relief of
		Cinquefoil (*Potentilla erecta*)	Diarrhea, symptomatic relief of Stomatitis
Camphor Tree (*Cinnamomum camphora*)	Anxiety disorders, management of Arrhythmias Bronchitis, acute Cough, symptomatic relief of Hypotension Rheumatic disorders, unspecified	**Clove** (*Syzygium aromaticum*)	Pain, dental Stomatitis
		Coffee (*Coffea arabica*)	Diarrhea, symptomatic relief of Stomatitis
Canadian Golden Rod (*Solidago canadensis*)	Infections, urinary tract Renal calculi	**Cola** (*Cola acuminata*)	Lack of stamina
Caraway (*Carum carvi*)	Digestive disorders, symptomatic relief of	**Colchicum** (*Colchicum autumnale*)	Brucellosis Gout, management of signs and symptoms
Cardamom (*Elettaria cardamomum*)	Digestive disorders, symptomatic relief of	**Colt's Foot** (*Tussilago farfara*)	Bronchitis, acute Cough, symptomatic relief of Stomatitis
Cascara Sagrada (*Rhamnus purshianus*)	Constipation	**Comfrey** (*Symphytum officinale*)	Trauma, blunt
Cayenne (*Capsicum annuum*)	Muscle tension Rheumatic disorders, unspecified	**Condurango** (*Marsdenia condurango*)	Appetite, stimulation of Digestive disorders, symptomatic relief of
Celandine (*Chelidonium majus*)	Liver and gallbladder complaints	**Coriander** (*Coriandrum sativum*)	Appetite, stimulation of Digestive disorders, symptomatic relief of
Centaury (*Centaurium erythraea*)	Appetite, stimulation of Digestive disorders, symptomatic relief of	**Cowslip** (*Primula veris*)	Bronchitis, acute Cough, symptomatic relief of

Herb	Indications	Herb	Indications
Curcuma *(Curcuma xanthorrhizia)*	Appetite, stimulation of Digestive disorders, symptomatic relief of	**Eucalyptus** *(Eucalyptus globulus)*	Bronchitis, acute Cough, symptomatic relief of Rheumatic disorders, unspecified
Dandelion *(Taraxacum officinale)*	Appetite, stimulation of Digestive disorders, symptomatic relief of Infections, urinary tract Liver and gallbladder complaints	**European Elder** *(Sambucus nigra)*	Bronchitis, acute Cold, common, symptomatic relief of Cough, symptomatic relief of Fever associated with common cold
Devil's Claw *(Harpagophytum procumbens)*	Appetite, stimulation of Digestive disorders, symptomatic relief of Rheumatic disorders, unspecified	**European Mistletoe** *(Viscum album)*	Rheumatic disorders, unspecified Tumor therapy adjuvant
Dill *(Anethum graveolens)*	Digestive disorders, symptomatic relief of	**European Sanicle** *(Sanicula europaea)*	Bronchitis, acute Cough, symptomatic relief of
Echinacea Pallida *(Echinacea pallida)*	Cold, common, symptomatic relief of Fever associated with common cold	**Fennel** *(Foeniculum vulgare)*	Bronchitis, acute Cough, symptomatic relief of Digestive disorders, symptomatic relief of
Echinacea Purpurea *(Echinacea purpurea)*	Bronchitis, acute Cold, common, symptomatic relief of Cough, symptomatic relief of Fever associated with common cold Infections, tendency to Infections, urinary tract Stomatitis Wound care, adjunctive therapy in	**Fenugreek** *(Trigonella foenum-graecum)*	Appetite, stimulation of Skin, inflammatory conditions
		Flax *(Linum usitatissimum)*	Constipation Skin, inflammatory conditions
English Hawthorn *(Crataegus laevigata)*	Cardiac output, low	**Frangula** *(Rhamnus frangula)*	Constipation
English Ivy *(Hedera helix)*	Bronchitis, acute Cough, symptomatic relief of	**Fumitory** *(Fumaria officinalis)*	Liver and gallbladder complaints
English Lavender *(Lavandula angustifolia)*	Anxiety disorders, management of Appetite, stimulation of Circulatory disorders Digestive disorders, symptomatic relief of Sleep, induction of	**Garlic** *(Allium sativum)*	Arteriosclerosis Hypercholesterolemia Hypertension
		German Chamomile *(Matricaria recutita)*	Bronchitis, acute Cold, common, symptomatic relief of Cough, symptomatic relief of Fever associated with common cold Infection, tendency to Skin, inflammatory conditions Stomatitis Wound care, adjunctive therapy in
English Plantain *(Plantago lanceolata)*	Bronchitis, acute Cold, common, symptomatic relief of Cough, symptomatic relief of Fever associated with common cold Skin, inflammatory conditions Stomatitis	**Ginger** *(Zingiber officinale)*	Appetite, stimulation of Digestive disorders, symptomatic relief of Motion sickness

Herb	Indications	Herb	Indications
Ginkgo (*Ginkgo biloba*)	Claudication, intermittent Organic brain dysfunction, symptomatic relief of Tinnitus Vertigo	**Iceland Moss** (*Cetraria islandica*)	Appetite, stimulation of Bronchitis, acute Cough, symptomatic relief of Digestive disorders, symptomatic relief of Stomatitis
Ginseng (*Panax ginseng*)	Lack of stamina	**Immortelle** (*Helichrysum arenarium*)	Digestive disorders, symptomatic relief of
Guaiac (*Guaiacum officinale*)	Rheumatic disorders, unspecified	**Jambolan** (*Syzygium cumini*)	Diarrhea, symptomatic relief of Skin, inflammatory conditions Stomatitis
Gumweed (*Grindelia* species)	Bronchitis, acute Cough, symptomatic relief of	**Japanese Mint** (*Mentha arvensis piperascens*)	Bronchitis, acute Cold, common, symptomatic relief of Cough, symptomatic relief of Fever associated with common cold Infection, tendency to Liver and gallbladder complaints Pain, unspecified Stomatitis
Haronga (*Haronga madagascariensis*)	Digestive disorders, symptomatic relief of		
Heartsease (*Viola tricolor*)	Skin, inflammatory conditions		
Hempnettle (*Galeopsis segetum*)	Bronchitis, acute Cough, symptomatic relief of	**Java Tea** (*Orthosiphon spicatus*)	Infections, urinary tract Renal calculi
Henbane (*Hyoscyamus niger*)	Digestive disorders, symptomatic relief of	**Juniper** (*Juniperus communis*)	Appetite, stimulation of Digestive disorders, symptomatic relief of
High Mallow (*Malva sylvestris*)	Bronchitis, acute Cough, symptomatic relief of Stomatitis	**Kava-Kava** (*Piper methysticum*)	Anxiety disorders, management of Sleep, induction of
Hops (*Humulus lupulus*)	Anxiety disorders, management of Sleep, induction of	**Knotweed** (*Polygonum aviculare*)	Bronchitis, acute Cough, symptomatic relief of Stomatitis
Horehound (*Marrubium vulgare*)	Appetite, stimulation of Digestive disorders, symptomatic relief of	**Lady's Mantle** (*Alchemilla vulgaris*)	Diarrhea, symptomatic relief of
Horse Chestnut (*Aesculus hippocastanum*)	Venous conditions	**Larch** (*Larix decidua*)	Blood pressure problems Bronchitis, acute Cold, common, symptomatic relief of Cough, symptomatic relief of Fever associated with common cold Infection, tendency to Rheumatic disorders, unspecified Stomatitis
Horseradish (*Armoracia rusticana*)	Bronchitis, acute Cough, symptomatic relief of Infections, urinary tract		
Horsetail (*Equisetum arvense*)	Infections, urinary tract Renal calculi Wound care, adjunctive therapy in	**Lemon Balm** (*Melissa officinalis*)	Anxiety disorders, management of Sleep, induction of

Herb	Indications	Herb	Indications
Lesser Galangal (*Alpinia officinarum*)	Appetite, stimulation of Digestive disorders, symptomatic relief of Stomatitis	**Mullein** (*Verbascum densiflorum*)	Bronchitis, acute Cough, symptomatic relief of
Licorice (*Glycyrrhiza glabra*)	Bronchitis, acute Cough, symptomatic relief of Gastritis	**Myrrh** (*Commiphora molmol*)	Stomatitis
Lily-of-the-Valley (*Convallaria majalis*)	Anxiety disorders, management of Arrhythmias Cardiac output, low	**Nasturtium** (*Tropaeolum majus*)	Bronchitis, acute Cough, symptomatic relief of Infections, urinary tract
Linden (*Tilia* species)	Bronchitis, acute Cough, symptomatic relief of	**Niauli** (*Melaleucea viridiflora*)	Bronchitis, acute Cough, symptomatic relief of
Lovage (*Levisticum officinale*)	Infections, urinary tract Renal calculi	**Oak** (*Quercus robur*)	Bronchitis, acute Cough, symptomatic relief of Diarrhea, symptomatic relief of Skin, inflammatory conditions Stomatitis
Ma-Huang (*Ephedra sinica*)	Bronchitis, acute Cough, symptomatic relief of Fever associated with common cold	**Oats** (*Avena sativa*)	Skin, inflammatory conditions Warts
Manna (*Fraxinus ornus*)	Constipation	**Onion** (*Allium cepa*)	Appetite, stimulation of Arteriosclerosis Bronchitis, acute Cold, common, symptomatic relief of Cough, symptomatic relief of Digestive disorders, symptomatic relief of Fever associated with common cold Hypertension Infection, tendency to Stomatitis
Marigold (*Calendula officinalis*)	Stomatitis Wound care, adjunctive therapy in		
Marshmallow (*Althaea officinalis*)	Bronchitis, acute Cough, symptomatic relief of		
Maté (*Ilex paraguariensis*)	Lack of stamina		
Mayapple (*Podophyllum peltatum*)	Warts	**Parsley** (*Petroselinum crispum*)	Infections, urinary tract Renal calculi
Meadowsweet (*Filipendula ulmaria*)	Bronchitis, acute Cold, common, symptomatic relief of Cough, symptomatic relief of Fever associated with common cold	**Passion Flower** (*Passiflora incarnata*)	Anxiety disorders, management of Sleep, induction of
Milk Thistle (*Silybum marianum*)	Digestive disorders, symptomatic relief of Liver and gallbladder complaints	**Peppermint** (*Mentha piperita*)	Bronchitis, acute Cold, common, symptomatic relief of Cough, symptomatic relief of Digestive disorders, symptomatic relief of Fever associated with common cold Infection, tendency to Liver and gallbladder complaints Stomatitis
Motherwort (*Leonurus cardiaca*)	Anxiety disorders, management of		

Herb	*Indications*	*Herb*	*Indications*
Petasites (*Petasites hybridus*)	Renal calculi	**Rosemary** (*Rosmarinus officinalis*)	Appetite, stimulation of Blood pressure problems Digestive disorders, symptomatic relief of Rheumatic disorders, unspecified
Pimpinella (*Pimpinella major*)	Cough, symptomatic relief of Bronchitis, acute		
Pineapple (*Ananas comosus*)	Wound care, adjunctive therapy in	**Sage** (*Salvia officinalis*)	Appetite, stimulation of Hyperhidrosis Stomatitis
Poplar (*Populus* species)	Hemorrhoids, symptomatic relief of Wound care, adjunctive therapy in	**Sandalwood** (*Santalum album*)	Infections, urinary tract
Potentilla (*Potentilla anserina*)	Diarrhea, symptomatic relief of Premenstrual syndrome, management of Stomatitis	**Saw Palmetto** (*Serenoa repens*)	Urinary frequency, symptomatic relief of Prostatic hyperplasia, benign, symptomatic treatment of
		Scopolia (*Scopolia carniolica*)	Liver and gallbladder complaints
Psyllium (*Plantago ovata*)	Constipation Diarrhea, symptomatic relief of Hemorrhoids Hypercholesterolemia, primary, adjunct to diet	**Scotch Broom** (*Cytisus scoparius*)	Hypertension Circulatory disorders
Psyllium Seed (*Plantago afra*)	Constipation Diarrhea, symptomatic relief of	**Scotch Pine** (*Pinus* species)	Blood pressure problems Bronchitis, acute Cold, common, symptomatic relief of
Pumpkin (*Cucurbita pepo*)	Urinary frequency, symptomatic relief of Prostatic hyperplasia, benign, symptomatic treatment of		Cough, symptomatic relief of Fever associated with common cold Infection, tendency to Pain, neurogenic Rheumatic disorders, unspecified Stomatitis
Quinine (*Cinchona pubescens*)	Appetite, stimulation of Digestive disorders, symptomatic relief of		
		Seneca Snakeroot (*Polygala senega*)	Bronchitis, acute Cough, symptomatic relief of
Radish (*Raphanus sativus*)	Bronchitis, acute Cough, symptomatic relief of Digestive disorders, symptomatic relief of	**Senna** (*Cassia senna*)	Constipation
Rauwolfia		**Shepherd's Purse** (*Capsella bursa-pastoris*)	Hemorrhage, nasal Premenstrual syndrome, management of Wound care, adjunctive therapy in
(*Rauwolfia serpentina*)	Anxiety disorders, management of Hypertension Sleep, induction of		
Rhatany (*Krameria triandra*)	Stomatitis	**Siberian Ginseng** (*Eleutherococcus senticosus*)	Infection, tendency to Lack of stamina
Rose (*Rosa centifolia*)	Stomatitis	**Sloe** (*Prunus spinosa*)	Stomatitis

Herb	Indications	Herb	Indications
Soapwort (*Saponaria officinalis*)	Bronchitis, acute Cough, symptomatic relief of	**Tolu Balsam** (*Myroxylon balsamum*)	Bronchitis, acute Cough, symptomatic relief of Hemorrhoids, symptomatic relief of Wound care, adjunctive therapy in
Soybean (*Glycine soja*)	Hypercholesterolemia, primary, adjunct to diet	**Triticum** (*Agropyron repens*)	Infections, urinary tract Renal calculi
Spiny Rest Harrow (*Ononis spinosa*)	Infections, urinary tract Renal calculi		
Spruce (*Picea* species)	Bronchitis, acute Cold, common, symptomatic relief of Cough, symptomatic relief of Fever associated with common cold Infection, tendency to Pain, neurogenic Rheumatic disorders, unspecified Stomatitis	**Turmeric** (*Curcuma domestica*)	Appetite, stimulation of Digestive disorders, symptomatic relief of
		Usnea (*Usnea* species)	Stomatitis
		Uva-Ursi (*Arctostaphylos uva-ursi*)	Infections, urinary tract
Squill (*Drimia maritima*)	Anxiety disorders, management of Arrhythmias Cardiac output, low	**Uzara** (*Xysmalobium undulatum*)	Diarrhea, symptomatic relief of
St. John's Wort (*Hypericum perforatum*)	Anxiety disorders, management of Depression, relief of symptoms Skin, inflammatory conditions Trauma, blunt Wound care, adjunctive therapy in	**Valerian** (*Valeriana officinalis*)	Anxiety disorders, management of Sleep, induction of
		Walnut (*Juglans regia*)	Hyperhidrosis Skin, inflammatory conditions
Star Anise (*Illicium verum*)	Appetite, stimulation of Bronchitis, acute Cough, symptomatic relief of	**Watercress** (*Nasturtium officinale*)	Bronchitis, acute Cough, symptomatic relief of
Stinging Nettle (*Urtica dioica*)	Infections, urinary tract Renal calculi Rheumatic disorders, unspecified Prostatic hyperplasia, benign, symptomatic treatment of Urinary frequency, symptomatic relief of	**White Fir** (*Abies alba*)	Pain, neurogenic Rheumatic disorders, unspecified
		White Mustard (*Sinapis alba*)	Bronchitis, acute Cold, common, symptomatic relief of Cough, symptomatic relief of Rheumatic disorders, unspecified
Sundew (*Drosera rotundifolia*)	Bronchitis, acute Cough, symptomatic relief of		
		White Nettle (*Lamium album*)	Bronchitis, acute Cough, symptomatic relief of Skin, inflammatory conditions Stomatitis
Sweet Clover (*Melilotus officinalis*)	Hemorrhoids, symptomatic relief of Trauma, blunt Venous conditions		
Sweet Orange (*Citrus sinensis*)	Appetite, stimulation of Digestive disorders, symptomatic relief of	**White Willow** (*Salix* species)	Pain, unspecified Rheumatic disorders, unspecified
		Wild Thyme (*Thymus serpyllum*)	Bronchitis, acute Cough, symptomatic relief of
Thyme (*Thymus vulgaris*)	Bronchitis, acute Cough, symptomatic relief of		

Herb	Indications	Herb	Indications
Witch Hazel (*Hamamelis virginiana*)	Hemorrhoids, symptomatic relief of Skin disorders Skin, inflammatory conditions Venous conditions Wound care, adjunctive therapy in	**Yarrow** (*Achillea millefolium*)	Appetite, stimulation of Digestive disorders, symptomatic relief of Liver and gallbladder complaints
Wormwood (*Artemisia absinthium*)	Appetite, stimulation of Digestive disorders, symptomatic relief of Liver and gallbladder complaints	**Yellow Gentian** (*Gentiana lutea*)	Appetite, stimulation of Digestive disorders, symptomatic relief of

PRODUCT IDENTIFICATION GUIDE

For quick identification, this section provides full-color reproductions of product packaging, as well as some actual-sized photographs of tablets and capsules. In all, the section contains some 600 photos.

Products in this section are arranged alphabetically by manufacturer. In some instances, not all dosage forms and sizes are pictured. For more information on any of the products in this section, please turn to the page indicated above the product's photo or check directly with the product's manufacturer.

While every effort has been made to guarantee faithful reproduction of the photos in this section, changes in size, color, and design are always a possibility. Be sure to confirm a product's identity with the manufacturer or your pharmacist.

MANUFACTURER'S INDEX

A & Z PHARMACEUTICAL INC.

A & Z Pharmaceutical Inc.
P. 796

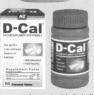

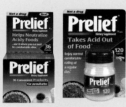

Calcium supplement with fruit flavor in packages of 30 and 60 caplets.

D-Cal™

AKPHARMA INC.

AkPharma Inc.
P. 796

Dietary Supplement Granulate and Tablets

Prelief®

AMERIFIT NUTRITION

Amerifit Nutrition
P. 797

Dietary Supplement
Estroven®

Amerifit Nutrition
P. 797

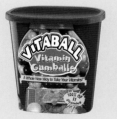

Multivitamin Supplement

**Vitaball®
Vitamin Gumballs**

AWARENESS CORPORATION

Awareness Corporation/AwarenessLife
P. 798

Experience®
Digestive/Weight

Daily Complete®
Vitamins/Minerals

Female Balance™
Menopause/PMS

Pure Gardens
Cream® Skin Care

**Awareness Natural
Dietary Supplements**

BAYER HEALTHCARE LLC

Bayer Healthcare LLC
P. 603

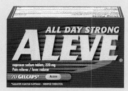

Tablets and Caplets available in 24, 50, 100 and 150 count.
Caplets also available in 200 count.
Gelcaps available in 20, 40 and 80 count.

Aleve®

Bayer Healthcare LLC
P. 604

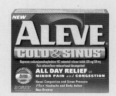

Aleve® Cold & Sinus

Bayer Healthcare LLC
P. 604

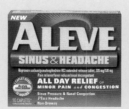

Aleve® Sinus & Headache

Bayer Healthcare LLC
P. 605

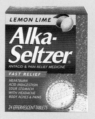

Lemon Lime Effervescent Antacid and Pain Reliever.
Also available in Original flavor and Extra Strength.

Alka-Seltzer®

Bayer Healthcare LLC
P. 606

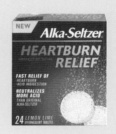

**Alka-Seltzer®
Heartburn Relief**

Bayer Healthcare LLC
P. 606

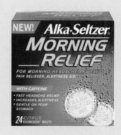

**Alka-Seltzer® Morning
Relief™**

Bayer Healthcare LLC
P. 607

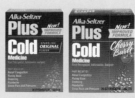

**Alka-Seltzer Plus®
Cold Medicine**

Bayer Healthcare LLC
P. 608

Cold, Cold & Cough, Flu, Cold & Sinus and Night-Time.

**Alka-Seltzer Plus®
Cold Medicine Liqui-Gels®**

Bayer Healthcare LLC
P. 609

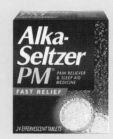

Alka-Seltzer PM®

Bayer Healthcare LLC
P. 613

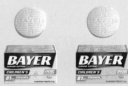

Low strength, chewable aspirin Cherry and Orange flavors

**Aspirin Regimen
BAYER® Children's**

Bayer Healthcare LLC
P. 612

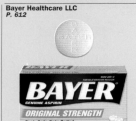

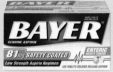

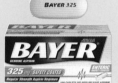

Genuine Bayer Tablets and Gelcaps
Aspirin Regimen 81 mg
Aspirin Regimen 325 mg

BAYER® Aspirin

Bayer Healthcare LLC
P. 617

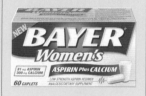

**BAYER® Women's
Aspirin Plus Calcium**

Bayer Healthcare LLC
P. 799

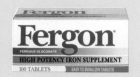

Ferrous Gluconate
Iron Supplement

Fergon®

Bayer Healthcare LLC
P. 799

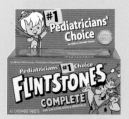

Also available in My First Flintstones
Chewable Tablets.

Flintstones® Complete

Bayer Healthcare LLC

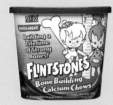

Also available in Scooby-Doo
Calcium Chews.

**Flintstones® Calcium
Chews**

Bayer Healthcare LLC
P. 619

Maximum Strength
Caplets and Gelcaps

Midol® Menstrual

Bayer Healthcare LLC
P. 619

Maximum Strength
Gelcaps and Caplets

Midol® PMS

Bayer Healthcare LLC

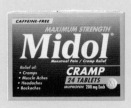

Maximum Strength Tablets

Midol® Cramp

Bayer Healthcare LLC
P. 620

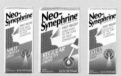

Nasal Decongestant
Spray and Drops
Available in Mild, Regular, Extra
Strength and Max 12-Hour Formula.

Neo-Synephrine®

Bayer Healthcare LLC
P. 621

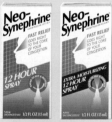

Nasal Spray available in 12 hour
and 12 hour Extra Moisturizing.

Neo Synephrine® 12 Hour

Bayer Healthcare LLC
P. 801

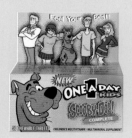

Kids Complete
Also available with calcium.

One-A-Day® Kids

Bayer Healthcare LLC

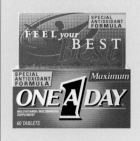

One-A-Day® Maximum

Bayer Healthcare LLC
P. 803

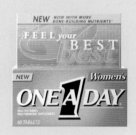

One-A-Day® Women's

Bayer Healthcare LLC
P. 803

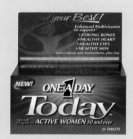

For active women 50 and over.

One-A-Day® Today™

Bayer Healthcare LLC
P. 802

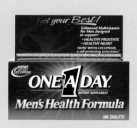

One-A-Day® Men's Health

Bayer Healthcare LLC
P. 803

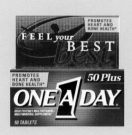

One-A-Day® 50+

Bayer Healthcare LLC
P. 622

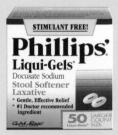

Stool Softener Laxative

Phillips'® Liqui-Gels

Bayer Healthcare LLC
P. 622

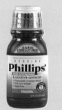

Original Flavor
Also available in
Fresh Mint, Cherry and
French Vanilla flavors.

**Phillips'®
Milk of Magnesia**

Bayer Healthcare LLC
P. 622

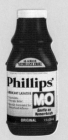

Lubricant Laxative in Original Formula.
Also available in refreshing Mint flavor.

Phillips'® M-O

Bayer Healthcare LLC
P. 623

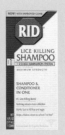

Also available in mousse form.

**Rid® Lice Killing
Shampoo**

BOEHRINGER INGELHEIM

Boehringer Ingelheim Consumer H.C.
P. 625

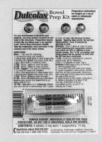

Dulcolax® Bowel Prep Kit
(bisacodyl USP)

Boehringer Ingelheim Consumer H.C.
P. 626

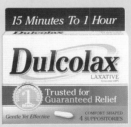

4 Comfort Shaped Suppositories

Dulcolax® Laxative

Boehringer Ingelheim Consumer H.C.
P. 626

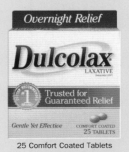

25 Comfort Coated Tablets

Dulcolax® Laxative

Boehringer Ingelheim Consumer H.C.
P. 627

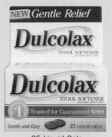

25 Liquid Gels
Blister pack of 10 and bottles of
25, 50 or 100 liquid gels

Dulcolax® Stool Softener

BRISTOL-MYERS SQUIBB CO.

Bristol-Myers Squibb Co.
P. 628

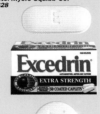
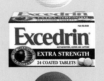

Bottles of 24, 50, 100
and 250 tablets, and pocket size
container of 10 tablets.
Bottles of 24, 50, 100, 250 caplets
and 24, 50 and 100 geltabs.

Excedrin® Extra Strength

FACED WITH AN
Rx SIDE EFFECT?

Turn to the
Companion Drug Index
(Green Pages)
for products that provide
symptomatic relief.

Bristol-Myers Squibb Co.
P. 629

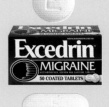
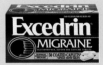

Bottles of 24, 50, 100
and 250 tablets.
Bottles of 24, 50 and 100 caplets.
Bottles of 24, 50 and 100 geltabs.

Excedrin® Migraine

Bristol-Myers Squibb Co.
P. 629

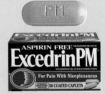

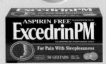

Tablets in bottles of 10.
Tablets and Caplets in bottles of
24, 50 and 100.
Geltabs in bottles of 24, 50 and 100.

Excedrin PM®

Bristol-Myers Squibb Co.
P. 630

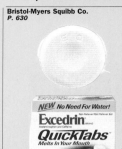

Peppermint flavor

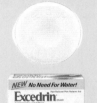

Spearmint flavor
Fast dissolving tablets in blister packs
of 16 and 32 per box.

Excedrin® QuickTabs™

Bristol-Myers Squibb Co.
P. 628

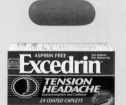

Caplets and Geltabs in bottles of
24, 50 and 100.

**Excedrin® Tension
Headache**

EFFCON

Effcon Laboratories
P. 631

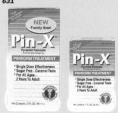

50 mg/mL
Oral Suspension available
in 60 mL and 30 mL.

Pin-X®
(pyrantel pamoate)

GLAXOSMITHKLINE
CONSUMER HEALTHCARE

GlaxoSmithKline Consumer Healthcare
P. 633

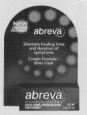

Cold Sore/Fever
Blister Treatment Cream

Abreva™

GlaxoSmithKline Consumer Healthcare
P. 633

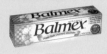

Available in 2 oz. and 4 oz. tubes
and 16 oz. jar.

**Balmex®
Diaper Rash Ointment**

GlaxoSmithKline Consumer Healthcare
P. 633

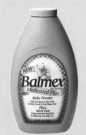

Available in 13 oz. bottle.

**Balmex® Medicated Plus
Baby Powder**

GlaxoSmithKline Consumer Healthcare
P. 634

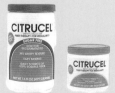

Fiber Therapy for Regularity
Sugar Free Orange available
in 8.6 oz., 16.9 oz., and 32 oz.
containers.
Regular Orange available in
16 oz., 30 oz., and 50 oz. containers.

Citrucel®

GlaxoSmithKline Consumer Healthcare
P. 636

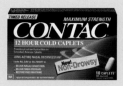

Nasal Decongestant/Antihistamine
Packages of 10 and 20
Maximum Strength Caplets.

Contac® 12 Hour Cold

GlaxoSmithKline Consumer Healthcare
P. 636

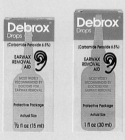

Multisymptom Cold & Flu Relief
Maximum Strength Formula in
packages of 16 and 30 caplets.
Non-Drowsy Formula
in packages of 16 caplets.

**Contac® Severe
Cold & Flu**

GlaxoSmithKline Consumer Healthcare
P. 637

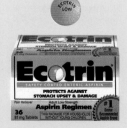

Drops
Available in ½ fl. oz. and 1 fl. oz.

Debrox®

GlaxoSmithKline Consumer Healthcare
P. 638

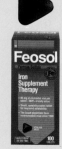

Adult Low Strength Tablets
in Bottles of 36
and 120 tablets.

Ecotrin®

GlaxoSmithKline Consumer Healthcare
P. 638

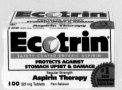

Regular Strength Tablets
in bottles of 100 and 250.

Ecotrin®

GlaxoSmithKline Consumer Healthcare
P. 638

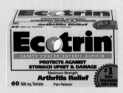

Maximum Strength Tablets
in bottles of 60 and 150.

Ecotrin®

GlaxoSmithKline Consumer Healthcare
P. 806

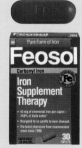

Packages of 30 caplets

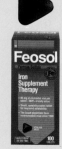

Packages of 100 tablets
Iron Supplement

Feosol®

GlaxoSmithKline Consumer Healthcare
P. 641

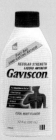

12 Fl. oz.

Gaviscon® Regular Strength Liquid Antacid

GlaxoSmithKline Consumer Healthcare
P. 640

Available in 100-tablet bottles and 30-tablet boxes.

Gaviscon® Regular Strength Antacid

GlaxoSmithKline Consumer Healthcare
P. 641

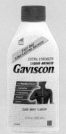

Extra Strength Formula
12 Fl. Oz.

Gaviscon® Extra Strength Liquid Antacid

GlaxoSmithKline Consumer Healthcare
P. 641

Extra Strength Formula
Available in 100-tablet bottles and 6 and 30-tablet boxes.

Gaviscon® Extra Strength Antacid

GlaxoSmithKline Consumer Healthcare
P. 641

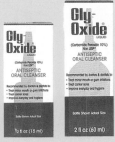

1/2 fl. oz.   2 fl. oz.

Gly-Oxide® Liquid

GlaxoSmithKline Consumer Healthcare
P. 643

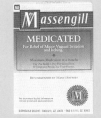

Medicated Disposable Douche With Povidone-Iodine.
Available in single or twin packs.

Massengill®

SEEKING AN ALTERNATIVE?

Check the Product Category Index, where you'll find alphabetical listings of all the products in each therapeutic class.

GlaxoSmithKline Consumer Healthcare
P. 644

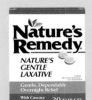

Available in packages of 15, 30 and 60 tablets.
A stimulant laxative with natural active ingredients.

Nature's Remedy® Nature's Gentle Laxative

GlaxoSmithKline Consumer Healthcare
P. 657

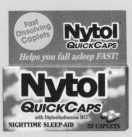

QuickCaps®

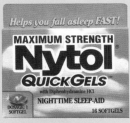

QuickGels™

Nytol®

GlaxoSmithKline Consumer Healthcare
P. 644

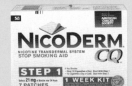

Step 1
Also available in 2 week kit.

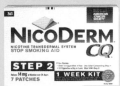

Step 2
Also available in 2 week kit.

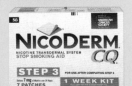

Step 3
Also available in 2 week kit.
Includes User's Guide, Audio Tape and Child Resistant Disposal Tray
Stop Smoking Aid
Nicotine Transdermal System

NicoDerm® CQ™

GlaxoSmithKline Consumer Healthcare
P. 653

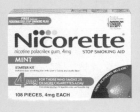

4 mg
Stop Smoking Aid in mint flavor
Nicotine Polacrilex Gum

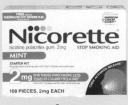

2 mg
Stop Smoking Aid in mint flavor
Nicotine Polacrilex Gum

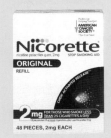

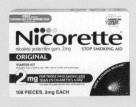

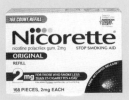

2 mg
Stop Smoking Aid in Original flavor
Nicotine Polacrilex Gum

Nicorette®

GlaxoSmithKline Consumer Healthcare
P. 807

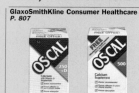

Calcium Supplement

Os-Cal®

GlaxoSmithKline Consumer Healthcare
P. 657

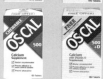

180 mg softgels

Gas Relief Phazyme®

GlaxoSmithKline Consumer Healthcare
P. 657

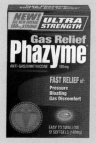

125 mg chewable tablets

**Quick Dissolve
Phazyme®**

GlaxoSmithKline Consumer Healthcare
P. 659

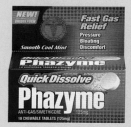

Acid Reducer
Packages of 6, 12, 18,
30, 50, 70 and 80 tablets.

Tagamet HB 200®

GlaxoSmithKline Consumer Healthcare
P. 659

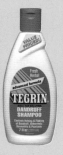

**Tegrin®
Dandruff Shampoo**

GlaxoSmithKline Consumer Healthcare
P. 660

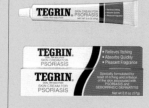

**Tegrin® Skin Cream
for Psoriasis**

GlaxoSmithKline Consumer Healthcare
P. 661

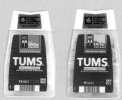

Peppermint and
Assorted flavors

Tums®

GlaxoSmithKline Consumer Healthcare
P. 661

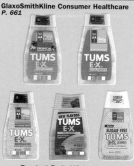

Tropical Fruit, Wintergreen,
Assorted Flavors, Assorted Berry
and SugarFree Orange Cream flavors

Tums E-X®

GlaxoSmithKline Consumer Healthcare
P. 661

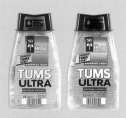

Assorted Mint and Fruit Flavors
Also available in Tropical Fruit,
Assorted Berries and
Spearmint flavors.

Tums® Ultra™

GlaxoSmithKline Consumer Healthcare
P. 661

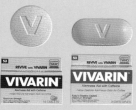

Alertness Aid with Caffeine
Available in tablets and caplets.

Vivarin®

GREEN PHARMACEUTICALS

Green Pharmaceuticals
P. 661

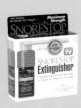

**SnoreStop® Extinguisher™
Oral Spray**

Green Pharmaceuticals
P. 662

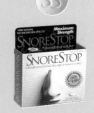

Box of 20 tablets.
Also available in box of 60 tablets.

**SnoreStop®
Maximum Strength
Chewable Tablets**

J&J-MERCK CONSUMER

J&J-Merck Consumer
P. 663

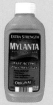

400 mg - 400 mg - 40 mg/5 mL

**Extra Strength
Fast-Acting Mylanta®**
(aluminum hydroxide/
magnesium hydroxide/simethicone)

J&J-Merck Consumer

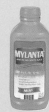

200 mg - 200 mg - 20 mg/5 mL

Fast-Acting Mylanta®
(aluminum hydroxide/magnesium
hydroxide/simethicone)

J&J-Merck Consumer
P. 664

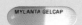

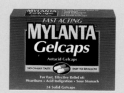

550 mg/125 mg

**Mylanta® Fast Acting
Gelcaps Antacid**
(calcium carbonate/
magnesium hydroxide)

J&J-Merck Consumer
P. 664

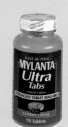

700 mg/300 mg

**Mylanta® Fast-Acting
Ultra Tabs**
(calcium carbonate/
magnesium hydroxide)

J&J-Merck Consumer
P. 664

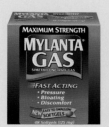

125 mg

Mylanta® Gas Maximum Strength
(simethicone)

J&J-Merck Consumer
P. 662

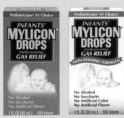

40 mg/0.6 mL

Infants Mylicon® Drops
(simethicone)

J&J-Merck Consumer
P. 665

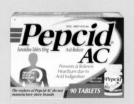

10 mg

Pepcid AC® Tablets
(famotidine)

J&J-Merck Consumer
P. 665

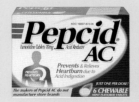

10 mg

Pepcid AC® Chewable Tablets
(famotidine)

J&J-Merck Consumer
P. 665

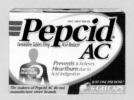

10 mg

Pepcid AC® Gelcaps
(famotidine)

J&J-Merck Consumer
P. 665

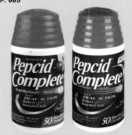

10 mg - 800 mg - 165 mg

Pepcid® Complete Chewable Tablets
(famotidine/calcium carbonate/ magnesium hydroxide)

KYOWA ENGINEERING-SUNDORY

Kyowa Engineering-Sundory
P. 809

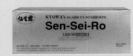

KYOWA's Agaricus Mushroom Extract
Dietary Supplement

Sen-Sei-Ro Liquid Gold™

Kyowa Engineering-Sundory
P. 810

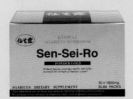

KYOWA's Agaricus Mushroom Powder
Dietary Supplement

Sen-Sei-Ro Powder Gold™

MANNATECH, INC.

Mannatech, Inc.
P. 811

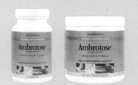

A Glyconutritional Dietary Supplement

Ambrotose®

Mannatech, Inc.
P. 812

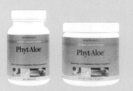

A Dietary Supplement of
Dried Fruits and Vegetables

Phyt•Aloe®

Mannatech, Inc.
P. 812

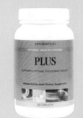

Dietary Supplement

PLUS with Ambrotose® complex

MATOL BOTANICAL INTERNATIONAL LTD.

Matol Botanical International Ltd.
P. 813

Dietary Supplement

Biomune OSF™ Plus

FACED WITH AN
Rx SIDE EFFECT?

Turn to the
Companion Drug Index
(Green Pages)
for products that provide
symptomatic relief.

MCNEIL

McNeil Consumer Healthcare
P. 666

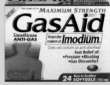

Softgels available in blister packs of
12 and 24.

Maximum Strength GasAid®

McNeil Consumer Healthcare
P. 666

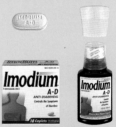

Available in 2 and 4 fl. oz. bottles
with a convenient dosage cup, and
caplets in 6's, 12's, 18's, 24's, 48's,
and 72's.

Imodium® A-D

McNeil Consumer Healthcare
P. 667

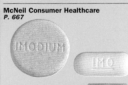

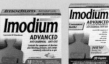

Vanilla mint chewable tablets
available in 12's, 18's,
30's and 42's. Caplets available
in 6's, 12's, 18's, and bottles of
30 and 42.

Imodium® Advanced

Lactaid Inc. Marketed By McNeil Consumer Healthcare
P. 814

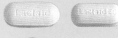
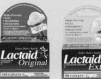

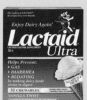

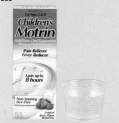

ORIGINAL STRENGTH available in bottles of 120.
EXTRA STRENGTH available in bottles of 50.
ULTRA CAPLETS available in single serve packets of 12, 32, 60 and 90 counts.
ULTRA CHEWABLE TABLETS available in single serve packets of 32 and 60 counts.

Lactaid® Caplets and Chewable Tablets

McNeil Consumer Healthcare
P. 669

Available in Berry flavor in 4 fl. oz. with child-resistant safety cap and convenient dosage cup.

Children's Motrin® Non-Staining Dye-Free Oral Suspension

McNeil Consumer Healthcare
P. 669

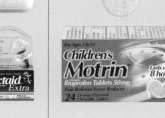
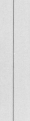
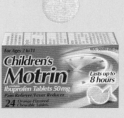

Available in Orange and Grape-Flavored Chewable Tablets of 50 mg.
Available in bottles of 24 with child-resistant safety cap.

Children's Motrin® Chewable Tablets

McNeil Consumer Healthcare
P. 669

Available in Berry, Bubble Gum and Grape flavors in 4 fl. oz. with child-resistant safety cap and convenient dosage cup.

Children's Motrin® Oral Suspension

McNeil Consumer Healthcare
P. 671

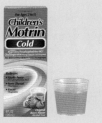
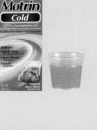

Available in Berry and Grape flavors in 4 fl. oz. with child-resistant safety cap and convenient dosage cup.
Berry Flavor also available in Non-Staining Dye-Free.

Children's Motrin® Cold Oral Suspension

McNeil Consumer Healthcare
P. 671

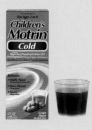

Available in Berry flavor in 4 fl. oz. with child-resistant safety cap and convenient dosage cup.

Children's Motrin® Cold Non-Staining Dye-Free Oral Suspension

McNeil Consumer Healthcare
P. 669

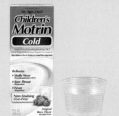
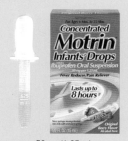

50 mg/1.25 mL
Available in 1/2 fl. oz. bottle.

Infants' Motrin® Concentrated Drops

McNeil Consumer Healthcare
P. 669

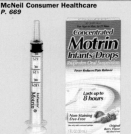

50 mg/1.25 mL
Available in 1 fl. oz. bottle.
New Syringe Dosing Device

Infants' Motrin® Non-Staining Dye-Free Concentrated Drops

McNeil Consumer Healthcare
P. 669

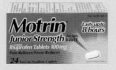

Available in bottles of 24 with child-resistant safety cap.

Junior Strength Motrin® Caplets

McNeil Consumer Healthcare
P. 669

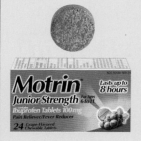
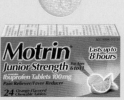

Available in Orange and Grape-flavored Chewable Tablets of 100 mg.
Available in bottles of 24 with child-resistant safety cap.

Junior Strength Motrin® Chewable Tablets

McNeil Consumer Healthcare
P. 668

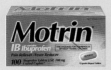

Gelcaps available in tamper evident packaging of 24, 50, and 100. Caplets available in tamper evident packaging of 24, 50, 100, 165, 250 and 300. Tablets available in tamper evident packaging of 24, 50, 100 and 165.

Motrin® IB

McNeil Consumer Healthcare
P. 669

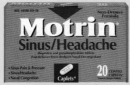

Caplets available in blister packs of 20's and 40's.

Motrin® Sinus/Headache

McNeil Consumer Healthcare
P. 671

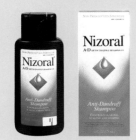

Available in 4 and 7 fl. oz. bottles.

Nizoral® A-D

McNeil Consumer Healthcare
P. 676

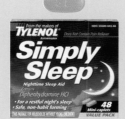

Mini-Caplets available in blister packs of 24, 48 and 72.

Simply-Sleep™

McNeil Consumer Healthcare
P. 686

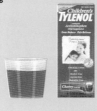

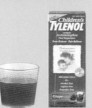

Available in Rich Cherry flavor in 2 and 4 fl. oz. bottles. Bubble Gum and Grape flavors in 4 fl. oz. with child-resistant safety cap and convenient dosage cup. Alcohol Free, 80 mg per 1/2 teaspoon.

Children's TYLENOL® Suspension Liquid

McNeil Consumer Healthcare
P. 688

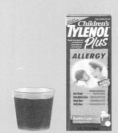

Available in Bubble Gum Blast flavor in child-resistant 4 fl. oz. bottles.

Children's TYLENOL® Plus Allergy Suspension Liquid

McNeil Consumer Healthcare
P. 686

Fruit flavor: bottles of 30 with child-resistant safety cap and blister packs of 60 and 96.
Bubble Gum and Grape flavor bottles: of 30 with child-resistant safety cap.

Children's TYLENOL® Soft Chews Chewable Tablets

McNeil Consumer Healthcare
P. 688

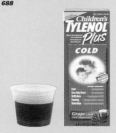

Available in 4 fl. oz. bottle with child-resistant safety cap and convenient dosage cup. Great Grape flavor.

Children's TYLENOL® Plus Cold Suspension Liquid

McNeil Consumer Healthcare
P. 688

Available in blister pack of 24 chewable tablets. Great Grape flavor.

Children's TYLENOL® Plus Cold Chewable Tablets

McNeil Consumer Healthcare
P. 688

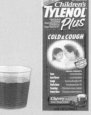

Available in 4 fl. oz. bottle with child-resistant safety cap and convenient dosage cup. Cherry flavor.

Children's TYLENOL® Plus Cold & Cough Suspension Liquid

McNeil Consumer Healthcare
P. 688

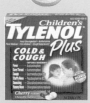

Available in blister pack of 24 chewable tablets. Cherry flavor.

Children's TYLENOL® Plus Cold & Cough Chewable Tablets

McNeil Consumer Healthcare
P. 690

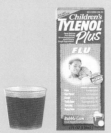

Available in Bubble Gum Blast flavor in child-resistant 4 fl. oz. bottles.

Children's TYLENOL® Plus Flu Suspension Liquid

McNeil Consumer Healthcare
P.690

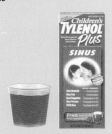

Available in Fruit Burst flavor in child-resistant 4 fl. oz. bottles.

Children's TYLENOL® Plus Sinus Suspension Liquid

McNeil Consumer Healthcare
P. 686

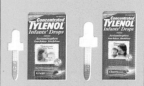

Available in Rich Cherry flavor and Rich Grape flavor 1/2 oz. bottle with child-resistant safety cap and calibrated dropper. Rich Grape Flavor, Alcohol Free, 80 mg per 0.8 mL. Cherry flavor also available in 1 oz. bottle.

Concentrated TYLENOL® Infants' Drops

McNeil Consumer Healthcare
P. 688

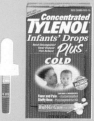

Available in 1/2 fl. oz. bottle with child-resistant safety cap and calibrated dropper. Bubble Gum flavor, Alcohol-free.

Concentrated TYLENOL® Infants' Drops Plus Cold

McNeil Consumer Healthcare
P. 688

Available in 1/2 fl. oz. bottle with child-resistant safety cap and calibrated dropper. Cherry flavor, Alcohol-free.

Concentrated TYLENOL® Infants' Drops Plus Cold & Cough

McNeil Consumer Healthcare
P. 686

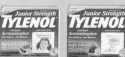

Available in blister pack of 24 chewable tablets. Fruit flavor and Grape flavor.

Junior Strength TYLENOL® Soft Chews Chewable Tablets

McNeil Consumer Healthcare
P. 677

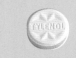

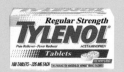

Tablets available in 100's.

Regular Strength TYLENOL®

McNeil Consumer Healthcare
P. 677

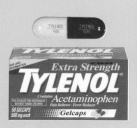

Extra Strength TYLENOL®

McNeil Consumer Healthcare
P. 677

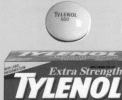

Gelcaps available in tamper-resistant bottles of 24's, 50's, 100's, 150's and 225's.

Geltabs available in tamper-resistant bottles of 24's, 50's, 100's and 150's.

Extra Strength TYLENOL®

McNeil Consumer Healthcare
P. 677

Geltabs available in tamper-evident bottles of 20, 40 and 80.

TYLENOL® 8 Hour Extended Release Geltabs

McNeil Consumer Healthcare
P. 677

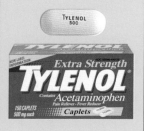

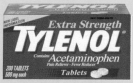

Caplets: tamper-resistant vials of 10 and bottles of 24's, 50's, 100's, 150's and 250's.

Tablets: tamper-resistant vials of 10 and bottles of 30's, 60's and 200's.

Liquid: tamper-evident bottles of 8 fl. oz.

Extra Strength TYLENOL®

McNeil Consumer Healthcare
P. 679

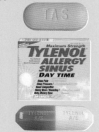

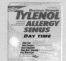

Caplets in blister packs of 24 & 48.
Gelcaps in blister packs of 24 & 48.
Geltabs in blister packs of 24 & 48.

Maximum Strength TYLENOL® Allergy Sinus Day Time

McNeil Consumer Healthcare
P. 679

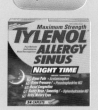

Caplets available in blister packs of 24's.

Maximum Strength TYLENOL® Allergy Sinus NightTime

McNeil Consumer Healthcare
P. 679

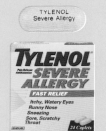

Caplets available in blister packs of 12's and 24's.

TYLENOL® Severe Allergy

McNeil Consumer Healthcare
P. 677

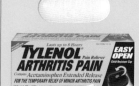

Caplets available in 24's, 50's, 100's, 150's, 250's and 290's.

TYLENOL® Arthritis Pain Extended Release

McNeil Consumer Healthcare
P. 681

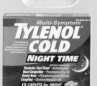
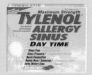

Caplets available in blister packs of 24.

Multi-Symptom TYLENOL® Cold Night Time

McNeil Consumer Healthcare
P. 681

Caplets available in
blister packs of 24.
Gelcaps available in
blister packs of 24.

**Multi-Symptom TYLENOL®
Cold Day Non-Drowsy**

McNeil Consumer Healthcare
P. 682

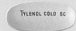

Available in blister
packs of 24.

**Multi-Symptom
TYLENOL® Cold Severe
Congestion Non-Drowsy**

McNeil Consumer Healthcare
P. 682

Gelcaps Available in
blister packs of 12's and 24's.

**Maximum Strength
TYLENOL® Flu NightTime**

McNeil Consumer Healthcare
P. 682

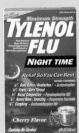

Available in 8 oz. bottles.

**Maximum Strength
TYLENOL® Flu
NightTime Liquid**

McNeil Consumer Healthcare
P. 682

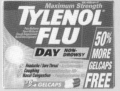

Gelcaps available in blister
packs of 24.

**Maximum Strength
TYLENOL® Flu Day
Non-Drowsy**

McNeil Consumer Healthcare
P. 684

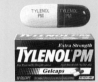

Geltabs available in tamper-resistant
bottles of 24, 50, 100 and 150.

Caplets available in tamper-resistant
bottles of 24, 50, 100, 150 and 225.

Gelcaps available in tamper-resistant
bottles of 24 and 50.

Geltabs, Caplets and Gelcaps
available in bottles of 50 for
households without children.

**Extra Strength
TYLENOL® PM**

McNeil Consumer Healthcare
P. 684

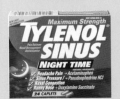

Available in blister packs of 24.

**Maximum Strength
TYLENOL® Sinus
Night Time**

McNeil Consumer Healthcare
P. 684

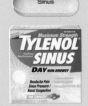

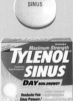

Caplets, Gelcaps and Geltabs
in blister packs of 24 and 48.

**Maximum Strength
TYLENOL® Sinus Day
Non-Drowsy**

McNeil Consumer Healthcare
P. 685

Cherry and Honey Lemon flavors
available in 8 fl. oz.

**Maximum Strength
TYLENOL® Sore Throat**

McNeil Consumer Healthcare
P. 686

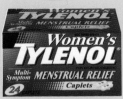

Caplets available in tamper-evident
bottles of 24.

**Women's TYLENOL®
Menstrual Relief**

Memory Secret
P. 815

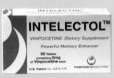

Powerful Memory Enhancer

Intelectol™

Novartis Consumer Health, Inc.
P. 816

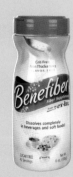

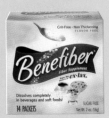

Available in 24 serving, 42 serving,
80 serving (club pack) bottles,
and 14 ct. packet carton.

**Benefiber®
Fiber Supplement**

Novartis Consumer Health, Inc.
P. 694

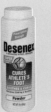 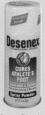
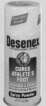

Powder   Spray Powder

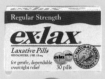

Antifungal Cream
Available in 12 g and 24 g.

Desenex®

Novartis Consumer Health, Inc.
P. 694

Available in Regular Strength
8's and 30's, Maximum Relief Formula
24's, 48's, and 90's, and
Chocolated Laxative 18's and 48's.

Ex•Lax®

Novartis Consumer Health, Inc.
P. 696

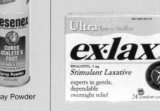

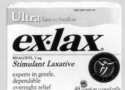

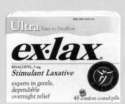

Ex•Lax® Ultra

Novartis Consumer Health, Inc.
P. 695

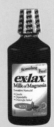

Mint Flavor
12 oz.

**Ex•Lax®
Milk of Magnesia**

Novartis Consumer Health, Inc.
P. 695

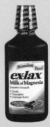

Chocolate Creme
12 oz.

**Ex•Lax®
Milk of Magnesia**

Novartis Consumer Health, Inc.
P. 695

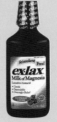

Raspberry Creme
12 oz.

**Ex•Lax®
Milk of Magnesia**

Novartis Consumer Health, Inc.
P. 696

125 mg
Available in Extra Strength Cherry 18 ct
and Extra Strength Peppermint 18 ct.

Gas-X®
(simethicone)

Novartis Consumer Health, Inc.
P. 696

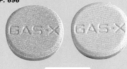

80 mg
Available in Cherry 36 ct and
Peppermint 36 ct.

Gas-X®
(simethicone)

Novartis Consumer Health, Inc.
P. 696

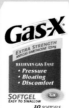

125 mg
Extra Strength Softgels
in packs of 10's, 30's, 50's, 60's.

Gas-X®
(simethicone)

Novartis Consumer Health, Inc.
P. 696

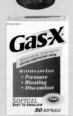

166 mg
Maximum Strength Softgels
in packs of 50's.

Gas-X®
(simethicone)

Novartis Consumer Health, Inc.
P. 696

125 mg/500 mg
Available in Extra Strength Wild Berry
8's and 24's and
Extra Strength Orange 8's and 24's.

Gas-X® with Maalox®
(simethicone/calcium carbonate)

Novartis Consumer Health, Inc.
P. 696

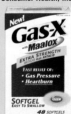

62.5 mg/250 mg
Extra Strength Softgels
in packs of 24's and 48's.

**Gas-X with
Maalox® Softgels**
(simethicone/calcium carbonate)

Novartis Consumer Health, Inc.
P. 697

Athlete's Foot Cream available in
12 g and 24 g.
Jock Itch Cream available in 12 g.

Lamisil ᴬᵀ® Cream

Novartis Consumer Health, Inc.
P. 697

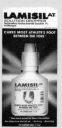

30 mL (1 oz)

**Lamisil AT®
Athlete's Foot
Solution Dropper**

Novartis Consumer Health, Inc.
P. 697

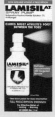

30 mL (1 oz)

**Lamisil AT®
Athlete's Foot
Spray Pump**

Novartis Consumer Health, Inc.
P. 697

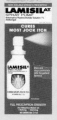

30 mL (1 oz)

**Lamisil AT®
Jock Itch
Spray Pump**

SEEKING AN
ALTERNATIVE?

Check the
Product Category Index,
where you'll find
alphabetical listings of
all the products in each
therapeutic class.

Novartis Consumer Health, Inc.
P. 698

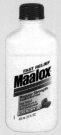

Cooling Mint Liquid
Also available in Smooth Cherry.
Bottles of 5 (Mint Only), 12 & 26 oz.

**Maalox® Antacid/Anti-Gas
Regular Strength**

Novartis Consumer Health, Inc.
P. 698

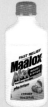

Cherry Liquid
Also available in Lemon (5, 12 & 26 oz.),
Cherry & Mint (12 & 26 oz.),
Vanilla Creme, Peaches N' Creme,
and Wild Berry (12 oz.).

**Maalox® Antacid/Anti-Gas
Maximum Strength**

Novartis Consumer Health, Inc.
P. 699

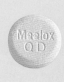

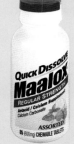

Assorted 85 ct
Wild Berry 45 ct
Lemon 85 ct

**Maalox® Quick Dissolve
Regular Strength Tablets
Antacid/Calcium
Supplement**

Novartis Consumer Health, Inc.
P. 699

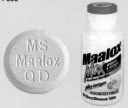

Assorted 35, 65, 90 ct
Wild Berry 35, 65 ct
Lemon 35, 65 ct

**Maalox® Max Quick
Dissolve Maximum
Strength Tablets
Antacid/AntiGas**

Novartis Consumer Health, Inc.
P. 699

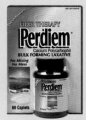

Available in 60 ct and
120 ct (club pak) blister card.

Perdiem Fiber Therapy

Novartis Consumer Health, Inc.
P. 700

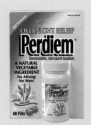

60 ct blister card

Perdiem Overnight Relief

Novartis Consumer Health, Inc.
P. 816

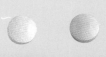

Slow Release Iron available
in 30, 60 and 90 ct.
Slow Release Iron & Folic Acid
available in 20 ct.

SLOW FE®

Novartis Consumer Health, Inc.
P. 700

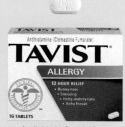

Available in 8 and 16 ct.

TAVIST® Allergy

Novartis Consumer Health, Inc.
P. 701

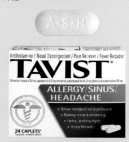

Available in 24 and 48 ct.

**TAVIST® Allergy/Sinus/
Headache**

Novartis Consumer Health, Inc.
P. 702

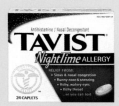

Available in 24 ct.

TAVIST® NightTime Allergy

Novartis Consumer Health, Inc.
P. 701

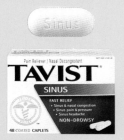

Available in 24 ct.

TAVIST® Sinus

Novartis Consumer Health, Inc.
P. 702

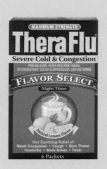

Flu & Congestion Non-Drowsy
Flu & Cough Night Time
Flu & Sore Throat Night Time
Severe Cold & Congestion Non-Drowsy
Cold & Sore Throat Night Time
Formulas above available in 6 ct.

Severe Cold & Congestion Night Time
Available in 6 ct. and 12 ct.

Cold & Cough Night Time
Available in 6 ct. and 12 ct.

Severe Cold & Congestion Night Time
Severe Cold & Congestion Non-Drowsy
Available in 12 ct. and 24 ct. caplets.

TheraFlu®

LOOKING FOR
A PARTICULAR
COMPOUND?

In the
Active Ingredients Index
(Yellow Pages),
you'll find all the
brands that contain it.

Novartis Consumer Health, Inc.
P. 707

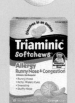

Allergy
Runny Nose &
Congestion
**Triaminic® Softchews®
Allergy**

Novartis Consumer Health, Inc.
P.707

Cold & Allergy

Cold & Cough   Cough &
Sore Throat

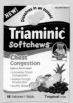

Chest Congestion

Triaminic® Softchews®

Novartis Consumer Health, Inc.
P. 709

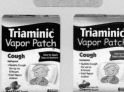

Menthol and
Mentholated Cherry Scents.

Triaminic® Vapor Patch

Novartis Consumer Health, Inc.
P. 704

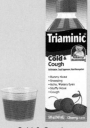

Cold & Cough

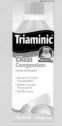

Chest Congestion

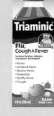

Cold & Allergy   Flu,
Cough & Fever

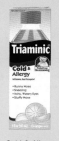
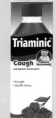

Cold & Night Time
Cough   Cough

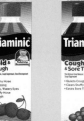

Cough & Congestion Cough & Sore
Throat

Triaminic®

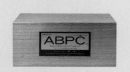

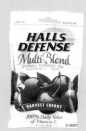

Pfizer Consumer Group, Pfizer Inc.
P. 710

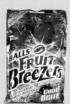

Pectin Throat Drops

Halls® Fruit Breezers

Pfizer Consumer Group, Pfizer Inc.
P. 711

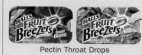

Honey-Lemon, Mentho-Lyptus® & Cherry

**Halls® Plus
Cough Suppressant/
Oral Anesthetic
Throat Drops
with Medicine Center**

Pfizer Consumer Group, Pfizer Inc.
P. 711

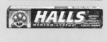

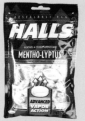

Cough Suppressant/
Oral Anesthetic Drops
Available in Spearmint,
Mentho-Lyptus®,
Ice Blue, Honey-Lemon,
Cherry and Strawberry Flavors.

Halls® Mentho-Lyptus®

Pfizer Consumer Group, Pfizer Inc.
P. 711

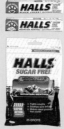

Cough Suppressant/
Oral Anesthetic Drops
Available in Black Cherry, Citrus Blend
and Mountain Menthol Flavors.

**Halls® Sugar Free
Squares Mentho-Lyptus®**

Pfizer Consumer Group, Pfizer Inc.
P. 712

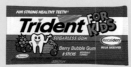

Sugarless Dental Gum available in
Berry Gum Flavor in a 8-stick pack.

**Trident for Kids™
with Recaldent™**

Pfizer Consumer Group, Pfizer Inc.
P. 712

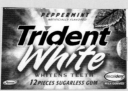

Available in Peppermint and
Wintergreen flavors in a 12-pellet
blister foil

**Trident White™
Sugarless Gum with
Recaldent™**

**PFIZER CONSUMER
HEALTHCARE, PFIZER INC.**

Pfizer Consumer Healthcare, Pfizer Inc.
P. 713

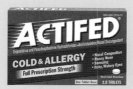

Available in boxes
of 12 and 24 tablets.

Actifed® Cold & Allergy

Pfizer Consumer Healthcare, Pfizer Inc.
P. 713

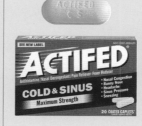

Actifed® Cold & Sinus

Pfizer Consumer Healthcare, Pfizer Inc.
P. 714

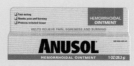

Ointment available in 1 oz. tubes.

Anusol® Ointment

Pfizer Consumer Healthcare, Pfizer Inc.
P. 714

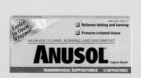

Suppositories available
in boxes of 12 and 24.

Anusol® Suppositories

Pfizer Consumer Healthcare, Pfizer Inc.
P. 714

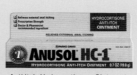

Anti-Itch Hydrocortisone Ointment
Available in 0.7 oz. tube.

Anusol HC-1™

Pfizer Consumer Healthcare, Pfizer Inc.
P. 715

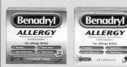

Tablets and Capsules
Available in boxes of 24 and 48
Tablets also available in
bottles of 100.

Benadryl® Allergy

Pfizer Consumer Healthcare, Pfizer Inc.
P. 715

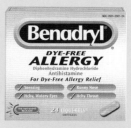

Available in boxes of 24 softgels.

**Benadryl® Dye-Free
Allergy Liqui-Gels®
Softgels**

Pfizer Consumer Healthcare, Pfizer Inc.
P. 716

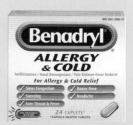

Available in boxes of 24 Tablets.

**Benadryl®
Allergy & Cold**

Pfizer Consumer Healthcare, Pfizer Inc.
P. 716

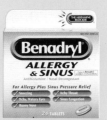

Available in boxes of 24 Tablets.

**Benadryl® Allergy &
Sinus**

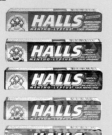

Pfizer Consumer Healthcare, Pfizer Inc.
P. 717

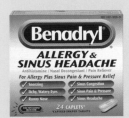

Available in boxes of 24 and 48 Caplets, and also available in boxes of 72 Gelcaps.

Benadryl® Allergy & Sinus Headache

Pfizer Consumer Healthcare, Pfizer Inc.
P. 717

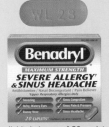

Available in boxes of 20 caplets.

Maximum Strength Benadryl® Severe Allergy & Sinus Headache

Pfizer Consumer Healthcare, Pfizer Inc.
P. 718

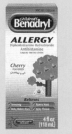

Available in boxes of 20 dissolving tablets.

Benadryl® Allergy & Sinus FASTMELT™

Pfizer Consumer Healthcare, Pfizer Inc.
P. 718

Available in 4 oz. and 8 oz. bottles.

Children's Benadryl® Allergy Liquid Medication

Pfizer Consumer Healthcare, Pfizer Inc.
P. 719

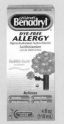

Available in 4 fl. oz. bottles.

Children's Benadryl® Dye-Free Allergy Liquid Medication

Pfizer Consumer Healthcare, Pfizer Inc.
P. 719

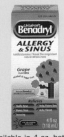

Available in 4 oz. bottles.

Children's Benadryl® Allergy & Sinus Liquid Medication

Pfizer Consumer Healthcare, Pfizer Inc.
P. 719

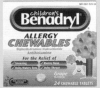

Available in boxes of 24 chewable Tablets.

Children's Benadryl® Allergy Chewables

Pfizer Consumer Healthcare, Pfizer Inc.
P. 720

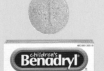

Available in boxes of 20 dissolving tablets.

Children's Benadryl® Allergy & Cold FASTMELT™

LOOKING FOR A PARTICULAR COMPOUND?

In the Active Ingredients Index (Yellow Pages), you'll find all the brands that contain it.

Pfizer Consumer Healthcare, Pfizer Inc.
P. 720

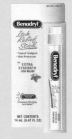

Extra Strength

Benadryl® Itch Relief Stick

Pfizer Consumer Healthcare, Pfizer Inc.
P. 721

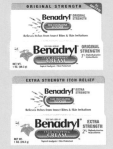

Original and Extra Strength

Benadryl® Itch Stopping Cream

Pfizer Consumer Healthcare, Pfizer Inc.
P. 722

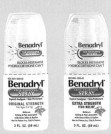

Original and Extra Strength

Benadryl® Itch Stopping Spray

Pfizer Consumer Healthcare, Pfizer Inc.
P. 722

Available in Arthritis Formula, Greaseless, Original Formula, Ultra Strength and Vanishing Scent.

BENGAY®

Pfizer Consumer Healthcare, Pfizer Inc.
P. 723

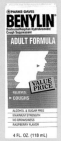

Available in 4 oz. bottles.

Benylin® Adult Cough Suppressant

Pfizer Consumer Healthcare, Pfizer Inc.
P. 723

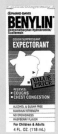

Available in 4 oz. bottles.

Benylin® Cough Suppressant Expectorant

Pfizer Consumer Healthcare, Pfizer Inc.
P. 724

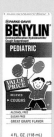

Available in 4 oz. bottles.

**Benylin® Pediatric
Cough Suppressant**

Pfizer Consumer Healthcare, Pfizer Inc.
P. 724

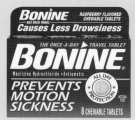

Available in 8 and 16
Chewable Tablets.

Bonine®

Pfizer Consumer Healthcare, Pfizer Inc.
P. 724

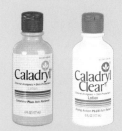

Itch Relief Plus Drying Action
Available in Lotion and Clear Lotion.

Caladryl®

Pfizer Consumer Healthcare, Pfizer Inc.
P. 725

Kids available in 1 oz. Creme
Cortizone•5 available in 1 oz.
and 2 oz. Creme and 1 oz. Ointment.

Cortizone•5®

Pfizer Consumer Healthcare, Pfizer Inc.
P. 726

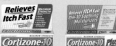

Cortizone•10 available in 1/2 oz.,
1 oz., and 2 oz. Creme and 1 oz.
and 2 oz. Ointment.
Cortizone•10 Plus available in
1 oz. and 2 oz. Creme.
Cortizone•10 Quick Shot Spray
available in 1.5 oz.

Cortizone•10®

Pfizer Consumer Healthcare, Pfizer Inc.
P. 727

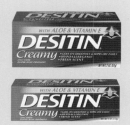

Diaper Rash Ointment

DESITIN® Creamy

Pfizer Consumer Healthcare, Pfizer Inc.
P. 728

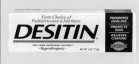
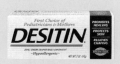

Diaper Rash Ointment

DESITIN®

Pfizer Consumer Healthcare, Pfizer Inc.
P. 728

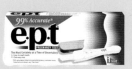

1, 2 and 3 Pregnancy Test Kits
Available
One Step. Easy to read.
99% accurate at detecting typical
pregnancy hormone levels.
Note, hormone levels may vary.
See insert.

e.p.t®

Pfizer Consumer Healthcare, Pfizer Inc.
P. 729

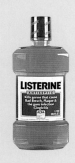

Listerine® Antiseptic

Pfizer Consumer Healthcare, Pfizer Inc.
P. 729

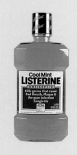

**Cool Mint
Listerine® Antiseptic**

Pfizer Consumer Healthcare, Pfizer Inc.
P. 729

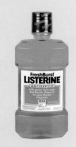

**FreshBurst Listerine®
Antiseptic**

Pfizer Consumer Healthcare, Pfizer Inc.
P. 729

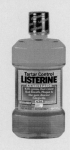

**Tartar Control Listerine®
Antiseptic**

Pfizer Consumer Healthcare, Pfizer Inc.
P. 730

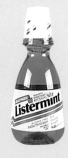

**Listermint®
Alcohol-Free Mouthwash**

Pfizer Consumer Healthcare, Pfizer Inc.
P. 730

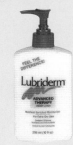

**Lubriderm® Advanced
Therapy Creamy Lotion**

Pfizer Consumer Healthcare, Pfizer Inc.
P. 730

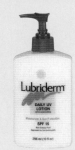

**Lubriderm® Daily UV
Lotion with Sunscreen**

Pfizer Consumer Healthcare, Pfizer Inc.
P. 730

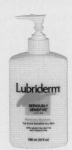

**Lubriderm® Seriously
Sensitive® Lotion**

Pfizer Consumer Healthcare, Pfizer Inc.
P. 730

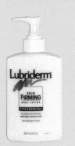

Lubriderm® Skin Firming Body Lotion

Pfizer Consumer Healthcare, Pfizer Inc.
P. 731

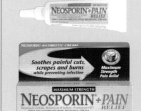

First Aid Antibiotic/
Pain Relieving Cream
Available in 1/2 oz. (14.2g) tubes.

NEOSPORIN®+ Pain Relief

Pfizer Consumer Healthcare, Pfizer Inc.
P. 733

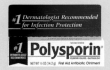

First Aid Antibiotic Powder & Ointment
Available in Powder, 0.35 oz. (10g)
and Ointment, 1/2 oz. (14.2g)
and 1 oz. (28.3g) tubes
and 1/32 oz (0.9g) foil packets.

Polysporin®

Pfizer Consumer Healthcare, Pfizer Inc.
P. 735

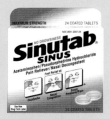

Maximum Strength
Without Drowsiness Formula
Available in 24 Caplets or Tablets.

Sinutab® Sinus

Pfizer Consumer Healthcare, Pfizer Inc.
P. 731

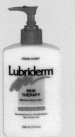

Available in Scented and
Fragrance Free.

Lubriderm® Lotion

Pfizer Consumer Healthcare, Pfizer Inc.
P. 731

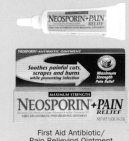

First Aid Antibiotic/
Pain Relieving Ointment
Available in 1/2 oz. (14.2g)
and 1 oz. (28.3g) tubes.

NEOSPORIN® + Pain Relief

Pfizer Consumer Healthcare, Pfizer Inc.
P. 734

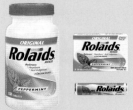

Fast, Effective Relief from
Heartburn, Acid Indigestion or
Sour Stomach.
Original Peppermint,
Spearmint, and Cherry Flavors.

Rolaids®

Pfizer Consumer Healthcare, Pfizer Inc.
P. 734

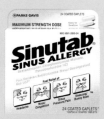

Maximum Strength Formula
Available in 24 Caplets or Tablets.

Sinutab® Sinus Allergy

Pfizer Consumer Healthcare, Pfizer Inc.
P.731

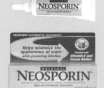

First Aid Antibiotic Ointment
Available in 1/2 oz. (14.2g) or 1 oz.
(28.3g) tubes; 1/32 oz. (0.9 g)
foil packets.

NEOSPORIN®

Pfizer Consumer Healthcare, Pfizer Inc.
P. 732

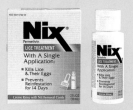

Lice Treatment Creme Rinse
2 fl. oz. (59 mL)
Also available in
2-bottle family pack.

Nix®

Pfizer Consumer Healthcare, Pfizer Inc.
P. 734

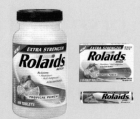

Cool Strawberry, Freshmint,
Fruit and Tropical Punch

Extra Strength Rolaids®

Pfizer Consumer Healthcare, Pfizer Inc.
P. 738

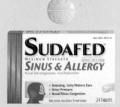

Available in boxes of 24.

Sudafed® Sinus & Allergy

Pfizer Consumer Healthcare, Pfizer Inc.
P. 731

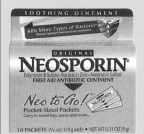

First Aid Antibiotic Ointment
Available in Individual Foil Packets.
1/32 oz. (0.9 g) 10 packets per Box.

NEOSPORIN® Neo to Go!™

Pfizer Consumer Healthcare, Pfizer Inc.
P. 733

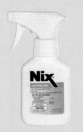

Lice Control Spray for
Bedding and Furniture.
*NOT FOR HUMAN USE

Nix®

Pfizer Consumer Healthcare, Pfizer Inc.
P. 734

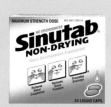

Available in Boxes of 24.

Sinutab® Non-Drying Liquid Caps

Pfizer Consumer Healthcare, Pfizer Inc.
P. 736

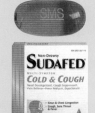

Available in 10 or 20 Liquid Caps.

Sudafed® Cold & Cough

Pfizer Consumer Healthcare, Pfizer Inc.
P. 738

Available in boxes of
10 and 20 liquid caps.

**Sudafed®
Sinus & Cold**

Pfizer Consumer Healthcare, Pfizer Inc.
P. 737

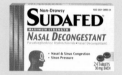

30 mg Tablets
Available in 24, 48 and 96 tablets.

**Sudafed®
Nasal Decongestant**

Pfizer Consumer Healthcare, Pfizer Inc.
P. 737

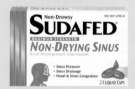

Available in 24 Liquid Caps.

**Sudafed® Non-Drying
Sinus Liquid Caps**

FACED WITH AN
Rx SIDE EFFECT?

Turn to the
Companion Drug Index
(Green Pages)
for products that provide
symptomatic relief.

Pfizer Consumer Healthcare, Pfizer Inc.
P. 737

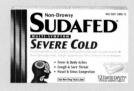

Pfizer Consumer Healthcare, Pfizer Inc.
P. 737

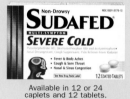

Available in 12 or 24
caplets and 12 tablets.

**Sudafed®
Severe Cold Formula**

Pfizer Consumer Healthcare, Pfizer Inc.
P. 735

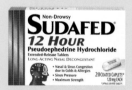

12 Hour Caplets
Available in 10 and 20 caplets.

Sudafed® 12 Hour

Pfizer Consumer Healthcare, Pfizer Inc.
P. 736

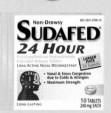

Available in boxes of 5 and 10 tablets.

Sudafed® 24 Hour

Pfizer Consumer Healthcare, Pfizer Inc.
P. 739

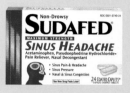

Pfizer Consumer Healthcare, Pfizer Inc.
P. 739

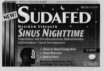

Available in 24 or 48 caplets and
24 tablets.

**Sudafed® Sinus
Headache**

Pfizer Consumer Healthcare, Pfizer Inc.
P. 739

Maximum Strength
Available in 12 tablets.

**Sudafed® Sinus
Nighttime**

Pfizer Consumer Healthcare, Pfizer Inc.
P. 740

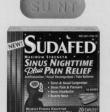

Maximum Strength
Available in 20 caplets.

**Sudafed® Sinus
Nighttime Plus Pain
Relief**

Pfizer Consumer Healthcare, Pfizer Inc.
P. 740

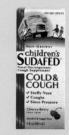

Available in 4 fl. oz. bottles.

**Children's Sudafed®
Cold & Cough
Liquid Medication**

Pfizer Consumer Healthcare, Pfizer Inc.
P. 741

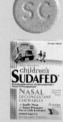

Available in boxes of
24 chewable tablets.

**Children's Sudafed®
Nasal Decongestant**

Pfizer Consumer Healthcare, Pfizer Inc.
P. 741

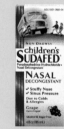

Available in 4 fl. oz. bottles.

**Children's Sudafed®
Nasal Decongestant
Liquid Medication**

Pfizer Consumer Healthcare, Pfizer Inc.
P. 741

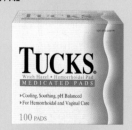

Pre-Moistened Pads
Available in 40 and 100 pad packages.
Tucks® Take Alongs available in 12
individually packed towelettes.

Tucks®

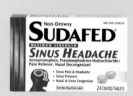

Pfizer Consumer Healthcare, Pfizer Inc.
P. 742

Nighttime Sleep Aid
SleepGels available in
8, 16 and 32 softgels.
SleepTabs available in
8, 16, 32 and 48 tablets.

Unisom®

Pfizer Consumer Healthcare, Pfizer Inc.
P. 742

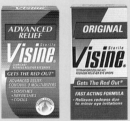

Visine®
Advanced Relief
Lubricant/Redness
Reliever Eye Drops

Visine®
Original
Redness Reliever
Eye Drops

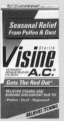

Visine A.C.®
Astringent/Redness
Reliever Eye Drops

Visine L.R.™
Redness Reliever
Eye Drops

Visine®

Pfizer Consumer Healthcare, Pfizer Inc.
P. 743

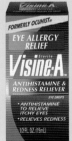

Visine-A®
Antihistamine and
Redness Reliever Eye Drops

Visine-A®

Pfizer Consumer Healthcare, Pfizer Inc.
P. 744

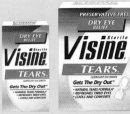

Visine Tears®
Lubricant
Eye Drops

Visine Tears®
Preservative Free
Lubricant Eye Drops

Visine Tears®

Pfizer Consumer Healthcare, Pfizer Inc.
P. 745

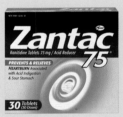

Available in boxes of
4, 10, 20, 30, 60, 80
and 110 tablets.

Zantac® 75

PROCTER & GAMBLE

Procter & Gamble
P. 751

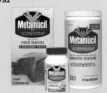

Available in 30, 48, 72, 114 and 180
dose canisters and cartons of 30
one-dose packets.
Also available in sugar free. Capsules
available in 100 ct. and 160 ct.
Cinnamon Spice and Apple Crisp
Wafers available in 12-dose cartons.

Metamucil®

Procter & Gamble
P. 753

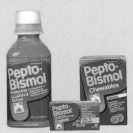

Also available in Maximum Strength
Liquid, Chewable Tablets and
Swallowable Caplets

Pepto-Bismol®

Procter & Gamble
P. 754

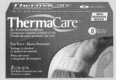

Back/Hip Wrap for Pain Relief
and Muscle Relaxation

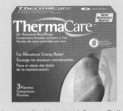

Patches For Menstrual Cramp Relief

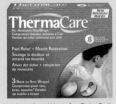

Neck to Arm Wrap for Pain Relief
and Muscle Relaxation

Air-Activated Heat Wraps

ThermaCare®

Procter & Gamble
P. 759

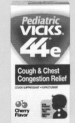

44®e
Cough & Chest Congestion Relief

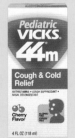

44®m
Cough & Cold Relief

Pediatric Vicks®

Procter & Gamble
P. 754

VICKS® 44®
Cough Relief

VICKS® 44®D
Cough & Head Congestion Relief

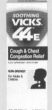

VICKS® 44® E
Cough & Chest Congestion Relief

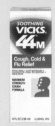

VICKS® 44® M
Cough, Cold & Flu Relief

VICKS®

Procter & Gamble
P. 757

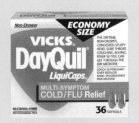

Multi-Symptom
Cold/Flu Relief
Also available as DayQuil Liquid.

**VICKS® DayQuil®
LiquiCaps®**

Procter & Gamble
P. 756

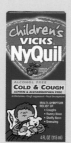

Cherry Flavor
Cold & Cough Relief

Children's VICKS® NyQuil®

Procter & Gamble
P. 758

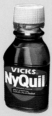

Multi-Symptom
Cold/Flu Relief
Also available as NyQuil LiquiCaps.

**VICKS® NyQuil®
Liquid**

Procter & Gamble
P. 758

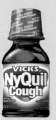

Cough Relief

**VICKS® NyQuil®
Cough**

PURDUE FREDERICK

The Purdue Frederick Company
P. 762

Maximum Strength Ointment

Antibiotics + Moisturizer

Antibiotics + Pain Reliever

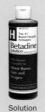

Solution

Betadine®

The Purdue Frederick Company
P. 764

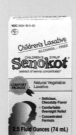

Natural Vegetable Laxative
Children's Syrup

Senokot®

The Purdue Frederick Company
P. 764

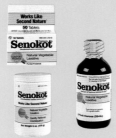

Natural Vegetable Laxative
Available in Tablets, Granules,
and Syrup.

Senokot®

The Purdue Frederick Company
P. 764

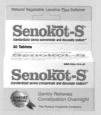

Natural Vegetable Laxative
Plus Softener Tablets

Senokot-S®

PURDUE PRODUCTS L.P.

Purdue Products L.P.
P. 763

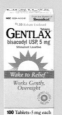

5 mg
100 Tablets

Gentlax®
(bisacodyl USP)

REXALL SUNDOWN

Rexall Sundown
P. 819

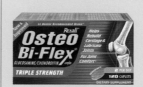

Osteo Bi-Flex®

SCHERING-PLOUGH

Schering-Plough HealthCare Products
P. 764

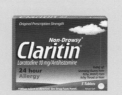

10 mg
Available in 5 ct, 10 ct and 20 ct.

Claritin® Tablets
(loratadine)

Schering-Plough HealthCare Products
P. 766

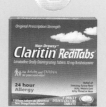

10 mg
Orally Disintegrating Tablets
Available in 4 ct and 10 ct.

Claritin® RediTabs®
(loratadine)

Schering-Plough HealthCare Products
P. 765

5 mg/120 mg
Available in 10 ct.

10 mg/240 mg
Available in 5 ct and 10 ct.
Available in 12 hour and
24 hour extended release tablets.

Claritin-D®
(loratadine/pseudoephedrine sulfate)

Schering-Plough HealthCare Products
P. 765

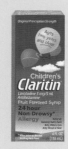

5 mg/5 mL
Available in 4 oz bottle.

Claritin® Children's Syrup
(loratadine)

Schering-Plough HealthCare Products
P. 766

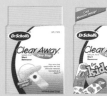

**Dr. Scholls®
Clear Away® One Step
Wart Removers**

Schering-Plough HealthCare Products
P. 767

Available as Athlete's Foot Cream,
Solution, and Jock Itch Cream.
Lotrimin® AF
(clotrimazole 1%)

Schering-Plough HealthCare Products
P. 767

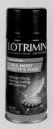 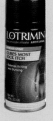

Available as Athlete's Foot
Spray Liquid, Powder and Deodorant
Powder, Athlete's Foot Powder
and Jock Itch Spray Powder.
Lotrimin® AF
(miconazole nitrate 2%)

Schering-Plough HealthCare Products
P. 768

Athlete's Foot Cream

Jock Itch Cream
Lotrimin Ultra®
(butenafine HCl 1%)

SUNPOWER

Sunpower Nutraceutical Inc.
P. 820

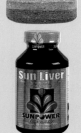

Sun Liver™

TAHITIAN NONI INTERNATIONAL

Tahitian Noni International
P. 820

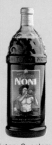

Dietary Supplement
Tahitian Noni® Juice

TOPICAL BIOMEDICS, INC.

Topical BioMedics, Inc.
P. 771

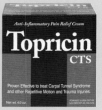

4 oz.
Also available in 2 oz. tube
and 32 oz. pump.
Topricin®

LOOKING FOR
A PARTICULAR
COMPOUND?

In the
Active Ingredients Index
(Yellow Pages),
you'll find all the
brands that contain it.

4LIFE RESEARCH™

4Life Research™
P. 805

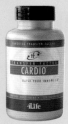

Dietary Supplement
Transfer Factor Cardio™

4Life Research™
P. 805

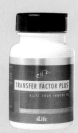

Dietary Supplement
Transfer Factor Plus™

NONPRESCRIPTION DRUG INFORMATION

This section presents information on nonprescription drugs, self-testing kits, and other medical products marketed for home use by consumers. It is made possible through the courtesy of the manufacturers whose products appear on the following pages. The information concerning each product has been prepared, edited, and approved by the manufacturer's professional staff.

Pharmaceutical product descriptions in this section must be in compliance with the Code of Federal Regulations' labeling requirements for over-the-counter drugs. The descriptions are designed to provide all information necessary for informed use, including, when applicable, active ingredients, inactive ingredients, indications, actions, warnings, cau-

tions, drug interactions, symptoms and treatment of oral overdosage, dosage and directions for use, professional labeling, and how supplied. In some cases, additional information has been supplied to complement the standard labeling.

In compiling this section, the publisher has emphasized the necessity of describing products comprehensively. The descriptions seen here include all information made available by the manufacturer. The publisher does not warrant or guarantee any product described here, and does not perform any independent analysis of the information provided. Inclusion of a product in this book does not represent an endorsement, and the publisher does not necessarily advocate the use of any product listed.

A.C. Grace Co.
1100 QUITMAN ROAD
P.O. BOX 570
BIG SANDY, TX 75755

Direct Inquiries to:
Inquiries: (903) 636-4368
Orders Only: 800-833-4368
www.acgrace.com

UNIQUE E®
NATURAL VITAMIN E COMPLEX
MIXED TOCOPHEROL CONCENTRATE

Description:
Established 1962... OUR ONLY PRODUCT.
WHY UNIQUE?
All NATURAL VITAMIN E COMPLEX.
NOT the *dl* SYNTHETIC CHEMICAL
form, *NOT ESTER*IFIED TOCOPH-
ERYL ACETATE (OR SUCCINATE),
NOT the ORDINARY SOY OIL
DILUTED MIXED TOCOPHEROLS OR
ADULTERATED FORMS.

Each soft easy-to-swallow high quality
GEL CAPSULE contains **ALL NATU-
RAL *UN*ESTERIFIED VITAMIN E
COMPLEX** providing **400 I.U. ANTI-
THROMBIC** function d-alpha tocoph-
erol with other naturally occuring **AN-
TIOXIDANT** tocopherols, **d-beta, d
GAMMA, d-delta** for maximum protec-
tion against *harmful* free radical dam-
age and inhibiting peroxynitrites dam-
aging to brain cells.

NO SOY or other OIL FILLER additives
which can turn rancid and cause harmful free radical damage even in sealed
gel capsules.

NO ALLERGY CAUSING PRESERVA-
TIVES, COLORS OR FLAVORINGS.

UNIQUE E® capsule potency is stabilized and Certified by Assay.

Dosage: Up to 6 capsules daily as
directed by your physician according to
individual weight or need, usually 1
capsule per each 40 lbs. of total body
weight. Best results when ENTIRE daily
dose is taken just before or with the
morning meal.

How Supplied:
Bottles of 180 and 90 easy-to-swallow
high quality gel capsules in safety sealed
light protected bottles.

UNKNOWN DRUG?
Consult the
Product Identification Guide
(Gray Pages)
for full-color photos of
leading over-the-counter
medications

Adams Laboratories, Inc.
14801 SOVEREIGN ROAD
FORT WORTH, TX 76155

Direct Inquiries to:
Medical Affairs 817-786-1200

MUCINEX™ 600 mg
(Guaifenesin Extended-Release Tablets)
MUCINEX™ 1200 mg
(Guaifenesin Extended-Release Tablets)

Drug Facts

Active Ingredient:
(in each extended-release tablet)

Purpose

MUCINEX™ 600 mg
Guaifenesin 600 mg .... Expectorant
MUCINEX™ 1200 mg
Guaifenesin 1200 mg .... Expectorant

Uses: Helps loosen phlegm (mucus)
and thin bronchial secretions to rid the
bronchial passageways of bothersome
mucus and make coughs more productive

Warnings:
Do not use
• for children under 12 years of age
Ask a doctor before use if you have
• persistent or chronic cough such as occurs with smoking, asthma, chronic
bronchitis, or emphysema
• cough accompanied by too much
phlegm (mucus)
Stop use and ask a doctor if
• cough lasts more than 7 days, comes
back, or occurs with fever, rash, or persistent headache. These could be signs
of a serious illness.
If pregnant or breast-feeding, ask a
health professional before use.
Keep out of reach of children. In case of
overdose, get medical help or contact a
Poison Control Center right away.

Directions:
• do not crush, chew, or break tablet
• take with a full glass of water
• this product can be administered without regard for the timing of meals
MUCINEX™ 600 mg
• adults and children 12 years of age
and over: one or two tablets every 12
hours. Do not exceed 4 tablets in 24
hours.
MUCINEX™ 1200 mg
• adults and children 12 years of age
and over: 1 tablet every 12 hours. Do
not exceed 2 tablets in 24 hours.
• children under 12 years of age: do not
use

Other Information:
• tamper evident: do not use if neckband
is broken
• store between 20–25°C (68–77°F)
• see bottom of bottle for lot code and expiration date

Inactive Ingredients: carbomer 934P,
NF; dyes; hydroxypropyl methylcellulose, USP; magnesium stearate, NF; microcrystalline cellulose, NF; sodium
starch glycolate, NF

How Supplied:
MUCINEX™ 600 mg
Bottles of 20 tablets, (NDC 63824-008-
20), 40 tablets (NDC 63824-008-40) and
sample bottles of 2 tablets (NDC 63824-
008-82). Round tablet debossed with "A"
on the light blue, marbled layer and
"600" on the white bi-layer. Each tablet
provides 600 mg guaifenesin.
MUCINEX™ 1200 mg
Tri Pack (NDC 63824-052-60) containing
3 bottles of 20 tablets (NDC 63824-052-
20) and sample bottles of 2 tablets (NDC
63824-052-82). Modified oval tablet debossed with "Adams" on the light green,
marbled layer and "1200" on the white
bi-layer. Each tablet provides 1200 mg
guaifenesin.
US Patent No. 6,372,252 B1
REV 0203

Alpharma
U.S. Pharmaceuticals
Division
7205 WINDSOR BOULEVARD
BALTIMORE, MD 21244

For General Inquiries Contact:
Customer Service
800-432-8534

PERMETHRIN LOTION 1%
Lice Treatment

Description:
EACH FLUID OUNCE CONTAINS: Active Ingredient: Permethrin 280 mg (1%).
Inactive Ingredients: Balsam fir canada,
cetyl alcohol, citric acid, FD&C Yellow
No. 6, fragrance, hydrolyzed animal protein, hydroxyethylcellulose, polyoxyethylene 10 cetyl ether, propylene glycol,
stearalkonium chloride, water, isopropyl
alcohol 5.6 g (20%), methylparaben
56 mg (0.2%), and propylparaben 22 mg
(0.08%).
Permethrin Lotion 1% kills lice and their
unhatched eggs with usually only one
application. Permethrin Lotion 1% protects against head lice reinfestation for
14 days. The creme rinse formula leaves
hair manageable and easy to comb.

Indications: For the treatment of
head lice. For prophylactic use during
head lice epidemics.

Warnings: For external use only. Keep
out of eyes when rinsing hair. Adults and
children: Close eyes and do not open eyes
until product is rinsed out. If product
gets into the eyes, immediately flush
with water. Do not use near the eyes or
permit contact with mucous membranes,
such as inside the nose, mouth, or vagina, as irritation may occur. Children:
Also protect children's eyes with a washcloth, towel or other suitable material or
method. This product should not be used
on pediatric patients less than 2 months

of age. Itching, redness, or swelling of the scalp may occur. If skin irritation persists or infection is present or develops, discontinue use and consult a doctor. Consult a doctor if infestation of eyebrows or eyelashes occurs. This product may cause breathing difficulty or an asthmatic episode in susceptible persons. As with any drug, if you are pregnant or nursing a baby, seek the advice of a health professional before using this product. Keep this and all drugs out of the reach of children. In case of accidental ingestion, seek professional assistance or contact a Poison Control Center immediately.

Dosage and Administration:
Treatment: Permethrin Lotion 1% should be used after hair has been washed with patient's regular shampoo, rinsed with water and towel dried. A sufficient amount should be applied to saturate hair and scalp (especially behind the ears and on the nape of the neck). Leave on hair for 10 minutes but not longer. Rinse with water. A single application is usually sufficient. If live lice are observed seven days or more after the first application of this product, a second treatment should be given. For proper head lice management, remove nits with the nit comb provided.

Head lice live on the scalp and lay small white eggs (nits) on the hair shaft close to the scalp. The nits are most easily found on the nape of the neck or behind the ears. All personal headgear, scarfs, coats, and bed linen should be disinfected by machine washing in hot water and drying, using the hot cycle of a dryer for at least 20 minutes. Personal articles of clothing or bedding that cannot be washed may be dry-cleaned, sealed in a plastic bag for a period of about 2 weeks, or sprayed with a product specifically designed for this purpose. Personal combs and brushes may be disinfected by soaking in hot water (above 130°F) for 5 to 10 minutes. Thorough vacuuming of rooms inhabited by infected patients is recommended.

Prophylaxis: Prophylactic use of Permethrin Lotion 1% is only recommended for individuals exposed to head lice epidemics in which at least 20% of the population at an institution are infested and for immediate household members of infested individuals. Casual use is strongly discouraged.

The method of application of Permethrin Lotion 1% for prophylaxis is identical to that described above for treatment of a lice infestation except nit removal is not required.

Directions For Use: One application of Permethrin Lotion 1% has been shown to protect greater than 95% of patients against reinfestation for at least two weeks. In epidemic settings, a second prophylactic application is recommended two weeks after the first because the life cycle of a head louse is approximately four weeks.

How Supplied: Bottles of 2 fl. oz. (59 mL) with nit removal comb and Family Pack of 2 bottles, 2 fl. oz. (59 mL) each, with 2 nit removal combs. Store at 15° to 25°C (59° to 77°F).
Manufactured by
Alpharma USPD Inc.
Baltimore, MD 21244
FORM NO. 5242   Rev. 9/99
VC1587

Bayer HealthCare LLC Consumer Care Division
**36 COLUMBIA ROAD
P.O. BOX 1910
MORRISTOWN, NJ 07962-1910**

Direct Inquiries to:
Consumer Relations
(800) 331-4536
www.bayercare.com

For Medical Emergency Contact:
Bayer HealthCare LLC
Consumer Care Division
(800) 331-4536

ALEVE®
**All Day Strong
naproxen sodium tablets, 220 mg
Pain reliever/fever reducer**

ALEVE® Caplets*, Gelcaps**, or Tablets
Naproxen Sodium Tablets, USP

Active Ingredient: **Purpose:**
(in each tablet/caplet/gelcap)
Naproxen sodium 220 mg (naproxen 200 mg) ...... Pain reliever/Fever reducer

Uses: Temporarily relieves minor aches and pains due to:
• headache
• muscular aches
• minor pain of arthritis
• toothache
• backache
• common cold
• menstrual cramps
temporarily reduces fever

---
* capsule-shaped tablet(s)
** gelatin coated capsule-shaped tablet(s)

Warnings: Allergy Alert: Naproxen sodium may cause a severe allergic reaction which may include:
• hives
• facial swelling
• asthma (wheezing)
• shock
Alcohol warning: If you consume 3 or more alcoholic drinks every day, ask your doctor whether you should take naproxen sodium or other pain relievers/fever reducers. Naproxen sodium may cause stomach bleeding.
Do not use if you have ever had an allergic reaction to any other pain reliever/fever reducer
Ask a doctor before use if you have had serious side effects from any pain reliever/fever reducer
Ask a doctor or pharmacist before use if you are
• under a doctor's care for any serious condition
• taking other drug
• taking any other product that contains naproxen sodium, or any other pain reliever/fever reducer
Stop use and ask a doctor if
• an allergic reaction occurs. Seek medical help right away.
• pain gets worse or lasts more than 10 days
• fever gets worse or lasts more than 3 days
• you have difficulty swallowing
• it feels like the pill is stuck in your throat
• you develop heartburn
• stomach pain occurs or lasts, even if symptoms are mild
• redness or swelling is present in the painful area
• any new symptoms appear
If pregnant or breast-feeding, ask a health professional before use. It is especially important not to use naproxen sodium during the last 3 months of pregnancy unless definitely directed to do so by a doctor because it may cause problems in the unborn child or complications during delivery.
Keep out of reach of children. In case of overdose, get medical help or contact a Poison Control Center right away.

Directions:
• **do not take more than directed**
• drink a full glass of water with each dose
[See table below]
Other Information:
• store at 20–25°C (68–77°F)

Continued on next page

Adults and children 12 years and older	• take 1 tablet (caplet, gelcap) every 8 to 12 hours while symptoms last • for the first dose you may take 2 tablets (caplets, gelcaps) within the first hour • the smallest effective dose should be used • do not exceed 2 tablets (caplets, gelcaps) in any 8- to 12-hour period • do not exceed 3 tablets (caplets, gelcaps) in a 24-hour period
Adults over 65 years	• do not take more than 1 tablet (caplet, gelcap) every 12 hours unless directed by a doctor
Children under 12 years	• ask a doctor

Aleve—Cont.

• avoid high humidity and excessive heat above 40°C (104°F)

ALEVE® Tablets, caplets, gelcaps
• **each contains:** sodium 20 mg

Aleve tablets, caplets:

Inactive Ingredients: FD&C blue #2 lake, hypromellose, magnesium stearate, microcrystalline cellulose, polyethylene glycol, povidone, talc, titanium dioxide

Aleve gelcaps:

Inactive Ingredients: D&C yellow #10 aluminum lake, EDTA disodium, edible ink, FD&C blue #1, FD&C yellow #6 aluminum lake, gelatin, glycerin, hypromellose, magnesium stearate, microcrystalline cellulose, polyethylene glycol, povidone, stearic acid, talc, titanium dioxide

How Supplied:
ALEVE® Caplets in boxes of 8, 24, 50, 100, 150, 200.
ALEVE® Gelcaps in boxes of 20, 40, 80.
ALEVE® Tablets in boxes of 24, 50, 100, 150.
Questions or comments? call **1-800-395-0689** or www.aleve.com
Do not use if carton is open or if foil seal imprinted with "Safety *SQUEASE®*" on bottle opening is missing or broken.
Distributed by
Bayer HealthCare LLC
PO Box 1910
Morristown, NJ 07962-1910 USA
B-R LLC
*Read Consumer
Leaflet Before Use*
*Shown in Product Identification
Guide, page 503*

ALEVE® COLD & SINUS
Pain reliever/fever reducer/nasal decongestant

Active ingredients:
(in each caplet)   **Purposes**
Naproxen sodium 220 mg
(naproxen 200 mg) ... Pain reliever/fever reducer
Pseudoephedrine HCl 120 mg, extended-release ..... Nasal decongestant
Uses: temporarily relieves these cold, sinus, and flu symptoms:
• sinus pressure
• minor body aches and pains
• headache
• nasal and sinus congestion (promotes sinus drainage and restores freer breathing through the nose)
• fever

Warnings:
Allergy alert: Naproxen sodium may cause a severe allergic reaction which may include:
• hives
• facial swelling
• asthma (wheezing)
• shock
Alcohol warning: If you consume 3 or more alcoholic drinks every day, ask your doctor whether you should take naproxen sodium or other pain relievers/

fever reducers. Naproxen sodium may cause stomach bleeding.

Do not use
• if you have ever had an allergic reaction to any other pain reliever/fever reducer
• if you are now taking a prescription monoamine oxidase inhibitor (MAOI) (certain drugs for depression, psychiatric, or emotional conditions, or Parkinson's disease), or for 2 weeks after stopping the MAOI drug. If you do not know if your prescription drug contains an MAOI, ask a doctor or pharmacist before taking this product.

Ask a doctor before use if you have
• heart disease
• high blood pressure
• thyroid disease
• diabetes
• trouble urinating due to an enlarged prostate gland
• had serious side effects from any pain reliever/fever reducer

Ask a doctor or pharmacist before use if you are
• using any other product containing naproxen or pseudoephedrine
• taking any other pain reliever/fever reducer or nasal decongestant
• under a doctor's care for any continuing medical condition
• taking other drugs on a regular basis

When using this product do not use more than directed.

Stop use and ask a doctor if
• an allergic reaction occurs. Seek medical help right away.
• you get nervous, dizzy, or sleepless
• you develop heartburn
• nasal congestion lasts more than 7 days
• symptoms continue or get worse
• you have trouble swallowing or the caplet feels stuck in your throat
• new or unexpected symptoms occur
• stomach pain occurs with use of this product or if even mild symptoms persist
• fever lasts for more than 3 days

If pregnant or breast-feeding, ask a health professional before use.
It is especially important not to use naproxen sodium during the last 3 months of pregnancy unless definitely directed to do so by a doctor because it may cause problems in the unborn child or complications during delivery.

Keep out of reach of children. In case of overdose, get medical help or contact a Poison Control Center right away.

Directions:
• **swallow whole;** do not crush or chew
• **drink a full glass of water with each dose**
• adults and children 12 years and older: **1 caplet every 12 hours;** do not take more than 2 caplets in 24 hours
• children under 12 years: ask a doctor

Other information:
• **each caplet contains:** sodium 20 mg
• store at 20 to 25° C (68–77°F)
• store in a dry place

Inactive Ingredients: colloidal silicon dioxide, FD&C blue #1 lake, hypromellose, lactose, magnesium stearate, microcrystalline cellulose, pharmaceutical glaze, polyethylene glycol, povidone, propylene glycol, talc, titanium dioxide

Questions or comments? 1-800-395-0689 or www.aleve.com

How Supplied: Boxes of 10, 20, or 30 caplets (capsule-shaped tablets)
Distributed by: Bayer Corporation
Consumer Care Division
Morristown, NJ 07960 USA   B-R LLC
*Shown in Product Identification
Guide, page 503*

ALEVE® SINUS & HEADACHE
Pain reliever/fever reducer/nasal decongestant

**Active ingredients
(in each caplet)**   **Purposes**
Naproxen sodium 220 mg
(naproxen 200 mg) ... Pain reliever/fever reducer
Pseudoephedrine HCl 120 mg, extended-release ..... Nasal decongestant

Uses: temporarily relieves these cold, sinus, and flu symptoms:
• sinus pressure
• minor body aches and pains
• headache
• nasal and sinus congestion (promotes sinus drainage and restores freer breathing through the nose)
• fever

Warnings: Allergy alert: Naproxen sodium may cause a severe allergic reaction which may include:
• hives
• facial swelling
• asthma (wheezing)
• shock
Alcohol warning: If you consume 3 or more alcoholic drinks every day, ask your doctor whether you should take naproxen sodium or other pain relievers/fever reducers. Naproxen sodium may cause stomach bleeding.

Do not use
• if you have ever had an allergic reaction to any other pain reliever/fever reducer
• if you are now taking a prescription monoamine oxidase inhibitor (MAOI) (certain drugs for depression, psychiatric or emotional conditions, or Parkinson's disease), or for 2 weeks after stopping the MAOI drug. If you do not know if your prescription drug contains an MAOI, ask a doctor or pharmacist before taking this product.

Ask a doctor before use if you have
• heart disease
• high blood pressure
• thyroid disease
• diabetes
• trouble urinating due to an enlarged prostate gland
• had serious side effects from any pain reliever/fever reducer

Ask a doctor or pharmacist before use if you are
• using any other product containing naproxen or pseudoephedrine
• taking any other pain reliever/fever reducer or nasal decongestant
• under a doctor's care for any continuing medical condition
• taking other drugs on a regular basis

When using this product do not use more than directed.

Stop use and ask a doctor if:
- an allergic reaction occurs. Seek medical help right away.
- you get nervous, dizzy, or sleepless
- you develop heartburn
- nasal congestion lasts more than 7 days
- symptoms continue or get worse
- you have trouble swallowing or the caplet feels stuck in your throat
- new or unexpected symptoms occur
- stomach pain occurs with use of this product or if even mild symptoms persist
- fever lasts for more than 3 days

If pregnant or breast-feeding, ask a health professional before use. It is especially important not to use naproxen sodium during the last 3 months of pregnancy unless definitely directed to do so by a doctor because it may cause problems in the unborn child or complications during delivery.

Keep out of reach of children. If case of overdose, get medical help or contact a Poison Control Center right away.

Directions:
- **swallow whole;** do not crush or chew
- **drink a full glass of water with each dose**
- adults and children 12 years and older: **1 caplet every 12 hours;** do not take more than 2 caplets in 24 hours
- children under 12 years: ask a doctor

Other information: • **each caplet contains:** sodium 20 mg
- store at 20 to 25°C (68–77°F)
- store in a dry place

Inactive Ingredients: colloidal silicon dioxide, D&C yellow #10 lake, FD&C blue #1 lake, hypromellose, lactose, magnesium stearate, microcrystalline cellulose, pharmaceutical glaze, polyethylene glycol, povidone, propylene glycol, talc, titanium dioxide

Questions or comments? 1-800-395-0689

How Supplied: Box of 10 or 20 Caplets (Capsule-Shaped Tablets).
Visit our website at www.aleve.com
Distributed by:
Bayer Corporation
Consumer Care Division
PO Box 1910
Morristown, NJ 07962-1910 USA
B-R LLC
154043

Shown in Product Identification Guide, page 503

ALKA-SELTZER® Original
ALKA-SELTZER® Cherry
ALKA-SELTZER® Extra Strength
ALKA-SELTZER® Lemon Lime
Effervescent Antacid Pain Reliever

Active Ingredients
(in each tablet): **Purpose:**
ALKA-SELTZER® Original, Cherry, and Lemon-Lime:
Aspirin 325 mg .... Analgesic
Citric acid
  1000 mg .... Antacid

- fully dissolve tablets in 4 ounces of water before taking

adults and children 12 years and over	2 tablets every 4 hours, or as directed by a doctor	do not exceed 8 tablets in 24 hours
adults 60 years and over	2 tablets every 4 hours, or as directed by a doctor	do not exceed 4 tablets in 24 hours

- fully dissolve tablets in 4 ounces of water before taking

adults and children 12 years and over	2 tablets every 6 hours, or as directed by a doctor	do not exceed 7 tablets in 24 hours
adults 60 years and over	2 tablets every 6 hours, or as directed by a doctor	do not exceed 4 tablets in 24 hours

Sodium bicarbonate (heat-treated)
  1916 mg .... Antacid
ALKA-SELTZER® Extra Strength:
Aspirin 500 mg .... Analgesic
Citric acid
  1000 mg .... Antacid
Sodium bicarbonate (heat-treated)
  1985 mg .... Antacid
ALKA-SELTZER® Cherry and Lemon-Lime:
Sodium bicarbonate (heat-treated)
  1700 mg .... Antacid

Uses: for the relief of:
ALKA-SELTZER® Original, Cherry and Lemon-Lime and ALKA-SELTZER® Extra Strength:
- heartburn, acid indigestion, and sour stomach when accompanied with headache or body aches and pains
- upset stomach with headache from overindulgence in food or drink
- pain alone (headache or body and muscular aches and pains)

Warnings:
ALKA-SELTZER® Original, Cherry, Lemon-Lime and Extra Strength:
Reye's syndrome: Children and teenagers should not use this medicine for chicken pox or flu symptoms before a doctor is consulted about Reye's syndrome, a rare but serious illness reported to be associated with aspirin.
Allergy alert: Aspirin may cause a severe allergic reaction which may include:
- hives • facial swelling • asthma (wheezing) • shock
Alcohol warning: If you consume 3 or more alcoholic drinks every day, ask your doctor whether you should take aspirin or other pain relievers/fever reducers. Aspirin may cause stomach bleeding.
Do not use if you have ever had an allergic reaction to aspirin or any other pain reliever/fever reducer
Ask a doctor before use if you have
- asthma
- ulcers
- bleeding problems
- stomach problems that last or come back frequently, such as heartburn, upset stomach, or pain
Ask a doctor or pharmacist before use if you are
- presently taking a prescription drug. Antacids may interact with certain prescription drugs.
- on a sodium-restricted diet
- taking a prescription drug for anticoagulation (blood thinning), diabetes, gout, or arthritis

When using this product do not exceed recommended dosage
Stop use and ask a doctor if
- an allergic reaction occurs. Seek medical help right away.
- symptoms get worse or last more than 10 days
- redness or swelling is present
- new symptoms occur
- ringing in the ears or loss of hearing occurs

If pregnant or breast-feeding, ask a health professional before use. **It is especially important not to use aspirin during the last 3 months of pregnancy unless definitely directed to do so by a doctor because it may cause problems in the unborn child or complications during delivery.**
Keep out of reach of children. In case of overdose, get medical help or contact a Poison Control Center right away.

Directions:
Alka Seltzer® Original, Cherry and Lemon-Lime:
[See first table above]
Alka Seltzer Extra Strength:
[See second table above]
Other Information:
- **each tablets contains:** sodium 567 mg (Original), sodium 503 mg (Cherry and Lemon-Lime) sodium 588 mg (Extra Strength)
- **phenylketonurics:** contains phenylalaline 12.3 mg (Cherry) and 9 mg (Lemon-Lime) per tablet
- protect from excessive heat
- Alka-Seltzer in water contains principally the antacid sodium citrate and the analgesic sodium acetylsalicylate

Inactive Ingredients:
Original: None
Cherry and Lemon-Lime: aspartame, dimethicone, docusate sodium, flavor, povidone, sodium benzoate
Extra Strength: Flavors

How Supplied: 2 effervescent tablets per foil pack
Original: Box of 12, 24, 36, 72, and 100 tablets
Lemon-Lime: Box of 12, 24, 36 tablets
Cherry and Extra Strenth: Box of 12 and 24 tablets
Questions or comments? 1-800-800-4793 or www.alka-seltzer.com
Shown in Product Identification Guide, page 503

Continued on next page

ALKA-SELTZER® HEARTBURN RELIEF
Antacid Medicine

Active ingredients: **Purpose:**
(in each tablet)
Citric acid 1000 mg .... antacid
Sodium bicarbonate (heat-treated) 1940 mg .... antacid

Inactive ingredients: acesulfame potassium, aspartame, flavor enhancer, flavors, magnesium stearate, mannitol

Uses:
for the relief of:
• heartburn
• acid indigestion
• upset stomach associated with these conditions

Warnings:
Do not use this product if you are on a sodium-restricted diet unless directed by a doctor.
Ask a doctor or pharmacist before use if you are presently taking a prescription drug. Antacids may interact with certain prescription drugs.
When using this product do not exceed recommended dosage.
Stop use and ask a doctor if symptoms last for more than 14 days.
If pregnant or breast-feeding, ask a health professional before use.
Keep out of reach of children.

Directions: Fully dissolve tablets in 4 ounces of water before taking. [See first table above]

Other Information:
• **each tablet contains:** sodium 578 mg.
• **phenylketonurics:** contains phenylalanine 5.6 mg per tablet
• protect from excessive heat
• Alka-Seltzer Heartburn Relief in water contains the antacid sodium citrate as the principal active ingredient.

How Supplied: Alka-Seltzer Heartburn Relief is available in 24 or 36 count packages in lemon lime flavor.
Questions or comments: 1-800-800-4793 or www.alka-seltzer.com
Bayer Corporation
Consumer Care Division
Morristown, NJ 07960
USA

Shown in Product Identification Guide, page 503

ALKA-SELTZER® MORNING RELIEF
Pain Reliever, Alertness Aid
For Morning Headache and Fatigue
with Caffeine
  • Fast Headache Relief
  • Increases Alertness
  • Gentle on your stomach

Active Ingredients: **Purposes:**
(in each tablet)
Aspirin 500 mg .... Analgesic
Caffeine 65 mg .... Alertness aid/ pain reliever aid

adults and children 12 years and over	2 tablets every 4 hours as needed, or as directed by a doctor.	do not exceed 8 tablets in 24 hours or as directed by a doctor.
adult 60 years of age and over	2 tablets every 4 hours as needed, or as directed by a doctor.	do not exceed 4 tablets in 24 hours or as directed by a doctor.
children under 12 years	Consult a doctor.	

adults and children 12 years and over	2 tablets every 6 hours, as needed, or as directed by a doctor	do not exceed 8 tablets in 24 hours
adults 60 years and over	2 tablets every 6 hours, as needed, or as directed by a doctor	do not exceed 4 tablets in 24 hours
children under 12 years	do not use	

Active Ingredients:

per tablet	Original	Cherry Burst	Orange Zest	Cold & Sinus	Cold & Cough	Night-Time	Flu	Nose & Throat
Aspirin 500 mg							√	
Acetaminophen 250 mg	√	√	√	√				√
Chlorpheniramine maleate 2 mg	√	√	√		√		√	√
Dextromethorphan HBr 10 mg					√	√		
Dextromethorphan HBr 15 mg							√	
Doxylamine succinate 6.25 mg						√		
Phenylephrine HCl 5 mg	√	√	√	√	√	√		√

Uses:
• for the temporary relief of minor aches and pains with fatigue or drowsiness associated with a hangover
• also effective for headaches, body aches and pains alone

Warnings:
Reye's syndrome: Children and teenagers should not use this medicine for chicken pox or flu symptoms before a doctor is consulted about Reye's syndrome, a rare but serious illness reported to be associated with aspirin.
Allergy alert: Aspirin may cause a severe allergic reaction which may include:
• hives • facial swelling • asthma (wheezing) • shock
Alcohol warning: If you consume 3 or more alcoholic drinks every day, ask your doctor whether you should take aspirin or other pain relievers/fever reducers. Aspirin may cause stomach bleeding.
Do not use
• if you have ever had an allergic reaction to any pain reliever/fever reducer
• this product if you are on a sodium-restricted diet unless directed by a doctor
• in children under 12 years of age

Ask a doctor before use if you have
• asthma • ulcers • bleeding problems • stomach problems that last or come back, such as heartburn, upset stomach, or pain

Ask a doctor or pharmacist before use if you are taking a prescription drug for
• anticoagulation (blood thinning) • gout • diabetes • arthritis

When using this product
• limit the use of caffeine-containing medications, foods or beverages because too much caffeine may cause nervousness, irritability, sleeplessness, and occasionally, rapid heart beat. The recommended dose of this product contains about as much caffeine as a cup of coffee.
• if fatigue or drowsiness persists or continues to recur, consult a doctor. For occasional use only. Not intended for use as a substitute for sleep.

Stop use and ask a doctor if
• allergic reaction occurs. Seek medical help right away.
• pain gets worse or lasts more than 10 days
• new symptoms occur

- redness or swelling is present
- ringing in the ears or loss of hearing occurs

If pregnant or breast-feeding, ask a health professional before use. **It is especially important not to use aspirin during the last 3 months of pregnancy unless definitely directed to do so by a doctor because it may cause problems in the unborn child or complications during delivery.**

Keep out of reach of children. In case of overdose, get medical help or contact a Poison Control Center right away.

Directions:
- do not exceed recommended dosage
- do not use for more than 2 days for hangover
- fully dissolve tablets in 4 ounces of water before taking
[See second table at top of previous page]

Other Information
- **each tablet contains:** sodium 410 mg
- **phenylketonurics:** contains phenylalanine 9 mg per tablet
- protect from excessive heat

Inactive Ingredients: acesulfame potassium, aspartame, citric acid, dimethicone, docusate sodium, flavor, mannitol, povidone, sodium benzoate, sodium bicarbonate

How Supplied: 2 Citrus effervescent tablets per foil pack in boxes of 12 and 24 tablets

Questions or comments? 1-800-800-4793 or www.alka-seltzer.com

Shown in Product Identification Guide, page 503

ALKA-SELTZER PLUS® COLD MEDICINE
Original, Cherry Burst and Orange Zest Flavors
Analgesic, Antihistamine, Nasal Decongestant

ALKA-SELTZER PLUS® COLD & SINUS MEDICINE
Non-Drowsy Medicine
Analgesic, Nasal Decongestant

ALKA-SELTZER PLUS® COLD & COUGH MEDICINE
Antihistamine, Cough Suppressant, Nasal Decongestant

ALKA-SELTZER PLUS® NIGHT-TIME COLD MEDICINE
Cough Suppressant, Antihistamine, Nasal Decongestant

ALKA-SELTZER PLUS® FLU MEDICINE
Analgesic, Cough Suppressant, Antihistamine

ALKA-SELTZER PLUS® NOSE & THROAT COLD MEDICINE
Analgesic, Nasal Decongestant, Cough Suppressant, Antihistamine

[See third table at top of previous page]
[See first table above]

Uses:
[See second table above]

Inactive Ingredients:

per tablet	Original	Cherry Burst	Orange Zest	Cold Sinus	Cold & Cough	Night-Time	Flu	Nose & Throat
FD&C Red #40		√	√				√	√
FD&C Yellow #6			√				√	
Carmel Color								√
Magnesium Stearate	√	√	√	√	√	√		√
acesulfame potassium	√	√	√			√	√	√
aspartame	√	√	√		√	√	√	√
citric acid	√	√	√	√	√	√	√	√
dimethicone							√	
docusate sodium							√	
flavors	√	√	√	√	√	√	√	√
fumaric acid	√	√	√	√	√	√	√	
glyceryl behenate	√	√	√	√	√	√	√	
maltodextrin	√	√	√	√	√	√		√
mannitol							√	
povidone							√	
poyethylene glycol behenate	√	√	√	√	√	√		
sodium benzoate							√	
sodium bicarbonate	√	√	√	√	√	√	√	√
sodium saccharin		√	√		√		√	√
sorbitol	√	√	√	√	√	√	√	√

per tablet	Original	Cherry Burst	Orange Zest	Cold & Sinus	Cold & Cough	Night-Time	Flu	Nose & Throat
body aches & pains	√	√	√				√	√
headache	√	√	√	√			√	√
coughing					√	√	√	√
fever	√	√	√	√			√	√
runny nose	√	√	√		√	√	√	√
sinus pain & pressure				√				
sneezing	√	√	√		√	√	√	√
nasal & sinus congestion	√	√	√	√	√	√	√	√
sore throat	√	√	√				√	√

Directions:
Do not take more than recommended dose.
[See first table at top of next page]
Alka-Seltzer Plus® Effervescent: Warnings and Other Information
1- Alka-Seltzer Plus Cold Medicine (all flavors)
2- **Alka-Seltzer Plus Cold & Sinus Medicine**
3- **Alka-Seltzer Plus Cold & Cough Medicine**
4- **Alka-Seltzer Plus Night-Time Cold Medicine**

Continued on next page

Alka-Seltzer Plus Cold—Cont.

5- Alka-Seltzer Plus Flu Medicine
6- Alka-Seltzer Plus Nose & Throat Cold Medicine

Warnings:
(The numbers following the warnings correspond to the products listed above.)
[See second table beginning on page 608 through 610]

Other Information:
(The numbers following the information correspond to the products listed above.)
[See second table at top of page 610]

How Supplied:
Specific to Cold Medicine: Contains 12, 20, and 36 Effervescent Tablets.
Specific to Cold & Sinus Medicine, Cold & Cough Medicine, Night-Time Cold Medicine, Flu Medicine: Contains 20 Effervescent Tablets.
Questions or comments?
1-800-800-4793 or
www.alka-seltzerplus.com
Bayer Corporation
Consumer Care Division
Morristown, NJ 07960 USA
Shown in Product Identification Guide, page 503

ALKA-SELTZER PLUS® COLD MEDICINE LIQUI-GELS®
Analgesic, Antihistamine, Nasal Decongestant

ALKA-SELTZER PLUS® COLD& SINUS MEDICINE LIQUI-GELS®
Analgesic, Nasal Decongestant

ALKA-SELTZER PLUS® COLD& COUGH MEDICINE LIQUI-GELS®
Analgesic, Antihistamine, Cough Suppressant, Nasal Decongestant

ALKA-SELTZER PLUS® NIGHT-TIME COLD MEDICINE LIQUI-GELS®
Analgesic, Cough Suppressant, Antihistamine, Nasal Decongestant

ALKA-SELTZER PLUS® FLU MEDICINE LIQUI-GELS®
Analgesic, Cough Suppressant, Nasal Decongestant

[See third table at top of page 610]
[See first table at top of page 611]
[See second table at top of page 611]
[See first table at top of page 612]

Alka-Seltzer Plus® Liqui-Gels®: Warnings and Other Information
1- Alka Seltzer Plus Cold Medicine Liqui-Gels
2- Alka Seltzer Plus Cold & Sinus Medicine Liqui-Gels
3- Alka Seltzer Plus Cold & Cough Medicine Liqui-Gels
4- Alka Seltzer Plus Night-Time Cold Medicine Liqui-Gels

ALKA-SELTZER PLUS® COLD MEDICINE (Original, Cherry Burst and Orange Zest)
ALKA-SELTZER PLUS® COLD & SINUS MEDICINE
ALKA-SELTZER PLUS® COLD & COUGH MEDICINE
ALKA-SELTZER PLUS® NOSE & THROAT MEDICINE

adults and children 12 years and over	take 2 tablets fully dissolved in 4 oz. of water every 4 hours	do not exceed 8 tablets in 24 hours or as directed by a doctor
children under 12 years	consult a doctor	

ALKA-SELTZER PLUS® NIGHT-TIME COLD MEDICINE

adults and children 12 years and over	take 2 tablets fully dissolved in 4 oz. of water at bedtime (may be taken every 4 hours)	do not exceed 8 tablets in 24 hours or as directed by a doctor
children under 12 years	consult a doctor	

ALKA-SELTZER PLUS® FLU MEDICINE

adults and children 12 years and over	take 2 tablets fully dissolved in 4 oz. of water every 6 hours	do not exceed 8 tablets in 24 hours or as directed by a doctor
children under 12 years	consult a doctor	

Reye's syndrome: Children and teenagers should not use this medicine for chicken pox or flu symptoms before a Doctor is consulted about Reye's syndrome, a rare but serious illness reported to be associated with aspirin.	5
Alcohol warning (acetaminophen): If you consume 3 or more alcoholic drinks every day, ask your doctor whether you should take acetaminophen or other pain relievers/fever reducers. Acetaminophen may cause liver damage.	1,2,6
Alcohol warning (aspirin): If you consume 3 or more alcoholic drinks every day, ask your doctor whether you should take aspirin or other pain relievers/fever reducers. Aspirin may cause stomach bleeding.	5
Sore throat warning: If sore throat is severe, persists for more than 3 days, is accompanied or followed by fever, headache, rash nausea, or vomiting, consult a doctor promptly.	1,5,6
Do not use:	
• If you are now taking a prescription Monamine Oxidase Inhibitor (MAOI) (certain drugs for depression, psychiatric or emotional conditions, or Parkinson's disease), or for 2 weeks after stopping the MAOI drug. If you are uncertain whether your prescription drug contains an MAOI, ask a doctor or pharmacist before taking this product.	ALL
• if you are allergic to aspirin or any other pain reliever/fever reducer.	5
• with any other products containing acetaminophen	1,2,6

(Table continued on next page)

5- **Alka Seltzer Plus Flu Medicine Liqui-Gels**

Warnings:
(The numbers following the warnings correspond to the products listed above.)
[See second table beginning on pages 612 and 613]

Other Information:
(The numbers following the warnings correspond to the products listed above.)
[See second table at top of page 613]

How Supplied: ALKA-SELTZER PLUS® Cold Medicine, ALKA-SELTZER PLUS® Cold & Cough Medicine, ALKA-SELTZER PLUS® Night-Time Cold Medicine: Carton of 20 softgels. ALKA-SELTZER PLUS® Cold & Sinus Medicine, ALKA-SELTZER PLUS® Flu Non-Drowsy Medicine: Carton of 12 softgels.

Questions or comments? 1-800-800-4793 or www.alka-seltzerplus.com

Ask a doctor before use if you have

•heart disease, high blood pressure, diabetes, thyroid disease	1,2,3,4,6
•glaucoma	1,3,4,5,6
•ulcers	5
•difficulty in urination due to enlargement of the prostate gland	ALL
•a breathing problem such as emphysema or chronic bronchitis	1,3,4,6
•persistent or chronic cough such as occurs with smoking, asthma, or emphysema	3,4,5,6
•cough with excessive phlegm (mucus)	3,4,5,6
•a breathing problem such as emphysema or chronic bronchitis, or asthma	5
•stomach problems that persist or recur	5

Ask a doctor or pharmacist before use if you are:

•taking sedatives or tranquilizers	1,3,4,5,6
•on a sodium restricted diet	ALL
•taking a prescription drug for anticoagulation (blood thinning), diabetes, gout, arthritis	5

When using this product:

•do not exceed recommended dosage	ALL
•you may get drowsy	1
•marked drowsiness may occur	3,4,5,6
•avoid alcoholic drinks	1,3,4,5,6
•excitability may occur, especially in children	1,3,4,5,6
•alcohol, sedatives, and tranquilizers may increase drowsiness	1,3,4,5,6
•be careful when driving a motor vehicle or operating machinery	1,3,4,5,6

Stop use and ask a doctor if:

•an allergic reaction occurs. Seek medical help right away	5
•nervousness, dizziness, or sleeplessness occurs	1,2,3,4,6
•new or unexpected symptoms occur	1,2,5,6
•symptoms do not improve within 7 days or are accompanied by a fever	1,2,3,4,6
•fever gets worse or lasts for more than 3 days	1,2,5,6
•pain gets worse or lasts more than 7 days	5
•redness or swelling is present	1,2,5,6
•cough persists for more than 7 days, tends to recur, or is accompanied by a fever, rash, or persistent headache. These may be signs of a serious condition.	3,4,5,6
•ringing in the ears or loss of hearing occurs	5

(Table continued on next page)

Distributed by:
Bayer Corporation
PO Box 1910
Morristown, NJ 07962-1910 USA

Liqui-Gels is a registered trademark of R.P. Scherer Corporation.

Shown in Product Identification Guide, page 503

ALKA-SELTZER PM™
[əl-ka sĕl-sur]
PAIN RELIEVER & SLEEP AID MEDICINE

Active ingredients: **Purpose:**
(in each tablet)
Aspirin 325 mg .... Pain reliever
Diphenhydramine citrate
   38 mg .... Nighttime sleep aid

Inactive Ingredients: acesulfame potassium, aspartame, citric acid, dimethicone, docusate sodium, flavors, povidone, sodium benzoate, sodium bicarbonate

Uses: temporarily relieves occasional headache and minor aches and pains with accompanying sleeplessness.

Warnings: Reye's syndrome: Children and teenagers should not use this medicine for chicken pox or flu symptoms before a doctor is consulted about Reye's syndrome, a rare but serious illness reported to be associated with aspirin.

Alcohol warning: If you consume 3 or more drinks every day, ask your doctor whether you should take aspirin or other pain relievers/fever reducers. Aspirin may cause stomach bleeding.

Do not use
• if you are allergic to aspirin or any other pain reliever/fever reducer
• in children under 12 years of age
• with any other product containing diphenhydramine, including one applied topically

Ask a doctor before use if you have:
• stomach problems (such as heartburn, upset stomach, or stomach pain) that continue or come back
• bleeding problems
• ulcers
• breathing problems such as emphysema, chronic bronchitis or asthma
• glaucoma
• trouble urinating due to enlargement of the prostate gland

Ask a doctor or pharmacist before use if you are:
• taking a prescription drug for
   • anticoagulation (blood thinning)
   • diabetes
   • gout
   • arthritis
• taking sedatives or tranquilizers
• on a sodium-restricted diet

When using this product avoid alcoholic drinks.

Stop use and ask a doctor if:
• an allergic reaction occurs. Seek medicial help right away.
• pain gets worse or lasts for more than 10 days.
• redness or swelling is present.
• new symptoms occur
• ringing in the ears or loss of hearing occurs.
• sleeplessness lasts for more than 2 weeks. Insomnia may be a symptom of a serious underlying medical illness.

If pregnant or breast-feeding, ask a health professional before use. **It is especially important not to use aspirin during the last 3 months of pregnancy unless definitely directed to do so by a**

Continued on next page

Alka-Seltzer PM—Cont.

doctor because it may cause problems in the unborn child or complications during delivery.
Keep out of reach of children. In case of overdose, get medical help or contact a Poison Control Center right away.

Directions:
- **do not exceed recommended dosage.**
- fully dissolve tablets in 4 ounces of water before taking.

adults and children 12 years and over	take 2 tablets with water at bedtime, if needed, or as directed by a doctor.
children under 12 years	do not use.

Other Information:
- **each tablet contains:** sodium 503 mg
- **phenylketonurics:** contains phenylalanine 4.0 mg per tablet.
- Protect from excessive heat

Place two (2) tablets in 4 oz of water. Dissolve tablets completely.

Drink Alka-Seltzer. You do not have to drink any of the residue that may be on the bottom of the glass. The medicines of Alka-Seltzer are in the water.

How Supplied Foil Packs of 24 Effervescent Tablets.
FOIL SEALED FOR YOUR SAFETY. DO NOT USE IF FOIL PACKS ARE TORN OR BROKEN.
Questions or comments?
1-800-800-4793 or www.alka-seltzer.com
For more information, visit our website at www.alka-seltzer.com
Questions or comments?
Please call 1-800-800-4793.
Made in the U.S.A.
Bayer Corporation
Consumer Care Division
P.O. Box 1910
Morristown, NJ 07962-1910 USA

Shown in Product Identification Guide, page 503

If pregnant or breast-feeding, ask a health professional before use.	ALL
If pregnant or breast-feeding, ask a health professional before use. **It is especially important not to use aspirin during the last 3 months of pregnancy unless definitely directed to do so by a doctor because it may cause problems in the unborn child or complications during delivery.**	5
Keep out of reach of children	ALL
Overdose warning (aspirin): In case of overdose, get medical help or contact a Poison Control Center right away.	5
Overdose warning (acetaminophen): Taking more than the recommended dose can cause serious health problems. In case of overdose, get medical help or contact a Poison Control Center right away. Quick medical attention is critical for adults as well as for children even if you do not notice any signs or symptoms.	1,2,3,4,6

•this product does not contain phenylpropanolamine (PPA)	ALL
•protect from excessive heat	ALL

	Sodium Content (per tablet)	Phenylketonurics: Phenylalanine Content (per tablet)
Original	475 mg	8.4 mg
Orange Zest	475 mg	4.2 mg
Cherry Burst	475 mg	5.6 mg
Cold & Sinus	475 mg	4.2 mg
Cold & Cough	504 mg	11 mg
Night-Time	474 mg	7.8 mg
Flu	386 mg	6.7 mg
Nose & Throat	360 mg	5.6 mg

Active Ingredients:

Per softgel	Cold	Cold & Sinus	Cold & Cough	Night-Time	Flu
Acetaminophen 325 mg	√	√	√	√	√
Chlorpheniramine maleate 2 mg	√		√		
Dextromethorphan hydrobromide 10 mg			√	√	√
Doxylamine succinate 6.25 mg				√	
Pseudophedrine HCl 30 mg	√	√	√	√	√

BACTINE® Antiseptic-Anesthetic First Aid Liquid

Product Information
Active Ingredients: **Purpose:**
Benzalkonium chloride
0.13% w/w .... First aid antiseptic
Lidocaine hydrochloride
2.5% w/w .... Pain reliever

Inactive Ingredients: Disodium EDTA, fragrances, octoxynol 9, propylene glycol, water.

Indications: First aid to help prevent bacterial contamination or skin infection and for the temporary relief of pain and itching in minor cuts, scrapes, and burns.

Directions: Adults and children 2 years of age and older: Clean the affected area. Apply a small amount of this product on the area 1 to 3 times daily. May be covered with a sterile bandage. If bandaged, let dry first. Children under 2 years of age: ask a doctor.

Other Information:
- protect from excessive heat

Warnings:
For external use only
Ask a doctor before use if you have
- deep or puncture wounds
- animal bites
- serious burns

When using this product:
- do not use in or near the eyes
- do not apply over large areas of the body or in large quantities
- do not apply over raw surfaces or blistered areas

Stop use and ask a doctor if:
- condition worsens
- symptoms persist for more than 7 days, or clear up and occur again within a few days

Keep out of reach of children. If swallowed, get medical help or contact a Poison Control Center right away

Protect from excessive heat.

How Supplied: Bactine Antiseptic-Anesthetic First Aid Liquid is available as 2 oz, 4 oz, and 16 oz. liquid with child resistant closures and 5.0 oz. pump spray.

Genuine BAYER® Aspirin
Caplets, Gelcaps, and Tablets

Active Ingredient: **Purposes:**
(in each caplet, gelcap, tablet)

Aspirin
   325 mg ..... pain reliever/fever reducer

Uses: Temporarily relieves:
- headache
- muscle pain
- toothache
- menstrual pain
- pain and fever of colds
- minor pain of arthritis

Warnings: Reye's syndrome: Children and teenagers should not use this medicine for chicken pox or flu symptoms before a doctor is consulted about Reye's syndrome, a rare but serious illness reported to be associated with aspirin.

Allergy alert: Aspirin may cause a severe allergic reaction which may include:
- hives
- facial swelling
- asthma (wheezing)
- shock

Alcohol warning: If you consume 3 or more alcoholic drinks every day, ask your doctor whether you should take aspirin or other pain relievers/fever reducers. Aspirin may cause stomach bleeding.

Do not use if you are allergic to aspirin or any other pain reliever/fever reducer.

Ask a doctor before use if you have:
- stomach problems (such as heartburn, upset stomach, or stomach pain) that continue or come back
- bleeding problems
- ulcers
- asthma

Ask a doctor or pharmacist before use if you are taking a prescription drug for
- anticoagulation (blood thinning)
- gout
- diabetes
- arthritis

Inactive Ingredients:

per softgel	Cold	Cold & Sinus	Cold & Cough	Night-Time	Flu
FD&C blue #1	√		√	√	
FD&C red #40	√	√			√
D&C red #33			√		
D&C yellow #10				√	
gelatin	√	√	√	√	√
glycerin	√	√	√	√	√
polyethylene glycol	√	√	√	√	√
polyvinyl acetate phthalate	√	√	√	√	√
potassium acetate	√	√	√	√	√
povidone	√	√	√	√	√
propylene glycol	√	√	√	√	√
sorbitol	√	√	√	√	√
titanium dioxide	√	√	√	√	√
Water	√	√	√	√	√

Uses:

	Cold	Cold & Sinus	Cold & Cough	Night-Time	Flu
body aches & pains	√		√	√	√
headache	√	√	√	√	√
coughing			√	√	√
fever	√		√	√	√
runny nose	√		√	√	
sinus pain & pressure		√			
sneezing	√		√	√	
nasal & sinus congestion	√	√	√	√	√
sore throat	√		√	√	√

Stop use and ask a doctor if:
- an allergic reaction occurs. Seek medical help right away.
- pain gets worse or lasts for more than 10 days
- fever lasts for more than 3 days
- new symptoms occur
- ringing in the ears or loss of hearing occurs
- redness or swelling is present

If pregnant or breast-feeding, ask a health professional before use. **It is especially important not to use aspirin during the last 3 months of pregnancy unless definitely directed to do so by a doctor because it may cause problems in the unborn child or complications during delivery.**

Keep out of reach of children. In case of overdose, get medical help or contact a Poison Control Center right away.

Directions:
- drink a full glass of water with each dose
- adults and children 12 years and over: take 1 or 2 caplets every 4 hours not to exceed 12 caplets in 24 hours
- children under 12 years: consult a doctor

Other Information:
- save carton for full directions and warnings
- store at room temperature

Inactive Ingredients:

BAYER® Genuine Aspirin Caplets: Cellulose, hypromellose, starch, triacetin

BAYER® Genuine Aspirin Gelcaps: butylparaben, cellulose, corn starch, D&C yellow #10 aluminum lake, FD&C blue #1 aluminum lake, gelatin, glycerin,

Continued on next page

Genuine Bayer—Cont.

hypromellose, methylparaben, povidone, propylene glycol, propylparaben, purified water, shellac, sodium lauryl sulfate, sorbitan trioleate, titanium dioxide, triacetin

BAYER® Genuine Aspirin Tablets: Cellulose, Hypromellose, Starch, Triacetin

How Supplied: BAYER® Genuine Aspirin Original Strength 325 mg is available in bottles of 100 coated caplets, in bottles of 80 Gelcaps, and in bottles of 100 coated tablets.

Questions or comments?
1-800-331-4536 or
www.bayeraspirin.com
Bayer Corporation
PO Box 1910
Morristown, NJ 07962-1910 USA
Shown in Product Identification Guide, page 504

ASPIRIN REGIMEN BAYER® 81 mg
ASPIRIN REGIMEN BAYER® 325 mg
Delayed Release Enteric Aspirin Adult Low Strength 81 mg Tablets and Regular Strength 325 mg Caplets

Active Ingredient:

(in each tablet)	Purpose:
Aspirin 81 mg	Pain reliever
Aspirin 325 mg	Pain reliever

Uses: For the temporary relief of minor aches and pains or as recommended by your doctor. **Because of its delayed action, this product will not provide fast relief of headaches or other symptoms needing immediate relief.**

Warnings: Reye's syndrome: Children and teenagers should not use this medicine for chicken pox or flu symptoms before a doctor is consulted about Reye's syndrome, a rare but serious illness reported to be associated with aspirin.

Allergy alert: Aspirin may cause a severe allergic reaction which may include: • hives • facial swelling • asthma (wheezing) • shock

Alcohol warning: If you consume 3 or more alcoholic drinks every day, ask your doctor whether you should take aspirin or other pain relievers/fever reducers. Aspirin may cause stomach bleeding.

Do not use if you are allergic to aspirin or any other pain reliever/fever reducer.

Ask a doctor before use if you have:
• stomach problems (such as heartburn, upset stomach, or stomach pain) that continue or come back
• bleeding problems
• ulcers
• asthma

Directions:

ALKA-SELTZER PLUS® COLD MEDICINE LIQUI-GELS®

adults and children 12 years and over	swallow 2 softgels with water every 4 hours	do not exceed 8 softgels in 24 hours or as directed by a doctor
children under 12 years	consult a doctor	

ALKA-SELTZER PLUS® NIGHT-TIME COLD MEDICINE LIQUI-GELS®

adults and children 12 years and over	swallow 2 softgels with water at bedtime (may be taken every 6 hours)	do not exceed 8 softgels in 24 hours or as directed by a doctor
children under 12 years	consult a doctor	

ALKA-SELTZER PLUS® COLD & SINUS MEDICINE LIQUI-GELS®
ALKA-SELTZER PLUS® COLD & COUGH MEDICINE LIQUI-GELS®
ALKA-SELTZER PLUS® FLU MEDICINE LIQUI-GELS®

adults and children 12 years and over	swallow 2 softgels with water every 4 hours	do not exceed 8 softgels in 24 hours or as directed by a doctor
children 6 to under 12 years	take 1 softgel with water every 4 hours	do not exceed 4 softgels in 24 hours or as directed by a doctor
children under 6 years	consult a doctor	

Alcohol warning: If you consume 3 or more alcoholic drinks every day, ask your doctor whether you should take acetaminophen or other pain relievers/fever reducers. Acetaminophen may cause liver damage.	**ALL**
Sore throat warning: If sore throat is severe, persists for more than 3 days, is accompanied or followed by fever, headache, rash nausea, or vomiting, consult a doctor promptly.	**1,3,4,5**

Do not use:

•with any other products containing acetaminophen	**ALL**
•If you are now taking a prescription Monamine Oxidase Inhibitor (MAOI) (certain drugs for depression, psychiatric or emotional conditions, or Parkinson's disease), or for 2 weeks after stopping the MAOI drug. If you are uncertain whether your prescription drug contains an MAOI, ask a doctor or pharmacist before taking this product.	**ALL**

Ask a doctor before use if you have

•heart disease, high blood pressure, diabetes, thyroid disease	**ALL**
•glaucoma	**1,3,4**
•difficulty in urination due to enlargement of the prostate gland	**ALL**
•a breathing problem such as emphysema or chronic bronchitis	**1,3,4**
•persistent or chronic cough such as occurs with smoking, asthma, or emphysema	**3,4,5**
•cough with excessive phlegm (mucus)	**3,4,5**

(Table continued on next page)

Ask a doctor or pharmacist before use if you are taking a prescription drug for
• anticoagulation (blood thinning)
• gout
• diabetes
• arthritis

Stop use and ask a doctor if
• an allergic reaction occurs. Seek medical help right away.
• pain gets worse or lasts for more than 10 days
• new symptoms occur

Ask a doctor or pharmacist before use if you are:	
• taking sedatives or tranquilizers	1,3,4
When using this product:	
• **do not exceed recommended dosage**	ALL
• you may get drowsy	1
• marked drowsiness may occur	3,4
• avoid alcoholic drinks	1,3,4
• excitability may occur, especially in children	1,3,4
• alcohol, sedatives, and tranquilizers may increase drowsiness	1,3,4
• be careful when driving a motor vehicle or operating machinery	1,3,4
Stop use and ask a doctor if:	
• nervousness, dizziness, or sleeplessness occurs	ALL
• new symptoms occur	ALL
• symptoms do not improve within 7 days (adults) or 5 days (children) or are accompanied by a fever	1,2,3,5
• symptoms do not improve within 7 days or are accompanied by a fever	4
• fever gets worse or lasts for more than 3 days	ALL
• redness or swelling is present	ALL
• cough persists for more than 7 days, tends to recur, or is accompanied by a fever, rash, or persistent headache. These may be signs of a serious condition.	3,4,5
If pregnant or breast-feeding, ask a health professional before use.	ALL
Keep out of reach of children	ALL
Overdose Warning: Taking more than the recommended dose can cause serious health problems. In case of overdose, get medical help or contact a Poison Control Center right away. Quick medical attention is critical for adults as well as for children even if you do not notice any signs or symptoms.	ALL

• this product does not contain phenylpropanolamine (PPA)	ALL
• store at room temperature and protect from excessive heat	ALL

Weight (lb)	Age (years)	Dosage	Maximum Dosage
under 32	children under 3	consult a doctor	
32 to 35	3 to under 4	2 tablets	repeat every 4 hours while symptoms persist up to a maximum of 5 doses in 24 hours or as directed by a doctor
36 to 45	4 to under 6	3 tablets	
46 to 65	6 to under 9	4 tablets	
66 to 76	9 to under 11	4 to 5 tablets	
77 to 83	11 to under 12	4 to 6 tablets	
	adults and children 12 years and over	5 to 8 tablets	

• ringing in the ears or loss of hearing occurs
• redness or swelling is present

If pregnant or breast-feeding, ask a health professional before use. **It is especially important not to use aspirin dur**ing the last 3 months of pregnancy unless definitely directed to do so by a doctor because it may cause problems in the unborn child or complications during delivery.
Keep out of reach of children. In case of overdose, get medical help or contact a Poison Control Center right away.

Directions:
ASPIRIN REGIMEN BAYER® 81 mg:
• drink a full glass of water with each dose
• adults and children 12 years and over: take 4 to 8 tablets every 4 hours not to exceed 48 tablets in 24 hours unless directed by a doctor
• children under 12 years: consult a doctor

ASPIRIN REGIMEN BAYER® 325 mg:
• drink a full glass of water with each dose
• adults and children 12 years and over: take 1 or 2 caplets every 4 hours not to exceed 12 caplets in 24 hours unless directed by a doctor
• children under 12 years: consult a doctor

Other Information:
• save carton for full directions and warnings
• store at room temperature

Inactive Ingredients:
ASPIRIN REGIMEN BAYER® 81 mg:
Carnauba wax, cellulose, croscarmellose sodium, D&C yellow #10 aluminum lake, FD&C yellow #6 aluminum lake, hypromellose, iron oxides, lactose, methacrylic acid copolymer, microcrystalline cellulose, polysorbate 80, propylene glycol, shellac, sodium lauryl sulfate, starch, titanium dioxide, triacetin
ASPIRIN REGIMEN BAYER® 325 mg:
Carnauba wax, cellulose, D&C yellow #10 aluminum lake, FD&C yellow #6 aluminum lake, hypromellose, iron oxides, methacrylic acid copolymer, polysorbate 80, propylene gylcol, shellac, sodium lauryl sulfate, starch, titanium dioxide, triacetin

How Supplied:
ASPIRIN REGIMEN BAYER® 81 mg: Bottle of 120 tablets delayed release enteric safety coated aspirin.
ASPIRIN REGIMEN BAYER® 325 mg: Bottle of 100 caplets delayed release enteric safety coated aspirin.
Questions or comments?
1-800-331-4536 or
www.bayeraspirin.com
Bayer Corporation
PO Box 1910
Morristown, NJ 07962-1910 USA
Shown in Product Identification Guide, page 504

BAYER® Children's Chewable Tablets
Genuine Aspirin
Cherry & Orange Flavored

Active Ingredient:
(in each tablet)   **Purposes:**
Aspirin
81 mg .... Pain reliever/fever reducer

Continued on next page

Bayer Children's—Cont.

Uses: For the temporary relief of:
• minor aches, pains, and headaches
• to reduce fever associated with colds, sore throats, and teething

Warnings: Reye's syndrome: Children and teenagers should not use this medicine for chicken pox or flu symptoms before a doctor is consulted about Reye's syndrome, a rare but serious illness reported to be associated with aspirin.

Allergy alert: Aspirin may cause a severe allergic reaction which may include:
• hives
• facial swelling
• asthma (wheezing)
• shock

Alcohol warning: If you consume 3 or more alcoholic drinks every day, ask your doctor whether you should take aspirin or other pain relievers/fever reducers. Aspirin may cause stomach bleeding.

Sore throat warning: If sore throat is severe, persists for more than 2 days, is accompanied or followed by fever, headache, rash, nausea, or vomiting, consult a doctor promptly.

Do not use:
• if you are allergic to aspirin or any other pain reliever/fever reducer
• for at least 7 days after tonsillectomy or oral surgery

Ask a doctor before use if you have:
• stomach problems (such as heartburn, upset stomach, or stomach pain) that continue or come back
• bleeding problems
• ulcers
• asthma
• a child experiencing arthritis pain

Ask a doctor or pharmacist before use if you are taking a prescription drug for
• anticoagulation (blood thinning)
• gout
• diabetes
• arthritis

Stop use and ask a doctor if:
• an allergic reaction occurs. Seek medical help right away.
• pain gets worse or lasts more than 10 days (for adults) or 5 days (for children)
• fever gets worse or lasts more than 3 days
• new symptoms occur
• ringing in the ears or loss of hearing occurs
• redness or swelling is present

If pregnant or breast-feeding, ask a health professional before use. **It is especially important not to use aspirin during the last 3 months of pregnancy unless definitely directed to do so by a doctor because it may cause problems in the unborn child or complications during delivery.**

Keep out of reach of children. In case of overdose, get medical help or contact a Poison Control Center right away.

Directions:
• drink a full glass of water with each dose
• to be administered only under adult supervision
• if possible use weight to dose. Otherwise use age.
[See third table at top of previous page]

Other Information:
• save carton for full directions and warnings.
• store at room temperature.

Inactive Ingredients:
BAYER® Children's Chewable: Cherry Flavored: D&C Red #27 Aluminum Lake, Dextrose, FD&C Red #40 Aluminum Lake, Flavor, Sodium, Saccharin, Starch
BAYER Children's Chewable: Orange Flavored: Dextrose, FD&C Yellow #6 Aluminum Lake, Flavor, Sodium Saccharin, starch

How Supplied: Bottle of 36 chewable tablets.
USE ONLY IF SEAL UNDER BOTTLE CAP WITH WHITE "Bayer Corporation" PRINT IS INTACT.
Questions or comments?
1-800-331-4536 or
www.bayeraspirin.com
Bayer Corporation
PO Box 1910
Morristown, NJ 07962-1910 USA
Shown in Product Identification Guide, page 503

PROFESSIONAL LABELING

Genuine Bayer Aspirin
Aspirin Regimen Bayer 325 mg
Aspirin Regimen Bayer 81 mg
Bayer Women's Aspirin with Calcium
Aspirin Regimen Bayer Childrens Chewable 81 mg

Professional Labeling:

Indications And Usage: Vascular Indications (Ischemic Stroke, TIA, Acute MI, Prevention of Recurrent MI, Unstable Angina Pectoris, and Chronic Stable Angina Pectoris): Aspirin is indicated to: (1) Reduce the combined risk of death and nonfatal stroke in patients who have had ischemic stroke or transient ischemia of the brain due to fibrin platelet emboli, (2) reduce the risk of vascular mortality in patients with a suspected acute MI, (3) reduce the combined risk of death and nonfatal MI in patients with a previous MI or unstable angina pectoris, and (4) reduce the combined risk of MI and sudden death in patients with chronic stable angina pectoris.

Revascularization Procedures (Coronary Artery Bypass Graft (CABG), Percutaneous Transluminal Coronary Angioplasty (PTCA), and Carotid Endarterectomy): Aspirin is indicated in patients who have undergone revascularization procedures (i.e., CABG, PTCA, or carotid endarterectomy) when there is a preexisting condition for which aspirin is already indicated.

Rheumatologic Disease Indications (Rheumatoid Arthritis, Juvenile Rheumatoid Arthritis, Spondyloarthropathies, Osteoarthritis, and the Arthritis and Pleurisy of Systemic Lupus Erythematosus (SLE)): Aspirin is indicated for the relief of the signs and symptoms of rheumatoid arthritis, juvenile rheumatoid arthritis, osteoarthritis, spondyloarthropathies, and arthritis and pleurisy associated with SLE.

Contraindications: Allergy: Aspirin is contraindicated in patients with known allergy to nonsteroidal anti-inflammatory drug products and in patients with the syndrome of asthma, rhinitis, and nasal polyps. Aspirin may cause severe urticaria, angioedema, or bronchospasm (asthma).

Reye's syndrome: Aspirin should not be used in children or teenagers for viral infections, with or without fever, because of the risk of Reye's syndrome with concomitant use of aspirin in certain viral illnesses.

Warnings: Alcohol Warning: Patients who consume three or more alcoholic drinks every day should be counseled about the bleeding risks involved with chronic, heavy alcohol use while taking aspirin.

Coagulation Abnormalities: Even low doses of aspirin can inhibit platelet function leading to an increase in bleeding time. This can adversely affect patients with inherited (hemophilia) or acquired (liver disease or vitamin K deficiency) bleeding disorders.

GI Side Effects: GI side effects include stomach pain, heartburn, nausea, vomiting, and gross GI bleeding. Although minor upper GI symptoms, such as dyspepsia, are common and can occur anytime during therapy, physicians should remain alert for signs of ulceration and bleeding, even in the absence of previous GI symptoms. Physicians should inform patients about the signs and symptoms of GI side effects and what steps to take if they occur.

Peptic Ulcer Disease: Patients with a history of active peptic ulcer disease should avoid using aspirin, which can cause gastric mucosal irritation and bleeding.

Precautions:

General: Renal Failure: Avoid aspirin in patients with severe renal failure (glomerular filtration rate less than 10 mL/minute).

Hepatic Insufficiency: Avoid aspirin in patients with severe hepatic insufficiency.

Sodium Restricted Diets: Patients with sodium-retaining states, such as congestive heart failure or renal failure, should avoid sodium-containing buffered aspirin preparations because of their high sodium content.

Laboratory Tests: Aspirin has been associated with elevated hepatic enzymes, blood urea nitrogen and serum creatinine, hyperkalemia, proteinuria, and prolonged bleeding time.

Drug Interactions: Angiotensin Converting Enzyme (ACE) Inhibitors: The hyponatremic and hypotensive effects of ACE inhibitors may be diminished by the concomitant administration of aspirin due to its indirect effect on the renin-angiotensin conversion pathway.

Acetazolamide: Concurrent use of aspirin and acetazolamide can lead to high serum concentrations of acetazolamide (and toxicity) due to competition at the renal tubule for secretion.

Anticoagulant Therapy (Heparin and Warfarin): Patients on anticoagulation therapy are at increased risk for bleeding because of drug-drug interactions and the effect on platelets. Aspirin can displace warfarin from protein binding sites, leading to prolongation of both the prothrombin time and the bleeding time. Aspirin can increase the anticoagulant activity of heparin, increasing bleeding risk.

Anticonvulsants: Salicylate can displace protein-bound phenytoin and valproic acid, leading to a decrease in the total concentration of phenytoin and an increase in serum valproic acid levels.

Beta Blockers: The hypotensive effects of beta blockers may be diminished by the concomitant administration of aspirin due to inhibition of renal prostaglandins, leading to decreased renal blood flow, and salt and fluid retention.

Diuretics: The effectiveness of diuretics in patients with underlying renal or cardiovascular disease may be diminished by the concomitant administration of aspirin due to inhibition of renal prostaglandins, leading to decreased renal blood flow and salt and fluid retention.

Methotrexate: Salicylate can inhibit renal clearance of methotrexate, leading to bone marrow toxicity, especially in the elderly or renal impaired.

Nonsteroidal Anti-inflammatory Drugs (NSAID's): The concurrent use of aspirin with other NSAID's should be avoided because this may increase bleeding or lead to decreased renal function.

Oral Hypoglycemics: Moderate doses of aspirin may increase the effectiveness of oral hypoglycemic drugs, leading to hypoglycemia.

Uricosuric Agents (Probenecid and Sulfinpyrazone): Salicylates antagonize the uricosuric action of uricosuric agents.

Carcinogenesis, Mutagenesis, Impairment of Fertility: Administration of aspirin for 68 weeks at 0.5 percent in the feed of rats was not carcinogenic. In the Ames Salmonella assay, aspirin was not mutagenic; however, aspirin did induce chromosome aberrations in cultured human fibroblasts. Aspirin inhibits ovulation in rats. (See Pregnancy.)

Pregnancy: Pregnant women should only take aspirin if clearly needed. Because of the known effects of NSAID's on the fetal cardiovascular system (closure of the ductus arteriosus), use during the third trimester of pregnancy should be avoided. Salicylate products have also been associated with alterations in maternal and neonatal hemostasis mechanisms, decreased birth weight, and with perinatal mortality.

Labor and Delivery: Aspirin should be avoided 1 week prior to and during labor and delivery because it can result in excessive blood loss at delivery. Prolonged gestation and prolonged labor due to prostaglandin inhibition have been reported.

Nursing Mothers: Nursing mothers should avoid using aspirin because salicylate is excreted in breast milk. Use of high doses may lead to rashes, platelet abnormalities, and bleeding in nursing infants.

Pediatric Use: Pediatric dosing recommendations for juvenile rheumatoid arthritis are based on well-controlled clinical studies. An initial dose of 90–130 mg/kg/day in divided doses, with an increase as needed for anti-inflammatory efficacy (target plasma salicylate levels of 150–300 mcg/mL) are effective. At high doses (i.e., plasma levels of greater than 200 mcg/mL), the incidence of toxicity increases.

Adverse Reactions: Many adverse reactions due to aspirin ingestion are dose-related. The following is a list of adverse reactions that have been reported in the literature. (See **Warnings**.)

Body as a Whole: Fever, hypothermia, thirst.

Cardiovascular: Dysrhythmias, hypotension, tachycardia.

Central Nervous System: Agitation, cerebral edema, coma, confusion, dizziness, headache, subdural or intracranial hemorrhage, lethargy, seizures.

Fluid and Electrolyte: Dehydration, hyperkalemia, metabolic acidosis, respiratory alkalosis.

Gastrointestinal: Dyspepsia, GI bleeding, ulceration and perforation, nausea, vomiting, transient elevations of hepatic enzymes, hepatitis, Reye's Syndrome, pancreatitis.

Hematologic: Prolongation of the prothrombin time, disseminated intravascular coagulation, coagulopathy, thrombocytopenia.

Hypersensitivity: Acute anaphylaxis, angioedema, asthma, bronchospasm, laryngeal edema, urticaria.

Musculoskeletal: Rhabdomyolysis.

Metabolism: Hypoglycemia (in children), hyperglycemia.

Reproductive: Prolonged pregnancy and labor, stillbirths, lower birth weight infants, antepartum and postpartum bleeding.

Respiratory: Hyperpnea, pulmonary edema, tachypnea.

Special Senses: Hearing loss, tinnitus. Patients with high frequency hearing loss may have difficulty perceiving tinnitus. In these patients, tinnitus cannot be used as a clinical indicator of salicylism.

Urogenital: Interstitial nephritis, papillary necrosis, proteinuria, renal insufficiency and failure.

Drug Abuse And Dependence: Aspirin is nonnarcotic. There is no known potential for addiction associated with the use of aspirin.

Overdosage: Salicylate toxicity may result from acute ingestion (overdose) or chronic intoxication. The early signs of salicylic overdose (salicylism), including tinnitus (ringing in the ears), occur at plasma concentrations approaching 200 mcg/mL. Plasma concentrations of aspirin above 300 mcg/mL are clearly toxic. Severe toxic effects are associated with levels above 400 mcg/mL. (See **Clinical Pharmacology**.) A single lethal dose of aspirin in adults is not known with certainty but death may be expected at 30 g. For real or suspected overdose, a Poison Control Center should be contacted immediately. Careful medical management is essential.

Signs and Symptoms: In acute overdose, severe acid-base and electrolyte disturbances may occur and are complicated by hyperthermia and dehydration. Respiratory alkalosis occurs early while hyperventilation is present, but is quickly followed by metabolic acidosis.

Treatment: Treatment consists primarily of supporting vital functions, increasing salicylate elimination, and correcting the acid-base disturbance. Gastric emptying and/or lavage is recommended as soon as possible after ingestion, even if the patient has vomited spontaneously. After lavage and/or emesis, administration of activated charcoal, as a slurry, is beneficial, if less than 3 hours have passed since ingestion. Charcoal adsorption should not be employed prior to emesis and lavage.

Severity of aspirin intoxication is determined by measuring the blood salicylate level. Acid-base status should be closely followed with serial blood gas and serum pH measurements. Fluid and electrolyte balance should aslo be maintained.

In severe cases, hyperthermia and hypovolemia are the major immediate threats to life. Children should be sponged with tepid water. Replacement fluid should be administered intravenously and augmented with correction of acidosis. Plasma electrolytes and pH should be monitored to promote alkaline diuresis of salicylate if renal function is normal. Infusion of glucose may be required to control hypoglycemia.

Hemodialysis and peritoneal dialysis can be performed to reduce the body drug content. In patients with renal insufficiency or in cases of life-threatening intoxication, dialysis is usually required. Exchange transfusion may be indicated in infants and young children.

Continued on next page

Bayer Prof Labeling—Cont.

Dosage and Administration: Each dose of aspirin should be taken with a full glass of water unless patient is fluid restricted. Anti-inflammatory and analgesic dosages should be individualized. When aspirin is used in high doses, the development of tinnitus may be used as a clinical sign of elevated plasma salicylate levels except in patients with high frequency hearing loss.

Ischemic Stroke and TIA: 50–325 mg once a day. Continue therapy indefinitely.

Suspected Acute MI: The initial dose of 160–162.5 mg is administered as soon as an MI is suspected. The maintenance dose of 160–162.5 mg a day is continued for 30 days post-infaction. After 30 days, consider further therapy based on dosage and administration for prevention of recurrent MI.

Prevention of Recurrent MI: 75–325 mg once a day. Continue therapy indefinitely.

Unstable Angina Pectoris: 75–325 mg once a day. Continue therapy indefinitely.

Chronic Stable Angina Pectoris: 75–325 mg once a day. Continue therapy indefinitely.

CABG: 325 mg daily starting 6 hours post-procedure. Continue therapy for 1 year post-procedure.

PTCA: The initial dose of 325 mg should be given 2 hours presurgery. Maintenance dose is 160–325 mg daily. Continue therapy indefinitely.

Carotid Endarterectomy: Doses of 80 mg once daily to 650 mg twice daily, started presurgery, are recommended. Continue therapy indefinitely.

Rheumatoid Arthritis: The initial dose is 3 g a day in divided doses. Increase as needed for anti-inflammatory efficacy with target plasma salicylate levels of 150–300 mcg/mL. At high doses (i.e., plasma levels of greater than 200 mcg/mL), the incidence of toxicity increases.

Juvenile Rheumatoid Arthritis: Initial dose is 90–130 mg/kg/day in divided doses. Increase as needed for anti-inflammatory efficacy with target plasma salicylate levels of 150–300 mcg/mL. At high doses (i.e., plasma levels of greater than 200 mcg/mL), the incidence of toxicity increases.

Spondyloarthropathies: Up to 4 g per day in divided doses.

Osteoarthritis: Up to 3 g per day in divided doses.

Arthritis and Pleurisy of SLE: The initial dose is 3 g a day in divided doses. Increase as needed for anti-inflammatory efficacy with target plasma salicylate levels of 150–300 mcg/mL. At high doses (i.e., plasma levels of greater than 200 mcg/mL), the incidence of toxicity increases.

Extra Strength BAYER® Aspirin Caplets, and Gelcaps

Active Ingredient: **Purposes:**
(in each caplet)
Aspirin
500 mg ...... Pain reliever/fever reducer

Uses: For the temporary relief of
• headache
• pain and fever of colds
• muscle pain
• menstrual pain
• toothache
• minor pain of arthritis

Warnings: Reye's syndrome: Children and teenagers should not use this medicine for chicken pox or flu symptoms before a doctor is consulted about Reye's syndrome, a rare but serious illness reported to be associated with aspirin.
Allergy alert: Aspirin may cause a severe allergic reaction which may include:
• hives • facial swelling • asthma (wheezing) • shock
Alcohol warning: If you consume 3 or more alcoholic drinks every day, ask your doctor whether you should take aspirin or other pain relievers/fever reducers. Aspirin may cause stomach bleeding.
Do not use if you are allergic to aspirin or any other pain reliever/fever reducer.
Ask a doctor before use if you have:
• stomach problems (such as heartburn, upset stomach, or stomach pain) that last or come back
• bleeding problems
• ulcers
• asthma
Ask a doctor or pharmacist before use if you are taking a prescription drug for
• anticoagulation (blood thinning)
• gout
• diabetes
• arthritis
Stop use and ask a doctor if:
• an allergic reaction occurs. Seek medical help right away.
• pain gets worse or lasts for more than 10 days
• fever lasts for more than 3 days
• new symptoms occur
• ringing in the ears or loss of hearing occurs
• redness or swelling is present
If pregnant or breast-feeding, ask a health professional before use. **It is especially important not to use aspirin during the last 3 months of pregnancy unless definitely directed to do so by a doctor because it may cause problems in the unborn child or complications during delivery.**
Keep out of reach of children. In case of overdose, get medical help or contact a Poison Control Center right away.

Directions:
• drink a full glass of water with each dose
• adults and children 12 years and over: take 1 or 2 caplets every 4 to 6 hours not to exceed 8 caplets in 24 hours
• children under 12 years: consult a doctor
Other Information:
• save carton for full directions and warnings
• store at room temperature

Inactive Ingredients: Extra Strength BAYER® Aspirin Caplets: Carnauba Wax, Cellulose, D&C Red #7 Calcium Lake, FD&C Blue #2 Aluminum Lake, FD&C Red #40 Aluminum Lake, Hypromellose, Propylene Glycol, Shellac, Starch, Titanium Dioxide, Triacetin
Extra Strength BAYER® Aspirin Gelcaps: Butylparaben, D&C Yellow #10 Aluminum Lake, FD&C Blue #1 Aluminum Lake, FD&C Red #40, Gelatin, Glycerin, Hypromellose, Methylparaben, Polyvinylpyrrolidone, Propylene Glycol, Propylparaben, Shellac, Sodium Lauryl Sulfate, Sorbitan Trioleate, Starch, Titanium Dioxide, Triacetin

How Supplied:
Extra Strength BAYER® Aspirin Caplets: Bottle of 50 coated caplets (500 mg).
Extra Strength BAYER® Aspirin Gelcaps: Bottle of 80 gelcaps (500 mg).
Questions or comments?
1-800-331-4536 or www.bayeraspirin.com
Bayer Corporation
PO Box 1910
Morristown, NJ 07962-1910 USA

Extra Strength BAYER® PLUS Buffered Aspirin Caplets

Active Ingredient:
(in each caplet) **Purposes**
Aspirin
500 mg .... Pain reliever/fever reducer

Uses: For the temporary relief of
• headache
• pain and fever of colds
• muscle pain
• menstrual pain
• toothache
• minor pain of arthritis

Warnings: Reye's syndrome: Children and teenagers should not use this medicine for chicken pox or flu symptoms before a doctor is consulted about Reye's syndrome, a rare but serious illness reported to be associated with aspirin.
Allergy alert: Aspirin may cause a severe allergic reaction which may include
• hives
• facial swelling
• asthma (wheezing)
• shock
Alcohol warning: If you consume 3 or more alcoholic drinks every day, ask your doctor whether you should take aspirin or other pain relievers/fever reducers. Aspirin may cause stomach bleeding.
Do not use if you are allergic to aspirin or any other pain reliever/fever reducer.
Ask a doctor before use if you have
• stomach problems (such as heartburn, upset stomach, or stomach pain) that continue or come back
• bleeding problems
• ulcers
• asthma
Ask a doctor or pharmacist before use if you are taking a prescription drug for
• anticoagulation (blood thinning)
• gout
• diabetes

- arthritis

Stop use and ask a doctor if

- an allergic reaction occurs. Seek medical help right away.
- pain gets worse or lasts more than 10 days
- fever lasts more than 3 days
- new symptoms occur
- ringing in the ears or loss of hearing occurs
- redness or swelling is present

If pregnant or breast-feeding, ask a health professional before use. **It is especially important not to use aspirin during the last 3 months of pregnancy unless definitely directed to do so by a doctor because it may cause problems in the unborn child or complications during delivery.**

Keep out of reach of children. In case of overdose, get medical help or contact a Poison Control Center right away.

Directions

- drink a full glass of water with each dose
- adults and children 12 years and over: take 1 or 2 caplets every 4 to 6 hours as needed, not to exceed 8 caplets in 24 hours
- children under 12 years: consult a doctor

Other Information

- contains calcium carbonate (350 mg = 140 mg elemental calcium)
- save carton for full directions and warnings
- store at room temperature

Inactive Ingredients: Calcium carbonate, carnauba wax, colloidal silicon dioxide, D&C red #7 calcium lake, FD&C blue #2 aluminum lake, FD&C red #40 aluminum lake, hypromellose, microcrystalline cellulose, propylene glycol, shellac, sodium starch glycolate, starch, titanium dioxide, zinc stearate

How Supplied: Bottle of 50 buffered caplets (500 mg).

Questions or comments?
1-800-331-4536 or
www.bayeraspirin.com
USE ONLY IF SEAL UNDER BOTTLE CAP WITH GREEN "Bayer Corporation" PRINT IS INTACT.
Bayer Corporation
PO Box 1910
Morristown, NJ 07962-1910 USA

**Extra Strength BAYER® PM
For Pain with Sleeplessness
Caplets**

**Active Ingredients:
(in each caplet)　　　　　　　Purpose**
Aspirin 500 mg .... Pain reliever
Diphenhydramine citrate
　38.3 mg .... Night time Sleep-aid

Uses: For the temporary relief of occasional headache and minor aches and pains with accompanying sleeplessness

Warnings: Reye's syndrome: Children and teenagers should not use this medicine for chicken pox or flu symptoms

before a doctor is consulted about Reye's syndrome, a rare but serious illness reported to be associated with aspirin.

Allergy alert: Aspirin may cause a severe allergic reaction which may include:

- hives
- facial swelling
- asthma (wheezing)
- shock

Alcohol warning: If you consume 3 or more alcoholic drinks every day, ask your doctor whether you should take aspirin or other pain relievers/fever reducers. Aspirin may cause stomach bleeding.

Do not use

- if you ever had an allergic reaction to any other pain reliever/fever reducer
- in children under 12 years of age
- with any other product containing diphenhydramine, including one applied topically

Ask a doctor before use if you have

- stomach problems (such as heartburn, upset stomach, or stomach pain) that continue or come back
- bleeding problems
- ulcers
- a breathing problem such as emphysema, chronic bronchitis, or asthma
- glaucoma
- trouble urinating due to enlargement of the prostate gland

Ask a doctor or pharmacist before use if you are

- taking sedatives or tranquilizers
- taking a prescription drug for
  - anticoagulation (blood thinning)
  - gout
  - diabetes
  - arthritis

When using this product avoid alcoholic drinks.

Stop use and ask a doctor if

- an allergic reaction occurs. Seek medical help right away.
- pain gets worse or lasts more than 10 days
- new symptoms occur
- ringing in the ears or loss of hearing occurs
- redness or swelling is present
- sleeplessness lasts for more than 2 weeks. Insomnia may be a symptom of a serious condition.

If pregnant or breast-feeding, ask a health professional before use. **It is especially important not to use aspirin during the last 3 months of pregnancy unless definitely directed to do so by a doctor because it may cause problems in the unborn child or complications during delivery.**

Keep out of reach of children. In case of overdose, get medical help or contact a Poison Control Center right away.

Directions

- do not exceed recommended dosage
- drink a full glass of water with each dose
- adults and children 12 years and over: take 2 caplets at bedtime, if needed, or as directed by a doctor.
- children under 12 years: consult a doctor

Other Information

- save carton for full directions and warnings
- store at room temperature

Inactive Ingredients: Carnauba wax, citric acid, colloidal silicon dioxide,

FD&C blue #1 aluminum lake, FD&C blue #2 aluminum lake, hypromellose, microcrystalline cellulose, propylene glycol, shellac, starch, titanium dioxide, zinc stearate

How Supplied: Bottle of 40 caplets.
Questions or comments?
1-800-331-4536 or
www.bayeraspirin.com
USE ONLY IF SEAL UNDER BOTTLE CAP WITH BLUE "Bayer Corporation" PRINT IS INTACT.
Bayer Corporation
PO Box 1910
Morristown, NJ 07962-1910 USA

BAYER® WOMEN'S ASPIRIN PLUS CALCIUM
Low Strength Aspirin Regimen
Analgesic/Dietary Supplement
81 mg Aspirin-300 mg Calcium

Directions: For calcium, take up to 4 caplets per day.

Serving Size: One Caplet

	Amount Per Serving	% Daily Value
Calcium (elemental)	300 mg	30%

Ingredients: Calcium Carbonate, Microcrystalline Cellulose, Aspirin, Lactose, Cellulose, Maltodextrin, Starch, Carnauba Wax, Hypromellose, Polydextrose, Titanium Dioxide, Triacetin, Sodium Starch Glycolate, Colloidal Silicon Dioxide, Zinc Stearate, Mineral Oil, Crospovidone, Magnesium Stearate, Stearic Acid.

What you should know about Osteoporosis
Menopausal women and women with a family history of the disease are groups at risk for developing osteoporosis. Adequate calcium intake throughout life, along with a healthy diet and regular exercise, builds and maintains good bone health and may reduce the risk of osteoporosis. While adequate calcium intake is important, daily intakes above 2,000 mg may not provide additional benefits.

**Active Ingredient:
(in each caplet)　　　　　　　Purpose**
Aspirin 81 mg .... Pain reliever

Uses: For the temporary relief of minor aches and pains or as recommended by your doctor

Warnings: Reye's syndrome: Children and teenagers should not use this medicine for chicken pox or flu symptoms before a doctor is consulted about Reye's syndrome, a rare but serious illness reported to be associated with aspirin.

Alcohol warning: If you consume 3 or more alcoholic drinks every day, ask your

Continued on next page

Bayer Women's—Cont.

doctor whether you should take aspirin or other pain relievers/fever reducers. Aspirin may cause stomach bleeding.

Allergy alert: Aspirin may cause a severe allergic reaction which may include:
- hives
- facial swelling
- asthma (wheezing)
- shock

Do not use if you are allergic to aspirin or any other pain reliever/fever reducer.

Ask a doctor before use if you have
- stomach problems (such as heartburn, upset stomach, or stomach pain) that continue or come back
- bleeding problems
- ulcers
- asthma

Ask a doctor or pharmacist before use if you are taking a prescription drug for
- anticoagulation (blood thinning)
- gout
- diabetes
- arthritis

Stop use and ask a doctor if
- an allergic reaction occurs. Seek medical help right away.
- pain gets worse or lasts more than 10 days
- new symptoms occur
- ringing in the ears or loss of hearing occurs
- redness or swelling is present

If pregnant or breast-feeding, ask a health professional before use. **It is especially important not to use aspirin during the last 3 months of pregnancy unless definitely directed to do so by a doctor because it may cause problems in the unborn child or complications during delivery.**

Keep out of reach of children. In case of overdose, get medical help or contact a Poison Control Center right away.

Directions:
- talk to your doctor about regimen use of aspirin
- drink a full glass of water with each dose
- for pain, adults and children 12 years and over: take 4 caplets not to exceed 4 caplets in 24 hours
- children under 12 years: consult a doctor

Other Information
- save carton for full directions and warnings
- store at room temperature

Inactive Ingredients: Calcium carbonate, carnauba wax, cellulose, colloidal silicon dioxide, crospovidone, hypromellose, lactose, magnesium stearate, maltodextrin, microcrystalline cellulose, mineral oil, polydextrose, sodium starch glycolate, starch, stearic acid, titanium dioxide, triacetin, zinc stearate.

How Supplied: Bottle of 90 Caplets

Aspirin is not appropriate for everyone, so be sure to talk to your doctor before you begin an aspirin regimen.

Ideal for women on an aspirin regimen, as directed by a doctor, who need a head start on their daily calcium requirements to help fight Osteoporosis.

For more information on how to fight heart disease and stroke, visit the American Heart Association Web Site at www.americanheart.org.

USE ONLY IF SEAL UNDER BOTTLE CAP WITH GREEN "Bayer Corporation" PRINT IS INTACT.

Questions or comments?
1-800-331-4536 or
www.bayeraspirin.com
Bayer Corporation
Consumer Care Division
PO Box 1910
Morristown, NJ 07962-1910 USA
Shown in Product Identification Guide, page 504

DOMEBORO® POWDER PACKETS
DOMEBORO® TABLETS

DOMEBORO® Powder Packets

Active Ingredient

(in each packet):	**Purpose:**

Aluminum acetate
648 mg .... Astringent
(Each powder packet, when dissolved in water and ready for use, provides the active ingredient aluminum acetate resulting from the reaction of hydrated calcium acetate 839 mg and aluminum sulfate 1191 mg.)

DOMEBORO® Tablets

Active Ingredient

(in each tablet):	**Purpose:**

Aluminum acetate
467 mg .... Astringent
(Each tablet, when dissolved in water and ready for use, provides the active ingredient aluminum acetate resulting from the reaction of hydrated calcium acetate 605 mg and aluminum sulfate 879 mg.)

Uses: temporarily relieves minor skin irritations due to:
- poison ivy
- poison oak
- poison sumac
- insect bites
- athlete's foot
- rashes caused by soaps, detergents, cosmetics, or jewelry

Warnings:

For external use only

When using this product
- avoid contact with the eyes
- do not cover compress or wet dressing with plastic to prevent evaporation

Stop use and ask a doctor if condition worsens or symptoms persist more than 7 days.

Keep out of reach of children. If swallowed, get medical help or contact a Poison Control Center right away.

Directions:

DOMEBORO® Powder Packets
- dissolve one, two, or three packets in 16 oz of water and stir the solution until fully dissolved to obtain the following modified Burow's Solution

Number of Packets	Dilution	% Aluminum acetate
one packet	1:40 dilution	0.14%
two packets	1:20 dilution	0.28%
three packets	1:13 dilution	0.42%

- do not strain or filter the solution
- can be used as a compress, wet dressing, or a soak.

DOMEBORO® Tablets
- dissolve one, two, or three tablets in 12 oz of water and stir the solution until fully dissolved to obtain the following modified Burow's Solution

Number of Tablets	Dilution	% Aluminum acetate
one tablet	1:40 dilution	0.13%
two tablets	1:20 dilution	0.26%
three tablets	1:13 dilution	0.39%

- do not strain or filter the solution
- can be used as a compress, wet dressing, or a soak

AS A COMPRESS OR WET DRESSING:
- saturate a clean, soft, white cloth (such as a diaper or torn sheet) in the solution
- gently squeeze and apply loosely to the affected area
- saturate the cloth in the solution every 15 to 30 minutes and apply to the affected area
- discard the solution after each use
- repeat as often as necessary

AS A SOAK:
- soak affected area in the solution for 15 to 30 minutes
- discard solution after each use
- repeat 3 times a day

Other Information: • protect from excessive heat

Inactive Ingredients:
DOMEBORO® Powder Packets
dextrin
DOMEBORO® Tablets:
dextrin, polyethylene glycol, sodium bicarbonate

How Supplied:
Tablets and Packets available in 12 and 100 count sizes
Questions or comments? **1-800-800-4793 or www.bayercare.com**

**Maximum Strength
MIDOL® Teen
Pain& Multi-Symptom Menstrual Relief
Aspirin Free/Caffeine Free
Caplet**

Midol. Because your period's more than a pain.™

Active Ingredients:
(in each caplet)   **Purpose:**
Acetaminophen
  500 mg .... Pain reliever
Pamabrom
  25 mg .... Diuretic

Uses: For the temporary relief of these symptoms associated with menstrual periods:
- cramps
- bloating
- water-weight gain
- headache
- backache
- muscle aches

Warnings: Alcohol warning: If you consume 3 or more alcoholic drinks every day, ask your doctor whether you should take acetaminophen or other pain relievers/fever reducers. Acetaminophen may cause liver damage.
Do not use with any other product containing acetaminophen.
Stop use and ask a doctor if
- new symptoms occur
- redness or swelling is present
- pain gets worse or lasts more than 10 days

If pregnant or breast-feeding, ask a health professional before use.
Keep out of reach of children.

Overdose warning: Taking more than the recommended dose can cause serious health problems. In case of overdose, get medical help or contact a Poison Control Center right away. Quick medical attenion is critical for adults as well as children even if you do not notice any signs or symptoms.

Directions
- do not take more than the recommended dose (see **Overdose Warning**)
- adults and children 12 years and older
  - take 2 caplets with water
  - repeat every 6 hours, as needed
  - do not exceed 8 caplets per day
- children under 12 years, consult a doctor

Other Information: Store at room temperature

Inactive Ingredients: Carnauba Wax, Croscarmellose sodium, D&C Red #7 calcium Lake, FD&C Blue #2 Aluminum Lake, hypromellose, Magnesium Stearate, Microcrystalline cellulose, Propylene glycol, Shellac, Starch, Titanium Dioxide, Triacetin.

How Supplied: Caplets-White capsule-shaped caplets available in packages of 24 caplets containing 3 blisters of 8 caplets each.
Questions or comments?
1-800-331-4536.
www.bayercare.com
ASPIRIN-FREE   CAFFEINE-FREE
Distributed by:
Bayer Corporation
Consumer Care Division
Morristown, NJ 07960 USA
Shown in Product Identification Guide, page 504

Maximum Strength
MIDOL® Menstrual
Pain & Multi-Symptom Menstrual Relief
Aspirin Free
Caplets and Gelcaps

Active Ingredients:
(in each caplet and gelcap)   Purpose:
Acetaminophen 500 mg .... Pain reliever
Caffeine 60 mg .... Stimulant
Pyrilamine maleate 15 mg .... Diuretic

Uses: For the temporary relief of these symptoms associated with menstrual periods:
- cramps
- bloating
- water-weight gain
- breast tenderness
- headache
- backache
- muscle aches
- fatigue

Warnings: Alcohol warning: If you consume 3 or more alcoholic drinks every day, ask your doctor whether you should take acetaminophen or other pain relievers/fever reducers. Acetaminophen may cause liver damage.
Do not use with any other product containing acetaminophen.
Ask a doctor before use if you have:
- glaucoma
- difficulty in urination due to enlargement of the prostate gland
- a breathing problem such as emphysema or chronic bronchitis
Ask a doctor or pharmacist before use if you are taking sedatives or tranquilizers.
When using this product:
- you may get drowsy
- avoid alcoholic drinks
- excitability may occur, especially in children
- alcohol, sedatives, and tranquilizers may increase drowsiness
- be careful when driving a motor vehicle or operating machinery
- limit the use of caffeine-containing medications, foods, or beverages. Too much caffeine may cause nervousness, irritability, sleeplessness, and occasionally, rapid heartbeat. The recommended dose of this product contains about as much caffeine as a cup of coffee.
Stop use and ask a doctor if:
- new symptoms occur
- redness or swelling is present
- pain gets worse or lasts for more than 10 days
If pregnant or breast-feeding, ask a health professional before use.
Keep out of reach of children.
Overdose warning: Taking more than the recommended dose can cause serious health problems. In case of overdose, get medical help or contact a Poison Control Center right away. Quick medical attention is critical for adults as well as children even if you do not notice any signs or symptoms.
Directions:
MIDOL® Extra Strength Caplets:
Do not take more than the recommended dose. (see **Overdose Warning**)

- adults and children 12 years and older
  - take 2 caplets with water
  - repeat every 4 hours, as needed
  - do not exceed 8 caplets per day
- children under 12 years, consult a doctor
Other Information:
- store at room temperature
MIDOL® Extra Strength Gelcaps:
Do not take more than the recommended dose. (see **Overdose Warning**)
- adults and children 12 years and older
  - take 2 gelcaps with water
  - repeat every 6 hours, as needed
  - do not exceed 8 gelcaps per day
- children under 12 years, consult a doctor

Other Information:
- store at room temperature
- avoid excessive heat 104°F (40°C)

Inactive Ingredients:
MIDOL® Extra Strength Caplets: Croscarmellose Sodium, FD&C Blue #2, Hypromellose, Magnesium Stearate, Microcrystalline Cellulose, Pregelatinized Starch, Triacetin.
MIDOL® Extra Strength Gelcaps: Carnauba Wax, Croscarmellose Sodium, D&C Red #33 Lake, Disodium EDTA, FD&C Blue #1 Lake, Gelatin, Glycerin, Hypromellose, Iron Oxide, Lecithin, Magnesium Stearate, Microcrystalline Cellulose, Pharmaceutical Glaze, Simethicone, Starch, Stearic Acid, Titanium Dioxide, Triacetin

How Supplied:
MIDOL® Extra Strength Caplets: Capsule-shaped caplets available in packages of 24 caplets containing 3 blisters of 8 capsules each.
MIDOL® Extra Strength Gelcaps: Capsule-shaped gelcaps available in packages of 24 gelcaps containing 3 blisters of 8 gelcaps each.
Use only if blister unit is unbroken.
Store at room temperature; avoid excessive heat 40°C (104°F).
Questions? Comments?
Please call 1-800-331-4536.
Visit our website at www.bayercare.com
ASPIRIN-FREE
B-R LLC
Distributed by:
Bayer Corporation
Consumer Care Division
Morristown, NJ 07960 USA
Shown in Product Identification Guide, page 504

Maximum Strength
MIDOL® PMS
Pain & Premenstrual Symptom Relief
Aspirin Free/Caffeine Free
Caplets and Gelcaps

Active Ingredients:
(in each caplet
and in each gelcap)   Purpose:
Acetaminophen 500 mg .... Pain reliever
Pamabrom 25 mg .... Diuretic
Pyrilamine maleate 15 mg .... Diuretic

Continued on next page

Midol PMS—Cont.

Uses: For the temporary relief of these symptoms associated with menstrual periods:
• bloating
• water-weight gain
• cramps
• breast tenderness
• headache
• backache

Warnings: Alcohol warning: If you consume 3 or more alcoholic drinks every day, ask your doctor whether you should take acetaminophen or other pain relievers/fever reducers. Acetaminophen may cause liver damage.

Do not use with any other product containing acetaminophen.

Ask a doctor before use if you have:
• glaucoma
• difficulty in urination due to enlargement of the prostate gland
• a breathing problem such as emphysema or chronic bronchitis

Ask a doctor or pharmacist before use if you are taking sedatives or tranquilizers.

When using this product:
• you may get drowsy
• excitability may occur, especially in children
• alcohol, sedatives, and tranquilizers may increase drowsiness
• avoid alcoholic drinks
• be careful when driving a motor vehicle or operating machinery

Stop use and ask a doctor if:
• new symptoms occur
• redness or swelling is present
• pain gets worse or lasts for more than 10 days

If pregnant or breast-feeding, ask a health professional before use.

Keep out of reach of children.

Overdose warning: Taking more than the recommended dose can cause serious health problems. In case of overdose, get medical help or contact a Poison Control Center right away. Quick medical attention is critical for adults as well as children even if you do not notice any signs or symptoms.

Directions:
MIDOL® Maximum Strength PMS Caplets:
Do not take more than the recommended dose. (see Overdose Warning)
• adults and children 12 years and older
  • take 2 caplets with water
  • repeat every 6 hours, as needed
  • do not exceed 8 caplets per day
• children under 12 years, consult a doctor
Other Information: Store at room temperature. Avoid excessive heat 104° F (40° C)
MIDOL® Maximum Strength PMS Gelcaps:
Do not take more than the recommended dose. (see Overdose Warning)
• adults and children 12 years and older
  • take 2 gelcaps with water
  • repeat every 6 hours, as needed
  • do not exceed 8 gelcaps per day
• children under 12 years, consult a doctor

Other Information: Store at room temperature. Avoid excessive heat 104° F (40° C)

Inactive Ingredients:
MIDOL® Maximum Strength PMS: Carnauba Wax, Croscarmellose Sodium, D&C Red #30 Aluminum Lake, D&C Yellow #10 Aluminum Lake, Hypromellose, Magnesium Stearate, Microcrystalline Cellulose, Propylene Glycol, Shellac, Starch, Titanium Dioxide, Triacetin
MIDOL® Maximum Strength PMS Gelcaps: Croscarmellose Sodium, D&C Red #27 Lake, EDTA Disodium, FD&C Blue #1, FD&C Red #40 Lake, Gelatin, Glycerin, Hypromellose, Iron Oxide, Magnesium Stearate, Microcrystalline Cellulose, Starch, Stearic Acid, Titanium Dioxide, Triacetin.

How Supplied:
MIDOL® Maximum Strength PMS Caplets: Capsule-shaped caplets available in packages of 24 caplets containing 3 blisters of 8 caplets each.
MIDOL® Maximum Strength PMS Gelcaps: Capsule-shaped gelcaps available in packages of 24 gelcaps containing 3 blisters of 8 gelcaps each.
Use only if blister unit is unbroken.
Store at room temperature; avoid excessive heat 40°C (104°F).
Questions? Comments?
Please call 1-800-331-4536.
Visit our website at
www.bayercare.com
ASPIRIN-FREE CAFFEINE-FREE
B-R LLC
Distributed by:
Bayer Corporation
Consumer Care Division
Morristown, NJ 07960 USA
Shown in Product Identification Guide, page 504

NEO-SYNEPHRINE®
Mild Formula, Regular Strength, Extra Strength

Active Ingredients:
Neo-Synephrine® Extra Strength Drops
Neo-Synephrine® Extra Strength Spray
Active Ingredient: **Purpose:**
Phenylephrine
Hydrochloride 1.0% .... Nasal decongestant
Neo-Synephrine® Regular Strength Drops
Neo-Synephrine® Regular Strength Spray
Active Ingredient: **Purpose:**
Phenylephrine
Hydrochloride 0.5% .... Nasal decongestant
Neo-Synephrine® Mild Formula Spray
Active Ingredient: **Purpose:**
Phenylephrine
Hydrochloride 0.25% .... Nasal decongestant

Uses: • Temporarily relieves nasal congestion:
— due to common cold
— due to hay fever or other respiratory allergies (allergic rhinitis)
— associated with sinusitis
• Temporarily relieves stuffy nose.
• Helps clear nasal passages; shrinks swollen membranes.
• Temporarily restores freer breathing through the nose.
• Helps decongest sinus openings and passages;
• temporarily relieves sinus congestion and pressure.

Warnings:
Ask a doctor before use if you have
• heart disease
• high blood pressure
• thyroid disease
• diabetes
• difficulty in urination due to enlargement of the prostate gland
When using this product
• **do not exceed recommended dosage**
• do not use more than 3 days. Frequent or prolonged use may cause nasal congestion to recur or worsen.
• temporary discomfort may occur such as burning, stinging, sneezing and increase in nasal discharge
• use by more than one person may spread infection.
Stop use and ask a doctor if symptoms persist more than 3 days.
If pregnant or breast-feeding, ask a health professional before use.
Keep out of reach of children. If swallowed, get medical help or contact a Poison Control Center right away.

Directions: use as directed.
Neo-Synephrine® Extra Strength Drops
Neo-Synephrine® Regular Strength Drops

Adults and children 12 years of age and over	2 or 3 drops in each nostril not more often than every 4 hours.
Children under 12 years	Ask a doctor.

Neo-Synephrine® Extra Strength Spray
Neo-Synephrine® Regular Strength Spray
To spray, squeeze bottle quickly and firmly.

Adults and children 12 years of age and over	2 or 3 sprays in each nostril not more often than every 4 hours.
Children under 12 years	Ask a doctor.

Neo-Synephrine® Mild Formula Spray
To spray, squeeze bottle quickly and firmly.

Adults and children 6 to under 12 years of age (with adult supervision)	2 or 3 sprays in each nostril not more often than every 4 hours.
Children under 6 years	Ask a doctor.

Other Information:
• Store at room temperature.
• Protect from light.

Inactive Ingredients: benzalkonium chloride, citric acid, sodium chloride, sodium citrate, water

How Supplied:
Neo-Synephrine® Regular Strength Drops;
Neo-Synephrine® Extra Strength Drops: 15 mL (0.5%).
DO NOT USE IF IMPRINTED BOTTLE OVERWRAP IS BROKEN OR MISSING.
Neo-Synephrine® Regular Strength Spray;
Neo-Synephrine® Extra Strength Spray: 15 mL (1.0%).
USE ONLY IF NECKBAND PRINTED WITH "Bayer" IS INTACT.
Neo-Synephrine® Mild Formula Spray: 15 mL (0.25%).
USE ONLY IF NECKBAND PRINTED WITH "Bayer" IS INTACT.
Questions or comments? 1-800-331-4536 or www.bayercare.com
Shown in Product Identification Guide, page 504

NEO-SYNEPHRINE®
12 Hour
(nasal spray)
12 Hour Extra Moisturizing
(nasal spray)

Active Ingredients:	**Purpose:**
Oxymetazoline hydrochloride 0.05%	Nasal decongestant

Uses: Temporarily relieves nasal congestion:
— due to common cold
— due to hay fever or other respiratory allergies (allergic rhinitis)
— associated with sinusitis
• temporarily relieves stuffy nose.
• helps clear nasal passages; shrinks swollen membranes.
• temporarily restores freer breathing through the nose.
• helps decongest sinus openings and passages; temporarily relieves sinus congestion and pressure.

Warnings:
Ask a doctor before use if you have
• heart disease
• high blood pressure
• thyroid disease
• diabetes
• difficulty in urination due to enlargement of the prostate gland
When using this product
• **do not exceed recommended dosage**
• do not use more than 3 days. Frequent or prolonged use may cause nasal congestion to recur or worsen.
• temporary discomfort such as burning, stinging, sneezing, and increase in nasal discharge may occur
• use by more than one person may spread infection
Stop use and ask a doctor if symptoms persist for more than 3 days.
If pregnant or breast-feeding, ask a health professional before use.
Keep out of reach of children. If swallowed, get medical help or contact a Poison Control Center right away.

Directions:
• use only as directed
• to spray, squeeze bottle quickly and firmly

adults and children 6 to under 12 years (with adult supervision)	2 to 3 sprays in each nostril not more often than every 10 to 12 hours. Do not exceed 2 doses in 24 hours.
children under 6 years	ask a doctor.

Other Information:
• store at room temperature.
• protect from light.

Inactive Ingredients:
NEO-SYNEPHRINE® 12 Hour Spray: benzalkonium chloride, disodium phosphate, EDTA disodium, sodium chloride, sodium phosphate, water
NEO-SYNEPHRINE® 12 Hour Extra Moisturizing Spray: Benzalkonium chloride, disodium phosphate, EDTA disodium, glycerin, sodium chloride, sodium phosphate, water

How Supplied: Plastic squeeze bottle of 15 ml (½ Fl oz).
USE ONLY IF NECKBAND PRINTED WITH "Bayer" IS INTACT.
Questions or comments? 1-800-331-4536 or www.bayercare.com
Shown in Product Identification Guide, page 504

PHILLIPS'® CHEWABLE TABLETS ANTACID-LAXATIVE STIMULANT FREE
Mint Flavor

Drug Facts

Active Ingredient (in each tablet):	**Purposes**
Magnesium hydroxide 311 mg	Saline laxative/antacid

Uses:
Laxative
• relieves occasional constipation (irregularity)

• this product usually causes bowel movement in ½ to 6 hours
Antacid
• relieves:
  • heartburn
  • acid indigestion
  • sour stomach
  • upset stomach associated with these symptoms

Warnings:
Ask a doctor before use if you have
• kidney disease
• stomach pain, nausea, or vomiting
• a sudden change in bowel habits that lasts over 14 days
Ask a doctor or pharmacist before use if you are taking a prescription drug. Antacids may interact with certain prescription drugs.
When using this product as an antacid, it may have a laxative effect.
Stop use and ask a doctor if
Laxative
• you have rectal bleeding or no bowel movement after using this product. These could be signs of a serious condition.
• you need to use a laxative for more than 1 week
Antacid
• you have taken the maximum dose for 2 weeks
If pregnant or breast-feeding, ask a health professional before use.
Keep out of reach of children. In case of overdose, get medical help or contact a Poison Control Center right away.

Directions:
• do not exceed the maximum recommended daily dose in a 24 hour period
[See table below]

Other information:
• store at room temperature

Inactive ingredients: colloidal silicon dioxide, dextrates, flavor, magnesium stearate, maltodextrin, starch, sucrose

Questions? call **1-800-331-4536** or www.bayercare.com

How Supplied: Bottles of 100 Tablets and 200 Tablets

Continued on next page

Laxative		Antacid	
• dose may be taken once in a 24 hour period preferably at bedtime, in divided doses, or as directed by a doctor • drink a full glass (8 oz) of liquid with each laxative dose		• take every 4 hours up to 4 times in a 24 hour period or as directed by a doctor	
adults and children 12 years and older	chew 8 tablets	adults and children 12 years and older	chew 2 to 4 tablets
children 6 to 11 years	chew 4 tablets	children under 12 years	ask a doctor
children 3 to 5 years	chew 2 tablets		
children under 3 years	ask a doctor		

PHILLIP'S® LIQUI-GELS®

Uses:
- For the relief of occasional constipation (irregularity).
- This product generally produces a bowel movement in 12–72 hours.

Active ingredient
(in each softgel):   Purpose:
Docusate sodium
100 mg .... Stool softener laxative

Inactive ingredients: FD&C blue #2 lake, gelatin, glycerin, methylparaben, polyethylene glycol, propylene glycol, propylparaben, shellac, sorbitol, titanium dioxide

Phillips' Liqui-Gels are a very low sodium product. Each softgel contains 5 mg of sodium.

Directions:
Take softgels with a full glass (8 oz) of water.

adults and children 12 years and over	Take 1 to 3 softgels daily or as directed by a doctor. This dose may be taken as a single daily dose or in divided doses.
children 6 to under 12 years	Take 1 softgel daily or as directed by a doctor.
children under 6 years of age	consult a doctor.

Warnings: Do not use laxative products for a period longer than 1 week unless directed by a doctor. **Ask a doctor before use if you have** abdominal pain, nausea, vomiting or if you have noticed a sudden change in bowel habits that persists over a period of 2 weeks. **Ask a doctor or pharmacist before use if you are** presently taking mineral oil. **Stop use and ask a doctor if** you have rectal bleeding or failure to have a bowel movement after use. These could be signs of a serious condition. **If pregnant or breast-feeding,** ask a health professional before use. **Keep out of reach of children**. In case of overdosage, get medical help or contact a Poison Control Center right away. **Storage:** Store at room temperature. Avoid excessive heat 104°F (40°C).
Questions? 1-800-331-4536 or www.bayercare.com

How Supplied: Blister packs of 10, 30 & 50 Liqui-Gels.

Liqui-Gels is a registered trademark of R.P. Scherer Corp.

Shown in Product Identification Guide, page 505

PHILLIPS'® MILK OF MAGNESIA
Original Formula
Cherry Formula
Mint Formula

Active Ingredient
(in each 5 mL tsp):   Purposes
Magnesium hydroxide
400 mg .... Saline laxative/ antacid

Uses:
Laxative • relieves occasional constipation (irregularity)
• this product usually causes bowel movement in ½ to 6 hours
Antacid • relieves: • heartburn • acid indigestion • sour stomach
• upset stomach associated with these symptoms

Warnings:
Ask a doctor before use if you have
• kidney disease • stomach pain, nausea, or vomiting
• a sudden change in bowel habits that lasts over 14 days
Ask a doctor or pharmacist before use if you are taking a prescription drug. Antacids may interact with certain prescription drugs.
When using this product as an antacid, it may have a laxative effect.
Stop use and ask a doctor if
Laxative • you have rectal bleeding or no bowel movement after using this product. These could be signs of a serious condition.
• you need to use a laxative for more than 1 week
Antacid • you have taken the maximum dose for 2 weeks
If pregnant or breast-feeding, ask a health professional before use.
Keep out of reach of children. In case of overdose, get medical help or contact a Poison Control Center right away.

Directions: • do not exceed the maximum recommended daily dose in a 24 hour period
• shake well before use
• laxative use:
• dose may be taken once a day preferably at bedtime, in divided doses, or as directed by a doctor. Drink a full glass (8 oz) of liquid with each laxative dose. Do not use dosage cup for children.
• antacid use:
• do not use dosage cup
[See table below]

Other Information:
• store at room temperature and avoid freezing • keep tightly closed

Inactive Ingredients:
Phillips' Milk of Magnesia Original Flavor
sodium hypochlorite, water
Phillips' Milk of Magnesia Cherry Flavor
carboxymethylcellulose sodium, citric acid, D&C red #28, flavor, glycerin, microcrystalline cellulose, sodium citrate, sodium hypochlorite, sucrose, water, xanthan gum
Phillips' Milk of Magnesia Fresh Mint
flavor, mineral oil, sodium hypochlorite, sodium saccharin, water

How Supplied:
Original, Fresh Mint and Wild Cherry are available in 4 fl. oz., 12 fl. oz. and 26 fl. oz. bottle. French Vanilla is available in a 12 fl. oz. bottle.
Questions:
1-800-331-4536 or www.bayercare.com
Shown in Product Identification Guide, page 505

PHILLIPS' MO
Lubricant Laxative
Original Formula
Refreshing Mint Formula

Active Ingredients:
(in each 5 mL tsp)   Purpose
Magnesium hydroxide
300 mg .... Saline laxative
Mineral oil
1.25 mL .... Lubricant laxative

Uses
• relieves occasional constipation (irregularity)
• this product usually causes bowel movement in ½ to 6 hours

Warnings
Do not use
• in children under 6 years, or if pregnant, bedridden, or have difficulty swallowing
• if you are presently taking a stool softener laxative
Ask a doctor before use if you have
• kidney disease
• stomach pain, nausea, or vomiting
• a sudden change in bowel habits that lasts over 14 days
Ask a doctor or pharmacist before use if you are taking a prescription drug. This product may interact with certain prescription drugs.

Age	Laxative	Antacid
adults and children 12 years and older	2 to 4 tablespoonsful	1 to 3 teaspoonsful every 4 hours up to 4 times a day or as directed by a doctor
children 6 to 11 years	1 to 2 tablespoonsful	ask a doctor
children 2 to 5 years	1 to 3 teaspoonsful	ask a doctor
children under 2 years	ask a doctor	ask a doctor

When using this product
- take only at bedtime. Do not use at any other time or administer to infants, except upon the advice of a physician.
- do not take with meals

Stop use and ask a doctor if
- you have rectal bleeding or no bowel movement after using this product. These could be signs of a serious condition.
- you need to use a laxative for more than 1 week

If breast-feeding, ask a health professional before use.

Keep out of reach of children. In case of overdose, get medical help or contact a Poison Control Center right away.

Directions
- shake well before use
- drink a full glass (8 oz) of liquid with each dose
- do not use dosage cup for children
- dose may be taken as a single dose, or in divided doses, or as directed by a doctor
- do not exceed the maximum recommended daily dose in a 24 hour period

adults and children 12 years and older	3 to 4 tablespoonsful
children 6 to 11 years	4 to 6 teaspoonsful
children under 6 years	ask a doctor

Other Information • store at room temperature and avoid freezing • keep tightly closed

Inactive Ingredients:
Phillips' MO Original
sodium citrate, sodium hypochlorite, water
Phillips' MO Mint Flavor
flavor, glycerin, microcrystalline cellulose, sodium carboxymethylcellulose, sodium citrate, sodium hypochlorite, sodium saccharin, water

How Supplied:
Original Flavor available in 12 fl. oz. bottle
Mint Flavor available in 12 and 26 fl. oz. bottles
Questions? **1-800-331-4536** or www.bayercare.com
Shown in Product Identification Guide, page 505

1-2-3 LICE ELIMINATION SYSTEM
LICE KILLING SHAMPOO
LICE TREATMENT
SHAMPOO & CONDITIONER IN ONE

- Kills lice and eggs
- Leaves no chemical residue
- Use on **DRY** hair
- Includes patented comb

Active Ingredients: **Purpose:**
Piperonyl butoxide
(4%) .... Lice Treatment
Pyrethrum extract (equivalent to 0.33% pyrethrins) .... Lice Treatment

Uses: Treats head, pubic (crab), and body lice

Warnings:
- **For external use only**
Do not use near the eyes or permit contact with the inside of the nose, mouth, or vagina. Irritation may occur.
Ask a doctor before use if you have an allergy to ragweed.
When using this product:
- keep out of eyes when rinsing hair
- close eyes tightly and do not open until product is rinsed out
- protect eyes with washcloth, towel, or other suitable method
- if product gets into the eyes, immediately flush with water
Stop use and ask a doctor if:
- skin irritation or infection is present or develops
- infestation of eyebrows or eyelashes occurs
Keep out of reach of children. If swallowed, get medical help or contact a Poison Control Center right away.

Directions:
- **Important: Read warnings and complete directions in the Consumer Information Insert before using.**
- Apply to **DRY HAIR** only. Massage until hair and scalp are thoroughly wet with product (see insert)
- After completing application, allow product to remain on hair for 10 minutes but no longer.
- Add sufficient warm water to form a lather and shampoo as usual. Rinse thoroughly.
- A fine-toothed comb or a special lice/nit removing comb (included) must be used to help remove dead lice, eggs, and nits from hair.
- **A second treatment must be done in 10 days to kill any newly hatched lice.**
Other Information:
- It is important to wash in hot water (130°F) all clothing, bedding, towels, and hair products (combs, brushes) used by infested persons.
- Dry clean non-washable fabrics.
- To eliminate infestation of furniture and bedding that cannot be washed or dry cleaned, a multi-use lice spray may be used.
- Store at room temperature: 59°–86°F (15°–30°C).
- Protect from excessive heat.

Inactive Ingredients Water, SD Alcohol, PEG-25 Hydrogenated Castor Oil, Ammonium Laureth Sulfate, Polyquaternium-10, Fragrance

RID® Lice Killing Shampoo will kill lice completely without leaving a chemical residue. To help prevent reinfestation, use it twice (Day 1 and Day 10). Amount of shampoo needed will vary by hair length. See below for guidelines:

Hair Length	Approximate Dosage for 1 Adult/Child:
Short (ear length or shorter)	Day 1: 1 oz - 2 oz Day 10: 1 oz - 2 oz Total: 2 oz - 4 oz
Medium (shoulder length)	Day 1: 2 oz - 3 oz Day 10: 2 oz - 3 oz Total: 4 oz - 6 oz
Long (past shoulder length)	Day 1: 3 oz - 4 oz Day 10: 3 oz - 4 oz Total: 6 oz - 8 oz

The patented RID® comb is proven 100% effective as demonstrated in laboratory studies performed by trained testers. Individual results may vary.

RID® 1-2-3 LICE Elimination System
Completely eliminate lice from your family and home.
Step 1—Kill Lice
- Apply RID® **Lice Killing Shampoo** according to label directions.
- Repeat this step 10 days later to help prevent reinfestation.
Step 2—Comb-Out Eggs & Nits
- After Step 1, apply RID® **Egg & Nit Comb-Out Gel** on damp hair to make removal faster and easier. *(Purchase separately)*
- Comb out the eggs and nits in the hair with a fine-toothed comb or with the RID® patented comb (included).
Step 3—Clean Home
- Use RID® **Home Lice Control Spray** to kill lice and their eggs on mattresses, furniture, car interiors, and other non-washable items. *(Purchase separately)*
- Wash bed linens, clothing, and other items in hot water and dry in high heat.

How Supplied: 6 FL OZ (177 ml), 1 Comb.

Questions or comments?
1-800-RID-LICE (1-800-743-5423)
www.ridlice.com

Distributed by: Bayer Corporation
Consumer Care Division
P.O. Box 1910
Morristown, NJ 07962-1910 USA
Shown in Product Identification Guide, page 505

1-2-3 LICE ELIMINATION SYSTEM
LICE KILLING NO-DRIP MOUSSE
pyrethrum extract*/piperonyl butoxide
aerosolized foam   Lice Treatment

- Kills lice completely
- Leaves no chemical residue
- Use on **DRY** hair
- Includes patented comb

Active Ingredients: **Purpose:**
(calculated without propellant)
Piperonyl butoxide
(4%) .... Lice Treatment
Pyrethrum extract* (equivalent to 0.33% pyrethrins) .... Lice Treatment

Uses: Treats head, pubic (crab), and body lice

Warnings:
- **For external use only**
- **Flammable:** Keep away from fire or flame
Do not use near the eyes or permit contact with the inside of the nose, mouth, or vagina. Irritation may occur.
Ask a doctor before use if you have an allergy to ragweed

Continued on next page

Rid Mousse—Cont.

When using this product:
- keep out of eyes when rinsing hair
- close eyes tightly and do not open eyes until product is rinsed out of hair
- protect eyes with washcloth, towel, or other suitable method
- if product gets into the eyes, immediately flush with water
- do not inhale; use in a well ventilated area
- do not puncture or incinerate. Contents under pressure.

Stop use and ask a doctor if:
- skin irritation or infection is present or develops
- infestation of eyebrows or eyelashes occurs

Keep out of reach of children. If swallowed, get medical help or contact a Poison Control Center right away.

Directions:
- **Important: Read warnings and complete directions in the Consumer Information Insert before using.**
- Shake well before using.
- Holding the can upside down, apply RID® No-Drip Mousse or other affected area. Massage until hair and scalp are thoroughly wet with product.
- After completing application, allow product to remain on the hair for 10 minutes but no longer.
- Rinse thoroughly with warm water and wash hair with soap or regular shampoo.
- A fine-toothed comb or a special lice/nit removing comb (included) must be used to help remove dead lice or their eggs (nits) from hair.
- A second treatment must be done in 7 to 10 days to kill any newly hatched lice.

Other Information:
- It is important to wash in hot water (130°F) all clothing, bedding, towels, and hair products (combs, brushes) used by infested persons.
- Dry clean non-washable fabrics.
- To eliminate infestation of furniture and bedding that cannot be washed or dry cleaned, a multi use lice spray may be used.
- Store at 20°–25°C (68°–77°F).
- Do not store at temperature above 43°C (110°F).
- Keep in a cool place out of the sun.

Inactive Ingredients: cetearyl alcohol, isobutane, PEG-20 stearate, propane, propylene glycol, purified water, quaternium-52, SD Alcohol 3-C (26.5% w/w)

Questions? call 1-800-RID-LICE (1-800-743-5423)

www.ridlice.com

RID Lice Killing No-Drip Mousse will kill lice completely without leaving a chemical residue. To help prevent reinfestation, use it **twice** (Day 1 and Day 10)†. Amount of Mousse needed will vary by hair length. See below for guidelines:

Hair Length	Approximate Dosage for 1 Adult/Child
Short (ear length or shorter)	Day 1: 1 oz – 2 oz / Day 10: 1 oz – 2 oz / **Total: 2 oz – 4 oz**
Medium (shoulder length)	Day 1: 2 oz – 3 oz / Day 10: 2 oz – 3 oz / **Total: 4 oz – 6 oz**
Long (past shoulder length)	Day 1: 3 oz – 4 oz / Day 10: 3 oz – 4 oz / **Total: 6 oz – 8 oz**

†While you must apply the 2nd application within 7–10 days of the 1st treatment, it is strongly recommended to wait until Day 10 for maximum effectiveness. Use RID Egg & Nit Comb-Out Gel after each treatment application to remove eggs & nits and help prevent reinfestation.

The patented RID® comb is proven 100% effective as demonstrated in laboratory studies performed by trained testers. Individual results may vary.

RID 1-2-3 LICE ELIMINATION SYSTEM
Completely eliminate lice from your family and home.
Step 1– Kill Lice
- Apply RID **Lice Killing Mousse** according to label directions.
- Repeat this step 7 to 10 days later to help prevent reinfestation.
Step 2– Comb-Out Eggs & Nits
- After Step 1, apply RID® Egg & Nit Comb-Out Gel on damp hair to make removal faster and easier. *(Purchase separately)*
- Comb out the eggs and nits in the hair with a fine-toothed comb or with the RID® patented comb (included).
Step 3– Clean Home
- Use RID® **Home Lice Control Spray** to kill lice and their eggs on mattresses, furniture, car interiors, and other non-washable items. *(Purchase separately)*
- Wash bed linens, clothing, and other items in hot water and dry in high heat.

How Supplied: 5.5 oz (156 g), 1 Comb.

---

*50% extract (not USP)
Distributed by:
Bayer Corporation
P.O. Box 1910
Morristown, NJ 07962-1910 USA

VANQUISH®
Extra Strength Pain Reliever Analgesic Caplets

Active Ingredients: **Purpose**
(in each caplet)
Acetaminophen 194 mg .... Pain reliever
Aspirin 227 mg .... Pain reliever
Caffeine 33 mg .... Pain reliever aid

Uses: Temporarily relieves minor pain due to
- headache
- backache
- menstrual cramps
- arthritis
- colds and flu
- muscle aches

Warnings: Reye's syndrome: Children and teenagers should not use this medicine for chicken pox or flu symptoms before a doctor is consulted about Reye's syndrome, a rare but serious illness reported to be associated with aspirin.
Alcohol warning: If you consume 3 or more alcoholic drinks every day, ask your doctor whether you should take acetaminophen and aspirin or other pain relievers/fever reducers. Acetaminophen and aspirin may cause liver damage and stomach bleeding.
Do not use
- if you have had an allergic reaction to any other pain reliever/fever reducer
- with any other product containing acetaminophen.
Ask a doctor before use if you have
- stomach problems (such as heartburn, upset stomach or stomach pain) that last or come back
- bleeding problems
- ulcers
- asthma
Ask a doctor or pharmacist before use if you are taking a prescription drug for
- anticoagulation (blood thinning)
- gout
- diabetes
- arthritis
Stop use and ask doctor if
- an allergic reaction occurs. Seek medical help right away.
- pain gets worse or lasts more than 10 days
- redness or swelling is present
- new symptoms occur
- ringing in the ears or loss of hearing occurs
If pregnant or breast-feeding, ask a health professional before use. **It is especially important not to use aspirin during the last 3 months of pregnancy unless definitely directed to do so by a doctor because it may cause problems in the unborn child or complications during delivery.**
Keep out of reach of children.

Overdose warning: Taking more than the recommended dose can cause serious health problems. In case of overdose, get medical help or contact a Poison Control Center right away. Prompt medical attention is critical for adults as well as children even if you do not notice any signs or symptoms.

Directions
- adults and children 12 years and over: take 2 caplets with water every 6 hours, not to exceed 8 caplets in 24 hours unless directed by a doctor
- children under 12 years: consult a doctor

Other Information
- save carton for full directions and warnings
- store at room temperature
- buffered with aluminum hydroxide and magnesium hydroxide

Inactive Ingredients: Aluminum hydroxide, colloidal silicon dioxide, hypromellose, magnesium hydroxide, microcrystalline cellulose, propylene glycol, starch, titanium dioxide, zinc stearate

How Supplied: Bottle of 100 analgesic caplets.
USE ONLY IF SEAL UNDER BOTTLE CAP WITH GREEN "Bayer Corporation" PRINT IS INTACT.
Questions or comments?
1-800-331-4536 or www.bayercare.com
Distributed by:
Bayer Corporation
PO Box 1910
Morristown, NJ 07962-1910

Beutlich LP Pharmaceuticals
**1541 SHIELDS DRIVE
WAUKEGAN, IL 60085-8304**

Direct Inquiries to:
847-473-1100
800-238-8542 in US & Canada
FAX 847–473-1122
www.beutlich.com
e-mail beutlich@beutlich.com

CEO–TWO® Evacuant
Laxative Adult Rectal Suppository

NDC #0283-0763-09

Composition: Each suppository contains sodium bicarbonate and potassium bitartrate in a special blend of water-soluble polyethylene glycols.

Indications: For relief of occasional constipation, irregularity or for bowel training programs. CEO-TWO generally produces a bowel movement in 5–30 minutes. The lubrication provided by the emollient base combined with the gentle pressure of the released carbon dioxide slowly distends the rectal ampulla stimulating peristalsis. CEO-TWO does not interfere with normal digestion, is not habit forming, won't cause cramping or irritation or alter the normal peristaltic reflex, and it leaves no residue.

Administration and Dosage: Adults and children over 12 years of age. Rectal dosage is one suppository containing 0.6 gram of sodium bicarbonate and 0.9 gram potassium bitartrate in a single daily dose. For children under 12 years of age: consult a doctor. For most effective results and ease of insertion, moisten a CEO-TWO suppository by placing it under a warm water tap for 30 seconds or in a cup of water for 10 seconds before insertion. Insert rectally past the largest diameter of the suppository. Patient should retain in the rectum as long as possible (usually about 5–30 minutes).

Warnings: For rectal use only. Do not use this product if you are on a low salt diet unless directed by a doctor. (172 milligrams of sodium per suppository) Do not lubricate with mineral oil or petrolatum prior to use. Do not use when abdominal pain, nausea or vomiting are present unless directed by a doctor. Laxative products should not be used for longer than one week unless directed by a doctor. If you have noticed a sudden change of bowel habits that persists over a period of 2 weeks, consult a doctor before using a laxative. Rectal bleeding or failure to have a bowel movement after use of a laxative may indicate a serious problem. Discontinue use and consult your doctor.

How Supplied: In box of 10 individually foil wrapped white opaque suppositories. Keep in cool dry place. **DO NOT REFRIGERATE**

HURRICAINE® TOPICAL ANESTHETIC

Composition: HURRICAINE contains 20% benzocaine in a flavored, water soluble polyethylene glycol base.

Action and Indications: HURRICAINE is a topical anesthetic that provides rapid anesthesia on all accessible mucous membrane in 15 to 30 seconds, short duration of 15 minutes, has virtually no systemic absorption, and tastes good. Hurricaine is used as a lubricant and topical anesthetic to facilitate passage of fiberoptic gastroscopes, laryngoscopes, proctoscopes and sigmoidoscopes. In addition, Hurricaine is effective in suppressing the pharyngeal and tracheal gag reflex during the placement of nasogastric tubes. Hurricaine is used to control pain and discomfort during certain gynecological procedures such as IUD insertion, vaginal speculum placement, and as a preinjection anesthesia prior to LEEP procedures and paracervical blocks. Hurricaine is also effective for the temporary relief of pain due to sore throat, stomatitis and mucositis. It is also effective in controlling various types of pain associated with dental procedures and the temporary relief of minor mouth irritations, canker sores and irritation to the mouth and gums caused by dentures or orthodontic appliances.

Contraindications: Patients with a known hypersensitivity to benzocaine should not use HURRICAINE. True allergic reactions are rare.

Adverse Reactions: Methemoglobinemia has been reported following the use of benzocaine on extremely rare occasions. Intravenous methylene blue is the specific therapy for this condition.

**Cautions: DO NOT USE IN THE EYES.
NOT FOR INJECTION.
KEEP THIS AND ALL DRUGS OUT OF THE REACH OF CHILDREN.**

Packaging Available
GEL
1 oz. Jar Fresh Mint NDC #0283-0998-31
1 oz. Jar Wild Cherry NDC #0283-0871-31
1 oz. Jar Pina Colada NDC #0283-0886-31
1 oz. Jar Watermelon NDC #0283-0293-31
1/6 oz. Tube Wild Cherry NDC #0283-0871-75
LIQUID
1 fl. oz. Jar Wild Cherry NDC #0283-0569-31
1 fl. oz. Jar Pina Colada NDC #0283-1886-31
.25 ml Dry Handle Swab Wild Cherry 100 Each Per Box NDC #0283-0693-01
.25 ml Dry Handle Swab Wild Cherry 6 Each Per Travel Pack NDC #0283-0693-36
SPRAY
2 oz. Aerosol Wild Cherry NDC #0283-0679-02
SPRAY KIT
2 oz. Aerosol Wild Cherry NDC #0283-0183-02 with 200 Disposable Extension Tubes

---

PERIDIN-C®

Composition: Each orange colored tablet contains 2 popular antioxidants; Vitamin C and Natural Bioflavonoids. Ascorbic Acid 200 mg. Hesperidin Complex 150 mg. Hesperidin Methyl Chalcone 50 mg. F.D. & C. #6. Sugar Free.

Dosage: 1 tablet daily or as directed.

How Supplied: In bottles of:
100 tablets NDC #0283-0597-01
500 tablets NDC #0283-0597-05

Boehringer Ingelheim Consumer Healthcare Products
Division of Boehringer Ingelheim Pharmceuticals Inc.
**900 RIDGEBURY ROAD
P.O. BOX 368
RIDGEFIELD, CT 06877**

For direct inquiries contact:
1-888-285-9159

DULCOLAX® Bowel Prep Kit
brand of bisacodyl USP

Drug Facts
Active Ingredient: **Purpose:**
Bisacodyl USP 5 mg
(in each tablet) .... Laxative
Bisacodyl USP 10 mg
(in each suppository) .... Laxative

Continued on next page

Dulcolax Bowel Prep—Cont.

Use: For use as part of a bowel cleansing regimen in preparing patients for surgery or for preparing the colon for x-ray or endoscopic examination.

Warnings:
Do not use:
• unless directed by a doctor.
• if you cannot swallow without chewing.
• in children under 6 years of age.
• within one hour after taking an antacid or milk.
When using this product:
• Do not chew or crush tablets.
• You may have stomach discomfort, faintness, rectal burning or cramps.
If pregnant or breast-feeding, ask a doctor before use. **Keep out of reach of children.** In case of overdose, get medical help or contact a Poison Control Center right away.

Directions:
• Read the entire label and directions at least 24 hours in advance of examination.
• Follow each step and complete all instructions or the entire x-ray or the endoscopic examination may have to be repeated.

Other Information:
• Store at controlled room temperature 20–25°C (68–77°F). Avoid excessive humidity.

Inactive Ingredients:
Tablets
Acacia, acetylated monoglyceride, carnauba wax, cellulose acetate phthalate, corn starch, dibutyl phthalate, docusate sodium, gelatin, glycerin, iron oxides, kaolin, lactose, magnesium stearate, methylparaben, pharmaceutical glaze, polyethylene glycol, povidone, propylparaben, Red No. 30 lake, sodium benzoate, sorbitan monooleate, sucrose, talc, titanium dioxide, white wax, Yellow No. 10 lake.
Suppository
Hydrogenated vegetable oil.

How Supplied: 4 tablets, 5 mg each and 1 suppository, 10 mg
Questions about Dulcolax
Call toll-free 1-888-285-9159
Distributed by:
Boehringer Ingelheim Consumer Healthcare Products
Division of Boehringer Ingelheim Pharmaceuticals, Inc. Ridgefield, CT 06877
©Boehringer Ingelheim Pharmaceuticals, Inc.
Shown in Product Identification Guide, page 505

DULCOLAX®
[dul 'cō-Lax]
brand of bisacodyl USP
Tablets of 5 mg
Laxative

Drug Facts
Active Ingredient:
(in each tablet)   **Purpose**
Bisacodyl USP, 5 mg .... Laxative

Uses:
• Relieves occasional constipation and irregularity.
• This product usually causes bowel movement in 6 to 12 hours.

Warnings:
Do not use • If you cannot swallow without chewing.
As a doctor before use if you have:
• Stomach pain, nausea or vomiting.
• A sudden change in bowel habits that lasts more than 2 weeks.
When using this product:
• Do not chew or crush tablet.
• Do not use within 1 hour after taking an antacid or milk.
• You may have stomach discomfort, faintness or cramps.
Stop use and ask a doctor if:
• You do not have a bowel movement within 12 hours or if rectal bleeding occurs. These could be signs of a serious condition.
• You need to use a laxative for more than 1 week.
If pregnant or breast-feeding, ask a doctor before use. **Keep out of reach of children.** In case of overdose, get medical help or contact a Poison Control Center right away.

Directions:

Adults and children 12 years and over	Take 1 to 3 tablets (usually 2) daily.
Children 6 to under 12 years	Take 1 tablet daily.
Children under 6 years	Ask a doctor.

Other Information • Store at 20–25°C (68–77°F). Avoid excessive humidity.

Inactive Ingredients: Acacia, acetylated monoglyceride, carnauba wax, cellulose acetate phthalate, corn starch, dibutyl phthalate, docusate sodium, gelatin, glycerin, iron oxides, kaolin, lactose, magnesium stearate, methylparaben, pharmaceutical glaze, polyethylene glycol, povidone, propylparaben, Red No. 30 lake, sodium benzoate, sorbitan monooleate, sucrose, talc, titanium dioxide, white wax, Yellow No. 10 lake.

How Supplied: Boxes of 25 Tablets.
Boehringer Ingelheim Consumer Healthcare Products.
Division of Boehringer Ingelheim
Pharmaceuticals, Inc., Ridgefield, CT 06877
Made in Mexico ©Boehringer Ingelheim Pharmaceuticals, Inc. 2002
Questions about DULCOLAX?
Call toll-free 1-888-285-9159
Shown in Product Identification Guide, page 505

DULCOLAX®
[dul' co-lax]
brand of bisacodyl USP
Suppositories of 10 mg
Laxative

Drug Facts:
Active Ingredient:
(in each suppository)   **Purpose:**
Bisacodyl USP, 10 mg .... Laxative

Uses:
• Relieves occasional constipation and irregularity.
• This product usually causes bowel movement in 15 minutes to 1 hour.

Warnings:
For rectal use only.
Do not use • When abdominal pain, nausea, or vomiting are present.
Ask a doctor before use if you have:
• Stomach pain, nausea or vomiting.
• A sudden change in bowel habits that lasts more than 2 weeks.
When using this product:
You may have abdominal discomfort, faintness, rectal burning and mild cramps.
Stop use and ask a doctor if:
• Rectal bleeding occurs or you fail to have a bowel movement after using a laxative. This may indicate a serious condition.
• You need to use a laxative for more than 1 week.
If pregnant or breast-feeding, ask a doctor before use. **Keep out of reach of children.** If swallowed, get medical help or contact a Poison Control Center right away.

Directions:

Adults and children 12 years and over	1 suppository once daily. Remove foil. Insert suppository well into rectum, pointed end first. Retain about 15 to 20 minutes.
Children 6 to under 12 years	1/2 suppository once daily.
Children under 6 years	Ask a doctor.

Other Information • Store at controlled room temperature 20–25°C (68–77°F)

Inactive Ingredients: Hydrogenated vegetable oil.

How Supplied: Boxes of 4 Comfort Shaped Suppositories
Boehringer Ingelheim Consumer Healthcare Products.
Division of Boehringer Ingelheim
Pharmaceuticals, Inc., Ridgefield, CT 06877   Made in Italy.

©Boehringer Ingelheim Pharmaceuticals, Inc. 2002
Questions? 1-888-285-9159
Shown in Product Identification Guide, page 505

DULCOLAX®
Stool Softener

Drug Facts:

Active Ingredient:
(in each softgel)   **Purpose:**
Docusate sodium USP,
100 mg .... Stool Softener

Uses:
• Temporary relief of occasional constipation.
• This product generally produces bowel movement within 12 to 72 hours.

Warnings:
Do not use:
• If abdominal pain, nausea or vomiting are present.
Ask a doctor before use if:
• You have noticed a sudden change in bowel habits that persists over a period of 2 weeks.
• You are presently taking mineral oil.
Stop use and ask a doctor if:
• Rectal bleeding or failure to have a bowel movement occur after use, which may indicate a serious condition.
• You need to use a laxative for more than 1 week.
If pregnant or breast-feeding, ask a health professional before use.
Keep out of reach of children. In case of overdose, get medical help or contact a Poison Control Center immediately.

Directions:

Adults and children 12 years and over.	Take 1 to 3 softgels daily.
Children 2 to under 12 years.	Take 1 softgel daily.
Children under 2 years.	Ask a doctor.

Other Information
• Each softgel contains: sodium, 5 mg
• Store at 15–30°C (59–86°F).
• Protect from excessive moisture.
Inactive Ingredients FD&C Red #40, FD&C Yellow #6, gelatin, glycerin, polyethylene glycol, propylene glycol, purified water and sorbitol special.
How Supplied: Blister Pack of 10, and bottles of 25, 50, or 100 liquid gels. Boehringer Ingelheim Consumer Healthcare Products. Division of Boehringer Ingelheim Pharmaceuticals, Inc., Ridgefield, CT 06877 ©Boehringer Ingelheim Pharmaceuticals, Inc. 2002
Questions about DULCOLAX?
Call toll-free 1-888-285-9159
*Among Stool Softener ingredients
Shown in Product Identification Guide, page 505

BOIRON
6 CAMPUS BLVD.
NEWTOWN SQUARE, PA 19073

Direct Inquiries and Medical Emergencies:
Boiron Information Center
info@boiron.com
(800)264-7661

OSCILLOCOCCINUM®
[oh-sill'o-cox-see'num']

Active Ingredients: Anas barbariae hepatis et cordis extractum 200CK. *Made according to the Homeopathic Pharmacopeia of the United States.*

Inactive Ingredients: sucrose, lactose.

Use: For temporary relief of symptoms of flu such as fever, chills, body aches and pains.

Directions: (Adults and children 2 years of age and older):
Take 1 dose at the onset of symptoms (dissolve entire contents of one tube in the mouth).
Repeat for 2 more doses at 6 hour intervals.

Warnings: Do not use if the label sealing the cap is broken.
Ask a doctor before use in children under 2 years of age.
Stop using this product and consult a doctor if symptoms persist for more than 3 days or worsen.
As with any drug, if pregnant or nursing a baby, ask a health professional before use.
Keep this and all medication out of reach of children.
Diabetics: this product contains sugar.

How Supplied: White pellets in unit dose containers of 0.04 oz. (1 gram) each. Supplied in boxes of 3 unit doses or 6 unit doses.
NDC #0220-9280-32 (3 doses) and NDC #0220-9280-33 (6 doses)
Made in France

FACED WITH AN Rx SIDE EFFECT?
Turn to the Companion Drug Index for products that provide symptomatic relief.

Bristol-Myers Squibb Company
345 PARK AVENUE
NEW YORK, NY 10154

Direct Inquiries to:
Bristol-Myers Squibb Company
Consumer Affairs Department
1350 Liberty Avenue
Hillside, NJ

Questions or Comments?
1-(800) 468-7746

OVERDOSE PROFESSIONAL INFORMATION FOR EXCEDRIN® PRODUCTS

All of the following listed Excedrin drug products contain acetaminophen. In case of overdose, please read the following Acetylcysteine information:

Overdose Information:
Acetylcysteine As An Antidote For Acetaminophen Overdose
Acetaminophen is rapidly absorbed from the upper gastrointestinal tract with peak plasma levels occurring between 30 and 60 minutes after therapeutic doses and usually within 4 hours following an overdose. The parent compound, which is nontoxic, is extensively metabolized in the liver to form principally the sulfate and glucuronide conjugates which are also nontoxic and are rapidly excreted in the urine. A small fraction of an ingested dose is metabolized in the liver by the cytochrome P-450 mixed function oxidase enzyme system to form a reactive, potentially toxic, intermediate metabolite which preferentially conjugates with hepatic glutathione to form the nontoxic cysteine and mercapturic acid derivatives which are then excreted by the kidney. Therapeutic doses of acetaminophen do not saturate the glucuronide and sulfate conjugation pathways and do not result in the formation of sufficient reactive metabolite to deplete glutathione stores. However, following ingestion of a large overdose (150 mg/kg or greater) the glucuronide and sulfate conjugation pathways are saturated resulting in a larger fraction of the drug being metabolized via the P-450 pathway. The increased formation of reactive metabolite may deplete the hepatic stores of glutathione with subsequent binding of the metabolite to protein molecules within the hepatocyte resulting in cellular necrosis. Acetylcysteine has been shown to reduce the extent of liver injury following acetaminophen overdose.
Early symptoms following a potentially hepatotoxic overdose may include: nausea, vomiting, diaphoresis and general malaise. Clinical and laboratory evidence of hepatic toxicity may not be ap-

Continued on next page

Excedrin-Prof. Info.—Cont.

parent until 48 to 72 hours postingestion. In most adults and adolescents, regardless of the quantity of acetaminophen reported to have been ingested, administer acetylcysteine immediately. Acetylcysteine therapy should be initiated and continued for a full course of therapy. Its effectiveness depends on early administration, with benefit seen principally in patients treated within 16 hours of the overdose.

If acetaminophen plasma assay capability is not available, and the estimated acetaminophen ingestion exceeds 150 mg/kg, acetylcysteine therapy should be initiated and continued for a full course of therapy.

For full prescribing information, refer to the acetylcysteine package insert. Do not await the results of assays for acetaminophen level before initiating treatment with acetylcysteine. The following additional procedures are recommended: the stomach should be emptied promptly by lavage or by induction of emesis with syrup of ipecac.

A serum acetaminophen assay should be obtained as early as possible, but no sooner than four hours following ingestion. Liver function studies should be obtained initially and repeated at 24-hour intervals.

For additional emergency information call your regional poison center or toll-free (1-800-525-6115) to the Rocky Mountain Poison Center for assistance in diagnosis and for directions in the use of acetylcysteine as an antidote.

Aspirin Free
EXCEDRIN® TENSION HEADACHE
Pain Reliever/Pain Reliever Aid

Active Ingredients: Each caplet and geltab contains Acetaminophen 500 mg and Caffeine 65 mg.

Inactive Ingredients: (caplet) benzoic acid, carnauba wax, corn starch, croscarmellose sodium, D&C red #27 lake, D&C yellow #10 lake, FD&C blue #1 lake, FD&C red #40, hypromellose, magnesium stearate, methylparaben*, microcrystalline cellulose, mineral oil, polysorbate 20, povidone, propylene glycol, propylparaben*, simethicone emulsion, sorbitan monolaurate, stearic acid, titanium dioxide

*may contain these ingredients

Inactive Ingredients: (geltab) benzoic acid, corn starch, croscarmellose sodium, FD&C blue #1, FD&C red #40, FD&C yellow #6, gelatin, glycerin, hypromellose, magnesium stearate, methylparaben*, microcrystalline cellulose, mineral oil, polysorbate 20, povidone, propylene glycol, propylparaben*, simethicone

emulsion, sorbitan monolaurate, stearic acid, titanium dioxide

*may contain these ingredients

Indications: • temporarily relieves minor aches and pains due to:
  • headache • muscular aches

Warnings

Alcohol warning: If you consume 3 or more alcoholic drinks every day, ask your doctor whether you should take acetaminophen or other pain relievers/fever reducers. Acetaminophen may cause liver damage.

Caffeine warning: The recommended dose of this product contains about as much caffeine as a cup of coffee. Limit the use of caffeine-containing medications, foods, or beverages while taking this product because too much caffeine may cause nervousness, irritability, sleeplessness, and, occasionally, rapid heart beat.

Do not use • with any other products containing acetaminophen. Taking more than directed may cause liver damage.

Stop use and ask a doctor if
• new symptoms occur
• symptoms do not get better or worsen
• painful area is red or swollen
• pain gets worse or lasts for more than 10 days
• fever gets worse or lasts more than 3 days

If pregnant or breast-feeding, ask a health professional before use.

Keep out of reach of children.

Overdose warning: Taking more than the recommended dose can cause serious health problems. In case of overdose, get medical help or contact a Poison Control Center right away. Quick medical attention is critical for adults as well as for children even if you do not notice any signs or symptoms.

Directions:
• do not use more than directed (see overdose warning)
• adults and children 12 years of age and over: take 2 caplets every 6 hours; not more than 8 caplets or geltabs in 24 hours
• children under 12 years of age: ask a doctor

Overdose: Acetylcysteine as an antidote for acetaminophen overdose.

See OVERDOSE PROFESSIONAL INFORMATION FOR EXCEDRIN PRODUCTS section at the beginning of the Bristol-Myers Squibb Co. listing.

How Supplied: EXCEDRIN® Tension Headache is supplied as: Coated red caplets with "ETH" debossed on one side in bottles of 24's, 50's, and 100's. Easy to swallow red geltabs with "Excedrin TH" printed in white on one side supplied in bottles of 24's, 50's, and 100's.

Store at room temperature.

Shown in Product Identification Guide, page 506

EXCEDRIN® Extra-Strength
Pain Reliever
[ĕx″cĕd′rin]

Active Ingredients: Each tablet, caplet, or geltab contains Acetaminophen 250 mg, Aspirin 250 mg, and Caffeine 65 mg.

Inactive Ingredients: (tablet, caplet) benzoic acid, carnauba wax, hydroxypropylcellulose, hydroxypropyl methylcellulose, microcrystalline cellulose, mineral oil, polysorbate 20, povidone, propylene glycol, simethicone emulsion, sorbitan monolaurate, stearic acid.
May also contain: FD&C blue # 1, titanium dioxide.

Inactive Ingredients: (geltab) benzoic acid, D&C yellow #10 lake, disodium EDTA, FD&C blue #1 lake, FD&C red #40 lake, ferric oxide, gelatin, glycerin, hydroxypropylcellulose, hydroxypropyl methylcellulose, maltitol solution, microcrystalline cellulose, mineral oil, pepsin, polysorbate 20, povidone, propylene glycol, propyl gallate, simethicone emulsion, sorbitan monolaurate, stearic acid, titanium dioxide.

Uses: For the temporary relief of minor aches and pains associated with headache, sinusitis, a cold, muscular aches, premenstrual and menstrual cramps, toothache, and for the minor pain from arthritis.

Warnings:
Warning: Children and teenagers should not use this medicine for chicken pox or flu symptoms before a doctor is consulted about Reye's syndrome, a rare but serious illness reported to be associated with aspirin.

Alcohol Warning: If you consume 3 or more alcoholic drinks every day, ask your doctor whether you should take acetaminophen and aspirin or other pain relievers/fever reducers. Acetaminophen and aspirin may cause liver damage and stomach bleeding.

Keep out of reach of children. In case of overdose, get medical help or contact a Poison Control Center right away. Do not take with any other products containing acetaminophen. Taking more than directed may cause liver damage. Prompt medical attention is critical for adults as well as for children even if you do not notice any signs or symptoms. As with any drug, if you are pregnant or nursing a baby, seek the advice of a health professional before using this product. IT IS ESPECIALLY IMPORTANT NOT TO USE ASPIRIN DURING THE LAST 3 MONTHS OF PREGNANCY UNLESS SPECIFICALLY DIRECTED TO DO SO BY A DOCTOR BECAUSE IT MAY CAUSE PROBLEMS IN THE UNBORN CHILD OR COMPLICATIONS DURING DELIVERY. Do not take this product for pain for more than 10 days or for fever for more than 3 days unless directed by a doctor. If pain or fever persists or gets worse, if new symptoms occur, or if redness or swelling is present, consult a doc-

tor because these could be signs of a serious condition. Consult a dentist promptly for toothache. Do not take this product if you are allergic to aspirin, have asthma, have stomach problems (such as heartburn, upset stomach or stomach pain) that persist or recur, or if you have ulcers or bleeding problems, unless directed by a doctor. If ringing in the ears or loss of hearing occurs, consult a doctor before taking any more of this product.

Drug Interaction Precaution: Do not take this product if you are taking a prescription drug for anticoagulation (thinning the blood), diabetes, gout or arthritis unless directed by a doctor.

Directions: Adults: 2 tablets, caplets or geltabs with water every 6 hours while symptoms persist, not to exceed 8 tablets, caplets or geltabs in 24 hours, or as directed by a doctor. Children under 12 years of age: consult a doctor.

Overdose: Acetylcysteine as an antidote for acetaminophen overdose. See OVERDOSE PROFESSIONAL INFORMATION FOR COMTREX AND EXCEDRIN PRODUCTS section at the beginning of the Bristol-Myers Products listing.

How Supplied: Extra Strength EXCEDRIN® is supplied as: Coated white circular tablet with letter "E" debossed on one side. Supplied in bottles of 12's, 24's, 50's, 100's, 175's, 275's. Coated white caplets with "E" debossed on one side. Supplied in bottles of 24's, 50's, 100's, 175's, 275's. Gel-coated round geltabs–green on one side, white on the other, printed with black "E" on one side. Supplied in bottles of 24's, 50's and 100's (2 bottles of 50 each). Store at room temperature.
Shown in Product Identification Guide, page 505

EXCEDRIN® MIGRAINE
[ĕx' cĕd' rin]
Pain Reliever/Pain Reliever Aid

Active Ingredients: Each tablet, caplet or geltab contains Acetaminophen 250 mg, Aspirin 250 mg and Caffeine 65 mg.

Inactive Ingredients: (tablet and caplet) benzoic acid, carnauba wax, hydroxypropylcellulose, hydroxypropyl methylcellulose, microcrystalline cellulose, mineral oil, polysorbate 20, povidone, propylene glycol, simethicone emulsion, sorbitan monolaurate, stearic acid, may also contain: FD&C blue no. 1, titanium dioxide.

Inactive Ingredients: (geltab) benzoic acid, D&C yellow #10 lake, disodium EDTA, FD&C blue #1 lake, FD&C red #40 lake, ferric oxide, gelatin, glycerin, hydroxypropylcellulose, hydroxypropyl

methylcellulose, maltitol solution, microcrystalline cellulose, mineral oil, pepsin, polysorbate 20, povidone, propylene glycol, propyl gallate, simethicone emulsion, sorbitan monolaurate, stearic acid, titanium dioxide.
Use: Treats migraine.

Warnings:
Reye's Syndrome: Children and teenagers should not use this drug for chicken pox, or flu symptoms before a doctor is consulted about Reye's syndrome, a rare but serious illness reported to be associated with aspirin.
Allergy alert: aspirin may cause a severe allergic reaction which may include: • hives • facial swelling • asthma (wheezing) • shock
Alcohol warning: If you consume 3 or more alcoholic drinks every day, ask your doctor whether you should take acetaminophen and aspirin or other pain relievers/fever reducers. Acetaminophen and aspirin may cause liver damage and stomach bleeding.
Caffeine warning: The recommended dose of this product contains about as much caffeine as a cup of coffee. Limit the use of caffeine-containing medications, foods, or beverages while taking this product because too much caffeine may cause nervousness, irritability, sleeplessness, and, occasionally, rapid heart beat.
Do not use • if you have ever had an allergic reaction to any other pain reliever/fever reducer
Ask a doctor before use if you have
• never had migraines diagnosed by a health professional
• a headache that is different from your usual migraines
• the worst headache of your life
• fever and stiff neck
• headaches beginning after or caused by head injury, exertion, coughing or bending
• experienced your first headache after the age of 50
• daily headaches
• asthma
• bleeding problems
• ulcers
• stomach problems such as heartburn, upset stomach, or stomach pain that do not go away or recur
• a migraine so severe as to require bed rest
• problems or serious side effects from taking pain relievers or fever reducers
Ask a doctor or pharmacist before use if you are taking a prescription drug for:
• anticoagulation (thinning of the blood)
• diabetes
• gout
• arthritis
Stop use and ask a doctor if
• an allergic reaction occurs. Seek medical help right away.
• your migraine is not relieved or worsens after first dose
• new or unexpected symptoms occur
• ringing in the ears or loss of hearing occurs
If pregnant or breast-feeding, ask a health professional before use. It is especially important not to use aspirin dur-

ing the last 3 months of pregnancy unless definitely directed to do so by a doctor because it may cause problems in the unborn child or complications during delivery.
Keep out of reach of children. In case of overdose, get medical help or contact a Poison Control Center right away. Quick medical attention is critical for adults as well as for children even if you do not notice any signs or symptoms.

Directions:
• adults: take 2 (tablets, caplets or geltabs) with a glass of water
• if symptoms persist or worsen, ask your doctor
• do not take more than 2 (tablets, caplets, or geltabs) in 24 hours, unless directed by a doctor
• under 18 years of age: ask a doctor
Overdose: Acetylcysteine as an antidote for acetaminophen overdose. See OVERDOSE PROFESSIONAL INFORMATION FOR COMTREX AND EXCEDRIN PRODUCTS section at the beginning of the Bristol-Myers Products listing.

How Supplied: EXCEDRIN® MIGRAINE is supplied as: Coated white circular tablets or coated white caplets with letter "E" debossed on one side. Supplied in bottles of 24's, 50's, 100's, and 175's. 275's (tablets) are available in club store packages. Coated round geltabs–green on one side, white on the other, printed with black "E" on one side. Supplied in bottles of 24's, 50's and 100's (2 bottles of 50 each).
Store at 20–25°C (68–77°F).
Shown in Product Identification Guide, page 505

EXCEDRIN® PM
[ĕx "cĕd 'rĭn]
Pain Reliever/Nighttime Sleep-Aid

Active Ingredients: Each tablet, caplet or geltab contains: Acetaminophen 500 mg and Diphenhydramine citrate 38 mg.

Inactive Ingredients: (Tablet and Caplet) benzoic acid, corn starch, D&C yellow #10 lake, FD&C blue #1 lake, hydroxypropyl methylcellulose, magnesium stearate, mineral oil, polysorbate 20, povidone, propylene glycol, simethicone emulsion, sodium citrate, sorbitan monolaurate, stearic acid, titanium dioxide, may also contain: carnauba wax, croscarmellose sodium, methylparaben, microcrystalline cellulose, propylparaben, sodium starch glycolate.
(Geltab) benzoic acid, corn starch, D&C red #33 lake, edetate disodium, FD&C blue #1, FD&C blue #1 lake, gelatin, glycerin, hydroxypropyl methylcellulose, magnesium stearate, mineral oil, polysorbate 20, povidone, propylene glycol, simethicone emulsion, sorbitan monolaurate, stearic acid, titanium dioxide,

Continued on next page

Excedrin PM—Cont.

may also contain: croscarmellose sodium, methylparaben, microcrystalline cellulose, propylparaben, sodium starch glycolate.

Uses: For temporary relief of occasional headaches and minor aches and pains with accompanying sleeplessness.

Warnings
Alcohol Warning: If you consume 3 or more alcoholic drinks every day, ask your doctor whether you should take acetaminophen or other pain relievers/fever reducers. Acetaminophen may cause liver damage.
Do not use
• in children under 12 years of age
• with other diphenhydramine products, including one applied topically
Ask a doctor before use if you have
• glaucoma
• a breathing problem such as emphysema or chronic bronchitis
• trouble urinating due to an enlarged prostate gland
Ask a doctor or pharmacist before use if you are taking sedatives or tranquilizers
When using this product
• avoid alcoholic drinks
Stop use and ask a doctor if
• new symptoms occur
• sleeplessness lasts continuously for more than 2 weeks. Insomnia may be a symptom of serious underlying medical illness.
• pain gets worse or lasts for more than 10 days
• redness or swelling is present
• fever gets worse or lasts for more than 3 days
If pregnant or breast-feeding, ask a health professional before use.
Keep out of reach of children. In case of overdose, get medical help or contact a Poison Control Center right away. Do not take with any other products containing acetaminophen. Taking more than directed may cause liver damage. Quick medical attention is critical for adults as well as for children even if you do not notice any signs or symptoms.

Directions
• children under 12 years of age: consult a doctor
• adults and children 12 years and over: take 2 tablets, caplets or geltabs at bedtime, if needed, or as directed by a doctor.

Overdose: Acetylcysteine as an antidote for acetaminophen overdose.
See OVERDOSE PROFESSIONAL INFORMATION FOR COMTREX AND EXCEDRIN PRODUCTS section at the beginning of the Bristol-Myers Products listing.

How Supplied: EXCEDRIN PM® is supplied as:
Light blue circular coated tablets with "PM" debossed on one side. Supplied in bottles of 10's, 24's, 50's, 100's.
Light blue coated caplet with "PM" debossed on one side. Supplied in bottles of 24's, 50's, 100's.

Gel coated-light blue and white geltabs with "PM" printed in black on one side. Supplied in bottles of 24's, 50's, 100's. Store at room temperature.
Shown in Product Identification Guide, page 505

EXCEDRIN® BRAND QUICKTABS™
Pain Reliever/Pain Reliever Aid

Active Ingredients: Each quicktab contains Acetaminophen 500 mg and Caffeine 65 mg.

Inactive Ingredients: aminoalkyl methacrylate copolymers, citric acid, colloidal silicon dioxide, crospovidone, distilled acetylated monoglycerides, ethylcellulose, flavors, magnesium stearate, mannitol, methacrylester copolymer, polyvinyl acetate, povidone, propylene glycol, propyl gallate, silica gel, sodium lauryl sulfate, sucralose, talc

Indications: • temporarily relieves minor aches and pains due to:
• headache • a cold • muscular aches
• arthritis • toothache • sinusitis
• premenstrual & menstrual cramps

Warnings:
Alcohol warning: If you consume 3 or more alcoholic drinks every day, ask your doctor whether you should take acetaminophen or other pain relievers/fever reducers. Acetaminophen may cause liver damage.
Do not use • with any other products containing acetaminophen. Taking more than directed may cause liver damage.
Stop use and ask a doctor if
• symptoms do not get better or worsen
• new symptoms occur
• pain gets worse or lasts for more than 10 days
• painful area is red or swollen
• fever gets worse or lasts more than 3 days
If pregnant or breast-feeding, ask a health professional before use.
Keep out of reach of children.
Overdose warning: Taking more than the recommended dose can cause serious health problems. In case of overdose, get medical help or contact a Poison Control Center right away. Quick medical attention is critical for adults as well as for children even if you do not notice any signs or symptoms.

Directions:
• do not use more than directed (see overdose warning)
• adults and children 12 years of age and over: allow 2 quicktabs to dissolve fully on the tongue every 6 hours; for best taste, do not chew
• do not take more than 8 quicktabs in 24 hours
• children under 12 years of age: ask a doctor

Other information:
• read all directions and warnings before use
• non-USP for dissolution
• Store at 20°–25° C (68°–77° F)
Overdose: Acetylcysteine as an antidote for acetaminophen overdose.

See OVERDOSE PROFESSIONAL INFORMATION FOR COMTREX AND EXCEDRIN PRODUCTS section at the beginning of the Bristol-Myers Squibb Co. listing.

How Supplied: EXCEDRIN® Brand QuickTabs™ are supplied as: Spearmint flavored, white, round, concave center, unscored tablets with "EQ" imprinted on one side supplied in blister packs of 4's, 16's and 32's. Peppermint flavored white, round, concave center, unscored tablets with "EQM" imprinted on one side, supplied in blister packs of 4's, 16's, and 32's.
Shown in Product Identification Guide, page 506

Celltech
Pharmaceuticals, Inc.
PO BOX 31710
ROCHESTER, NY 14603

Direct Inquiries to:
Customer Service Department
P.O. Box 31766
Rochester, NY 14603
(585) 274-5300
(888) 963-3382

DELSYM®
(dextromethorphan polistirex)
Extended-Release Suspension
12-Hour Cough Suppressant

Active Ingredient (in each 5 mL teaspoonful): dextromethorphan polistirex equivalent to 30 mg dextromethorphan hydrobromide.

Purpose: Cough suppressant

Use: Temporarily relieves cough due to minor throat and bronchial irritation as may occur with the common cold or inhaled irritants.

Warnings: Do not use if you are now taking a prescription monoamine oxidase inhibitor (MAOI) (certain drugs for depression, psychiatric or emotional conditions, or Parkinson's disease), or for 2 weeks after stopping the MAOI drug. If you do not know if your prescription drug contains an MAOI, ask a doctor or pharmacist before taking this product.
Ask a doctor before use if you have
• chronic cough that lasts as occurs with smoking, asthma or emphysema
• cough that occurs with too much phlegm (mucus)
Stop use and ask a doctor if cough lasts more than 7 days, cough comes back, or occurs with fever, rash or headache that lasts. These could be signs of a serious condition.
If pregnant or breast-feeding, ask a health professional before use.
Keep out of reach of children. In case of overdose, get medical help or contact a Poison Control Center right away.

Directions:
- shake bottle well before use
- dose as follows or as directed by a doctor

adults and children 12 years of age and over	2 teaspoonfuls every 12 hours, not to exceed 4 teaspoonfuls in 24 hours
children 6 to under 12 years of age	1 teaspoonful every 12 hours, not to exceed 2 teaspoonfuls in 24 hours
children 2 to under 6 years of age	½ teaspoonful every 12 hours, not to exceed 1 teaspoonful in 24 hours
children under 2 years of age	consult a doctor

Other Information:
- **each 5 mL teaspoonful contains:** sodium 5 mg
- store at 20°–25°C (68°–77°F)

Inactive Ingredients: alcohol 0.26%, citric acid, ethycellulose, FD&C Yellow No. 6, flavor, high fructose corn syrup, methylparaben, polyethylene glycol 3350, polysorbate 80, propylene glycol, propylparaben, purified water, sucrose, tragacanth, vegetable oil, xanthan gum.

How Supplied:

89 mL (3 fl oz.) bottles

NDC 53014-842-61

148 ml (5 fl oz.) bottles

NDC 53014-842-56

Celltech Pharmaceuticals, Inc.

Rochester, NY 14623 USA

®Celltech Manufacturing, Inc.

Chattem, Inc.
1715 WEST 38th STREET
CHATTANOOGA, TN 37409

Direct Inquiries to:

(423) 821-2037

DEXATRIM RESULTS
DEXATRIM RESULTS, Ephedrine Free Formula

DEXATRIM RESULTS:
Supplement Facts:
[See first table above]

Other Ingredients: Dicalcium phosphate, microcrystalline cellulose, croscarmellose sodium, stearic acid, magnesium stearate, silica, and coating ingredients (mono- and diglycerides, hypromellose, hydroxypropyl cellulose, and PEG 400)

	Amount Per Caplet	% Daily Value
Vitamin B6	2 mg	100
Calcium	15 mg	2
Proprietary herbal blend:	725 mg	Not established

Green tea leaf standardized extract (180 mg antioxidant polyphenols, 90 mg epigallocatechin gallate (EGCG), 50 mg naturally occurring caffeine), Asian ginseng root standardized and 5-hydroxytryptophan (5-HTP) from Griffonia simplicifolia seed.

	Amount Per Caplet	% Daily Value
Vitamin C	10 mg	17
Vitamin E	5 IU	17
Vitamin B6	2 mg	100
Pantothenic acid	5 mg	50
Calcium	90 mg	9
Phosphorous	70 mg	7
Magnesium	6.7 mg	2
Zinc	2.5 mg	17
Manganese	0.67 mg	34
Chromium	40 mcg	33
Proprietary herbal blend #1:	202 mg	Not established

Bitter orange peel extract, yohimbe bark, eleuthero root, licorice root, rutin, kelp, fenugreek seed, hesperidin complex

Proprietary herbal blend #2:	130 mg	Not established

Cocoa extract (CocoGen™), caffeine, green tea leaf extract.

DEXATRIM RESULTS, Ephedrine Free Formula:
Supplement Facts:
[See second table above]

Other Ingredients: Gelatin, microcrystalline cellulose, croscarmellose sodium, stearic acid, silicon dioxide, pharmaceutical glaze, carnauba wax.

Warnings: FOR ADULT USE ONLY. NOT FOR USE BY INDIVIDUALS UNDER 18 YEARS OF AGE. Do not take more than three caplets per day (24 HOURS). Do not exceed recommended serving size. Exceeding the recommended dose has not been shown to result in greater effectiveness. Do not use if pregnant or nursing. Consult a physician or licensed qualified health care professional before using this product if you have, or have a family history of heart disease, thyroid disease, diabetes, high blood pressure, recurrent headaches, depression or other psychiatric condition, glaucoma, difficulty in urination, prostate enlargement, or seizure disorder, if you are using a monoamine oxidase inhibitor (MAOI) or any other dietary supplement, prescription drug or over-the-counter drug containing ephedrine, pseudoephedrine, or phenylpropanolamine (ingredients found in certain allergy, asthma, cough/cold and weight control products). Discontinue use and call a physician or licensed qualified health care professional immediately if you experience rapid heartbeat, dizziness, severe headache, shortness of breath, or other similar symptoms. INDIVIDUALS WHO CONSUME CAFFEINE WITH THIS PRODUCT MAY EXPERIENCE SERIOUS ADVERSE HEALTH EFFECTS. EXCEEDING RECOMMENDED SERVING MAY CAUSE SERIOUS ADVERSE HEALTH EFFECTS INCLUDING HEART ATTACK AND STROKE.
KEEP OUT OF REACH OF CHILDREN.
DEXATRIM RESULTS: This product contains 50 mg of naturally-occurring caffeine per serving (little over one-half cup of coffee).
DEXATRIM RESULTS, Ephedrine Free Formula: This product contains 40 mg of naturally occurring caffeine per serving (equivalent to one-half cup of coffee). Improper use of these products may be hazardous to a person's health.

Suggested Use: Take one caplet 3 times per day.

How Supplied: Tamper-resistant bottles of 60 caplets.
Product Identification: DEXATRIM RESULTS: natural light brown oblong caplet with a clear film coating.
DEXATRIM RESULTS, Ephedrine Free Formula: natural brown caplet-shaped tablet with pharmaceutical glaze.

Effcon™ Laboratories, Inc.
P.O. BOX 7499
MARIETTA, GA 30065-1499

Address inquiries to:
Brad Rivet
(800-722-2428)
Fax: (770-428-6811)

For Medical Emergency Contact:
Brad Rivet
(800-722-2428)
Fax: (770-428-6811)

PIN-X®
Pinworm Treatment

Description: Each 1 mL of liquid for oral administration contains:
Pyrantel base .... 50 mg
   (as Pyrantel Pamoate)

Continued on next page

Pin-X—Cont.

Indication: For the treatment of pinworms.

Warnings: Keep this and all drugs out of the reach of children. In case of accidental overdose, seek professional assistance or contact a poison control center immediately.
If you are pregnant or have liver disease, do not take this product unless directed by a doctor.

Directions for Use: Adults and children 2 years to under 12 years of age: oral dosage is a single dose of 5 milligrams of pyrantel base per pound, or 11 milligrams per kilogram, of body weight not to exceed 1 gram. Dosage information is summarized on the following dosing schedule:

Weight		Dosage
		(taken as a single dose)
25 to 37 lbs.	=	$^1/_2$ tsp.
38 to 62 lbs.	=	1 tsp.
63 to 87 lbs.	=	$1^1/_2$ tsp.
88 to 112 lbs.	=	2 tsp.
113 to 137 lbs.	=	$2^1/_2$ tsp.
138 to 162 lbs.	=	3 tsp. (1 tbsp.)
163 to 187 lbs.	=	$3^1/_2$ tsp.
188 lbs. & over	=	4 tsp.

SHAKE WELL BEFORE USING

How Supplied: Pin-X is supplied as a tan to yellowish, caramel-flavored suspension which contains 50 mg of pyrantel base (as pyrantel pamoate) per mL, in bottles of 30 mL (1 fl oz). NDC 55806-024-10 and in bottles of 60 mL (2 fl oz) NDC 55806-024-11
Store at controlled room temperature 15°–30°C (59°–86°F).
Manufactured for:
Effcon™ Laboratories Inc.
Marietta, GA 30065-1499
Rev. 1/89
Code 587A00
Shown in Product Identification Guide, page 506

EDUCATIONAL MATERIAL

Patient Education Brochures—Pin-X® Pinworm Treatment

Effcon Laboratories provides complimentary Patient Education Brochures for patient counseling regarding the treatment and prevention of pinworm infestation. Brochures are available for all healthcare professionals and may be requested by phone (800-722-2428); fax (770-428-6811); or through Effcon's web page (www.effcon.com).

Fleming & Company
1600 FENPARK DR.
FENTON, MO 63026

Direct Inquiries to:
Tom Fleming
636 343-8200
FAX (636) 343-9865
e-mail: info@flemingcompany.com

CHLOR–3
Medicinal Condiment

DESCRIPTION
Medical condiment containing sodium chloride 50%; potassium chloride 30%; magnesium chloride 20%.

Active Ingredients: A mixture of sodium chloride (50% 24.3 mEq/half tsp. iodized); potassium chloride (30% 11.5 mEq/half tsp.); magnesium chloride (20% 5.7 mEq/half tsp.).

Indications: The first medicinal condiment to restore needed K^+ & Mg^{++} lost during diuresis, at the expense of Na^+. To restore electrolytes lost by overcooking foods, or to add to diets that lack green vegetables, bananas, etc. And to replace conventional salting of foods in culinary and gourmet arts.

Symptoms and Treatment of Oral Overdosage: Hyperkalemia and hypermagnesemia are not end-stage results of usage.

How Supplied: In 8-oz plastic shaker, tamper-evident bottles.

OCEAN Hypertonic Nasal Irrigant

Description: Buffered USP sodium chloride in an 8 fluid ounce bottle to which water is added. When shaken and dissolved, a 3% saline solution is prepared.

Ingredients: Sodium Chloride, USP, and Sodium Phosphate

Action and Uses: For irrigating the nasal membranes and sinus cavities which may contribute to reducing dust and allergens, preventing bleeding, decreasing swelling, or liquefying and flushing mucus from the nose. In the hospital setting, it can be used post surgically.

Administration and Dosage: After water is added and the salt is dissolved, lean over a sink or go into a shower. Tilt the head slightly away from the nostril being irrigated. The solution is sprayed into each nostril allowing for drainage from both sides. The tip is adjustable to control the amount of solution entering the nasal membrane. Use as much of the salt solution as needed. May be repeated several times daily.

How Supplied: Plastic bottle containing the correct amount of sodium chloride and sodium phosphate. Fill with 8 ounces of water to form saline solution.

OCEAN® Nasal Spray
(buffered isotonic saline)

Description: A 0.65% special saline made isotonic by the addition of a dual preservative system and buffering excipients prevent nasal irritation.
Ingredients: 0.65% Sodium Chloride and Phenylcarbinol and Benzalkonium Chloride as preservatives.

Action and Uses: For dry nasal membranes including rhinitis medicamentosa, rhinitis sicca and atrophic rhinitis. For patients 'hooked on nose drops' and glaucoma patients on diuretics having dry nasal capillaries. OCEAN® may also be used as a mist or drop. Upright delivers a spray; horizontally a stream; upside down a drop.

Administration and Dosage: For dry nasal membranes, two squeezes in each nostril P.R.N.

Supplied: Plastic 45cc spray bottles and pints.

PURGE
(Flavored Castor Oil Stimulant Laxative)

Composition: Contains 95% castor oil (USP) in a sweetened lemon flavored base that completely masks the odor and taste of the oil.

Indications: Preparation of the bowel for x-ray, surgery and proctological procedures, IVPs, and constipation.

Dosage: Adults and children 12 years of age and over: 15–60 mL (1–4 tbsp) in a single dose. Children 2 to under 12 years of age: 5–15 mL (1–3 tsp) in a single dose. Children under 2 years: consult a physician.

Precaution: Not indicated when nausea, vomiting, abdominal pain or symptoms of appendicitis occur. Pregnancy, use only on advice of physician.

Supplied: Plastic 1 oz. & 2 oz. bottles.

UNKNOWN DRUG?
Consult the
Product Identification Guide
(Gray Pages)
for full-color photos of
leading over-the-counter
medications

GlaxoSmithKline Consumer Healthcare, L.P.

P.O. BOX 1467
PITTSBURGH, PA 15230

Direct Inquiries to:
Consumer Affairs
1-800-245-1040

For Medical Emergencies Contact:
Consumer Affairs
1-800-245-1040

ABREVA™
Cold Sore/Fever Blister Treatment Cream
Docosanol 10% Cream

Uses:
- Treats cold sore/fever blisters on the face or lips
- Shortens healing time and duration of symptoms: tingling, pain, burning, and/or itching

Active Ingredient: **Purpose:**
Docosanol 10% ... Cold sore/fever blister treatment

Inactive Ingredients: Benzyl alcohol, light mineral oil, propylene glycol, purified water, sucrose distearate, sucrose stearate.

Directions:
- **adults and children 12 years or over:**
  - wash hands before and after applying cream
  - apply to affected area on face or lips at the first sign of cold sore/fever blister (tingle). **Early treatment ensures the best results.**
  - rub in gently but completely
  - use 5 times a day until healed
- **children under 12 years:** ask a doctor

Warnings:
For external use only.
Do not use
- if you are allergic to any ingredient in this product
When using this product
- apply only to affected areas
- do not use in or near the eyes
- avoid applying directly inside your mouth
- do not share this product with anyone. This may spread infection.
Stop use and ask a doctor if
- your cold sore gets worse or the cold sore is not healed within 10 days
- **Keep out of reach of children.** If swallowed, get medical help or contact a poison control center right away.
Other Information:
- store at 20°–25°C (68°–77°F)
- do not freeze

How Supplied: Abreva Cream is supplied in 2.0 g [.07 oz] tubes.
Question? Call 1-877-709-3539 weekdays
Shown in Product Identification Guide, page 506

BALMEX®
Medicated Plus™ Baby Powder

Description: Balmex® Medicated Plus™ Baby Powder helps prevent and treat diaper rash with cornstarch (86.9%) and zinc oxide (10%), plus it contains WATER LOCK®, a patented, safe, super absorbing ingredient that helps keep your baby dry.

Indications and Uses: Balmex Medicated Plus Baby Powder helps treat and prevent diaper rash, protects chafed skin associated with diaper rash and helps protect from wetness. The cornstarch and zinc oxide based formulation provides a protective barrier on the skin against the natural causes of irritation, a super absorbing starch copolymer which allows our formula to absorb 2 times more moisture than cornstarch alone.

Directions: Change wet and soiled diapers promptly, cleanse the diaper area, and allow to dry. Apply powder liberally as often as necessary, with each diaper change, especially at bedtime or anytime when exposure to wet diapers may be prolonged. Apply powder close to the body away from the child's face. Carefully shake the powder into the diaper or into the hand and apply to diaper area.

Warnings: Avoid contact with eyes. Keep powder away from child's face to avoid inhalation, which can cause breathing problems. For external use only. Do not use on broken skin. If condition worsens or does not improve within 7 days, contact a physician. Keep out of reach of children. If swallowed, get medical help or contact a Poison Control Center right away.

Active Ingredients: Topical starch (cornstarch) 86.9%. zinc oxide 10%.

Inactive Ingredients: Fragrance, Starch Copolymer (WATER LOCK®), Tribasic Calcium Phosphate

How Supplied: 13 oz. (368g.) Bottle
WATER LOCK® is a registered trademark of Grain Processing Corporation
Shown in Product Identification Guide, page 506

BALMEX®
Diaper Rash Ointment (Zinc Oxide) With Aloe & Vitamin E

Description: Balmex® Diaper Rash Ointment with Aloe & Vitamin E contains Zinc Oxide (11.3%) in a unique formulation including balsan (specially purified balsam peru) suitable for topical application for the treatment and prevention of diaper rash.

Indications and Uses: Balmex helps treat and prevent diaper rash while it moisturizes and nourishes the skin. The zinc oxide based formulation provides a protective barrier on the skin against the natural causes of irritation. Balmex spreads on smooth and wipes off the baby easily, without causing irritation to the affected area. Balmex tactile properties promote compliance amongst mothers.

Directions: Change wet and soiled diapers promptly, cleanse the diaper area, and allow to dry. Apply ointment liberally as often as necessary, with each diaper change, especially at bedtime or anytime when exposure to wet diapers may be prolonged.

Warnings:
For external use only
When using this product avoid contact with eyes
Stop use and ask a doctor if condition worsens or does not improve within 7 days. This may be a sign of a serious condition.
Keep out of reach of children. If swallowed, get medical help or contact a Poison Control Center right away.

Active Ingredient: Zinc Oxide (11.3%).

Inactive Ingredients: Aloe Vera Gel, Balsan (Specially Purified Balsam Peru), Beeswax, Benzoic Acid, Dimethicone, Methylparaben, Mineral Oil, Propylparaben, Purified Water, Sodium Borate, Tocopheryl (Vitamin E Acetate).

How Supplied: 2 oz. (57g.) and 4 oz. (113g.) tubes and 16 oz. (454g.) jar.
Shown in Product Identification Guide, page 506

BC® POWDER
ARTHRITIS STRENGTH BC® POWDER
BC® COLD POWDER LINE

Description: BC® POWDER: **Active Ingredients**: Each powder contains Aspirin 650 mg, Salicylamide 195 mg and Caffeine 33.3 mg. **Inactive Ingredients:** Docusate Sodium, Fumaric Acid, Lactose Monohydrate and Potassium Chloride. ARTHRITIS STRENGTH BC® POWDER: **Active Ingredients:** Each powder contains Aspirin 742 mg, Salicylamide 222 mg and Caffeine 38 mg. **Inactive Ingredients:** Docusate Sodium, Fumaric Acid, Lactose Monohydrate and Potassium Chloride.

BC® ALLERGY SINUS COLD POWDER

Active Ingredients: Aspirin 650 mg, Pseudoephedrine Hydrochloride 60 mg and Chlorpheniramine Maleate 4 mg per powder. **Inactive Ingredients:** Fumaric Acid, Glycine, Lactose, Potassium Chloride, Silica, Sodium Lauryl Sulfate. BC® SINUS COLD POWDER. **Active Ingredients:** Aspirin 650 mg and Pseudoephedrine Hydrochloride 60 mg. per powder. **Inactive Ingredients:** Colloidal Silicon Dioxide, Microcrystalline Cellu-

Continued on next page

BC Powders—Cont.

lose, Povidone, Pregelatinized Starch, Stearic Acid.

Indications: BC Powder is for relief of simple headache; for temporary relief of minor arthritic pain, for relief of muscular aches, discomfort and fever of colds; and for relief of normal menstrual pain and pain of tooth extraction.

Arthritis Strength BC Powder is specially formulated to fight occasional minor pain and inflammation of arthritis. Like Original Formula BC, Arthritis Strength BC provides fast temporary relief of minor arthritis pain and inflammation, relief of muscular aches, discomfort and fever of colds; and pain of tooth extraction.

BC Allergy Sinus Cold Powder is for relief of multiple symptoms such as body aches, fever, nasal congestion, sneezing, running nose, and watery itchy eyes associated with allergy and sinus attacks and the onset of colds. BC Sinus Cold Powder is for relief of such symptoms as body aches, fever, and nasal congestion.

BC Powder®, Arthritis
Strength BC® Powder and BC Cold Powder Line:

Warnings: Children and teenagers should not use this medicine for chicken pox or flu symptoms before a doctor is consulted about Reye's Syndrome, a rare but serious illness reported to be associated with aspirin. Keep this and all medicines out of children's reach. In case of accidental overdose, contact a physician or poison control center immediately.

As with any drug, if you are pregnant or nursing a baby seek the advice of a health professional before using this product.

IT IS ESPECIALLY IMPORTANT NOT TO USE ASPIRIN DURING THE LAST 3 MONTHS OF PREGNANCY UNLESS SPECIFICALLY DIRECTED TO DO SO BY A DOCTOR BECAUSE IT MAY CAUSE PROBLEMS IN THE UNBORN CHILD OR COMPLICATIONS DURING DELIVERY.

Alcohol Warning: If you consume 3 or more alcoholic drinks every day, ask your doctor whether you should take aspirin or other pain relievers/fever reducers. Aspirin may cause stomach bleeding.

Allergy Alert: Aspirin may cause a severe allergic reaction which may include hives, facial swelling, shock or asthma (wheezing). **Ask a doctor before use if you have** asthma, ulcers, a bleeding problem, stomach problems that last or come back such as heartburn, upset stomach or pain. **Ask a doctor or pharmacist before use** if you are taking a prescription drug for gout, diabetes, arthritis or anticoagulation (blood thinning). **Stop use and ask a doctor if** an allergic reaction occurs, ringing in ears or loss of hearing occurs, pain gets worse or persists for more than 10 days, fever

lasts more than 3 days, redness or swelling is present, or new symptoms occur. For BC Powder and Arthritis Strength BC Powder:

When using these products limit the use of caffeine containing drugs, foods, or drinks, because too much caffeine may cause nervousness, irritability, sleeplessness, and occasionally, rapid heartbeat. For BC Cold Powder Line:

Do not exceed recommended dosage. If nervousness, dizziness, or sleeplessness occur, discontinue use and consult a doctor. If symptoms do not improve within 7 days, or are accompanied by fever that lasts more than 3 days, or if new symptoms occur, consult a physician before continuing use. Do not take BC if you are sensitive to aspirin, or have heart disease, high blood pressure, thyroid disease, diabetes, asthma, glaucoma, emphysema, chronic pulmonary disease, shortness of breath, difficulty in breathing or difficulty in urination due to enlargement of the prostate gland, or if you are presently taking a prescription antihypertensive or antidepressant drug unless directed by a doctor. *"Drug interaction precaution.* Do not use this product if you are now taking a prescription monoamine oxidase inhibitor (MAOI) (certain drugs for depression, psychiatric or emotional conditions, or Parkinson's disease), or for 2 weeks after stopping the MAOI drug. If you are uncertain whether your prescription drug contains an MAOI, consult a health professional before taking this product." BC Allergy Sinus Cold Powder with antihistamine may cause drowsiness. Avoid alcoholic beverages when taking this product because it may increase drowsiness. Use caution when driving a motor vehicle or operating machinery. May cause excitability, especially in children.

Overdosage: In case of accidental overdosage, contact a physician or poison control center immediately.

Dosage and Administration: BC® Powder, Arthritis Strength BC® Powder, BC® Cold Powder Line:
Place one powder on tongue and follow with liquid. If you prefer, stir powder into glass of water or other liquid. For BC Powder and Arthritis Strength BC Powder:
Adults and children 12 years and over: Take one powder every 3–4 hours not to exceed 4 powders in 24 hours.
For BC Cold Powder Line:
Adults and children 12 years and over: Take one powder every 6 hours not to exceed 4 powders in 24 hours. For children under 12, consult a physician.

How Supplied: BC Powder: Available in tamper evident overwrapped envelopes of 2 or 6 powders, as well as tamper evident boxes of 24 and 50 powders.
Arthritis Strength BC Powder: Available in tamper evident over wrapped envelopes of 6 powders, and tamper evident overwrapped boxes of 24 and 50 powders.

BC Cold Powder Line:
Available in tamper-evident overwrapped envelopes of 6 powders, as well as tamper-evident boxes of 12 powders (For BC Allergy Sinus Cold Powder only).

Orange Flavor
CITRUCEL®
[sĭt 'rə-sĕl]
(Methylcellulose)
Bulk-forming Fiber Laxative

Description: Each 19 g adult dose (approximately one heaping measuring tablespoonful) contains Methylcellulose 2 g. Each 9.5 g child's dose (one-half the adult dose) contains Methylcellulose 1 g. Methylcellulose is a nonallergenic fiber. Also contains: Citric Acid, FD&C Yellow No. 6 Lake, Orange Flavors (natural and artificial), Potassium Citrate, Riboflavin, Sucrose, and other ingredients. Each adult dose contains approximately 3 mg of sodium and contributes 60 calories from Sucrose.

Actions: Promotes elimination by providing additional fiber (bulk) to the diet. This product generally produces bowel movement in 12 to 72 hours.

Indications: For relief of constipation (irregularity). May also be used for relief of constipation associated with other bowel disorders such as irritable bowel syndrome, diverticular disease, and hemorrhoids as well as for bowel management during postpartum, postsurgical, and convalescent periods when recommended by a physician.

Contraindications: Intestinal obstruction, fecal impaction, known hypersensitivity to formula ingredients.

Warnings: Patients should be instructed to consult their physician before using any laxative if they have noticed a sudden change in bowel habits which persists for two weeks. Unless directed by a physician, patients should be advised not to use laxative products when abdominal pain, nausea, or vomiting is present. Patients should also be advised to discontinue use and consult a physician if rectal bleeding or failure to have a bowel movement occurs after use of any laxative product. Unless recommended by a physician, patients should not exceed the recommended maximum daily dose. Patients should not use laxative products for a period longer than one week unless directed by a physician. **TAKING THIS PRODUCT WITHOUT ADEQUATE FLUID MAY CAUSE IT TO SWELL AND BLOCK YOUR THROAT OR ESOPHAGUS AND MAY CAUSE CHOKING. DO NOT TAKE THIS PRODUCT IF YOU HAVE DIFFICULTY IN SWALLOWING. IF YOU EXPERIENCE CHEST PAIN, VOMITING, OR DIFFICULTY IN SWALLOWING OR BREATHING AFTER TAKING THIS PRODUCT, SEEK IMMEDIATE**

MEDICAL ATTENTION. KEEP THIS AND ALL DRUGS OUT OF THE REACH OF CHILDREN.

Dosage and Administration: Adult Dose: dissolve one leveled scoop (one heaping tablespoon – 19g) in 8 ounces of cold water up to three times daily at the first sign of constipation. Children age 6 to 12 years of age: *one-half the adult dose* stirred briskly in 8 ounces of cold water, once daily at the first sign of constipation. The mixture should be administered promptly and drinking another glass of water is highly recommended (see warnings). Children under 6 years of age: *Use only as directed by a physician.* Continued use for 12 to 72 hours may be necessary for full benefit.

TAKE THIS PRODUCT (CHILD OR ADULT DOSE) WITH AT LEAST 8 OZ. (A FULL GLASS) OF WATER OR OTHER FLUID. TAKING THIS PRODUCT WITHOUT ENOUGH LIQUID MAY CAUSE CHOKING. SEE WARNINGS.

How Supplied: 16 oz., 30 oz., and 50 oz. containers. Boxes of 20-single-dose packets. Store below 86°F (30°C). Protect contents from humidity; keep tightly closed.
Shown in Product Identification Guide, page 506

Sugar Free Orange Flavor
CITRUCEL®
[sĭt ′rə-sĕl]
(Methylcellulose)
Bulk-forming Fiber Laxative

Description: Each 10.2 g adult dose (approximately one rounded measuring tablespoonful) contains Methylcellulose 2 g. Each 5.1 g child's dose (one-half the adult dose) contains Methylcellulose 1 g. Methylcellulose is a nonallergenic fiber. Also contains: Aspartame, Dibasic Calcium Phosphate, FD&C Yellow No. 6 Lake, Malic Acid, Maltodextrin, Orange Flavors (natural and artificial), Potassium Citrate, and Riboflavin. Each 10.2 g dose contains approximately 3 mg of sodium and contributes 24 calories from Maltodextrin.

Actions: Promotes elimination by providing additional fiber (bulk) to the diet. This product generally produces bowel movement in 12 to 72 hours.

Indications: For relief of constipation (irregularity). May also be used for relief of constipation associated with other bowel disorders such as irritable bowel syndrome, diverticular disease, and hemorrhoids as well as for bowel management during postpartum, postsurgical, and convalescent periods when recommended by a physician.

Contraindications and Warnings: See entry for "Orange Flavor Citrucel".

Phenylketonurics: CONTAINS PHENYLALANINE 52 mg per adult dose. Individuals with phenylketonuria and other individuals who must restrict their intake of phenylalanine should be warned that each 10.2 g adult dose contains aspartame which provides 52 mg of phenylalanine.

Dosage and Administration: Adult Dose: dissolve one leveled scoop (one rounded measuring tablespoon – 10.2 g) in 8 ounces of cold water up to three times daily at the first sign of constipation. Children age 6 to 12 years of age: *one-half the adult dose* stirred briskly into at least 8 ounces of cold water, once daily at the first sign of constipation. The mixture should be administered promptly and drinking another glass of water is highly recommended (see warnings). Children under 6 years of age: *Use only as directed by a physician.* Continued use for 12 to 72 hours may be necessary for full benefit.

TAKE THIS PRODUCT (CHILD OR ADULT DOSE) WITH AT LEAST 8 OZ. (A FULL GLASS) OF WATER OR OTHER FLUID. TAKING THIS PRODUCT WITHOUT ENOUGH LIQUID MAY CAUSE CHOKING. SEE WARNINGS.

How Supplied:
8.6 oz, 16.9 oz, and 32 oz containers. Boxes of 20 single-dose packets. Store below 86°F (30°C). Protect contents from humidity; keep tightly closed.
Shown in Product Identification Guide, page 506

CITRUCEL®
(methylcellulose)
Soluble Fiber Caplet
Bulk-Forming Fiber Laxative

Uses: Helps restore and maintain regularity. Helps relieve constipation. Also useful in treatment of constipation (irregularity) associated with other bowel disorders when recommended by a physician. This product generally produces a bowel movement in 12 to 72 hours.

Active Ingredient: Each caplet contains 500mg Methylcellulose.

Inactive Ingredients: Crospovidone, Dibasic Calcium Phosphate, FD&C Yellow No. 6 Aluminum Lake, Magnesium Stearate, Maltodextrin, Povidone, Sodium Lauryl Sulfate.

Directions: Adult dose: Take two caplets as needed with 8 ounces of liquid, up to six times daily. Children (6–12 years): Take one caplet with 8 ounces of liquid, up to six times per day. The dosage requirement may vary according to the severity of constipation. Children under 6 years: consult a physician. TAKE THIS PRODUCT (CHILD OR ADULT DOSE) WITH AT LEAST 8 OUNCES (A FULL GLASS) OF WATER OR OTHER FLUID. TAKING THIS PRODUCT WITHOUT ENOUGH LIQUID MAY CAUSE CHOKING. SEE WARNINGS.

Directions for Use: Take each dose with 8oz. of liquid.

Age	Dose	Daily Maximum
Adults & Children over 12 years	2 Caplets	Up to 6 times daily*
Children (6 to 12 years)	1 Caplet	Up to 6 times daily*
Children under 6 years	Consult a physician	

*Refer to directions below.

Warnings: Consult a physician before using any laxative product if you have noticed a sudden change in bowel habits which persists for two weeks. Unless directed by a physician, do not use laxative products when abdominal pain, nausea, or vomiting are present. Discontinue use and consult a physician if rectal bleeding or failure to produce a bowel movement occurs after use of any laxative product. Unless recommended by a physician, do not exceed recommended maximum daily dose. Laxative products should not be used for a period longer than a weak unless directed by a physician. If sensitive to any of the ingredients, do not use. TAKING THIS PRODUCT WITHOUT ADEQUATE FLUID MAY CAUSE IT TO SWELL AND BLOCK YOUR THROAT OR ESOPHAGUS AND MAY CAUSE CHOKING. DO NOT TAKE THIS PRODUCT IF YOU HAVE DIFFICULTY IN SWALLOWING. IF YOU EXPERIENCE CHEST PAIN, VOMITING, OR DIFFICULTY IN SWALLOWING OR BREATHING AFTER TAKING THIS PRODUCT, SEEK IMMEDIATE MEDICAL ATTENTION. KEEP THIS AND ALL DRUGS OUT OF THE REACH OF CHILDREN.

Store at room temperature 15–30°C (59–86°F). Protect contents from moisture.

Tamper evident feature: Bottle sealed with printed foil under cap. Do not use if foil is torn or broken.

How Supplied: Bottles of 100 and 164 caplets

Questions or comments?

Call toll-free 1-800-897-6081 weekdays.

Patents Pending

The various Citrucel Logos and design elements of the packaging are Registered Trademarks of GlaxoSmithKline.

©2001 GlaxoSmithKline

Distributed by:

GlaxoSmithKline Consumer Healthcare

GlaxoSmithKline Consumer Healthcare, L.P.

Pittsburgh, PA 15230, Made in Canada.

Continued on next page

CONTAC® Non-Drowsy
Decongestant
12 Hour Cold Caplets

Product Information: Each Maximum Strength Contac 12 Hour Cold Caplet provides up to 12 hours of relief. Part of the caplet goes to work right away for fast relief; the rest is released gradually to provide up to 12 hours of prolonged relief. With just one caplet in the morning and one at bedtime, you feel better all day, sleep better at night, breathing freely without congestion or sinus pressure.

Indications: Temporarily relieves nasal congestion due to the common cold, hay fever or other upper respiratory allergies and associated with sinusitis. Helps decongest sinus openings and passages; temporarily relieves sinus congestion and pressure.

Directions: Adults and children over 12 years of age: One caplet every 12 hours, not to exceed 2 caplets in 24 hours, or as directed by a doctor. Children under 12 years of age: consult a doctor.

TAMPER-EVIDENT PACKAGING FEATURES FOR YOUR PROTECTION:
Each caplet is encased in a plastic cell with a foil back; do not use if cell or foil is broken.

Warnings: Do not exceed the recommended dosage. If nervousness, dizziness, or sleeplessness occur, discontinue use and consult a doctor. If symptoms do not improve within 7 days or are accompanied by high fever, consult a doctor. Do not take this product, unless directed by a doctor, if you have heart disease, high blood pressure, thyroid disease, diabetes, glaucoma or difficulty in urination due to enlargement of the prostate gland. KEEP THIS AND ALL DRUGS OUT OF REACH OF CHILDREN. IN CASE OF ACCIDENTAL OVERDOSE, SEEK PROFESSIONAL ASSISTANCE OR CONTACT A POISON CONTROL CENTER IMMEDIATELY. As with any drug, if you are pregnant or nursing a baby, seek the advice of a health professional before using this product.

Drug Interaction Precaution: Do not use this product if you are now taking a prescription monoamine oxidase inhibitor (MAOI) (certain drugs for depression, psychiatric or emotional conditions, or Parkinson's disease), or for 2 weeks after stopping the MAOI drug. If you are uncertain whether your prescription drug contains an MAOI, consult a health professional before taking this product.

Active Ingredient: Pseudoephedrine Hydrochloride 120 mg.

Store at 15° to 25°C (59° to 77°F) in a dry place and protest from light.

Each Caplet Also Contains: Carnauba Wax, Colloidal Silicon Dioxide, Dibasic Calcium Phosphate, Hypromellose, Magnesium Stearate, Microcrystalline Cellulose, Polyethylene Glycol, Polysorbate 80, Titanium Dioxide.

How Supplied: Consumer packages of 10 and 20 caplets.
Note: There are other CONTAC products. Make sure this is the one you are interested in. See the table below for all of the products in the CONTAC line.
Shown in Product Identification Guide, page 506

CONTAC® Non-Drowsy
Timed Release-Maximum Strength
12 Hour Cold Caplets

Indications: For the temporary relief of nasal congestion due to the common cold, hay fever or other upper respiratory allergies, and nasal congestion associated with sinusitis. Promotes nasal and/or sinus drainage; temporarily relieves sinus congestion and pressure. Temporarily restores freer breathing through the nose.

Each Maximum Strength Contac 12-Hour Cold caplet provides up to 12 hours of relief. Part of the caplet goes to work right away for fast relief; the rest is released gradually to provide up to 12 hours of prolonged relief. With just one caplet in the morning and one at bedtime, you feel better all day, sleep better at night, breathing freely without congestion or sinus pressure.

Active Ingredient: Each coated extended-release caplet contains Pseudoephedrine Hydrochloride 120 mg.

Inactive Ingredients: carnauba wax, collodial silicon dioxide, dibasic calcium phosphate, hypromellose, magnesium stearate, microcrystalline cellulose, polyethylene glycol, polysorbate 80, titanium dioxide.

Directions: Adults and children 12 years of age and over – One caplet every 12 hours, not to exceed two caplets in 24 hours. This product is not recommended for children under 12 years of age.

Warnings: Do not exceed recommended dosage. If nervousness, dizziness, or sleeplessness occur, discontinue use and consult a doctor. If symptoms do not improve within 7 days or are accompanied by fever, consult a doctor. Do not take this product if you have heart disease, high blood pressure, thyroid disease, diabetes, or difficulty in urination due to enlargement of the prostate gland unless directed by a doctor. As with any drug, if you are pregnant or nursing a baby, seek the advice of a health professional before using this product.

Drug Interaction Precaution: Do not use this product if you are now taking a prescription monoamine oxidase inhibitor (MAOI) (certain drugs for depression, psychiatric or emotional conditions, or Parkinson's disease), or for 2 weeks after stopping the MAOI drug. If you are uncertain whether your prescription contains an MAOI, consult a health professional before taking this product.
KEEP THIS AND ALL DRUGS OUT OF THE REACH OF CHILDREN. In case of accidental overdose, seek professional assistance or contact a Poison Control Center immediately.
Store at 15° to 25°C (59° to 77°F) in a dry place and protect from light.

How Supplied: Packets of 10 and 20 Caplets
U.S. Patent No. 5,895,663
Comments or questions?
Call toll-free 1-800-245-1040 weekdays.

CONTAC®
Severe Cold and Flu
Caplets Maximum Strength
Analgesic• Decongestant
Antihistamine• Cough Suppressant
CONTAC®
Severe Cold and Flu
Caplets Non-Drowsy
Nasal Decongestant • Analgesic•
Cough Suppressant

Active Ingredients: Each *Non-Drowsy Caplet* contains Acetaminophen 325 mg, Psudoephedrine HCl 30 mg and Dextromethorphan Hydrobromide 15 mg.
Each *Maximum Strength Caplet* contains Acetaminophen 500 mg, Dextromethorphan Hydrobromide 15 mg, Pseudoephedrine HCl 30 mg and chlorpheniromine Maleate 2 mg.

Product Information: Two caplets every 6 hours to help relieve the discomforts of severe colds with flu-like symptoms.

Indications: *Non-Drowsy & Maximum Strength Caplets:* Temporarily relieves nasal congestion & coughing due to the common cold. Provides temporary relief of fever, sore throat, headache & minor aches associated with the common cold or the flu.
Maximum Strength Caplets: Temporarily relieves runny nose, sneezing, itchy and watery eyes due to the common cold.

Directions: Adults (12 years and older): Two caplets every 6 hours, not to exceed 8 caplets in any 24-hour period, or as directed by a doctor. Children under 12 years of age: consult a doctor.
TAMPER-EVIDENT PACKAGING FEATURES FOR YOUR PROTECTION:
Caplets are encased in a plastic cell with a foil back; do not use if cell or foil is broken. The letters ND SCF for non-drowsy and SCF for maximum strength appear on each caplet; do not use this product if these letters are missing.

Warnings: For *Non-Drowsy and Maximum Strength Caplets:* Do not exceed recommended dosage. If nervousness, dizziness, or sleeplessness occur, discontinue use and consult a doctor.

PDR For Nonprescription Drugs

	CONTAC Non-Drowsy 12 Hour Cold Caplets	CONTAC 12 Hour Cold Capsules	CONTAC Severe Cold and Flu Caplets Maximum Strength (each 2 caplet dose)	CONTAC Severe Cold and Flu Non-Drowsy Caplets (each 2 caplet dose)	CONTAC Day & Night Cold & Flu	
					Day Caplets	Night Caplets
Phenylpropanolamine HCl	—	75.0 mg	—	—	—	—
Chlorpheniramine Maleate	—	8.0 mg	4.0 mg	—	—	—
Pseudoephedrine HCl	120 mg	—	60 mg	60.0 mg	60.0 mg	60.0 mg
Acetaminophen	—	—	1000.0 mg	650.0 mg	650.0 mg	650.0 mg
Dextromethorphan Hydrobromide	—	—	30.0 mg	30.0 mg	30.0 mg	—
Diphenhydramine HCl	—	—	—	—	—	50.0 mg

If symptoms do not improve or are accompanied by fever that lasts for more than 3 days, or if new symptoms occur, consult a doctor. If sore throat is severe, persists for more than 2 days, is accompanied or followed by fever, headache, rash, nausea, or vomiting, consult a doctor promptly. A persistent cough may be a sign of a serious condition. If cough persists for more than 7 days, tends to recur, or is accompanied by rash, persistent headache, fever that lasts for more than 3 days, or if new symptoms occur, consult a doctor. Do not take this product for persistent or chronic cough such as occurs with smoking, asthma, emphysema, or if cough is accompanied by excessive phlegm (mucus) unless directed by a doctor. Do not take this product if you have heart disease, high blood pressure, thyroid disease, diabetes, glaucoma or difficulty in urination due to enlargement of the prostate gland unless directed by a doctor. **Alcohol Warning:** If you consume 3 or more alcoholic drinks every day, ask your doctor whether you should take acetaminophen or other pain relievers/fever reducers. Acetaminophen may cause liver damage. **KEEP THIS AND ALL DRUGS OUT OF THE REACH OF CHILDREN.** Prompt medical attention is critical for adults as well as for children even if you do not notice any signs or symptoms. In case of accidental overdose, seek professional assistance or contact a Poison Control Center immediately. As with any drug, if you are pregnant or nursing a baby, seek the advice of a health professional before using this product.
Additional Warnings for *Maximum Strength Caplets:* May cause excitability especially in children. Do not take this product, unless directed by a doctor, if you have a breathing problem such as emphysema or chronic bronchitis. May cause marked drowsiness: alcohol, sedatives, and tranquilizers may increase the drowsiness effect. Avoid taking alcoholic beverages while taking this product. Do not take this product if you are taking sedatives or tranquilizers, without first consulting your doctor. Use caution when driving a motor vehicle or operating machinery.

Drug Interaction Precaution: Do not use this product if you are now taking a prescription monoamine oxidase inhibitor (MAOI) (certain drugs for depression, psychiatric or emotional conditions, or Parkinson's disease), or for 2 weeks after stopping the MAOI drug. If you are uncertain whether your prescription drug contains an MAOI, consult a health professional before taking this product.

Inactive Ingredients: Each ***Non-Drowsy and Maximum Strength Caplet*** contains: Carnauba Wax, Colloidal Silicon Dioxide, Hypromellose, Magnesium stearate, Microcrystalline Cellulose, Polyethylene Glycol, Polysorbate 80, Starch, Stearic Acid, Titanium Dioxide.
Each ***Maximum Strength Caplet*** also contains: FD&C Blue #1 Al Lake.

Avoid storing at high temperature (greater than 100°F).

How Supplied: ***Non-Drowsy:*** Consumer packages of 16.
Maximum Strength: Consumer packages of 16 & 30.
Shown in Product Identification Guide, page 506

Product Change: Maximum Strength Caplets now with new decongestant (pseudoephedrine HCl).

Note: There are other CONTAC products. Make sure this is the one you are interested in. See the table below for all of the products in the CONTAC line.
[See table above]

DEBROX® Drops
Ear Wax Removal Aid

Active Ingredient: **Purpose:**
Carbamide peroxide
  6.5% non USP* .. Earwax removal aid

Actions: DEBROX®, used as directed, cleanses the ear with sustained microfoam. DEBROX Drops foam on contact with earwax due to the release of oxygen (there may be an associated crackling sound). DEBROX Drops provide a safe, nonirritating method of softening and removing ear wax.

Uses: For occasional use as an aid to soften, loosen, and remove excessive earwax.

Directions: Adults and children over 12 years of age: tilt head sideways and place 5 to 10 drops into ear. Tip of applicator should not enter ear canal. Keep drops in ear for several minutes by keeping head tilted or placing cotton in the ear. Use twice daily for up to four days if needed, or as directed by a doctor. Any wax remaining after treatment may be removed by gently flushing the ear with warm water, using a soft rubber bulb ear syringe. Children under 12 years of age: consult a doctor.

Warnings: FOR USE IN THE EAR ONLY. Do not use if you have ear drainage or discharge, ear pain, irritation or rash in the ear, or are dizzy; consult a doctor. Do not use if you have an injury or perforation (hole) of the eardrum or after ear surgery unless directed by a doctor. Do not use for more than four days. If excessive earwax remains after use of this product, consult a doctor. Avoid contact with the eyes. In case of accidental ingestion, seek professional assistance or contact a poison control center immediately.

Other Information: Avoid exposing bottle to excessive heat and direct sunlight. Keep tip on bottle when not in use. Product foams on contact with earwax due to release of oxygen. There may be an associated "crackling" sound. Keep this and all drugs out of the reach of children.

Inactive Ingredients: citric acid, flavor, glycerin, propylene glycol, sodium lauroyl sarcosinate, sodium stannate, water

How Supplied: DEBROX Drops are available in ½-fl-oz or 1-fl-oz (15 or 30 ml) plastic squeeze bottles with applicator spouts.
Questions or comments? 1-800-245-1040 weekdays.

Shown in Product Identification Guide, page 506

Continued on next page

ECOTRIN

Enteric-Coated Aspirin
Antiarthritic, Antiplatelet
COMPREHENSIVE PRESCRIBING
INFORMATION

Description: Ecotrin enteric coated aspirin (acetylsalicylic acid) tablets available in 81mg, 325mg and 500 mg tablets for oral administration. The 325 mg and 500 mg tablets contain the following inactive ingredients: Carnuba Wax, Colloidal Silicon Dioxide, FD&C Yellow No. 6, Hypromellose, Methacrylic Acid Copolymer, Microcrystalline Cellulose, Pregelatinized Starch, Propylene Glycol, Simethicone, Sodium Starch Glycolate, Stearic Acid, Talc, Titanium Dioxide, and Triethyl Citrate. The 81 mg tablets contain Carnuba Wax, Corn Starch, D&C Yellow No. 10, FD&C Yellow No. 6, Hypromellose, Methacrylic Acid Copolymer, Microcrystalline Cellulose, Propylene Glycol, Simethicone, Stearic Acid, Talc and Triethyl Citrate.

Aspirin is an odorless white, needle-like crystalline or powdery substance. When exposed to moisture, aspirin hydrolyzes into salicylic and acetic acids, and gives off a vinegary-odor. It is highly lipid soluble and slightly soluble in water.

Clinical Pharmacology: Mechanism of Action: Aspirin is a more potent inhibitor of both prostaglandin synthesis and platelet aggregation than other salicylic acid derivatives. The differences in activity between aspirin and salicylic acid are thought to be due to the acetyl group on the aspirin molecule. This acetyl group is responsible for the inactivation of cyclooxygenase via acetylation.

PHARMACOKINETICS

Absorption: In general, immediate release aspirin is well and completely absorbed from the gastrointestinal (GI) tract. Following absorption, aspirin is hydrolyzed to salicylic acid with peak plasma levels of salicylic acid occurring within 1–2 hours of dosing (see Pharmacokinetics—Metabolism). The rate of absorption from the GI tract is dependent upon the dosage form, the presence or absence of food, gastric pH (the presence or absence of GI antacids or buffering agents), and other physiologic factors. Enteric coated aspirin products are erratically absorbed from the GI tract.

Distribution: Salicylic acid is widely distibuted to all tissues and fluids in the body including the central nervous system (CNS), breast milk, and fetal tissues. The highest concentrations are found in the plasma, liver, renal cortex, heart, and lungs. The protein binding of salicylate is concentration-dependent, i.e., non-linear. At low concentrations (< 100 mcg/mL) approximately 90 percent of plasma salicylate is bound to albumin while at higher concentrations (> 400 mcg/mL), only about 75 percent is bound. The early signs of salicylic overdose (salicylism), including tinnitus (ringing in the ears), occur at plasma concentrations approximating 200 mcg/mL. Severe toxic effects are associated with levels > 400 mcg/mL (See Adverse Reactions and Overdosage.)

Metabolism: Aspirin is rapidly hydrolyzed in the plasma to salicylic acid such that plasma levels of aspirin are essentially undetectable 1–2 hours after dosing. Salicylic acid is primarily conjugated in the liver to form salicyluric acid, a phenolic glucuronide, an acyl glucuronide, and a number of minor metabolites. Salicylic acid has a plasma half-life of approximately 6 hours. Salicylate metabolism is saturable and total body clearance decreases at higher serum concentrations due to the limited ability of the liver to form both salicyluric acid and phenolic glucuronide. Following toxic doses (10–20 grams (g)), the plasma half-life may be increased to over 20 hours.

Elimination: The elimination of salicylic acid follows zero order pharmacokinetics; (i.e., the rate of drug elimination is constant in relation to plasma concentration). Renal excretion of unchanged drug depends upon urine pH. As urinary pH rises above 6.5, the renal clearance of free salicylate increases from < 5 percent to > 80 percent. Alkalinization of the urine is a key concept in the management of salicylate overdose. (See Overdosage.) Following therapeutic doses, approximately 10 percent is found excreted in the urine as salicylic acid, 75 percent as salicyluric acid, and 10 percent phenolic and 5 percent acyl glucuronides of salicylic acid.

Pharmacodynamics: Aspirin affects platelet aggregation by irreversibly inhibiting prostaglandin cyclo-oxygenase. This effect lasts for the life of the platelet and prevents the formation of the platelet aggregating factor thromboxane A2. Non-acetylated salicylates do not inhibit this enzyme and have no effect on platelet aggregation. At somewhat higher doses, aspirin reversibly inhibits the formation of prostaglandin 1_2 (prostacyclin), which is an arterial vasodilator and inhibits platelet aggregation.

At higher doses aspirin is an effective anti-inflammatory agent, partially due to inhibition of inflammatory mediators via cyclooxygenase inhibition in peripheral tissues. In vitro studies suggest that other mediators of inflammation may also be suppressed by aspirin administration, although the precise mechanism of action has not been elucidated. It is this non-specific suppression of cyclooxygenase activity in peripheral tissues following large doses that leads to its primary side effect of gastric irritation. (See Adverse Reactions.)

Clinical Studies: Ischemic Stroke and Transient Ischemic Attack (TIA): In clinical trials of subjects with TIA's due to fibrin platelet emboli or ischemic stroke, aspirin has been shown to significantly reduce the risk of the combined endpoint of stroke or death and the combined endpoint of TIA, stroke, or death by about 13–18 percent.

Suspect Acute Myocardial Infarction (MI): In a large, multi-center study of aspirin, streptokinase, and the combination of aspirin and streptokinase in 17,187 patients with suspected acute MI, aspirin treatment produced a 23-percent reduction in the risk of vascular mortality. Aspirin was also shown to have an additional benefit in patients given a thrombolytic agent.

Prevention of Recurrent MI and Unstable Angina Pectoris: These indications are supported by the results of six large, randomized, multi-center, placebo-controlled trials of predominantly male post-MI subjects and one randomized placebo-controlled study of men with unstable angina pectoris. Aspirin therapy in MI subjects was associated with a significant reduction (about 20 percent) in the risk of the combination endpoint of subsequent death and/or nonfatal reinfarction in these patients. In aspirin-treated unstable angina patients the event rate was reduced to 5 percent from the 10 percent rate in the placebo group.

Chronic Stable Angina Pectoris: In a randomized, multi-center, double-blind trial designed to assess the role of aspirin for prevention of MI in patients with chronic stable angina pectoris, aspirin significantly reduced the primary combined endpoint of nonfatal MI, fatal MI, and sudden death by 34 percent. The secondary endpoint for vascular events (first occurrence of MI, stroke, or vascular death) was also significantly reduced (32 percent).

Revascularization Procedures: Most patients who undergo coronary artery revascularization procedures have already had symptomatic coronary artery disease for which aspirin is indicated. Similarly, patients with lesions of the carotid bifurcation sufficient to require carotid endarterectomy are likely to have had a precedent event. Aspirin is recommended for patients who undergo revascularization procedures if there is a pre-existing condition for which aspirin is already indicated.

Rheumatologic Diseases: In clinical studies in patients with rheumatoid arthritis, juvenile rheumatoid arthritis, ankylosing spondylitis and osteoarthritis, aspirin has been shown to be effective in controlling various indices of clinical disease activity.

Animal Toxicology: The acute oral 50 percent lethal dose in rats is about 1.5 g/kg and in mice 1.1 g/kg. Renal papillary necrosis and decreased urinary concentrating ability occur in rodents chronically administered high doses. Dose-dependent gastric mucosal injury occurs in rats and humans. Mammals may develop aspirin toxicosis associated with GI symptoms, circulatory effects, and central nervous system depression. (See Overdosage.)

Indications and Usage: Vascular Indications (Ischemic Stroke, TIA, Acute MI, Prevention of Recurrent MI, Unstable Angina Pectoris, and Chronic Stable

Angina Pectoris): Aspirin is indicated to: (1) Reduce the combined risk of death and nonfatal stroke in patients who have had ischemic stroke or transient ischemia of the brain due to fibrin platelet emboli, (2) reduce the risk of vascular mortality in patients with a suspected acute MI, (3) reduce the combined risk of death and nonfatal MI in patients with a previous MI or unstable angina pectoris, and (4) reduce the combined risk of MI and sudden death in patients with chronic stable angina pectoris.

Revascularization Procedures (Coronary Artery Bypass Graft (CABG), Percutaneous Transluminal Coronary Angioplasty (PTCA), and Carotid Endarterectomy): Aspirin is indicated in patients who have undergone revascularization procedures (i.e., CABG, PTCA, or carotid endarterectomy) when there is a preexisting condition for which aspirin is already indicated.

Rheumatologic Disease Indications (Rheumatoid Arthritis, Juvenile Rheumatoid Arthritis, Spondyloarthropathies, Osteoarthritis, and the Arthritis and Pleurisy of Systemic Lupus Erythematosus (SLE)): Aspirin is indicated for the relief of the signs and symptoms of rheumatoid arthritis, juvenile rheumatoid arthritis, osteoarthritis, spondyloarthropathies, and arthritis and pleurisy associated with SLE.

Contraindications: Allergy: Aspirin is contraindicated in patients with known allergy to nonsteroidal anti-inflammatory drug products and in patients with the syndrome of asthma, rhinitis, and nasal polyps. Aspirin may cause severe urticaria, angioedema, or bronchospasm (asthma).

Reye's Syndrome: Aspirin should not be used in children or teenagers for viral infections, with or without fever, because of the risk of Reye's syndrome with concomitant use of aspirin in certain viral illnesses.

Warnings: Alcohol Warning: Patients who consume three or more alcoholic drinks every day should be counseled about the bleeding risks involved with chronic, heavy alcohol use while taking aspirin.

Coagulation Abnormalities: Even low doses of aspirin can inhibit platelet function leading to an increase in bleeding time. This can adversely affect patients with inherited (hemophilia) or acquired (liver disease or vitamin K deficiency) bleeding disorders.

GI Side Effects: GI side effects include stomach pain, heartburn, nausea, vomiting, and gross GI bleeding. Although minor upper GI symptoms, such as dyspepsia, are common and can occur anytime during therapy, physicians should remain alert for signs of ulceration and bleeding, even in the absence of previous GI symptoms. Physicians should inform patients about the signs and symptoms of GI side effects and what steps to take if they occur.

Peptic Ulcer Disease: Patients with a history of active peptic ulcer disease should avoid using aspirin, which can cause gastric mucosal irritation and bleeding.

Precautions
General
Renal Failure: Avoid aspirin in patients with severe renal failure (glomerular filtration rate less than 10 mL/minute).

Hepatic Insufficiency: Avoid aspirin in patients with severe hepatic insufficiency.

Sodium Restricted Diets: Patients with sodium-retaining states, such as congestive heart failure or renal failure, should avoid sodium-containing buffered aspirin preparations because of their high sodium content.

Laboratory Tests: Aspirin has been associated with elevated hepatic enzymes, blood urea nitrogen and serum creatinine, hyperkalemia, proteinuria, and prolonged bleeding time.

Drug Interactions
Angiotensin Converting Enzyme (ACE) Inhibitors: The hyponatremic and hypotensive effects of ACE inhibitors may be diminished by the concomitant administration of aspirin due to its direct effect on the renin-angiotensin conversion pathway.

Acetazolamide: Concurrent use of aspirin and acetazolamide can lead to high serum concentrations of acetazolamide (and toxicity) due to competition at the renal tubule for secretion.

Anticoagulant Therapy (Heparin and Warfarin): Patients on anticoagulation therapy are at increased risk for bleeding because of drug-drug interactions and the effect on platelets. Aspirin can displace warfarin from protein binding sites, leading to prolongation of both the prothrombin time and the bleeding time. Aspirin can increase the anticoagulant activity of heparin, increasing bleeding risk.

Anticonvulsants: Salicylate can displace protein-bound phenytoin and valproic acid, leading to a decrease in the total concentration of phenytoin and an increase in serum valproic acid levels.

Beta Blockers: The hypotensive effects of beta blockers may be diminished by the concomitant administration of aspirin due to inhibition of renal prostaglandins, leading to decreased renal blood flow, and salt and fluid retention.

Diuretics: The effectiveness of diuretics in patients with underlying renal or cardiovascular disease may be diminished by the concomitant administration of aspirin due to inhibition of renal prostaglandins, leading to decreased renal blood flow and salt and fluid retention.

Methotrexate: Salicylate can inhibit renal clearance of methotrexate, leading to bone marrow toxicity, especially in the elderly or renal impaired.

Nonsteroidal Anti-inflammatory Drugs (NSAID's): The concurrent use of aspirin with other NSAID's should be

avoided because this may increase bleeding or lead to decreased renal function.

Oral Hypoglycemics: Moderate doses of aspirin may increase the effectiveness of oral hypoglycemic drugs, leading to hypoglycemia.

Uricosuric Agents (Probenecid and Sulfinpyrazone): Salicylates antagonize the uricosuric action of uricosuric agents.

Carcinogenesis, Mutagenesis, Impairment of Fertility: Administration of aspirin for 68 weeks at 0.5 percent in the feed of rats was not carcinogenic. In the Ames Salmonella assay, aspirin was not mutagenic; however, aspirin did induce chromosome aberrations in cultured human fibroblasts. Aspirin inhibits ovulation in rats. (See Pregnancy.)

Pregnancy: Pregnant women should only take aspirin if clearly needed. Because of the known effects of NSAID's on the fetal cardiovascular system (closure of the ductus arteriosus), use during the third trimester of pregnancy should be avoided. Salicylate products have also been associated with alterations in maternal and neonatal hemostasis mechanisms, decreased birth weight, and with perinatal mortality.

Labor and Delivery: Aspirin should be avoided 1 week prior to and during labor and delivery because it can result in excessive blood loss at delivery. Prolonged gestation and prolonged labor due to prostaglandin inhibition have been reported.

Nursing Mothers: Nursing mothers should avoid using aspirin because salicylate is excreted in breast milk. Use of high doses may lead to rashes, platelet abnormalities, and bleeding in nursing infants.

Pediatric Use: Pediatric dosing recommendations for juvenile rheumatoid arthritis are based on well-controlled clinical studies. An initial dose of 90–130 mg/kg/day in divided doses, with an increase as needed for anti-inflammatory efficacy (target plasma salicylate levels of 150–300 mcg/mL) are effective. At high doses (i.e., plasma levels of greater than 200 mg/mL), the incidence of toxicity increases.

Adverse Reactions: Many adverse reactions due to aspirin ingestion are dose-related. The following is a list of adverse reactions that have been reported in the literature. (See Warnings.)

Body as a Whole: Fever, hypothermia, thirst.

Cardiovascular: Dysrhythmias, hypotension, tachycardia.

Central Nervous System: Agitation, cerebral edema, coma, confusion, dizziness, headache, subdural or intracranial hemorrhage, lethargy, seizures.

Fluid and Electrolyte: Dehydration, hyperkalemia, metabolic acidosis, respiratory alkalosis.

Gastrointestinal: Dyspepsia, GI bleeding, ulceration and perforation, nausea,

Continued on next page

Ecotrin—Cont.

vomiting, transient elevations of hepatic enzymes, hepatitis, Reye's Syndrome, pancreatitis.
Hematologic: Prolongation of the prothrombin time, disseminated intravascular coagulation, coagulopathy, thrombocytopenia.
Hypersensitivity: Acute anaphylaxis, angioedema, asthma, bronchospasm, laryngeal edema, urticaria.
Musculoskeletal: Rhabdomyolysis.
Metabolism: Hypoglycemia (in children), hyperglycemia.
Reproductive: Prolonged pregnancy and labor, stillbirths, lower birth weight infants, antepartum and postpartum bleeding.
Respiratory: Hyperpnea, pulmonary edema, tachypnea.
Special Senses: Hearing loss, tinnitus. Patients with high frequency hearing loss may have difficulty perceiving tinnitus. In these patients, tinnitus cannot be used as a clinical indicator of salicylism.
Urogenital: Interstitial nephritis, papillary necrosis, proteinuria, renal insufficiency and failure.

Drug Abuse and Dependence: Aspirin is non-narcotic. There is no known potential for addiction associated with the use of aspirin.

Overdosage: Salicylate toxicity may result from acute ingestion (overdose) or chronic intoxication. The early signs of salicylic overdose (salicylism), including tinnitus (ringing in the ears), occur at plasma concentrations approaching 200 mcg/mL. Plasma concentrations of aspirin above 300 mcg/mL are clearly toxic. Severe toxic effects are associated with levels above 400 mcg/mL. (See Clinical Pharmacology.) A single lethal dose of aspirin in adults is not known with certainty but death may be expected at 30 g. For real or suspected overdose, a Poison Control Center should be contacted immediately. Careful medical management is essential.
Signs and Symptoms: In acute overdose, severe acid-base and electrolyte disturbances may occur and are complicated by hyperthermia and dehydration. Respiratory alkalosis occurs early while hyperventilation is present, but is quickly followed by metabolic acidosis.
Treatment: Treatment consists primarily of supporting vital functions, increasing salicylate elimination, and correcting the acid-base disturbance. Gastric emptying and/or lavage is recommended as soon as possible after ingestion, even if the patient has vomited spontaneously. After lavage and/or emesis, administration of activated charcoal, as a slurry, is beneficial, if less than 3 hours have passed since ingestion. Charcoal adsorption should not be employed prior to emesis and lavage.
Severity of aspirin intoxication is determined by measuring the blood salicylate level. Acid-base status should be closely followed with serial blood gas and serum pH measurements. Fluid and electrolyte balance should be maintained.
In severe cases, hyperthermia and hypovolemia are the major immediate threats to life. Children should be sponged with tepid water. Replacement fluid should be administered intravenously and augmented with correction of acidosis. Plasma electrolytes and pH should be monitored to promote alkaline diuresis of salicylate if renal function is normal. Infusion of glucose may be required to control hypoglycemia.
Hemodialysis and peritoneal dialysis can be performed to reduce the body drug content. In patients with renal insufficiency or in cases of life-threatening intoxication, dialysis is usually required. Exchange transfusion may be indicated in infants and young children.

Dosage and Administration: Each dose of aspirin should be taken with a full glass of water unless patient is fluid restricted. Anti-inflammatory and analgesic dosages should be individualized. When aspirin is used in high doses, the development of tinnitus may be used as a clinical sign of elevated plasma salicylate levels except in patients with high frequency hearing loss.
Ischemic Stroke and TIA: 50–325 mg once a day. Continue therapy indefinitely.
Suspected Acute MI: The initial dose of 160–162.5 mg is administered as soon as an MI is suspected. The maintenance dose of 160–162.5 mg a day is continued for 30 days post infarction. After 30 days, consider further therapy based on dosage and administration for prevention of recurrent MI.
Prevention of Recurrent MI: 75–325 mg once a day. Continue therapy indefinitely.
Unstable Angina Pectoris: 75–325 mg once a day. Continue therapy indefinitely.
Chronic Stable Angina Pectoris: 75–325 mg once a day. Continue therapy indefinitely.
CABG: 325 mg daily starting 6 hours post-procedure. Continue therapy for 1 year post-procedure.
PTCA: The initial dose of 325 mg should be given 2 hours pre-surgery. Maintenance dose is 160–325 mg daily. Continue therapy indefinitely.
Carotid Endarterectomy: Doses of 80 mg once daily to 650 mg twice daily, started presurgery, are recommended. Continue therapy indefinitely.
Rheumatoid Arthritis: The initial dose is 3 g a day in divided doses. Increase as needed for anti-inflammatory efficacy with target plasma salicylate levels of 150–300 mcg/mL. At high doses (i.e., plasma levels of greater than 200 mg/mL), the incidence of toxicity increases.
Juvenile Rheumatoid Arthritis: Initial dose is 90–130 mg/kg/day in divided doses. Increase as needed for anti-inflammatory efficacy with target plasma salicylate levels of 150–300 mcg/mL. At high doses (i.e., plasma levels of greater than 200 mg/mL), the incidence of toxicity increases.
Spondyloarthropathies: Up to 4 g per day in divided doses.
Osteoarthritis: Up to 3 g per day in divided doses.
Arthritis and Pleurisy of SLE: The initial dose is 3 g a day in divided doses. Increase as needed for anti-inflammatory efficacy with target plasma salicylate levels of 150–300 mcg/mL. At high doses (i.e., plasma levels of greater than 200 mg/mL), the incidence of toxicity increases.

How Supplied: 81 mg convex orange film coated tablet with ECOTRIN LOW printed in black ink on one side of the tablet. Available as follows
NDC 0108-0117-82 Bottle of 36 tablets
NDC 0108-0117-83 Bottle of 120 tablets
325 mg convex orange film coated tablet with ECOTRIN REG printed in black ink on one side of the tablet. Available as follows:
NDC 0108-0014-26 Bottle of 100 tablets
NDC 0108-0014-29 Bottle of 250 tablets
500 mg convex orange film coated tablet with ECOTRIN MAX printed in black ink on one side of the tablet. Available as follows:
NDC 0108-0016-23 Bottle of 60 tablets
NDC 0108-0016-27 Bottle of 150 tablets
Store in a tight container at 25°C (77° F); excursions permitted to 15–30° C (59–86° F).
Shown in Product Identification Guide, page 506

GAVISCON® Regular Strength Antacid Tablets
[găv 'ĭs-kŏn]

Composition: Each chewable tablet contains the following active ingredients: Aluminum hydroxide dried gel... 80 mg Magnesium trisilicate .... 20 mg and the following inactive ingredients: alginic acid, calcium stearate, flavor, sodium bicarbonate, starch (may contain corn starch), and sucrose.

Actions: Unique formulation produces soothing foam which floats on stomach contents. Foam containing antacid precedes stomach contents into the esophagus when reflux occurs to help protect the sensitive mucosa from further irritation. GAVISCON® acts locally without neutralizing entire stomach contents to help maintain integrity of the digestive process. Endoscopic studies indicate that GAVISCON Antacid Tablets are equally as effective in the erect or supine patient.

Indications: GAVISCON is specifically formulated for the temporary relief of heartburn (acid indigestion) due to acid reflux. GAVISCON is not indicated for the treatment of peptic ulcers.

Directions: Chew 2 to 4 tablets four times a day or as directed by a physician. Tablets should be taken after meals and

at bedtime or as needed. For best results follow by a half glass of water or other liquid. DO NOT SWALLOW WHOLE.

Warnings: Do not take more than 16 tablets in a 24-hour period or 16 tablets daily for more than 2 weeks, except under the advice and supervision of a physician. Do not use this product except under the advice and supervision of a physician if you are on a sodium-restricted diet. Each GAVISCON Tablet contains approximately 19 mg of sodium.

Drug Interaction Precaution: Antacids may interact with certain prescription drugs. If you are presently taking a prescription drug, do not take this product without checking with your physician or other health professional.
Store at a controlled room temperature in a dry place.

Keep this and all drugs out of the reach of children. In case of accidental overdose, seek professional assistance or contact a poison control center immediately.

How Supplied: Bottles of 100 tablets and in foil-wrapped 2s in boxes of 30 tablets.
Shown in Product Identification Guide, page 507

GAVISCON® EXTRA STRENGTH
Antacid Tablets
[găv 'ĭs-kŏn]

Composition: Each chewable tablet contains the following active ingredients:
Aluminum hydroxide .... 160 mg
Magnesium carbonate .... 105 mg
and the following inactive ingredients: alginic acid, calcium stearate, flavor, sodium bicarbonate, and sucrose. May contain stearic acid. Contains sorbitol or mannitol. May contain starch.

Actions: Gavison's unique antacid foam barrier neutralizes stomach acid.

Indications: For the relief of heartburn, sour stomach, acid indigestion and upset stomach associated with these conditions.

Directions: Chew 2 to 4 tablets four times a day or as directed by a physician. Tablets should be taken after meals and at bedtime or as needed. For best results follow by a half glass of water or other liquid. DO NOT SWALLOW WHOLE.

Warnings: Do not take more than 16 tablets in a 24-hour period or 16 tablets daily for more than 2 weeks, except under the advice and supervision of a physician. Do not use this product except under the advice and supervision of a physician if you are on a sodium-restricted diet. Each Extra Strength Gaviscon tablet contains approximately 19 mg of sodium.

Drug Interaction Precaution: Antacids may interact with certain prescription drugs. If you are presently taking a prescription drug, do not take this prod-

uct without checking with your physician or other health professional.

Store at a controlled room temperature in a dry place.

Keep this and all drugs out of the reach of children. In case of accidental overdose, seek professional assistance or contact a poison control center immediately.

How Supplied: Bottles of 100 tablets and in foil-wrapped 2s in boxes of 6 and 30 tablets.
Shown in Product Identification Guide, page 507

GAVISCON® Regular Strength
Liquid Antacid
[găv 'ĭs-kŏn]

Composition: Each tablespoonful (15 ml) contains the following active ingredients:
Aluminum hydroxide .... 95 mg
Magnesium carbonate .... 358 mg
and the following inactive ingredients: Benzyl alcohol, D&C Yellow #10, edetate disodium, FD&C Blue #1, flavor, glycerin, saccharin sodium, sodium alginate, sorbitol solution, water, and xanthan gum.

Actions: Gaviscon's unique antacid foam barrier neutralizes stomach acid.

Indications: For the relief of heartburn, sour stomach, acid indigestion and upset stomach associated with these conditions.

Directions: SHAKE WELL BEFORE USING. Take 1 or 2 tablespoonfuls four times a day or as directed by a physician. GAVISCON Regular Strength Liquid should be taken after meals and at bedtime. Dispense product only by spoon or other measuring device.

Warnings: Except under the advice and supervision of a physician, do not take more than 8 tablespoonfuls in a 24-hour period or 8 tablespoonfuls daily for more than 2 weeks. May have laxative effect. Do not use this product if you have a kidney disease. Do not use this product if you are on a sodium-restricted diet except under the advice and supervision of a physician. Each tablespoonful of GAVISCON Regular Strength Liquid contains approximately 1.7 mEq sodium.

Keep this and all drugs out of the reach of children. In case of accidental overdose, seek professional assistance or contact a poison control center immediately.

Drug Interaction Precaution: Antacids may interact with certain prescription drugs. If you are presently taking a prescription drug, do not take this product without checking with your physician or other health professional.

Keep tightly closed. Avoid freezing. Store at a controlled room temperature.

How Supplied: 12 fluid oz (355 ml) bottles.
Shown in Product Identification Guide, page 507

GAVISCON® EXTRA STRENGTH
Liquid Antacid
[găv 'ĭs-kŏn]

Composition: Each 2 teaspoonfuls (10 mL) contains the following active ingredients:
Aluminum hydroxide .... 508 mg
Magnesium carbonate .... 475 mg
and the following inactive ingredients: Benzyl alcohol, edetate disodium, flavor, glycerin, saccharin sodium, simethicone emulsion, sodium alginate, sorbitol solution, water, and xanthan gum.

Actions: Gaviscon's unique antacid foam barrier neutralizes stomach acid.

Indications: For the relief of heartburn, sour stomach, acid indigestion and upset stomach associated with these conditions.

Directions: SHAKE WELL BEFORE USING. Take 2 to 4 teaspoonfuls four times a day or as directed by a physician. GAVISCON Extra Strength Liquid should be taken after meals and at bedtime. Dispense product only by spoon or other measuring device.

Warnings: Except under the advice and supervision of a physician, do not take more than 16 teaspoonfuls in a 24-hour period or 16 teaspoonfuls daily for more than 2 weeks. May have laxative effect. Do not use this product if you have a kidney disease. Do not use this product if you are on a sodium-restricted diet except under the advice and supervision of a physician. Each teaspoonful contains approximately 0.9 mEq sodium.

Keep this and all drugs out of the reach of children. In case of accidental overdose, seek professional assistance or contact a poison control center immediately.

Drug Interaction Precaution: Antacids may interact with certain prescription drugs. If you are presently taking a prescription drug, do not take this product without checking with your physician or other health professional.

Keep tightly closed. Avoid freezing. Store at a controlled room temperature.

How Supplied: 12 fl oz (355 mL) bottles.
Shown in Product Identification Guide, page 507

GLY-OXIDE® Liquid

Description/Active Ingredient: GLY-OXIDE® Liquid contains carbamide peroxide 10%.

Actions: Gly-Oxide is specially formulated to release peroxide and oxygen bubbles in your mouth. The peroxide and oxygen-rich microfoam help:
• gently remove unhealthy tissue, then cleanse and soothe canker sores and minor wounds and inflammations so natural healing can better occur.

Continued on next page

Gly-Oxide—Cont.

- kill odor-forming germs.
- foam and flush out food particles ordinary brushing can miss.
- clean stains from orthodontics/dentures/bridgework/etc. better than brushing alone.

Indications For Temporary Use: Gly-Oxide liquid is for temporary use in cleansing canker sores and minor wound or gum inflammation resulting from minor dental procedures, dentures, orthodontic appliances, accidental injury, or other irritations of the mouth and gums. Gly-Oxide can also be used to guard against the risk of infections in the mouth and gums.

Everyday Uses: Gly-Oxide may be used routinely to improve oral hygiene as an aid to regular brushing or when regular brushing is inadequate or impossible such as total care geriatrics, etc. Gly-Oxide kills germs to reduce mouth odors and/or odors on dental appliances. Gly-Oxide penetrates between teeth and other areas of the mouth to flush out food particles ordinary brushing can miss. This can be especially useful when brushing is made more difficult by the presence of orthodontics or other dental appliances. Plus, Gly-Oxide helps remove stains on dental appliances to improve appearance.

Directions For Temporary Use: Do not dilute. Replace tip on bottle when not in use. **Adults and children 2 years of age and older:** Apply several drops directly from bottle onto affected area; spit out after 2 to 3 minutes. Use up to four times daily after meals and at bedtime or as directed by dentist or doctor. OR place 10 drops on tongue, mix with saliva, swish for several minutes, and then spit out. Use by children under 12 years of age should be supervised. **Children under 2 years of age:** Consult a dentist or doctor.

Directions For Everyday Use: The product may be used following the temporary use directions above. OR apply Gly-Oxide to the toothbrush (it will sink into the brush), cover with toothpaste, brush normally, and spit out.

Warnings: Severe or persistent oral inflammation, denture irritation, or gingivitis may be serious. If sore mouth symptoms do not improve in 7 days, or if irritation, pain, or redness persists or worsens, or if swelling, rash, or fever develops, discontinue use of product and see your dentist or doctor promptly. Avoid contact with eyes. **KEEP THIS AND ALL DRUGS OUT OF THE REACH OF CHILDREN.** In case of accidental overdose, seek professional assistance or contact a poison control center immediately.

Inactive Ingredients: Citric Acid, Flavor, Glycerin, Propylene Glycol, Sodium Stannate, Water, and Other Ingredients.

Protect from excessive heat and direct sunlight.

How Supplied: GLY-OXIDE® Liquid is available in $\frac{1}{2}$-fl-oz and 2-fl-oz plastic squeeze bottles with applicator spouts. Comments or Questions? Call Toll-free 1-800-245-1040 Weekdays SmithKline Beecham Consumer Healthcare, L.P.
Pittsburgh, PA 15230   Made in U.S.A.
Shown in Product Identification Guide, page 507

GOODY'S
Body Pain Formula Powder

Indications: For temporary relief of minor body aches & pains due to muscular aches, arthritis & headaches.

Directions: Adults: Place one powder on tongue and follow with liquid, or stir powder into a glass of water or other liquid. May be repeated in 4 to 6 hours. Do not take more than 4 powders in any 24-hour period. Children under 12 years of age: Consult a doctor.

Warnings: Children and teenagers should not use this medicine for chicken pox or flu symptoms before a doctor is consulted about Reye's Syndrome, a rare but serious illness reported to be associated with aspirin. Do not use with any other product containing acetaminophen. **Ask a doctor before use if you have** asthma, ulcers, a bleeding problem, stomach problems that last or come back such as heartburn, upset stomach or pain. **Ask a doctor or pharmacist before use if** you are taking a prescription drug for gout, diabetes, arthritis or anticoagulation (blood thinning). **Stop use and ask a doctor if** an allergic reaction occurs, ringing in ears or loss of hearing occurs, pain gets worse or persists for more than 10 days, fever lasts more than 3 days, redness or swelling is present, or new symptoms occur. As with any drug, if you are pregnant, or nursing a baby, seek the advice of a health professional before using this product.
IT IS ESPECIALLY IMPORTANT NOT TO USE ASPIRIN DURING THE LAST 3 MONTHS OF PREGNANCY UNLESS SPECIFICALLY DIRECTED TO DO SO BY A DOCTOR BECAUSE IT MAY CAUSE PROBLEMS IN THE UNBORN CHILD OR COMPLICATIONS DURING DELIVERY.
Alcohol Warning: If you consume 3 or more alcoholic drinks every day, ask your doctor whether you should take acetaminophen and aspirin or other pain relievers/fever reducers. Acetaminophen and aspirin may cause liver damage and stomach bleeding.
Keep this and all medicines out of the reach of children. Overdose warning: Taking more than the recommended dose can cause serious health problems. In case of overdose, contact a doctor or poison control center immediately.

Active ingredients: Each powder contains: 500 mg. aspirin and 325 mg. acetaminophen.

Inactive Ingredients: Each powder contains: Lactose Monohydrate and Potassium Chloride.

GOODY'S®
Extra Strength Headache Powder

Indications: For Temporary Relief of Minor Aches & Pains Due to Headaches, Arthritis, Colds & Fever

Directions: Adults: Place one powder on tongue and follow with liquid or stir powder into a glass of water or other liquid. May be repeated in 4 to 6 hours. Do not take more than 4 powders in any 24-hour period. Children under 12 years of age: Consult a doctor.

Warnings: Children and teenagers should not use this medicine for chicken pox or flu symptoms before a doctor is consulted about Reye's Syndrome, a rare but serious illness reported to be associated with aspirin. Do not use with any other product containing acetaminophen. **Ask a doctor before use if you have** asthma, ulcers, a bleeding problem, stomach problems that last or come back such as heartburn, upset stomach or pain. **Ask a doctor or pharmacist before use if** you are taking a prescription drug for gout, diabetes, arthritis or anticoagulation (blood thinning). **When using this product** limit the use of caffeine containing drugs, foods, or drinks, because too much caffeine may cause nervousness, irritability, sleeplessness, and occasionally, rapid heartbeat. **Stop use and ask a doctor if** an allergic reaction occurs, ringing in ears or loss of hearing occurs, pain gets worse or persists for more than 10 days, fever lasts for more than 3 days, redness or swelling is present, or new symptoms occur. As with any drug, if you are pregnant, or nursing a baby, seek the advice of a health professional before using this product.
IT IS ESPECIALLY IMPORTANT NOT TO USE ASPIRIN DURING THE LAST 3 MONTHS OF PREGNANCY UNLESS SPECIFICALLY DIRECTED TO DO SO BY A DOCTOR BECAUSE IT MAY CAUSE PROBLEMS IN THE UNBORN CHILD OR COMPLICATIONS DURING DELIVERY.
Alcohol Warning: If you consume 3 or more alcoholic drinks every day, ask your doctor whether you should take acetaminophen and aspirin or other pain relievers/fever reducers. Acetaminophen and aspirin may cause liver damage and stomach bleeding. **Keep this and all medicines out of the reach of children. Overdose warning:** Taking more than the recommended dose can cause serious health problems. In case of overdose, contact a doctor or poison control center immediately.

Active Ingredients: Each Powder contains 520 mg. aspirin in combination with 260 mg. acetaminophen and 32.5 mg. caffeine.

Inactive Ingredients: Lactose Monohydrate and Potassium Chloride.

GOODY'S®
Extra Strength Pain Relief Tablets

Indications: Goody's EXTRA STRENGTH tablets are a specially developed pain reliever that provide fast & effective temporary relief from minor aches & pain due to headaches, arthritis, colds or "flu," muscle strain, backache & menstrual discomfort. It is recommended for temporary relief of toothaches and to reduce fever.

Dosage: Adults: Two tablets with water or other liquid. May be repeated in 4 to 6 hours. Do not take more than 8 tablets in any 24-hour period. Children under 12 years of age: Consult a doctor.

Warnings: Children and teenagers should not use this medicine for chicken pox or flu symptoms before a doctor is consulted about Reye's Syndrome, a rare but serious illness reported to be associated with aspirin. Do not use with any other product containing acetaminophen. **Ask a doctor before use if you have** asthma, ulcers, a bleeding problem, stomach problems that last or come back such as heartburn, upset stomach or pain. **Ask a doctor or pharmacist before use** if you are taking a prescription drug for gout, diabetes, arthritis or anticoagulation (blood thinning) **When using this product** limit the use of caffeine containing drugs, foods, or drinks, because too much caffeine may cause nervousness, irritability, sleeplessness, and occasionally, rapid heartbeat. **Stop use and ask a doctor if** an allergic reaction occurs, ringing in ears or loss of hearing occurs, pain gets worse or persists for more than 10 days, fever lasts more than 3 days, redness or swelling is present, or new symptoms occur.

As with any drug, if you are pregnant, or nursing a baby, seek the advice of a health professional before using this product. IT IS ESPECIALLY IMPORTANT NOT TO USE ASPIRIN DURING THE LAST 3 MONTHS OF PREGNANCY UNLESS SPECIFICALLY DIRECTED TO DO SO BY A DOCTOR BECAUSE IT MAY CAUSE PROBLEMS IN THE UNBORN CHILD OR COMPLICATIONS DURING DELIVERY. **Alcohol Warning:** If you consume 3 or more alcoholic drinks every day, ask your doctor whether you should take acetaminophen and aspirin or other pain relievers/ fever reducers. Acetaminophen and aspirin may cause liver damage and stomach bleeding. **Keep this and all medicines out of the reach of children. Overdose warning:** Taking more than the recommended dose can cause serious health problems. In case of overdose, contact a doctor or poison control center immediately.

Active Ingredients: Each tablet contains 260 mg. aspirin in combination with 130 mg. acetaminophen and 16.25 mg. caffeine. **Inactive Ingredients:** Corn Starch, Crospovidone, Povidone, Pregelatinized Starch and Stearic Acid.

GOODY'S PM® POWDER
For Pain with Sleeplessness

Indications: For temporary relief of occasional headaches and minor aches and pains with accompanying sleeplessness.

Directions: Adults and children 12 years of age and older: One dose (2 powders). Take both powders at bedtime, if needed, or as directed by a doctor. Place powders on tongue and follow with liquid. If you prefer, stir powders into glass of water or other liquid.

Warnings: Keep this and all medicines out of the reach of children. Overdose Warning: Taking more than the recommended dose can cause serious health problems. In case of accidental overdose, contact a doctor or poison control center immediately. Prompt medical attention is critical for adults as well as for children even if you do not notice any signs or symptoms.
As with any drug, if you are pregnant or nursing a baby, seek the advice of a health professional before using this product. Do not give this product to children under 12 years of age. Do not use for more than 10 days or for fever for more than 3 days unless directed by a doctor. Consult your doctor if redness or swelling is present, symptoms persist or get worse or new ones occur. If sleeplessness persists continuously for more than 2 weeks consult your doctor. Insomnia may be a symptom of serious underlying medical illness. Do not take this product, unless directed by a doctor, if you have a breathing problem such as emphysema or chronic bronchitis or if you have glaucoma or difficulty in urination due to enlargement of the prostate gland. **Do Not Use** with any other product containing diphenhydramine, including one applied topically, or with any other product containing acetaminophen. Avoid alcoholic beverages while taking this product. Do not use this product if you are taking sedatives or tranquilizers without first consulting your doctor. **Alcohol Warning:** If you consume 3 or more alcoholic drinks every day, ask your doctor whether you should take acetaminophen or other pain relievers/fever reducers. Acetaminophen may cause liver damage.

Caution: This product will cause drowsiness. Do not drive a motor vehicle or operate machinery after use.

Active Ingredients: Each powder contains 500 mg. Acetaminophen and 38 mg. Diphenhydramine Citrate.

Inactive Ingredients: Citric Acid, Docusate Sodium, Fumaric Acid, Glycine, Lactose Monohydrate, Magnesium Stearate, Potassium Chloride, Silica Gel, Sodium Citrate Dihydrate.

MASSENGILL®
[*mas 'sen-gil*]
Baby Powder Scent Soft Cloth Towelette

Ingredients: Purified Water, Octoxynol-9, Lactic Acid, Disodium Edta, Fragrance, Potassium Sorbate, Cetylpyridinium Chloride, and Sodium Bicarbonate.

Indications: For cleansing and refreshing the external vaginal area.

Actions: Massengill Baby Powder Scent Soft Cloth Towelette safely cleanse the external vaginal area. The towelette delivery system makes the application soft and gentle.

Directions: Remove towelette from foil packet, unfold, and gently wipe from front to back. After towelette has been used once, return towelette to foil packet and throw it away. Safe to use daily as often as needed. For external use only.

How Supplied: 50 individually sealed soft cloth towelettes per carton. Comments, questions or for information about STD's and vaginal health, call toll free 1-800-245-1040 weekdays.

MASSENGILL Feminine Cleansing Wash, Floral
[*mas 'sen-gil*]

Ingredients: Purified Water, sodium laureth sulfate, magnesium laureth sulfate, sodium laureth-8 sulfate, magnesium laureth-8 sulfate, sodium oleth sulfate, magnesium oleth sulfate, lauramidopropyl betaine, myristamine oxide, lactic acid, PEG-120 methyl glucose dioleate, fragrance, sodium methylparaben, sodium ethylparaben, sodium propylparaben, methylchloroisothiazolinone, methylisothiazolinone, D&C Red #33.

Indications: For cleansing and refreshing of external vaginal area.

Actions: Massengill feminine cleansing wash safely and gently cleanses the external vaginal area.

Directions: Pour small amount into palm of hand or wash cloth and lather into wet skin. Rinse clean. Safe to use daily. For external use only.

How Supplied: 8 fl. oz plastic flip-top bottle.

> ### EDUCATIONAL MATERIAL

"The facts about Vaginal Infections and STDs"
A guide for women on vaginal infections and sexually transmitted diseases (STDs).

Continued on next page

Massengil Educ.—Cont.

Free to physicians, pharmacists and patients in limited quantities by writing GlaxoSmithKline Consumer Healthcare, L.P. PO Box 1469, Pittsburgh, PA 15230 or calling 1-800-366-8900. GlaxoSmithKline Consumer Healthcare, L.P.
1000 GSK Drive
Moon Township, PA 15108

NATURE'S REMEDY®
Nature's Gentle Laxative

Description: Nature's Remedy® is a stimulant laxative with an active ingredient, Sennosides, that gently stimulates the body's natural function.

Indication: For relief of occasional constipation. Nature's Remedy tablets generally produce bowel movement in 6 to 12 hours.

Active Ingredients:
(in each tablet): **Purpose:**
Sennosides, USP,
  8.6 mg .... Stimulant laxative

Inactive Ingredients: FD&C blue #2 aluminum lake, FD&C yellow #6 aluminum lake, hydroxypropyl cellulose, hydroxypropyl methylcellulose, lactose, microcrystalline cellulose, polyethylene glycol, pregelatinized starch, silicon dioxide stearic acid, titanium dioxide

Directions:
[See table below]

Warnings: Keep out of reach of children. Do not use laxative products when abdominal pain, nausea, or vomiting are present unless directed by a doctor. If you have noticed a sudden change in bowel habits that persists over a period of 2 weeks, consult a doctor before using a laxative. Laxative products should not be used for a period longer than 1 week unless directed by a doctor. Rectal bleeding or failure to have a bowel movement after use of a laxative may indicate a serious condition. Discontinue use and consult your doctor. In case of accidental overdose, seek professional assistance or contact a Poison Control Center immediately. As with any drug, if you are pregnant or nursing a baby, seek the advice of a health professional before using this product.

Adults and children 12 years of age and over	2 Tablets once or twice daily with water, not to exceed 4 tablets twice a day
Children 6 to under 12 years of age	1 Tablet once or twice daily with water, not to exceed 2 tablets twice a day
Children 2 to under 6 years of age	1/2 Tablet once or twice daily with water, not to exceed 1 tablet twice a day
Children under 2 years of age	Consult a doctor

Store at room temperature, avoid excessive heat (greater than 100°F) or high humidity.

How Supplied: Beige, film-coated tablets with foil-backed blister packaging in boxes of 15, 30 and 60.
Shown in Product Identification Guide, page 507

NICODERM® CQ®
Nicotine Transdermal System/Stop Smoking Aid

Formerly available only by prescription
Available as:

  Step 1 - 21 mg/24 hours
  Step 2 - 14 mg/24 hours
  Step 3 - 7 mg/24 hours

If you smoke:
More than 10 Cigarettes per Day: Start with Step 1
10 Cigarettes a Day or Less: Start with Step 2

WHAT IS THE NICODERM CQ PATCH AND HOW IS IT USED?

NicoDerm CQ is a small, nicotine containing patch. When you put on a NicoDerm CQ patch, nicotine passes through the skin and into your body. NicoDerm CQ is very thin and uses special material to control how fast nicotine passes through the skin. Unlike the sudden jolts of nicotine delivered by cigarettes, the amount of nicotine you receive remains relatively smooth throughout the 24 or 16 hours period you wear the NicoDerm CQ patch. This helps to reduce cravings you may have for nicotine.

Active Ingredient: Nicotine

Purpose: Stop Smoking Aid

Use: reduces withdrawal symptoms, including nicotine craving, associated with quitting smoking

Directions:
* **if you are under 18 years of age, ask a doctor before use**
* before using this product, read the enclosed user's guide for complete directions and other information
* stop smoking completely when you begin using the patch
* **if you smoke more than 10 cigarettes per day,** use according to the following 10 week schedule:

STEP 1	STEP 2	STEP 3
Use one 21 mg patch/day	Use one 14 mg patch/day	Use one 7 mg patch/day
Weeks 1–6	Weeks 7–8	Weeks 9–10

* if you smoke **10 or less cigarettes per day,** do not use **STEP 1 (21 mg)**. Start with **STEP 2 (14 mg)** for 6 weeks, then **STEP 3 (7 mg)** for two weeks and then stop.
* steps 2 and 3 allow you to gradually reduce your level of nicotine. Completing the full program will increase your chances of quitting successfully.
* apply one new patch every 24 hours on skin that is dry, clean and hairless
* remove backing from patch and immediately press onto skin. Hold for 10 seconds.
* wash hands after applying or removing patch. Throw away the patch in the enclosed disposal tray. See enclosed user's guide for safety and handling.
* you may wear the patch for 16 or 24 hours
* if you crave cigarettes when you wake up, wear the patch for 24 hours
* if you have vivid dreams or other sleep disturbances, you may remove the patch at bedtime and apply a new one in the morning
* the used patch should be removed and a new one applied to a different skin site at the same time each day
* do not wear more than one patch at a time
* do not cut patch in half or into smaller pieces
* do not leave patch on for more than 24 hours because it may irritate your skin and loses strength after 24 hours
* stop using the patch at the end of 10 weeks. If you started with **STEP 2**, stop using the patch at the end of 8 weeks. If you still feel the need to use the patch talk to your doctor.

Warnings:
If you are pregnant or breast-feeding, only use this medicine on the advice of your health care provider. Smoking can seriously harm your child. Try to stop smoking without using any nicotine replacement medicine. This medicine is believed to be safer than smoking. However, the risks to your child from this medicine are not fully known.
Do Not Use
* if you continue to smoke, chew tobacco, use snuff, or use a nicotine gum or other nicotine containing products
Ask a doctor before use if you have
* heart disease, recent heart attack, or irregular heartbeat. Nicotine can increase your heart rate.
* high blood pressure not controlled with medication. Nicotine can increase your blood pressure.
* an allergy to adhesive tape or skin problems because you are more likely to get rashes
Ask a doctor or pharmacist before use if you are
* using a non-nicotine stop smoking drug
* taking a prescription medication for depression or asthma. Your prescription dose may need to be adjusted.

When using this product
- do not smoke even when not wearing the patch. The nicotine in your skin will still be entering your blood stream for several hours after you take off the patch.
- if you have vivid dreams or other sleep disturbances remove this patch at bedtime

Stop use and ask a doctor if
- skin redness caused by the patch does not go away after four days, or if skin swells, or you get a rash
- irregular heartbeat or palpitations occur
- you get symptoms of nicotine overdose such as nausea, vomiting, dizziness, weakness and rapid heartbeat

Keep out of reach of children and pets. Used patches have enough nicotine to poison children and pets. If swallowed, get medical help or contact a Poison Control Center right away. Dispose of the used patches by folding sticky ends together and inserting in disposal tray in this box.

READ THE LABEL
Read the carton and the User's Guide before using this product. Keep the carton and User's Guide. They contain important information.

Inactive Ingredients: Ethylene vinyl acetate-copolymer, polyisobutylene and high density polyethylene between pigmented and clear polyester backings. Store at 20–25°C (68–77°F)

TO INCREASE YOUR SUCCESS IN QUITTING:
1. You must be motivated to quit.
2. Complete the full treatment program, applying a new patch every day.
3. Use with a support program as described in the Users Guide.

NicoDerm CQ User's Guide
KEYS TO SUCCESS
1) You must really want to quit smoking for **NicoDerm® CQ®** to help you.
2) Complete the full program, applying a new patch every day.
3) **NicoDerm CQ** works best when used together with a support program: See page 3 for details.
4) If you have trouble using **NicoDerm CQ**, ask your doctor or pharmacist or call GlaxoSmithKline 1-800-834-5895 weekdays (10:00 am 4:30 pm EST).

SO, YOU'VE DECIDED TO QUIT.
Congratulations. Your decision to stop smoking is one of the most important things you can do to improve your health. Quitting smoking is a two-part process that involves:
1) overcoming your physical need for nicotine, and
2) breaking your smoking habit.

NicoDerm CQ helps smokers quit by reducing nicotine withdrawal symptoms.

Many NicoDerm CQ users will be able to stop smoking for a few days but often will start smoking again. Most smokers have to try to quit several times before they completely stop.

Your own chances of quitting smoking depend on how strongly you are addicted to nicotine, how much you want to quit, and how closely you follow a quitting plan like the one that comes with NicoDerm CQ.

QUITTING SMOKING IS HARD!
If you find you cannot stop or if you start smoking again after using NicoDerm CQ please talk to a health care professional who can help you find a program that may work better for you. Breaking this addiction doesn't happen overnight.
Because NicoDerm CQ provides some nicotine, the NicoDerm CQ patch will help you stop smoking by reducing nicotine withdrawal symptoms such as nicotine craving, nervousness and irritability.
This User's Guide will give you support as you become a non-smoker. It will answer common questions about NicoDerm CQ and give tips to help you stop smoking, and should be referred to often.

WHERE TO GET HELP.
You are more likely to stop smoking by using NicoDerm CQ with a support program that helps you break your smoking habit. There may be support groups in your area for people trying to quit. Call your local chapter of the American Lung Association, American Cancer Society or American Heart Association for further information. Toll free phone numbers are printed on the wallet card on the back cover of this User's Guide.
If you find you cannot stop smoking or if you start smoking again after using NicoDerm CQ, remember breaking this addiction doesn't happen overnight. You may want to talk to a health care professional who can help you improve your chances of quitting the next time you try NicoDerm CQ or another method.

LET'S GET ORGANIZED.
Your reason for quitting may be a combination of concerns about health, the effect of smoking on your appearance, and pressure from your family and friends to stop smoking. Or maybe you're concerned about the dangerous effect of second-hand smoke on the people you care about.
All of these are good reasons. You probably have others. Decide your most important reasons, and write them down on the wallet card inside the back cover of this User's Guide. Carry this card with you. In difficult moments, when you want to smoke, the card will remind you why you are quitting.

WHAT YOU'RE UP AGAINST.
Smoking is addictive in two ways. Your need for nicotine has become both physical and mental. You must overcome both addictions to stop smoking. So while NicoDerm CQ will lessen your body's craving for nicotine, you've got to want to quit smoking to overcome the mental dependence on cigarettes. Once you've decided that you're going to quit, it's time to get started. But first, there are some important cautions you should consider.

SOME IMPORTANT WARNINGS.
This product is only for those who want to stop smoking.

Do not use
- if you continue to smoke, chew tobacco, use snuff or use a nicotine gum or other nicotine products.

Ask a doctor before use if you have:
- heart disease, recent heart attack, or irregular heartbeat, Nicotine can increase your heart rate.
- high blood pressure not controlled with medication. Nicotine can increase your blood pressure.
- an allergy to adhesive tape or have skin problems because you are more likely to get rashes.

Ask a doctor or pharmacist before use if you are
- using a non-nicotine stop smoking drug
- taking a prescription medication for asthma or depression. Your prescription dose may need to be adjusted.

When using this product:
- do not smoke even when not wearing the patch. The nicotine in your skin will still be entering your bloodstream for several hours after you take off the patch.
- you have vivid dreams or other sleep disturbances remove this patch at bedtime.

Stop use and ask a doctor if:
- skin redness caused by the patch does not go away after four days, or if your skin swells or you get a rash.
- irregular heartbeat or palpitations occur
- you get symptoms of nicotine overdose, such as nausea, vomiting, dizziness, weakness and rapid heartbeat.

If you are pregnant or breast-feeding, only use this medicine on the advice of your health care provider. Smoking can seriously harm your child. Try to stop smoking without using any nicotine replacement medicine. This medicine is believed to be safer than smoking. However, the risks to your child from this medicine are not fully known.

Keep out of reach of children and pets. Used patches have enough nicotine to poison children and pets. If swallowed, get medical help or contact a Poison Control Center right away. Dispose of the used patches by folding sticky ends together and inserting in the disposal tray in this box.

LET'S GET STARTED.
If you are under 18 years of age, ask a doctor before use.
Becoming a non-smoker starts today. Your first step is to read through this entire User's Guide carefully.
First, check that you bought the right starting dose.
If you smoke more than 10 cigarettes a day, begin with Step 1 (21 mg). As the carton indicates, people who smoke 10 or less cigarettes per day should not use Step 1 (21 mg). They should start with Step 2 (14 mg). Throughout this User's Guide we will give specific instructions for people who smoke 10 or less cigarettes per day.
Next, set your personalized quitting schedule.
Take out a calendar that you can use to track your progress. Pick a quit date, and mark this on your calendar using the stickers in the middle of this User's Guide, as described below.

Continued on next page

Nicoderm CQ—Cont.

DIRECTIONS: FOR PEOPLE WHO SMOKE MORE THAN 10 CIGARETTES PER DAY

STEP 1. **(Weeks 1–6). Your quit date (and the day you'll start using NicoDerm CQ patch).**

Choose your quit date (it should be soon).

This is the day you will quit smoking cigarettes entirely and begin using NicoDerm CQ to reduce your cravings for nicotine. Place the Step 1 sticker on this date. For the first six weeks, you'll use the highest-strength (21 mg) NicoDerm CQ patches. Be sure to follow the directions on page 10.

Completing the full program will increase your chances of quitting successfully. This is done by changing over to the Step 2 (14mg) patch for 2 weeks followed by a final 2 weeks with the Step 3 (7mg) patch. The Step 2 and Step 3 treatment periods allow you to gradually reduce the amount of nicotine you get, rather than stopping suddenly, and will increase your chances of quitting.

STEP 2. **(Weeks 7–8). The day you'll start reducing your use of NicoDerm CQ patch.**

Switching to Step 2 (14mg) patches after 6 weeks begins to gradually reduce your nicotine usage. Place the Step 2 sticker on this date (the first day of week seven). Use the 14mg patches for two weeks.

STEP 3. **(Weeks 9–10). The day you'll further start reducing your use of Nico-Derm CQ patch.**

After eight weeks, nicotine intake is further reduced by moving down to Step 3 (7mg) patches. Place the Step 3 sticker on this date (the first day of week nine). Use the 7 mg patches for two weeks.

THE NICODERM CQ PROGRAM

STEP 1	STEP 2	STEP 3
Use one 21 mg patch/day Weeks 1–6	Use one 14 mg patch/day Weeks 7–8	Use one 7 mg patch/day Weeks 9–10

STOP USING NICODERM CQ AT THE END OF WEEK 10. If you still feel the need to use the patch after Week 10, talk with your doctor or health professional.

DIRECTIONS: FOR PEOPLE WHO SMOKE 10 OR LESS CIGARETTES PER DAY

Do not use Step 1 (21 mg).

Begin with STEP 2 – Initial Treatment Period (Weeks 1–6): 14mg patches.

Choose our quit date (it should be soon). This is the Day you will quit smoking cigarettes entirely and begin using NicoDerm CQ to reduce your cravings for nicotine. Place the Step 2 sticker on this date. For the first six weeks, you'll use the Step 2 (14mg) NicoDerm CQ patches. Be sure to follow the directions on page 10.

Continue with STEP 3 – Step Down Treatment Period (Weeks 7–8): 7mg patches.

Completing the full program will increase your chances of quitting successfully. This is done by changing over to the Step 3 (7mg) patches for 2 weeks. The two week step down treatment period allows you to gradually reduce the amount of nicotine you get, rather than stopping suddenly, and will increase your chances of quitting. Place the Step 3 sticker on the first day of week seven. Use the 7mg patches for two weeks. People who smoke 10 or less cigarettes per day should not use NicoDerm CQ for longer than 8 weeks. If you still feel the need to use NicoDerm CQ after 8 weeks, talk with your doctor.

PLAN AHEAD.

Because smoking is an addiction, it is not easy to stop. After you've given up nicotine, you may still have a strong urge to smoke. Plan ahead NOW for these times, so you're not tempted to start smoking again in a moment of weakness. The following tips may help:

• Keep the phone numbers of supportive friends and family members handy.
• Keep a record of your quitting process. Track whether you feel a craving for cigarettes. In the event that you slip, immediately stop smoking and resume your quit attempt with the NicoDerm CQ patch. If you smoke at all, write down what you think caused the slip.
• Put together an Emergency Kit that includes items that will help take your mind off occasional urges to smoke. You might include cinnamon gum or lemon drops to suck on, a relaxing cassette tape, and something for your hands to play with, like a smooth rock, rubber band or small metal balls.
• Set aside some small rewards, like a new magazine or a gift certificate from your favorite store, which you'll "give" yourself after passing difficult hurdles.
• Think now about the times when you most often want a cigarette, and then plan what else you might do instead of smoking. For instance, you might plan to take your coffee break in a new location, or take a walk right after dinner, so you won't be tempted to smoke.

HOW NICODERM CQ WORKS.

NicoDerm CQ patches provide nicotine to your system. They work as a temporary aid to help you quit smoking by reducing nicotine withdrawal symptoms, including nicotine craving. NicoDerm CQ provides a lower level of nicotine to your blood than cigarettes, and allows you to gradually do away with your body's need for nicotine.

Because NicoDerm CQ does not contain the tar or carbon monoxide of cigarette smoke, it does not have the same health dangers as tobacco. However, it still delivers nicotine, the addictive part of cigarette smoke. Nicotine can cause side effects such as headache, nausea, upset stomach, and dizziness.

HOW TO USE NICODERM CQ PATCHES.

Read all the following instructions, and the instructions on the outer carton, before using NicoDerm CQ. Refer to them often to make sure you're using NicoDerm CQ correctly. Please refer to the CD for additional help.

1) Stop smoking completely before you start using NicoDerm CQ.
2) To reduce nicotine craving and other withdrawal symptoms, use NicoDerm CQ according to the directions on pages 6–8.
3) Insert used NicoDerm CQ patches in the child resistant disposal tray provided in the box – safely away from children and pets.

When to apply and remove NicoDerm CQ patches.

Each day apply a new patch to a different place on skin that is dry, clean and hairless. **You can wear a NicoDerm CQ patch for either 16 or 24 hours.** If you crave cigarettes when you wake up, wear the patch for 24 hours. If you begin to have vivid dreams or other disruptions of your sleep while wearing the patch 24 hours, try taking the patch off at bedtime (after about 16 hours) and putting on a new one when you get up the next day.

PLACE THESE STICKERS ON YOUR CALENDAR

STEP 1	STEP 2
A new 21 mg patch every day AT THE BEGINNING OF WEEK #1 (QUIT DAY)	A new 14 mg patch every day AT THE BEGINNING OF WEEK #7

For people who smoke 10 or less cigarettes per day: Do not use STEP 1 (21 mg). Use STEP 2 (14 mg) at the beginning of week #1 and STEP 3 (7 mg) at the beginning of week #7.

PLACE THESE STICKERS ON YOUR CALENDAR

STEP 3	EX-SMOKER
A new 7 mg patch every day AT THE BEGINNING OF WEEK #9	WHEN YOU HAVE COMPLETED YOUR QUITTING PROGRAM

Do not smoke even when you are not wearing the patch.

Remove the used patch and put on a new patch at the same time every day. Applying the patch at about the same time each day (first thing in the morning, for instance) will help you remember when to put on a new patch. Do not leave the same NicoDerm CQ patch on for more than 24 hours because it may irritate your skin and because it loses strength after 24 hours.

Do not use NicoDerm CQ continuously for more than 10 weeks (8 weeks for people who smoke 10 or less cigarettes per day).

How to apply a NicoDerm CQ patch.

1. Do not remove the NicoDerm CQ patch from its sealed protective pouch until you are ready to use it. NicoDerm CQ patches will lose nicotine to the air if you store them out of the pouch.
2. Choose a non-hairy, clean, dry area of skin. Do not put a NicoDerm CQ patch on skin that is burned, broken out, cut, or irritated in any way. Make sure your skin is free of lotion and soap before applying a patch.

3. A clear, protective liner covers the sticky back side of the NicoDerm CQ patch—the side that will be put on your skin. The liner has a slit down the middle to help you remove it from the patch. With the sticky back side facing you, pull half the liner away from the NicoDerm CQ patch starting at the middle slit, as shown in the illustration above. Hold the NicoDerm CQ patch at one of the outside edges (touch the sticky side as little as possible), and pull off the other half of the protective liner.

Place this liner in the slot in the disposable tray provided in the NicoDerm CQ package where it will be out of reach of children and pets.

4. Immediately apply the sticky side of the NicoDerm CQ patch to your skin. **Press the patch firmly on your skin with the heel of your hand for at least 10 seconds.** Make sure it sticks well to your skin, especially around the edges.

5. Wash your hands when you have finished applying the NicoDerm CQ patch. Nicotine on your hands could get into your eyes and nose, and cause stinging, redness, or more serious problems.

6. After 24 or 16 hours, remove the patch you have been wearing. Fold the used NicoDerm CQ patch in half with the sticky side together. Carefully dispose of the used patch in the slot of the disposal tray provided in the NicoDerm CQ package where it will be out of the reach of children and pets. Even used patches have enough nicotine to poison children and pets. Wash your hands.

7. Chose a different place on your skin to apply the next NicoDerm CQ patch and repeat Steps 1 to 6. Do not apply a new patch to a previously used skin site for at least one week.

If your NicoDerm CQ patch gets wet during wearing.

Water will not harm the NicoDerm CQ patch you are wearing if applied properly. You can bathe, swim, or shower for short periods while you are wearing the NicoDerm CQ patch.

If your NicoDerm CQ patch comes off while wearing.

NicoDerm CQ patches generally stick well to most people's skin. However, a patch may occasionally come off. If your NicoDerm CQ patch falls off during the day, put on a new patch, making sure you select a non-hairy, non-irritated area of the skin that is clean and dry.

If the soap you use has lanolin or moisturizers, the patch may not stick well. Using a different soap may help. Body creams, lotions and sunscreens can also cause problems with keeping your patch on. Do not apply creams or lotions to the place on your skin where you will put the patch.

If you have followed the directions and the patch still does not stick to you, try using medical adhesive tape over the patch.

Disposing of NicoDerm CQ patches.

Fold the used patch in half with the sticky side together.

Carefully dispose of the patch in the disposal slot of the tray provided in the NicoDerm CQ package where it will be out of the reach of children and pets.

Small amounts of nicotine, even from a used patch, can poison children and pets. **Keep all nicotine patches away from children and pets.** Wash your hands after disposing of the patch.

If your skin reacts to the NicoDerm CQ patch.

When you first put on a NicoDerm CQ patch, mild itching, burning, or tingling is normal and should go away within an hour. After you remove a NicoDerm CQ patch, the skin under the patch might be somewhat red. Your skin should not stay red for more than a day after removing the patch. **Stop use and ask a doctor if skin redness caused by the patch does not go away after four days, or if your skin swells, or you get a rash. Do not put on a new patch.**

Storage Instructions

Keep each NicoDerm CQ patch in its protective pouch, unopened, until you are ready to use it, because the patch will lose nicotine to the air if it's outside the pouch.

Store NicoDerm CQ patches at 20–25 C (68–77 F) because they are sensitive to heat. Remember, the inside of your car can reach temperatures much higher than this. A slight yellowing of the sticky side of the patch is normal. Do not use NicoDerm CQ patches stored in pouches that are open or torn.

TIPS TO MAKE QUITTING EASIER.

Within the first few weeks of giving up smoking, you may be tempted to smoke for pleasure, particularly after completing a difficult task, or at a party or bar. Hear are some tips to help get you through the important first stages of becoming a nonsmoker:

On Your Quit Date:

Ask your family, friends and co-workers to support you in your efforts to stop smoking.

- Throw away all your cigarettes, matches, lighters, ashtrays, etc.
- Keep busy on your quit day. Exercise. Go to a movie. Take a walk. Get together with friends.
- Figure out how much money you'll save by not smoking. Most ex-smokers can save more than $1,000 a year on the price of cigarettes alone.
- Write down what you will do with the money you save.
- Know your high risk situations and plan ahead how you will deal with them.
- Visit your dentist and have your teeth cleaned to get rid of the tobacco stains.

Right after Quitting:

- During the first few days after you've stopped smoking, spend as much time as possible at places where smoking is not allowed.
- Drink large quantities of water and fruit juices.
- Try to avoid alcohol, coffee and other beverages you associate with smoking.
- Remember that temporary urges to smoke will pass, even if you don't smoke a cigarette.
- Keep your hands busy with something like a pencil or a paper clip.
- Find other activities that help you relax without cigarettes. Swim, jog, take a walk, play basketball.

- Don't worry too much about gaining weight. Watch what you eat, take time for daily exercise, and change your eating habits if you need to.
- Laughter helps. Watch or read something funny

WHAT TO EXPECT.

The First Few Days.

Your body is now coming back into balance. During the first few days after you stop smoking, you might feel edgy and nervous and have trouble concentrating. You might get headaches, feel dizzy and a little out of sorts, feel sweaty or have stomach upsets. You might even have trouble sleeping at first. These are typical nicotine withdrawal symptoms that will go away with time. Your smoker's cough will get worse before it gets better. But don't worry, that's a good sign. Coughing helps clear the tar deposits out of your lungs.

After A Week Or Two.

By now you should be feeling more confident that you can handle those smoking urges. Many of your nicotine withdrawal symptoms have left by now, and you should be noticing some positive signs: less coughing, better breathing and an improved sense of taste and smell, to name a few.

After A Month.

You probably have the urge to smoke much less often now. But urges may still occur, and when they do, they are likely to be powerful ones that come out of nowhere. Don't let them catch you off guard. Plan ahead for these difficult times.

Concentrate on the ways non-smokers are more attractive than smokers. Their skin is less likely to wrinkle. Their teeth are whiter, cleaner. Their breath is fresher.

Their hair and clothes smell better. That cough that seems to make even a laugh sound more like a rattle is a thing of the past. Their children and others around them are healthier, too.

What To Do About Relapse.

What should you do if you slip and start smoking again? The answer is simple. A lapse of one or two or even a few cigarettes should not spoil your efforts! Throw away your cigarettes, forgive yourself and continue with the program. Listen to the CD again and re-read the User's Guide to ensure that you're using NicoDerm CQ correctly and following the other important tips for dealing with the mental and social dependence on nicotine. Your doctor, pharmacist or other health professional can also provide useful counseling on the importance of stopping smoking. You should consider them partners in your quit attempt.

What To Do About Relapse After a Successful Quit Attempt.

If you have taken up regular smoking again, don't be discouraged. Research shows that the best thing you can do is try again, since several quitting attempts may be needed before you're suc

Continued on next page

cessful. And your chances of quitting successfully increase with each quit attempt.

The important thing is to learn from your last attempt.

- Admit that you've slipped, but don't treat yourself as a failure.
- Try to identify the "trigger" that caused you to slip, and prepare a better plan for dealing with this problem next time.
- Talk positively to yourself – tell yourself that you have learned something from this experience.
- Make sure you used NicoDerm CQ patches correctly
- Remember that it takes practice to do anything, and quitting smoking is no exception.

WHEN THE STRUGGLE IS OVER.

Once you've stopped smoking, take a second and pat yourself on your back. Now do it again. You deserve it. Remember now why you decided to stop smoking in the first place. Look at your list of reasons. Read them again. And smile.

Now think about all the money you are saving and what you'll do with it. All the non-smoking places you can go, and what you might do there. All those years you may have added to your life, and what you'll do with them. Remember that temptation may not be gone forever. However, the hard part is behind you so look forward with a positive attitude, and enjoy your new life as a non-smoker.

QUESTIONS & ANSWERS

1. How will I feel when I stop smoking and start using NicoDerm CQ?
You'll need to prepare yourself for some nicotine withdrawal symptoms. These begin almost immediately after you stop smoking, and are usually at their worst during the first three or four days. Understand that any of the following is possible:

- craving for nicotine
- anxiety, irritability, restlessness, mood changes, nervousness
- disruptions of your sleep
- drowsiness
- trouble concentrating
- increased appetite and weight gain headaches, muscular pain, constipation, fatigue.

NicoDerm CQ reduces nicotine withdrawal symptoms such as irritability and nervousness, as well as the craving for nicotine you used to satisfy by having a cigarette.

2. Is NicoDerm CQ just substituting one form of nicotine for another?
NicoDerm CQ does contain nicotine. The purpose of NicoDerm CQ is to provide you with enough nicotine to reduce the physical withdrawal symptoms so you can deal with the mental aspects of quitting.

3. Can I be hurt by using NicoDerm CQ?
For most adults, the amount of nicotine delivered from the patch is less than from smoking. If you believe you may be sensitive to even this amount of nicotine, you should not use this product without advice from your doctor. There are also some important warnings in this User's Guide (See page 4).

4. Will I gain weight?
Many people do tend to gain a few pounds the first 8–10 weeks after they

stop smoking. This is a very small price to pay for the enormous gains that you will make in your overall health and attractiveness. If you continue to gain weight after the first two months, try to analyze what you're doing differently. Reduce your fat intake, choose healthy snacks, and increase your physical activity to burn off the extra calories. Drink lots of water. This is good for your body and skin, and also helps to reduce the amount you eat.

5. Is NicoDerm CQ more expensive than smoking?
The total cost of NicoDerm CQ program is similar to what a person who smokes one and a half packs of cigarettes a day would spend on cigarettes for the same period of time. Also, use of NicoDerm CQ is only a short-term cost, while the cost of smoking is a long-term cost, including the health problems smoking causes.

6. What if I slip up?
Discard your cigarettes, forgive yourself and then get back on track. Don't consider yourself a failure or punish yourself. In fact, people who have already tried to quit are more likely to be successful the next time.

GOOD LUCK!
WALLET CARD
My most important reasons to quit smoking are:
WALLET CARD
Where to call for Help:

American Lung Association	American Cancer Society	American Heart Association
800-586-4872	800-227-2345	800-242-8721

For people who smoke more than 10 cigarettes per day:

STEP 1	STEP 2	STEP 3
Use one 21 mg patch/day Weeks 1–6	Use one 14 mg patch/day Weeks 7–8	Use one 7 mg patch/day Weeks 9–10

People who smoke 10 or less cigarettes per day. Do not use STEP 1 (21 mg). Use STEP 2 (14 mg) for six weeks and STEP 3 (7 mg) for two weeks and then stop.

Copyright © 2002 GlaxoSmithKline
For your family's protection, NicoDerm CQ patches are supplied in child resistant pouches. Do not use if individual pouch is open or torn.
Manufactured by ALZA Corporation, Mountain View, CA 94043 for GlaxoSmithKline Consumer Healthcare, L.P. Comments or Questions? Call 1–800–834–5895 Weekdays. (10 a.m.–4:30 p.m. EST).

- **Not for sale to those under 18 years of age.**
- **Proof of age required.**
- **Not for sale in vending machines or from any source where proof of age cannot be verified.**

Available as
NicoDerm CQ Step 1 (21 mg/24 hours)–7 Patches*
NicoDerm CQ Step 1 (21 mg/24 hours)–14 Patches*

NicoDerm CQ Step 2 (14 mg/24 hours)–7 Patches*
NicoDerm CQ Step 2 (14 mg/24 hours)–14 Patches*
NicoDerm CQ Step 3 (7 mg/24 hours)–7 Patches**
NicoDerm CQ Step 3 (7 mg/24 hours)–14 Patches**
NicoDerm CQ Clear Step 1 (21 mg/24 hours)–7 Patches*
NicoDerm CQ Clear Step 1 (21 mg/24 hours)–14 Patches*
NicoDerm CQ Clear Step 1 (21 mg/24 hours)–21 Patches*
NicoDerm CQ Clear Step 2 (14 mg/24 hours)–14 Patches*
NicoDerm CQ Clear Step 3 (7 mg/24 hours)–14 Patches**
*   User's Guide, CD & Child Resistant Disposal Tray
** User's Guide, & Child Resistant Disposal Tray
Shown in Product Identification Guide, page 507

NICODERM® CQ® CLEAR
Nicotine Transdermal System/Stop Smoking Aid

Formerly available only by prescription Available as:

Step 1 -	21 mg/24 hours
Step 2 -	14 mg/24 hours
Step 3 -	7 mg/24 hours

If you smoke:
More than 10 Cigarettes per Day: Start with Step 1
10 Cigarettes a Day or Less: Start with Step 2
WHAT IS THE NICODERM CQ PATCH AND HOW IS IT USED?
NicoDerm CQ is a small, nicotine containing patch. When you put on a NicoDerm CQ patch, nicotine passes through the skin and into your body. NicoDerm CQ is very thin and uses special material to control how fast nicotine passes through the skin. Unlike the sudden jolts of nicotine delivered by cigarettes, the amount of nicotine you receive remains relatively smooth throughout the 24 or 16 hours period you wear the NicoDerm CQ patch. This helps to reduce cravings you may have for nicotine.

Active Ingredient: Nicotine

Purpose: Stop Smoking Aid

Use: reduces withdrawal symptoms, including nicotine craving, associated with quitting smoking

Directions:
- **if you are under 18 years of age, ask a doctor before use**
- before using this product, read the enclosed user's guide for complete directions and other information
- stop smoking completely when you begin using the patch
- **if you smoke more than 10 cigarettes per day,** use according to the following 10 week schedule:

STEP 1	STEP 2	STEP 3
Use one 21 mg patch/day	Use one 14 mg patch/day	Use one 7 mg patch/day
Weeks 1–6	Weeks 7–8	Weeks 9–10

- if you smoke **10 or less cigarettes per day**, do not use **STEP 1 (21 mg)**. Start with **STEP 2 (14 mg)** for 6 weeks, then **STEP 3 (7 mg)** for two weeks and then stop.
- steps 2 and 3 allow you to gradually reduce your level of nicotine. Completing the full program will increase your chances of quitting successfully.
- apply one new patch every 24 hours on skin that is dry, clean and hairless
- remove backing from patch and immediately press onto skin. Hold for 10 seconds.
- wash hands after applying or removing patch. Throw away the patch in the enclosed disposal tray. See enclosed user's guide for safety and handling.
- you may wear the patch for 16 or 24 hours
- if you crave cigarettes when you wake up, wear the patch for 24 hours
- if you have vivid dreams or other sleep disturbances, you may remove the patch at bedtime and apply a new one in the morning
- the used patch should be removed and a new one applied to a different skin site at the same time each day
- do not wear more than one patch at a time
- do not cut patch in half or into smaller pieces
- do not leave patch on for more than 24 hours because it may irritate your skin and loses strength after 24 hours
- stop using the patch at the end of 10 weeks. If you started with **STEP 2**, stop using the patch at the end of 8 weeks. If you still feel the need to use the patch talk to your doctor.

Warnings:

If you are pregnant or breast-feeding, only use this medicine on the advice of your health care provider. Smoking can seriously harm your child. Try to stop smoking without using any nicotine replacement medicine. This medicine is believed to be safer than smoking. However, the risks to your child from this medicine are not fully known.

Do Not Use
- if you continue to smoke, chew tobacco, use snuff, or use a nicotine gum or other nicotine containing products

Ask a doctor before use if you have
- heart disease, recent heart attack, or irregular heartbeat. Nicotine can increase your heart rate.
- high blood pressure not controlled with medication. Nicotine can increase your blood pressure.
- an allergy to adhesive tape or skin problems because you are more likely to get rashes

Ask a doctor or pharmacist before use if you are
- using a non-nicotine stop smoking drug
- taking a prescription medication for depression or asthma. Your prescription dose may need to be adjusted.

When using this product
- do not smoke even when not wearing the patch. The nicotine in your skin will still be entering your blood stream for several hours after you take off the patch.
- if you have vivid dreams or other sleep disturbances remove this patch at bedtime

Stop use and ask a doctor if
- skin redness caused by the patch does not go away after four days, or if skin swells, or you get a rash
- irregular heartbeat or palpitations occur
- you get symptoms of nicotine overdose such as nausea, vomiting, dizziness, weakness and rapid heartbeat

Keep out of reach of children and pets. Used patches have enough nicotine to poison children and pets. If swallowed, get medical help or contact a Poison Control Center right away. Dispose of the used patches by folding sticky ends together and inserting in disposal tray in this box.

READ THE LABEL
Read the carton and the User's Guide before using this product. Keep the carton and User's Guide. They contain important information.

Inactive Ingredients: Ethylene vinyl acetate-copolymer, polyisobutylene and high density polyethylene between clear polyester backings.

Store at 20–25°C (68–77°F)

TO INCREASE YOUR SUCCESS IN QUITTING:
1. You must be motivated to quit.
2. Complete the full treatment program, applying a new patch every day.
3. Use with a support program as described in the Users Guide.

NicoDerm CQ User's Guide
KEYS TO SUCCESS
1) You must really want to quit smoking for **NicoDerm® CQ®** to help you.
2) Complete the full program, applying a new patch every day.
3) **NicoDerm CQ** works best when used together with a support program: See page 3 for details.
4) If you have trouble using **NicoDerm CQ**, ask your doctor or pharmacist or call GlaxoSmithKline 1-800-834-5895 weekdays (10:00 am 4:30 pm EST).

SO, YOU'VE DECIDED TO QUIT.
Congratulations. Your decision to stop smoking is one of the most important things you can do to improve your health. Quitting smoking is a two-part process that involves:
1) overcoming your physical need for nicotine, and
2) breaking your smoking habit.
NicoDerm CQ helps smokers quit by reducing nicotine withdrawal symptoms.
Many NicoDerm CQ users will be able to stop smoking for a few days but often will start smoking again. Most smokers have to try to quit several times before they completely stop.
Your own chances of quitting smoking depend on how strongly you are addicted to nicotine, how much you want to quit, and how closely you follow a quitting plan like the one that comes with NicoDerm CQ.

QUITTING SMOKING IS HARD!
If you find you cannot stop or if you start smoking again after using NicoDerm CQ please talk to a health care professional who can help you find a program that may work better for you. Breaking this addiction doesn't happen overnight.
Because NicoDerm CQ provides some nicotine, the NicoDerm CQ patch will help you stop smoking by reducing nicotine withdrawal symptoms such as nicotine craving, nervousness and irritability.
This User's Guide will give you support as you become a non-smoker. It will answer common questions about NicoDerm CQ and give tips to help you stop smoking, and should be referred to often.

WHERE TO GET HELP.
You are more likely to stop smoking by using NicoDerm CQ with a support program that helps you break your smoking habit. There may be support groups in your area for people trying to quit. Call your local chapter of the American Lung Association, American Cancer Society or American Heart Association for further information. Toll free phone numbers are printed on the wallet card on the back cover of this User's Guide.
If you find you cannot stop smoking or if you start smoking again after using NicoDerm CQ, remember breaking this addiction doesn't happen overnight. You may want to talk to a health care professional who can help you improve your chances of quitting the next time you try NicoDerm CQ or another method.

LET'S GET ORGANIZED.
Your reason for quitting may be a combination of concerns about health, the effect of smoking on your appearance, and pressure from your family and friends to stop smoking. Or maybe you're concerned about the dangerous effect of second-hand smoke on the people you care about.
All of these are good reasons. You probably have others. Decide your most important reasons, and write them down on the wallet card inside the back cover of this User's Guide. Carry this card with you. In difficult moments, when you want to smoke, the card will remind you why you are quitting.

WHAT YOU'RE UP AGAINST.
Smoking is addictive in two ways. Your need for nicotine has become both physical and mental. You must overcome both addictions to stop smoking. So while NicoDerm CQ will lessen your body's craving for nicotine, you've got to want to quit smoking to overcome the mental dependence on cigarettes. Once you've decided that you're going to quit, it's time to get started. But first, there are some important cautions you should consider.

SOME IMPORTANT WARNINGS.
This product is only for those who want to stop smoking.

Do not use
- if you continue to smoke, chew tobacco, use snuff or use a nicotine gum or other nicotine products.

Continued on next page

Nicoderm CQ Clear—Cont.

Ask a doctor before use if you have:

- heart disease, recent heart attack, or irregular heartbeat, Nicotine can increase your heart rate.
- high blood pressure not controlled with medication. Nicotine can increase your blood pressure.
- an allergy to adhesive tape or have skin problems because you are more likely to get rashes.

Ask a doctor or pharmacist before use if you are

- using a non-nicotine stop smoking drug
- taking a prescription medication for asthma or depression. Your prescription dose may need to be adjusted.

When using this product:

- do not smoke even when not wearing the patch. The nicotine in your skin will still be entering your bloodstream for several hours after you take off the patch.
- you have vivid dreams or other sleep disturbances remove this patch at bedtime.

Stop use and ask a doctor if:

- skin redness caused by the patch does not go away after four days, or if your skin swells or you get a rash.
- irregular heartbeat or palpitations occur
- you get symptoms of nicotine overdose, such as nausea, vomiting, dizziness, weakness and rapid heartbeat.

If you are pregnant or breast-feeding, only use this medicine on the advice of your health care provider. Smoking can seriously harm your child. Try to stop smoking without using any nicotine replacement medicine. This medicine is believed to be safer than smoking. However, the risks to your child from this medicine are not fully known.

Keep out of reach of children and pets. Used patches have enough nicotine to poison children and pets. If swallowed, get medical help or contact a Poison Control Center right away. Dispose of the used patches by folding sticky ends together and inserting in the disposal tray in this box.

LET'S GET STARTED.

If you are under 18 years of age, ask a doctor before use.

Becoming a non-smoker starts today. Your first step is to read through this entire User's Guide carefully.

First, check that you bought the right starting dose.

If you smoke more than 10 cigarettes a day, begin with Step 1 (21 mg). As the carton indicates, people who smoke 10 or less cigarettes per day should not use Step 1 (21 mg). They should start with Step 2 (14 mg). Throughout this User's Guide we will give specific instructions for people who smoke 10 or less cigarettes per day.

Next, set your personalized quitting schedule.

Take out a calendar that you can use to track your progress. Pick a quit date, and mark this on your calendar using the stickers in the middle of this User's Guide, as described below.

DIRECTIONS: FOR PEOPLE WHO SMOKE MORE THAN 10 CIGARETTES PER DAY

STEP 1. (Weeks 1–6). Your quit date (and the day you'll start using NicoDerm CQ patch).

Choose your quit date (it should be soon).

This is the day you will quit smoking cigarettes entirely and begin using NicoDerm CQ to reduce your cravings for nicotine. Place the Step 1 sticker on this date. For the first six weeks, you'll use the highest-strength (21 mg) NicoDerm CQ patches. Be sure to follow the directions on page 10.

Completing the full program will increase your chances of quitting successfully. This is done by changing over to the Step 2 (14mg) patch for 2 weeks followed by a final 2 weeks with the Step 3 (7mg) patch. The Step 2 and Step 3 treatment periods allow you to gradually reduce the amount of nicotine you get, rather than stopping suddenly, and will increase your chances of quitting.

STEP 2. (Weeks 7–8). The day you'll start reducing your use of NicoDerm CQ patch.

Switching to Step 2 (14mg) patches after 6 weeks begins to gradually reduce your nicotine usage. Place the Step 2 sticker on this date (the first day of week seven). Use the 14mg patches for two weeks.

STEP 3. (Weeks 9–10). The day you'll further start reducing your use of NicoDerm CQ patch.

After eight weeks, nicotine intake is further reduced by moving down to Step 3 (7mg) patches. Place the Step 3 sticker on this date (the first day of week nine). Use the 7 mg patches for two weeks.

THE NICODERM CQ PROGRAM

STEP 1	STEP 2	STEP 3
Use one	Use one	Use one
21 mg	14 mg	7 mg
patch/day	patch/day	patch/day
Weeks 1–6	Weeks 7–8	Weeks 9–10

STOP USING NICODERM CQ AT THE END OF WEEK 10. If you still feel the need to use the patch after Week 10, talk with your doctor or health professional.

DIRECTIONS: FOR PEOPLE WHO SMOKE 10 OR LESS CIGARETTES PER DAY

Do not use Step 1 (21 mg).

Begin with STEP 2 – Initial Treatment Period (Weeks 1–6): 14mg patches.

Choose our quit date (it should be soon). This is the Day you will quit smoking cigarettes entirely and begin using NicoDerm CQ to reduce your cravings for nicotine. Place the Step 2 sticker on this date. For the first six weeks, you'll use the Step 2 (14mg) NicoDerm CQ patches. Be sure to follow the directions on page 10.

Continue with STEP 3 – Step Down Treatment Period (Weeks 7–8): 7mg patches.

Completing the full program will increase your chances of quitting successfully. This is done by changing over to the Step 3 (7mg) patches for 2 weeks.

The two week step down treatment period allows you to gradually reduce the amount of nicotine you get, rather than stopping suddenly, and will increase your chances of quitting. Place the Step 3 sticker on the first day of week seven. Use the 7mg patches for two weeks. People who smoke 10 or less cigarettes per day should not use NicoDerm CQ for longer than 8 weeks. If you still feel the need to use NicoDerm CQ after 8 weeks, talk with your doctor.

PLAN AHEAD.

Because smoking is an addiction, it is not easy to stop. After you've given up nicotine, you may still have a strong urge to smoke. Plan ahead NOW for these times, so you're not tempted to start smoking again in a moment of weakness. The following tips may help:

- Keep the phone numbers of supportive friends and family members handy.
- Keep a record of your quitting process. Track whether you feel a craving for cigarettes. In the event that you slip, immediately stop smoking and resume your quit attempt with the NicoDerm CQ patch. If you smoke at all, write down what you think caused the slip.
- Put together an Emergency Kit that includes items that will help take your mind off occasional urges to smoke. You might include cinnamon gum or lemon drops to suck on, a relaxing cassette tape, and something for your hands to play with, like a smooth rock, rubber band or small metal balls.
- Set aside some small rewards, like a new magazine or a gift certificate from your favorite store, which you'll "give" yourself after passing difficult hurdles.
- Think now about the times when you most often want a cigarette, and then plan what else you might do instead of smoking. For instance, you might plan to take your coffee break in a new location, or take a walk right after dinner, so you won't be tempted to smoke.

HOW NICODERM CQ WORKS.

NicoDerm CQ patches provide nicotine to your system. They work as a temporary aid to help you quit smoking by reducing nicotine withdrawal symptoms, including nicotine craving. NicoDerm CQ provides a lower level of nicotine to your blood than cigarettes, and allows you to gradually do away with your body's need for nicotine.

Because NicoDerm CQ does not contain the tar or carbon monoxide of cigarette smoke, it does not have the same health dangers as tobacco. However, it still delivers nicotine, the addictive part of cigarette smoke. Nicotine can cause side effects such as headache, nausea, upset stomach, and dizziness.

HOW TO USE NICODERM CQ PATCHES.

Read all the following instructions, and the instructions on the outer carton, before using NicoDerm CQ. Refer to them often to make sure you're using NicoDerm CQ correctly. Please refer to the CD for additional help.

1) Stop smoking completely before you start using NicoDerm CQ.

2) To reduce nicotine craving and other withdrawal symptoms, use NicoDerm CQ according to the directions on pages 6–8.

3) Insert used NicoDerm CQ patches in the child resistant disposal tray provided in the box – safely away from children and pets.

When to apply and remove NicoDerm CQ patches.

Each day apply a new patch to a different place on skin that is dry, clean and hairless. **You can wear a NicoDerm CQ patch for either 16 or 24 hours.** If you crave cigarettes when you wake up, wear the patch for 24 hours. If you begin to have vivid dreams or other disruptions of your sleep while wearing the patch 24 hours, try taking the patch off at bedtime (after about 16 hours) and putting on a new one when you get up the next day.

PLACE THESE STICKERS ON YOUR CALENDAR

STEP 1	STEP 2
A new 21 mg patch every day AT THE BEGINNING OF WEEK #1 (QUIT DAY)	A new 14 mg patch every day AT THE BEGINNING OF WEEK #7

For people who smoke 10 or less cigarettes per day: Do not use STEP 1 (21 mg). Use STEP 2 (14 mg) at the beginning of week #1 and STEP 3 (7 mg) at the beginning of week #7.

PLACE THESE STICKERS ON YOUR CALENDAR

STEP 3	EX-SMOKER
A new 7 mg patch every day AT THE BEGINNING OF WEEK #9	WHEN YOU HAVE COMPLETED YOUR QUITTING PROGRAM

Do not smoke even when you are not wearing the patch.

Remove the used patch and put on a new patch at the same time every day. Applying the patch at about the same time each day (first thing in the morning, for instance) will help you remember when to put on a new patch. Do not leave the same NicoDerm CQ patch on for more than 24 hours because it may irritate your skin and because it loses strength after 24 hours.

Do not use NicoDerm CQ continuously for more than 10 weeks (8 weeks for people who smoke 10 or less cigarettes per day).

How to apply a NicoDerm CQ patch.

1. Do not remove the NicoDerm CQ patch from its sealed protective pouch until you are ready to use it. NicoDerm CQ patches will lose nicotine to the air if you store them out of the pouch.

2. Choose a non-hairy, clean, dry area of skin. Do not put a NicoDerm CQ patch on skin that is burned, broken out, cut, or irritated in any way. Make sure your skin is free of lotion and soap before applying a patch.

3. A clear, protective liner covers the sticky back side of the NicoDerm CQ patch—the side that will be put on your skin. The liner has a slit down the middle to help you remove it from the patch. With the sticky back side facing you, pull half the liner away from the NicoDerm CQ patch starting at the middle slit, as shown in the illustration above. Hold the NicoDerm CQ patch at one of the outside edges (touch the sticky side as little as possible), and pull off the other half of the protective liner.

Place this liner in the slot in the disposable tray provided in the NicoDerm CQ package where it will be out of reach of children and pets.

4. Immediately apply the sticky side of the NicoDerm CQ patch to your skin. **Press the patch firmly on your skin with the heel of your hand for at least 10 seconds.** Make sure it sticks well to your skin, especially around the edges.

5. Wash your hands when you have finished applying the NicoDerm CQ patch. Nicotine on your hands could get into your eyes and nose, and cause stinging, redness, or more serious problems.

6. After 24 or 16 hours, remove the patch you have been wearing. Fold the used NicoDerm CQ patch in half with the sticky side together. Carefully dispose of the used patch in the slot of the disposal tray provided in the NicoDerm CQ package where it will be out of the reach of children and pets. Even used patches have enough nicotine to poison children and pets. Wash your hands.

7. Chose a different place on your skin to apply the next NicoDerm CQ patch and repeat Steps 1 to 6. Do not apply a new patch to a previously used skin site for at least one week.

If your NicoDerm CQ patch gets wet during wearing.

Water will not harm the NicoDerm CQ patch you are wearing if applied properly. You can bathe, swim, or shower for short periods while you are wearing the NicoDerm CQ patch.

If your NicoDerm CQ patch comes off while wearing.

NicoDerm CQ patches generally stick well to most people's skin. However, a patch may occasionally come off. If your NicoDerm CQ patch falls off during the day, put on a new patch, making sure you select a non-hairy, non-irritated area of the skin that is clean and dry.

If the soap you use has lanolin or moisturizers, the patch may not stick well. Using a different soap may help. Body creams, lotions and sunscreens can also cause problems with keeping your patch on. Do not apply creams or lotions to the place on your skin where you will put the patch.

If you have followed the directions and the patch still does not stick to you, try using medical adhesive tape over the patch.

Disposing of NicoDerm CQ patches.

Fold the used patch in half with the sticky side together.

Carefully dispose of the patch in the disposal slot of the tray provided in the NicoDerm CQ package where it will be out of the reach of children and pets. Small amounts of nicotine, even from a used patch, can poison children and pets.

Keep all nicotine patches away from children and pets. Wash your hands after disposing of the patch.

If your skin reacts to the NicoDerm CQ patch.

When you first put on a NicoDerm CQ patch, mild itching, burning, or tingling is normal and should go away within an hour. After you remove a NicoDerm CQ patch, the skin under the patch might be somewhat red. Your skin should not stay red for more than a day after removing the patch. **Stop use and ask a doctor if skin redness caused by the patch does not go away after four days, or if your skin swells, or you get a rash. Do not put on a new patch.**

Storage Instructions

Keep each NicoDerm CQ patch in its protective pouch, unopened, until you are ready to use it, because the patch will lose nicotine to the air if it's outside the pouch.

Store NicoDerm CQ patches at 20–25 C (68–77 F) because they are sensitive to heat. Remember, the inside of your car can reach temperatures much higher than this. A slight yellowing of the sticky side of the patch is normal. Do not use NicoDerm CQ patches stored in pouches that are open or torn.

TIPS TO MAKE QUITTING EASIER.

Within the first few weeks of giving up smoking, you may be tempted to smoke for pleasure, particularly after completing a difficult task, or at a party or bar. Hear are some tips to help get you through the important first stages of becoming a nonsmoker:

On Your Quit Date:

Ask your family, friends and co-workers to support you in your efforts to stop smoking.

- Throw away all your cigarettes, matches, lighters, ashtrays, etc.
- Keep busy on your quit day. Exercise. Go to a movie. Take a walk. Get together with friends.
- Figure out how much money you'll save by not smoking. Most ex-smokers can save more than $1,000 a year on the price of cigarettes alone.
- Write down what you will do with the money you save.
- Know your high risk situations and plan ahead how you will deal with them.
- Visit your dentist and have your teeth cleaned to get rid of the tobacco stains.

Right after Quitting:

- During the first few days after you've stopped smoking, spend as much time as possible at places where smoking is not allowed.
- Drink large quantities of water and fruit juices.
- Try to avoid alcohol, coffee and other beverages you associate with smoking.
- Remember that temporary urges to smoke will pass, even if you don't smoke a cigarette.
- Keep your hands busy with something like a pencil or a paper clip.
- Find other activities that help you relax without cigarettes. Swim, jog, take a walk, play basketball.

Continued on next page

Nicoderm CQ Clear—Cont.

- Don't worry too much about gaining weight. Watch what you eat, take time for daily exercise, and change your eating habits if you need to.
- Laughter helps. Watch or read something funny

WHAT TO EXPECT.
The First Few Days.

Your body is now coming back into balance. During the first few days after you stop smoking, you might feel edgy and nervous and have trouble concentrating. You might get headaches, feel dizzy and a little out of sorts, feel sweaty or have stomach upsets. You might even have trouble sleeping at first. These are typical nicotine withdrawal symptoms that will go away with time. Your smoker's cough will get worse before it gets better. But don't worry, that's a good sign. Coughing helps clear the tar deposits out of your lungs.

After A Week Or Two.

By now you should be feeling more confident that you can handle those smoking urges. Many of your nicotine withdrawal symptoms have left by now, and you should be noticing some positive signs: less coughing, better breathing and an improved sense of taste and smell, to name a few.

After A Month.

You probably have the urge to smoke much less often now. But urges may still occur, and when they do, they are likely to be powerful ones that come out of nowhere. Don't let them catch you off guard. Plan ahead for these difficult times.

Concentrate on the ways non-smokers are more attractive than smokers. Their skin is less likely to wrinkle. Their teeth are whiter, cleaner. Their breath is fresher.

Their hair and clothes smell better. That cough that seems to make even a laugh sound more like a rattle is a thing of the past. Their children and others around them are healthier, too.

What To Do About Relapse.

What should you do if you slip and start smoking again? The answer is simple. A lapse of one or two or even a few cigarettes should not spoil your efforts! Throw away your cigarettes, forgive yourself and continue with the program. Listen to the CD again and re-read the User's Guide to ensure that you're using NicoDerm CQ correctly and following the other important tips for dealing with the mental and social dependence on nicotine. Your doctor, pharmacist or other health professional can also provide useful counseling on the importance of stopping smoking. You should consider them partners in your quit attempt.

What To Do About Relapse After a Successful Quit Attempt.

If you have taken up regular smoking again, don't be discouraged. Research shows that the best thing you can do is try again, since several quitting attempts may be needed before you're successful. And your chances of quitting successfully increase with each quit attempt.

The important thing is to learn from your last attempt.
- Admit that you've slipped, but don't treat yourself as a failure.
- Try to identify the "trigger" that caused you to slip, and prepare a better plan for dealing with this problem next time.
- Talk positively to yourself – tell yourself that you have learned something from this experience.
- Make sure you used NicoDerm CQ patches correctly
- Remember that it takes practice to do anything, and quitting smoking is no exception.

WHEN THE STRUGGLE IS OVER.

Once you've stopped smoking, take a second and pat yourself on your back. Now do it again. You deserve it. Remember now why you decided to stop smoking in the first place. Look at your list of reasons. Read them again. And smile.

Now think about all the money you are saving and what you'll do with it. All the non-smoking places you can go, and what you might do there. All those years you may have added to your life, and what you'll do with them. Remember that temptation may not be gone forever. However, the hard part is behind you so look forward with a positive attitude, and enjoy your new life as a non-smoker.

QUESTIONS & ANSWERS
1. How will I feel when I stop smoking and start using NicoDerm CQ?

You'll need to prepare yourself for some nicotine withdrawal symptoms. These begin almost immediately after you stop smoking, and are usually at their worst during the first three or four days. Understand that any of the following is possible:
- craving for nicotine
- anxiety, irritability, restlessness, mood changes, nervousness
- disruptions of your sleep
- drowsiness
- trouble concentrating
- increased appetite and weight gain headaches, muscular pain, constipation, fatigue

NicoDerm CQ reduces nicotine withdrawal symptoms such as irritability and nervousness, as well as the craving for nicotine you used to satisfy by having a cigarette.

2. Is NicoDerm CQ just substituting one form of nicotine for another?

NicoDerm CQ does contain nicotine. The purpose of NicoDerm CQ is to provide you with enough nicotine to reduce the physical withdrawal symptoms so you can deal with the mental aspects of quitting.

3. Can I be hurt by using NicoDerm CQ?

For most adults, the amount of nicotine delivered from the patch is less than from smoking. If you believe you may be sensitive to even this amount of nicotine, you should not use this product without advice from your doctor. There are also some important warnings in this User's Guide (See page 4).

4. Will I gain weight?

Many people do tend to gain a few pounds the first 8–10 weeks after they stop smoking. This is a very small price to pay for the enormous gains that you will make in your overall health and attractiveness. If you continue to gain weight after the first two months, try to analyze what you're doing differently. Reduce your fat intake, choose healthy snacks, and increase your physical activity to burn off the extra calories. Drink lots of water. This is good for your body and skin, and also helps to reduce the amount you eat.

5. Is NicoDerm CQ more expensive than smoking?

The total cost of NicoDerm CQ program is similar to what a person who smokes one and a half packs of cigarettes a day would spend on cigarettes for the same period of time. Also, use of NicoDerm CQ is only a short-term cost, while the cost of smoking is a long-term cost, including the health problems smoking causes.

6. What if I slip up?

Discard your cigarettes, forgive yourself and then get back on track. Don't consider yourself a failure or punish yourself. In fact, people who have already tried to quit are more likely to be successful the next time.

GOOD LUCK!
WALLET CARD

My most important reasons to quit smoking are:

WALLET CARD

Where to call for Help:

| American Lung Association 800-586-4872 | American Cancer Society 800-227-2345 | American Heart Association 800-242-8721 |

For people who smoke more than 10 cigarettes per day:

| STEP 1 Use one 21 mg patch/day Weeks 1–6 | STEP 2 Use one 14 mg patch/day Weeks 7–8 | STEP 3 Use one 7 mg patch/day Weeks 9–10 |

People who smoke 10 or less cigarettes per day. Do not use STEP 1 (21 mg). Use STEP 2 (14 mg) for six weeks and STEP 3 (7 mg) for two weeks and then stop.

Copyright © 2002 GlaxoSmithKline

For your family's protection, NicoDerm CQ patches are supplied in child resistant pouches. Do not use if individual pouch is open or torn.

Manufactured by ALZA Corporation, Mountain View, CA 94043 for GlaxoSmithKline Consumer Healthcare, L.P.

Comments or Questions? Call 1–800–834–5895 Weekdays. (10 a.m.– 4:30 p.m. EST).

- **Not for sale to those under 18 years of age.**
- **Proof of age required.**
- **Not for sale in vending machines or from any source where proof of age cannot be verified.**

Available as

NicoDerm CQ Step 1 (21 mg/24 hours)–7 Patches*

NicoDerm CQ Step 1 (21 mg/24 hours)–14 Patches*

NicoDerm CQ Step 2 (14 mg/24 hours)–7 Patches*

NicoDerm CQ Step 2 (14 mg/24 hours)–14 Patches*

NicoDerm CQ Step 3 (7 mg/24 hours)–7 Patches**

NicoDerm CQ Step 3 (7 mg/24 hours)–14 Patches**

NicoDerm CQ Clear Step 1 (21 mg/24 hours)–7 patches*

NicoDerm CQ Clear Step 1 (21 mg/24 hours)–14 patches*

NicoDerm CQ Clear Step 1 (21 mg/24 hours)–21 patches*

NicoDerm CQ Clear Step 2 (14 mg/24 hours)–14 patches*

NicoDerm CQ Clear Step 3 (7 mg/24 hours)–14 patches**

*   User's Guide, CD & Child Resistant Disposal Tray

** User's Guide, & Child Resistant Disposal Tray

NICORETTE®

Nicotine Polacrilex Gum/Stop Smoking Aid
Available in Original 2mg and 4mg Strengths,
Mint 2mg and 4mg Strengths and Orange 2mg and 4mg Strengths

If you smoke:

LESS THAN 25 CIGARETTES A DAY: Use 2 mg

25 OR MORE CIGARETTES A DAY: Use 4 mg

Action: Stop Smoking Aid

Drug Facts:

Active Ingredient: **Purpose:**
(In each chewing piece)

Nicotine polacrilex,
2 or 4 mg .... Stop smoking aid

Use:
- reduces withdrawal symptoms, including nicotine craving, associated with quitting smoking

Warnings:
- **If you are pregnant or breast-feeding, only use this medicine on the advice of your health care provider.** Smoking can seriously harm your child. Try to stop smoking without using any nicotine replacement medicine. This medicine is believed to be safer than smoking. However, the risks to your child from this medicine are not fully known.

Weeks 1 to 6	Weeks 7 to 9	Weeks 10 to 12
1 piece every 1 to 2 hours	1 piece every 2 to 4 hours	1 piece every 4 to 8 hours

Do not use:
- if you continue to smoke, chew tobacco, use snuff, or use a nicotine patch or other nicotine containing products

Ask a doctor before use if you have:
- heart disease, recent heart attack, or irregular heartbeat. Nicotine can increase your heart rate.
- high blood pressure not controlled with medication. Nicotine can increase blood pressure.
- stomach ulcer or diabetes

Ask a doctor or pharmacist before use if you are:
- using a non-nicotine stop smoking drug
- taking prescription medicine for depression or asthma. Your prescription dose may need to be adjusted.

Stop use and ask a doctor if:
- mouth, teeth or jaw problems occur
- irregular heartbeat or palpitations occur
- you get symptoms of nicotine overdose such as nausea, vomiting, dizziness, diarrhea, weakness and rapid heartbeat

Keep out of reach of children and pets. Pieces of nicotine gum may have enough nicotine to make children and pets sick. Wrap used pieces of gum in paper and throw away in the trash. In case of overdose, get medical help or contact a Poison Control Center right away.

Directions:
- **if you are under 18 years of age, ask a doctor before use**
- before using this product, read the enclosed User's Guide for complete directions and other important information
- stop smoking completely when you begin using the gum
- **if you smoke 25 or more cigarettes a day;** use 4 mg nicotine gum
- **if you smoke less than 25 cigarettes a day;** use 2 mg nicotine gum use according to the following 12 week schedule:

[See table above]

- nicotine gum is a medicine and must be used a certain way to get the best results
- chew the gum slowly until it tingles. Then park it between your cheek and gum. When the tingle is gone, begin chewing again, until the tingle returns.
- repeat this process until most of the tingle is gone (about 30 minutes)
- do not eat or drink for 15 minutes before chewing the nicotine gum, or while chewing a piece
- to improve your chances of quitting, use at least 9 pieces per day for the first 6 weeks
- if you experience strong or frequent cravings, you may use a second piece within the hour. However, do not continuously use one piece after another since this may cause you hiccups, heartburn, nausea or other side effects.
- do not use more than 24 pieces a day

- stop using the nicotine gum at the end of 12 weeks. If you still feel the need to use nicotine gum, talk to your doctor.

To remove the gum, tear off single unit.

Peel off backing starting at corner with loose edge.

Push gum through foil.

TO INCREASE YOUR SUCCESS IN QUITTING:
1. **You must be motivated to quit.**
2. **Use Enough**—Chew **at least 9 pieces** of Nicorette per day during the first six weeks.
3. **Use Long Enough**—Use Nicorette for the full 12 weeks.
4. **Use with a support program** as described in the enclosed User's Guide.

*GlaxoSmithKline Consumer Healthcare, L.P. makes an annual grant to the American Cancer Society for cancer research and education for the use of their seal.

READ THE LABEL
Read the carton and the User's Guide before taking this product. Do not discard carton or User's Guide. They contain important information.

Other Information:
- store at 20–25°C (68–77°F)
- protect from light

Inactive Ingredients:
Original [2 mg] Inactive Ingredients: Flavors, glycerin, gum base, sodium carbonate, sorbitol, sodium bicarbonate.

Continued on next page

Nicorette—Cont.

Original [4 mg] Inactive Ingredients: Flavors, glycerin, gum base, sodium carbonate, sorbitol, D&C Yellow 10.

Mint 2 mg Inactive Ingredients: Gum base, magnesium oxide, menthol, peppermint oil, sodium bicarbonate, sodium carbonate, xylitol.

Mint 4 mg Inactive Ingredients: Gum base, magnesium oxide, menthol, peppermint oil, sodium carbonate, xylitol, D&C yellow #10 Al. lake.

Orange [2 mg] Inactive Ingredients: Flavor, gum base, magnesium oxide, sodium bicarbonate, sodium carbonate, xylitol

Orange [4 mg] Inactive Ingredients: Flavor, gum base, magnesium oxide, sodium carbonate, xylitol, D&C Yellow #10 Al. lake.

How Supplied: Nicorette Original, Mint, and Orange are available in:
2 mg or 4 mg Starter kit*—108 pieces
2 mg or 4 mg Refill—48 pieces
Nicorette Original & Mint are also available in 168 & 192 count refills
*User's Guide and Audio Tape included in kit
Blister packaged for your protection. **Do not use if individual seals are open or torn.**
Questions or comments? call **1-800-419-4766** weekdays (10:00 a.m.– 4:30 p.m. EST)
- not for sale to those under 18 years of age
- proof of age required
- not for sale in vending machines or from any source where proof of age cannot be verified
Manufactured by Pharmacia AB, Stockholm, Sweden for
GlaxoSmithKline Consumer Healthcare, L.P.
Pittsburgh, PA 15230
©2001 GlaxoSmithKline

USER'S GUIDE:
HOW TO USE NICORETTE TO HELP YOU QUIT SMOKING
KEYS TO SUCCESS:
1) You must really want to quit smoking for Nicorette to help you.
2) You can greatly increase your chances for success by using at least 9 to 12 pieces every day when you start using Nicorette.
3) You should continue to use Nicorette as explained in the User's Guide for 12 full weeks.
4) Nicorette works best when used together with a support program.
5) If you have trouble using Nicorette, ask your doctor or pharmacist or call GlaxoSmithKline at 1-800-419-4766 weekdays (10:00am–4:30pm EST).

SO YOU DECIDED TO QUIT
Congratulations. Your decision to stop smoking is an important one. That's why you've made the right choice in choosing Nicorette gum. Your own chances of quitting smoking depend on how much you want to quit, how strongly you are addicted to tobacco, and how closely you follow a quitting program like the one that comes with Nicorette.

QUITTING SMOKING IS HARD!
If you've tried to quit before and haven't succeeded, don't be discouraged! Quitting isn't easy. It takes time, and most people try a few times before they are successful. The important thing is to try again until you succeed. This User's Guide will give you support as you become a non-smoker. It will answer common questions about Nicorette and give tips to help you stop smoking, and should be referred to often.

WHERE TO GET HELP
You are more likely to stop smoking by using Nicorette with a support program that helps you break your smoking habit. There may be support groups in your area for people trying to quit. Call your local chapter of the American Lung Association (1-800-586-4872), American Cancer Society (1-800-227-2345) or American Heart Association (1-800-242-8721) for further information. If you find you cannot stop smoking or if you start smoking again after using Nicorette, remember breaking this addiction doesn't happen overnight. You may want to talk to a health care professional who can help you improve your chances of quitting the next time you try Nicorette or another method.

LET'S GET ORGANIZED
Your reason for quitting may be a combination of concerns about health, the effect of smoking on your appearance, and pressure from your family and friends to stop smoking. Or maybe you're concerned about the dangerous effect of second-hand smoke on the people you care about. All of these are good reasons. You probably have others. Decide your most important reasons, and write them down on the wallet card inside the back cover of the User's Guide. Carry this card with you. In difficult moments, when you want to smoke, the card will remind you why you are quitting.

WHAT YOU'RE UP AGAINST
Smoking is addictive in two ways. Your need for nicotine has become both physical and mental. You must overcome both addictions to stop smoking. So while Nicorette will lessen your body's physical addiction to nicotine, you've got to want to quit smoking to overcome the mental dependence on cigarettes. Once you've decided that you're going to quit, it's time to get started. But first, there are some important cautions you should consider.

SOME IMPORTANT WARNINGS. This product is only for those who want to stop smoking.

If you are pregnant or breast-feeding, only use this medicine on the advice of your health care provider. Smoking can seriously harm your child. Try to stop smoking without using any nicotine replacement medicine. This medicine is believed to be safer than smoking. However, the risks to your child from this medicine are not fully known.

Do not use
- if you continue to smoke, chew tobacco, use snuff, or use a nicotine patch or other nicotine containing products.

Ask a doctor before use if you have
- heart disease, recent heart attack, or irregular heartbeat. Nicotine can increase your heart rate.
- high blood pressure not controlled with medication. Nicotine can increase your blood pressure.
- stomach ulcer or diabetes

Ask a doctor or pharmacist before use if you are
- using a non-nicotine stop smoking drug
- taking a prescription medicine for depression or asthma. Your prescription dose may need to be adjusted.

Stop use and ask a doctor if
- mouth, teeth or jaw problems occur
- irregular heartbeat or palpitations occur
- you get symptoms of nicotine overdose such as nausea, vomiting, dizziness, diarrhea, weakness and rapid heartbeat

Keep out of reach of children and pets. Pieces of nicotine gum may have enough nicotine to make children and pets sick. Wrap used pieces of gum in paper and throw away in the trash. In case of overdose, get medical help or contact a Poison Control Center right away.

LET'S GET STARTED
Becoming a non-smoker starts today. First, check that you bought the right starting dose next, read through the entire User's Guide carefully. **Then, set your personalized quitting schedule.** Take out a calendar that you can use to track your progress, and identify four dates, using the stickers in the User's Guide.

STEP 1: (Weeks 1–6) Your quit date (and the day you'll start using Nicorette gum). Choose your quit date (it should be soon). This is the day you will quit smoking cigarettes entirely and begin using Nicorette to satisfy your craving for nicotine. For the first six weeks, you'll use a piece of Nicorette every hour or two. Be sure to follow the directions on pages 8 and 11 of the User's Guide. Place the Step 1 sticker on this date.

STEP 2: (Weeks 7–9) The day you'll start reducing your use of Nicorette. After six weeks, you'll begin gradually reducing your Nicorette usage to one piece every two to four hours. Place the Step 2 sticker on this date (the first day of week seven).

STEP 3: (Weeks 10–12) The day you'll further reduce your use of Nicorette. Nine weeks after you begin using Nicorette, you will further reduce your nicotine intake by using one piece every four to eight hours. Place the Step 3 sticker on this date (the first day of week ten). For the next three weeks, you'll use a piece of Nicorette every four to eight hours. **End of treatment: The day you'll complete Nicorette therapy.**

Nicorette should not be used for longer than twelve weeks. Identify the date thirteen weeks after the date you chose in Step 1 and place the "EX-Smoker" sticker on your calendar.

PLAN AHEAD

Because smoking is an addiction, it is not easy to stop. After you've given up cigarettes, you will still have a strong urge to smoke. Plan ahead NOW for these times, so you're not defeated in a moment of weakness. The following tips may help:

- Keep the phone numbers of supportive friends and family members handy.
- Keep a record of your quitting process. Track the number of Nicorette pieces you use each day, and whether you feel a craving for cigarettes. If you smoke at all, write down what you think caused the slip.
- Put together an Emergency Kit that includes items that will help take your mind off occasional urges to smoke. Include cinnamon gum or lemon drops to suck on, a relaxing cassette tape and something for your hands to play with, like a smooth rock, rubber band or small metal balls.
- Set aside some small rewards, like a new magazine or a gift certificate from your favorite store, which you'll 'give' yourself after passing difficult hurdles.
- Think now about the times when you most often want a cigarette, and then plan what else you might do instead of smoking. For instance, you might plan to take your coffee break in a new location, or take a walk right after dinner, so you won't be tempted to smoke.

HOW NICORETTE GUM WORKS

Nicorette's sugar-free chewing pieces provide nicotine to your system—they work as a temporary aid to help you quit smoking by reducing nicotine withdrawal symptoms. Nicorette provides a lower level of nicotine to your blood than cigarettes, and allows you to gradually do away with your body's need for nicotine. Because Nicorette does not contain the tar or carbon monoxide of cigarette smoke, it does not have the same health dangers as tobacco. However, it still delivers nicotine, the addictive part of cigarette smoke. Nicotine can cause side effects such as headache, nausea, upset stomach and dizziness.

HOW TO USE NICORETTE GUM

If you are under 18 years of age, ask a doctor before use.

Before you can use Nicorette correctly, you have to practice! That sounds silly, but it isn't.

Nicorette isn't like ordinary chewing gum. It's a medicine, and must be chewed a certain way to work right. Chewed like ordinary gum, Nicorette won't work well and can cause side effects. An overdose can occur if you chew more than one piece of Nicorette at the same time, or if you chew many pieces one after another. Read all the following instructions before using Nicorette. Refer to them often to make sure you're using Nicorette gum correctly. If you chew too fast, or do not chew correctly, you may get hiccups, heartburn, or other stomach problems.

1. Stop smoking completely before you start using Nicorette.
2. To reduce craving and other withdrawal symptoms, use Nicorette according to the dosage schedule on page 11 of the User's Guide.

The following chart lists the recommended usage schedule for Nicorette:

Weeks 1 through 6	Weeks 7 through 9	Weeks 10 through 12
1 piece every 1 to 2 hours	1 piece every 2 to 4 hours	1 piece every 4 to 8 hours

DO NOT USE MORE THAN 24 PIECES PER DAY.

3. Chew each Nicorette piece <u>very slowly several times.</u>
4. Stop chewing when you notice a peppery taste, or a slight tingling in your mouth. (This usually happens after about 15 chews, but may vary from person to person.)
5. "PARK" the Nicorette piece between your cheek and gum and leave it there.
6. When the peppery taste or tingle is almost gone (in about a minute), start to chew a few times slowly again. When the taste or tingle returns, stop again.
7. Park the Nicorette piece again (in a different place in your mouth).
8. Repeat steps 3 to 7 (chew, chew, park) until most of the nicotine is gone from the Nicorette piece (usually happens in about half an hour; the peppery taste or tingle won't return).
9. Wrap the used Nicorette in paper and throw away in the trash.

See the chart in the **"DIRECTIONS"** section above for the recommended usage schedule for Nicorette.

[See table above]

To improve your chances of quitting, use at least 9 pieces of Nicorette a day. Heavier smokers may need more pieces to reduce their cravings. Don't eat or drink for 15 minutes before using Nicorette or while chewing a piece. The effectiveness of Nicorette may be reduced by some foods and drinks, such as coffee, juices, wine or soft drinks.

HOW TO REDUCE YOUR NICORETTE USAGE

The goal of using Nicorette is to slowly reduce your dependence on nicotine. The schedule for using Nicorette will help you reduce your nicotine craving gradually. Here are some tips to help you cut back during each step:

- After a while, start chewing each Nicorette piece for only 10 to 15 minutes, instead of half an hour. Then gradually begin to reduce the number of pieces used.
- Or, try chewing each piece for longer than half an hour, but reduce the number of pieces you use each day.
- Substitute ordinary chewing gum for some of the Nicorette pieces you would normally use. Increase the number of pieces of ordinary gum as you cut back on the Nicorette pieces.

STOP USING NICORETTE AT THE END OF WEEK 12.

If you still feel the need to use Nicorette after Week 12, talk with your doctor.

TIPS TO MAKE QUITTING EASIER

Within the first few weeks of giving up smoking, you may be tempted to smoke for pleasure, particularly after completing a difficult task, or at a party or bar. Here are some tips to help get you through the important first stages of becoming a non-smoker:

On your Quit Date:

- Ask your family, friends, and co-workers to support you in your efforts to stop smoking.
- Throw away all your cigarettes, matches, lighters, ashtrays, etc.
- Keep busy on your quit day. Exercise. Go to a movie. Take a walk. Get together with friends.
- Figure out how much money you'll save by not smoking. Most ex-smokers can save more than $1,000 a year.
- Write down what you will do with the money you save.
- Know your high risk situations and plan ahead how you will deal with them.
- Keep Nicorette gum near your bed, so you'll be prepared for any nicotine cravings when you wake up in the morning.
- Visit your dentist and have your teeth cleaned to get rid of the tobacco stains.

Right after Quitting:

- During the first few days after you've stopped smoking, spend as much time as possible at places where smoking is not allowed.
- Drink large quantities of water and fruit juices.
- Try to avoid alcohol, coffee and other beverages you associate with smoking.
- Remember that temporary urges to smoke will pass, even if you don't smoke a cigarette.
- Keep your hands busy with something like a pencil or a paper clip.
- Find other activities which help you relax without cigarettes. Swim, jog, take a walk, play basketball.
- Don't worry too much about gaining weight. Watch what you eat, take time for daily exercise, and change your eating habits if you need to.
- Laughter helps. Watch or read something funny.

WHAT TO EXPECT

Your body is now coming back into balance. During the first few days after you stop smoking, you might feel edgy and nervous and have trouble concentrating. You might get headaches, feel dizzy and a little out of sorts, feel sweaty or have stomach upsets. You might even have trouble sleeping at first. These are typical withdrawal symptoms that will go away with time. Your smoker's cough will get worse before it gets better. But don't worry, that's a good sign. Coughing helps clear the tar deposits out of your lungs.

After a Week or Two.

By now you should be feeling more confident that you can handle those smoking urges. Many of your withdrawal

Continued on next page

Nicorette—Cont.

symptoms have left by now, and you should be noticing some positive signs: less coughing, better breathing and an improved sense of taste and smell, to name a few.

After a Month.

You probably have the urge to smoke much less often now. But urges may still occur, and when they do, they are likely to be powerful ones that come out of nowhere. Don't let them catch you off guard. Plan ahead for these difficult times. Concentrate on the ways nonsmokers are more attractive than smokers. Their skin is less likely to wrinkle. Their teeth are whiter, cleaner. Their breath is fresher. Their hair and clothes smell better. That cough seems to make even a laugh sound more like a rattle is a thing of the past. Their children and others around them are healthier, too.

What To Do About Relapse.

What should you do if you slip and start smoking again? The answer is simple. A lapse of one or two or even a few cigarettes has not spoiled your efforts! Discard your cigarettes, forgive yourself and try again. If you start smoking again, keep your box of Nicorette for your next quit attempt. If you have taken up regular smoking again, don't be discouraged. Research shows that the best thing you can do is to try again. The important thing is to learn from your last attempt.

- Admit that you've slipped, but don't treat yourself as a failure.
- Try to identify the 'trigger' that caused you to slip, and prepare a better plan for dealing with this problem next time.
- Talk positively to yourself—tell yourself that you have learned something from this experience.
- Make sure you used Nicorette gum correctly over the full 12 weeks to reduce your craving for nicotine.
- Remember that it takes practice to do anything, and quitting smoking is no exception.

WHEN THE STRUGGLE IS OVER

Once you've stopped smoking, take a second and pat yourself on the back. Now do it again. You deserve it. Remember now why you decided to stop smoking in the first place. Look at your list of reasons. Read them again. And smile. Now think about all the money you are saving and what you'll do with it. All the non-smoking places you can go, and what you might do there. All those years you may have added to your life, and what you'll do with them. Remember that temptation may not be gone forever. However, the hard part is behind you, so look forward with a positive attitude and enjoy your new life as a non-smoker.

QUESTIONS & ANSWERS

1. How will I feel when I stop smoking and start using Nicorette? You'll need to prepare yourself for some nicotine withdrawal symptoms. These begin almost immediately after you stop smoking, and are usually at their worst during the first three to four days. Understand that any of the following is possible:

- craving for cigarettes
- anxiety, irritability, restlessness, mood changes, nervousness
- drowsiness
- trouble concentrating
- increased appetite and weight gain
- headaches, muscular pain, constipation, fatigue

Nicorette can help provide relief from withdrawal symptoms such as irritability and nervousness, as well as the craving for nicotine you used to satisfy by having a cigarette.

2. Is Nicorette just substuting one form of nicotine for another? Nicorette does contain nicotine. The purpose of Nicorette is to provide you with enough nicotine to help control the physical withdrawal symptoms so you can deal with the mental aspects of quitting. During the 12 week program, you will gradually reduce your nicotine intake by switching to fewer pieces each day. Remember, don't use Nicorette together with nicotine patches or other nicotine containing products.

3. Can I be hurt by using Nicorette? For most adults, the amount of nicotine in the gum is less than from smoking. Some people will be sensitive to even this amount of nicotine and should not use this product without advice from their doctor. Because Nicorette is a gum-based product, chewing it can cause dental fillings to loosen and aggravate other mouth, tooth and jaw problems. Nicorette can also cause hiccups, heartburn and other stomach problems especially if chewed too quickly or not chewed correctly.

4. Will I gain weight? Many people do tend to gain a few pounds in the first 8–10 weeks after they stop smoking. This is a very small price to pay for the enormous gains that you will make in your overall health and attractiveness. If you continue to gain weight after the first two months, try to analyze what you're doing differently. Reduce your fat intake, choose healthy snacks, and increase your physical activity to burn off the extra calories.

5. Is Nicorette more expensive than smoking? The total cost of Nicorette for the twelve week program is about equal to what a person who smokes one and a half packs of cigarettes a day would spend on cigarettes for the same period of time. Also use of Nicorette is only a short-term cost, while the cost of smoking is a long-term cost, because of the health problems smoking causes.

6. What if I slip up? Discard your cigarettes, forgive yourself and then get back on track. Don't consider yourself a failure or punish yourself. In fact, people who have already tried to quit are more likely to be successful the next time.

GOOD LUCK!

[End User's Guide]

Copyright © 1999 SmithKline Beecham

To remove the gum, tear off a single unit.

Peel off backing starting at corner with loose edge.

Push gum through foil.

Blister packaged for your protection. Do not use if individual seals are broken.

Manufactured by Pharmacia & Upjohn AB, Stockholm, Sweden for SmithKline Beecham Consumer Healthcare, LP Pittsburgh, PA 15230
Comments or Questions? Call 1-800-419-4766 weekdays.
(10 a.m.–4:30 p.m. EST).

- **Not for sale to those under 18 years of age.**
- **Proof of age required.**
- **Not for sale in vending machines or from any source where proof of age cannot be verified.**

Nicorette Original, Mint, and Orange are available in:

2 mg or 4 mg Starter kit*—108 pieces
2 mg or 4 mg Refill—48 pieces
*User's Guide and Audio Tape included in kit

Shown in Product Identification Guide, page 507

Maximum Strength NYTOL® QUICKGELS® SOFTGELS

Indication: For relief of occasional sleeplessness.

Directions: Adults and children 12 years of age and over: oral dosage is one softgel (50 mg) at bedtime if needed, or as directed by a doctor.

Warnings: Do not give to children under 12 years of age. If sleeplessness persists continuously for more than two weeks, consult your doctor. Insomnia may be a symptom of serious underlying medical illness. **Do not take this product, unless directed by a doctor, if you have a breathing problem such as emphysema or chronic bronchitis, or if you have glaucoma or difficulty in urination due to enlargement of the prostate gland. Do not use** with any other product containing diphenhydramine, including one applied topically. Avoid alcoholic beverages while taking this product. Do not take this product if you are taking sedatives or tranquilizers, without first consulting your doctor. In case of accidental overdose, seek professional assistance or contact a Poison Control Center immediately. As with any drug, if you are pregnant or nursing a baby, seek the advice of a health professional before using this product. Keep out of reach of children.

Drug Interactions: Alcohol and other drugs which cause CNS depression will heighten the depressant effect of this product. Monoamine oxidase (MAO) inhibitors will prolong and intensify the anticholinergic effects of antihistamines.

Symptoms and Treatment of Oral Overdosage: In adults overdose may cause CNS depression resulting in hypnosis and coma. In children CNS hyperexcitability may follow sedation; the stimulant phase may bring tremor, delirium and convulsions. Gastrointestinal reactions may include dry mouth, appetite loss, nausea and/or vomiting. Respiratory distress and cardiovascular com-

plications (hypotension) may be evident. Treatment includes inducing emesis and controlling symptoms.

Active Ingredient: Diphenhydramine Hydrochloride 50 mg per softgel.

Inactive Ingredients: Edible Ink, Gelatin, Glycerin, Polyethylene Glycol, Purified Water, Sorbitol.

How Supplied: Available in packages of 8 and 16 softgels.
Shown in Product Identification Guide, page 508

NYTOL® QUICKCAPS® CAPLETS

Indication: For relief of occasional sleeplessness.

Directions: Adults and children 12 years of age and over: oral dosage is two caplets (50 mg) at bedtime if needed, or as directed by a doctor.

Warnings: Do not give to children under 12 years of age. If sleeplessness persists continuously for more than two weeks, consult your doctor. Insomnia may be a symptom of serious underlying medical illness. **Do not take this product, unless directed by a doctor, if you have a breathing problem such as emphysema or chronic bronchitis, or if you have glaucoma or difficulty in urination due to enlargement of the prostate gland. Do not use** with any other product containing diphenhydramine, including one applied topically. Avoid alcoholic beverages while taking this product. Do not take this product if you are taking sedatives or tranquilizers, without first consulting your doctor. In case of accidental overdose, seek professional assistance or contact a Poison Control Center immediately. As with any drug, if you are pregnant or nursing a baby, seek the advice of a health professional before using this product. Keep out of reach of children.
Drug Interactions: Alcohol and other drugs which cause CNS depression will heighten the depressant effect of this product. Monoamine oxidase (MAO) inhibitors will prolong and intensify the anticholinergic effects of antihistamines.
Symptoms and Treatment of Oral Overdosage: In adults, overdose may cause CNS depression resulting in hypnosis and coma. In children, CNS hyperexcitability may follow sedation; the stimulant phase may bring tremor, delirium and convulsions. Gastrointestinal reactions may include dry mouth, appetite loss, nausea and/or vomiting. Respiratory distress and cardiovascular complications (hypotension) may be evident. Treatment includes inducing emesis and controlling symptoms.

Active Ingredient: Diphenhydramine Hydrochloride 25 mg per caplet.

Inactive Ingredients: Corn Starch, Lactose, Microcrystalline Cellulose, Silica, Stearic Acid.

How supplied: Available in tamper-evident packages of 16, 32 and 72 caplets.
Shown in Product Identification Guide, page 507

Quick Dissolve
PHAZYME®–125 MG Chewable Tablets
[fay-zime]

Description: A great tasting, smooth cool mint chewable tablet containing simethicone, an antiflatulent to alleviate or relieve the symptoms referred to as gas. Uniquely formulated to dissolve quickly and completely in your mouth. It has no known side effects or drug interactions.

Active Ingredient: Each tablet contains simethicone 125 mg.

Inactive Ingredients: Aspartame, citricacid, colloidal silicon dioxide, crospovidone, dextrates, maltodextrin, mannitol, peppermint flavor, pregelatinized starch, sodium bicarbonate, sorbitol, talc, tribasic calcium phosphate.

Actions: Simethicone minimizes gas formation and relieves gas entrapment in both the stomach and the lower G.I. tract. This action combats the distress due to gastrointestinal gas.
Other Information: Each tablet contains sodium 8 mg. Phenylketonurics: contains phenylalanine 0.4 mg per tablet.

Indication: Relieves pressure, bloating or fullness commonly referred to as gas.

Warnings: Keep this and all drugs out of the reach of children. If condition persists, consult your physician.
Store at room temperature 59°–86°F (15°–30°C).

Dosage: Directions: Chew one or two tablets thoroughly, as needed after a meal. Do not exceed four tablets per day except under the advice and supervision of a physician.

How Supplied: White, bevel-edged tablets imprinted with "Phazyme 125" in 18 count and 48 count bottles.
Shown in Product Identification Guide, page 508

Ultra Strength
PHAZYME®–180 MG Softgels
[fay-zime]

Description: An orange, easy to swallow softgel, containing simethicone, an antiflatulent to alleviate or relieve the symptoms referred to as gas. It has no known side effects or drug interactions.
Active Ingredient: Each softgel contains simethicone 180 mg.
Inactive Ingredients: FD&C Yellow No. 6, gelatin, glycerin, and white edible ink.

Actions: Simethicone minimizes gas formation and relieves gas entrapment in both the stomach and the lower G.I. tract. This action combats the distress due to gastrointestinal gas.

Indication: Relieves pressure, bloating or fullness commonly referred to as gas.

Warnings: Keep this and all drugs out of the reach of children. If condition persists, consult your physician.
Store at room temperature 59°–86°F (15°–30°C).

Dosage: Directions: Swallow one or two softgels as needed after a meal. Do not exceed two softgels per day except under the advice and supervision of a physician.

How Supplied: Orange softgel imprinted with "PZ 180" in 12 count and 36 count blister pack, 60 count and 100 count bottles.
Shown in Product Identification Guide, page 508

SENSODYNE® FRESH MINT
SENSODYNE® FRESH IMPACT
SENSODYNE® COOL GEL
SENSODYNE® WITH BAKING SODA
SENSODYNE® TARTAR CONTROL
SENSODYNE® TARTAR CONTROL PLUS WHITENING
SENSODYNE® ORIGINAL FLAVOR
SENSODYNE® EXTRA WHITENING
Anticavity toothpaste for sensitive teeth

Active Ingredients: "Fresh Impact" Potassium Nitrate 5% Sodium Fluoride 0.15% w/v fluoride ion 5% Potassium Nitrate and 0.15% w/v Sodium Monofluorophosphate (Extra Whitening) or Sodium Fluoride (Fresh Mint, 0.15% w/v; Baking Soda, 0.15% w/v; Cool Gel, 0.13% w/v; Tartar Control, 0.13% w/v; Tartar Control Plus Whitening 0.145% w/v; Original Flavor, 0.13% w/v), or Sodium Fluoride 0.15% w/v fluoride ion (Fresh Impact). Sensodyne Fresh Mint, Sensodyne Fresh Impact, Sensodyne Cool Gel, Sensodyne with Baking Soda, Sensodyne Tartar Control, Sensodyne Tartar Control Plus Whitening, Sensodyne Original Flavor and Sensodyne Extra Whitening contain fluoride for cavity prevention and Potassium Nitrate clinically proven to reduce pain sensitivity for relief of dentinal hypersensitivity resulting from the exposure of tooth dentin due to periodontal surgery, cervical (gum line) erosion, abrasion or recession which causes pain on contact with hot, cold, or tactile stimuli.

Inactive Ingredients: *Baking Soda:* Flavor, Glycerin, Hydrated Silica, Hydroxyethylcellulose, Methylparaben, Propylparaben, Silica, Sodium Bicarbon-

Continued on next page

Extra Whitening: Calcium Peroxide, Flavor, Glycerin, Hydrated Silica, PEG-12, PEG-75, Silica, Sodium Carbonate, Sodium Lauryl Sulfate, Sodium Saccharin, Titanium Dioxide, Water.

Tartar Control: Cellulose Gum, Cocamidopropyl Betaine, Flavor, Glycerin, Hydrated Silica, Silica, Sodium Bicarbonate, Sodium Saccharin, Tetrapotassium Pyrophosphate, Titanium Dioxide, Water.

Tartar Control Plus Whitening: Cellulose Gum, Flavor, Glycerin, Polyethylene Glycol, Silica, Sodium Lauryl Sulfate, Sodium Saccharin, Tetrapotassium Pyrophosphate, Titanium Dioxide, Water.

Cool Gel: Cellulose Gum, FD&C Blue #1, Flavor, Glycerin, Hydrated Silica, Silica, Sodium Methyl Cocoyl Taurate, Sodium Saccharin, Sorbitol, Trisodium Phosphate, Water. **Fresh Impact:** D&C yellow #10 lake, FD&C blue #1 lake, flavor, glycerin, hydrated silica, sodium benzoate, sodium hydroxide, sodium lauryl sulfate, sodium saccharin, sorbitol, titanium dioxide, water, xanthan gum

Fresh Mint: Inactive Ingredients: Carbomer, cellulose gum, D&C yellow #10, FD&C blue #1, flavor, glycerin, hydrated silica, octadecene/MA copolymer, poloxamer 407, potassium hydroxide, sodium lauroyl sarcosinate, sodium saccharin, sorbitol, titanium dioxide, water, xanthan gum.

Original Flavor: Cellulose Gum, D&C Red No. 28, Glycerin, Hydrated Silica, Peppermint Oil, Silica, Sodium Methyl Cocoyl Taurate, Sodium Saccharin, Sorbitol, Titanium Dioxide, Trisodium Phosphate, Water.

Actions: All Sensodyne Formulas significantly reduce tooth hypersensitivity, with response to therapy evident after two weeks of use. Controlled double-blind clinical studies provide substantial evidence of the safety and effectiveness of Potassium Nitrate. The current theory on mechanism of action is that potassium nitrate has an effect on neural transmission, interrupting the signal which would result in the sensation of pain. Fluorides are anticariogenic, forming fluoroapatite in the outer surface of the dental enamel which is resistant to acids and caries.

Warnings: Sensitive teeth may indicate a serious problem that may need prompt care by a dentist. See your dentist if the problem persists or worsens. Do not use this product longer than 4 weeks unless recommended by a dentist or physician. Keep this and all drugs out of the reach of children. If you accidentally swallow more than used for brushing, seek professional assistance or contact a Poison Control Center immediately.

Dosage and Administration: Adults and children 12 years of age and older: Apply a 1-inch strip of the product onto a soft bristle toothbrush. Brush teeth thoroughly for at least 1 minute twice a day (morning and evening) or as recommended by a dentist or physician. Make sure to brush all sensitive areas of the teeth. Children under 12 years of age: consult a dentist or physician.

How Supplied: All Sensodyne formulas are supplied in 2.1 oz. (60g), 4.0 oz. (113g) and 6.0 oz. (170g) tubes. Sensodyne Cool Gel is supplied in 4.0 oz. and 6.0 oz. tubes. Sensodyne Baking Soda is supplied in 4.0 oz and 6.0 oz. only.

**SINGLET® For Adults
Nasal Decongestant/Antihistamine/
Analgesic (pain reliever)/Antipyretic
(fever reducer)**

Indications: For temporary relief of nasal congestion and sinus and headache pain associated with sinusitis or due to a cold, hay fever or other upper respiratory allergies. Also temporarily relieves nasal congestion, sinus headache, runny nose, sneezing, itching of the nose or throat, and itchy, watery eyes due to hay fever or other upper respiratory allergies. Also temporarily relieves fever due to the common cold.

Directions: Adults (12 years and older): 1 caplet every 4 to 6 hours, **not to exceed 4 caplets in any 24-hour period,** or as directed by a doctor. Children under 12 years of age: Consult a doctor.

Warnings: Do not exceed recommended dosage. If nervousness, dizziness, or sleeplessness occur, discontinue use and consult a doctor. Do not take this product for more than 10 days. If symptoms do not improve or are accompanied by fever that lasts for more than 3 days, or if new symptoms occur, consult a doctor. Do not take this product, unless directed by a doctor, if you have a breathing problem such as emphysema or chronic bronchitis, or if you have heart disease, high blood pressure, thyroid disease, diabetes, glaucoma or difficulty in urination due to enlargement of the prostate gland. May cause excitability especially in children. May cause drowsiness; alcohol, sedatives, and tranquilizers may increase the drowsiness effect. Avoid alcoholic beverages while taking this product. Do not take this product if you are taking sedatives or tranquilizers, without first consulting your doctor. Use caution when driving a motor vehicle or operating machinery. **KEEP THIS AND ALL DRUGS OUT OF THE REACH OF CHILDREN.** Prompt medical attention is critical for adults as well as for children even if you do not notice any signs or symptoms. In case of accidental overdose, seek professional assistance or contact a Poison Control Center immediately. As with any drug, if you are pregnant or nursing a baby, seek the advice of a health professional before using this product.

Alcohol Warning: If you consume 3 or more alcoholic drinks every day, ask your doctor whether you should take acetaminophen or other pain reliever/fever reducers. Acetaminophen may cause liver damage.

Drug Interaction Precaution: Do not use this product if you are now taking a prescription monoamine oxidase inhibitor (MAOI) (certain drugs for depression, psychiatric or emotional conditions, or Parkinson's disease), or for 2 weeks after stopping the MAOI drug. If you are uncertain whether your prescription drug contains an MAOI, consult a health professional before taking this product.

Active Ingredients: Each caplet contains: Pseudoephedrine Hydrochloride 60 mg, Chlorpheniramine Maleate 4 mg, Acetaminophen 650 mg.

Inactive Ingredients: D&C Red 27, D&C Yellow 10, FD&C Blue 1, Hydroxypropyl Cellulose, Hypromellose, Magnesium Stearate, Microcrystalline Cellulose, Polyethylene Glycol, Pregelatinized Corn Starch, Sodium Starch Glycolate, Sucrose and Titanium Dioxide.
Store at room temperature (59°–86°F). Avoid excessive heat and humidity.
Comments or Questions? Call toll-free 1-800-245-1040 weekdays
Distributed by: GlaxoSmithKline Consumer Healthcare, L.P.
Pittsburgh, PA 15230. Made in U.S.A.

**SOMINEX Original Formula
Nighttime Sleep Aid
Doctor-preferred sleep ingredient**

Indications: Helps to reduce difficulty falling asleep.

Directions: Adults and children 12 years and over: Take 2 tablets at bedtime if needed, or as directed by a doctor. For best results, take recommended dose. This will provide approximately six to eight hours of restful sleep.

Warnings: Do not give to children under 12 years of age. If sleeplessness persists continually for more than 2 weeks, consult your doctor. Insomnia may be a symptom of serious underlying medical illness. Do not take this product, unless directed by a doctor, if you have a breathing problem such as emphysema or chronic bronchitis, or if you have glaucoma or difficulty in urination due to enlargement of the prostate gland. Avoid alcoholic beverages while taking this product. Do not take this product if you are taking sedatives or tranquilizers, without first consulting your doctor. As with any drug, if you are pregnant or nursing a baby, seek the advice of a health professional before using this product. **Keep this and all drugs out of the reach of children.** In case of accidental overdose, seek professional assistance or contact a poison control center immediately.

Active Ingredients: Each tablet contains 25 mg Diphenhydramine HCl.

Inactive Ingredients: Dibasic Calcium Phosphate, FD&C Blue #1, Magnesium Stearate, Microcrystalline Cellulose, Silicon Dioxide, Starch.

Tamper Evident Feature: Individually sealed in foil for your protection. Do not use if foil or plastic bubble is torn or punctured.

Store at room temperature, avoid excessive heat (greater than 100°F) or humidity.

How Supplied: Consumer Packages of 16, 32 and 72 tablets

Also Available in Maximum Strength Formula.

Comments or Questions? Call Toll-Free 1-800-245-1040 Weekdays.

GlaxoSmithKline Consumer Healthcare, L.P.

Pittsburgh, PA 15230. Made in U.S.A.

TAGAMET HB® 200
Cimetidine Tablets 200 mg/
Acid Reducer

Tagamet HB® 200 relieves and prevents heartburn, acid indigestion and sour stomach when used as directed. It contains the same ingredient found in prescription strength Tagamet. Tagamet HB 200 reduces the production of stomach acid.

Active Ingredient: Cimetidine, 200 mg.

Inactive Ingredients: Cellulose, cornstarch, hypromellose, magnesium stearate, polyethylene glycol, polysorbate 80, povidone, sodium lauryl sulfate, sodium starch glycolate, titanium dioxide.

Uses:
• For relief of heartburn associated with acid indigestion and sour stomach.
• For prevention of heartburn associated with acid indigestion and sour stomach brought on by eating or drinking certain food and beverages.

Directions:
• For **relief** of symptoms, swallow 1 tablet with a glass of water.
• For **prevention** of symptoms, swallow 1 tablet with a glass of water **right before or anytime up to 30 minutes before** eating food or drinking beverages that cause heartburn.
• Tagamet HB 200 can be used up to twice daily (up to 2 tablets in 24 hours).
• This product should not be given to children under 12 years old unless directed by a doctor.

Warnings:
Allergy Warning: Do not use if you are allergic to Tagamet HB 200 (cimetidine) or other acid reducers.
Ask a Doctor Before Use If You are Taking:
 • theophylline (oral asthma medicine)
 • warfarin (blood thinning medicine)
 • phenytoin (seizure medicine)
If you are not sure whether your medication contains one of these drugs or have any other questions about medicines you are taking, call our consumer affairs specialist at 1-800-482-4394.

• Do not take the maximum daily dosage for more than 2 weeks continuously except under the advice and supervision of a doctor.
• If you have trouble swallowing, or persistent abdominal pain, see your doctor promptly. You may have a serious condition that may need a different treatment.
• As with any drug, if you are pregnant or nursing a baby, seek the advice of a health professional before using this product.
• Keep this and all medications out of the reach of children.
• In case of accidental overdose, seek professional assistance or contact a poison control center immediately.

READ THE LABEL
Read the directions and warnings before taking this medication.
Store at 15°–30°C (59°–86°F).
Comments or questions? Call Toll-Free 1-800-482-4394 weekdays.

PHARMACOKINETIC INTERACTIONS
Cimetidine at prescription doses is known to inhibit various P450 metabolizing isoenzymes, which could affect metabolism of other drugs and increase their blood concentration. Investigation of pharmacokinetic interactions at the recommended OTC doses of cimetidine have thus far shown only small effects. A pharmacokinetic study conducted in 26 normal male subjects (mean age, 38 years) at steady state using the maximum recommended OTC dose level (200 mg twice a day), showed that Tagamet HB 200, on average, increased the 24 hour AUC of theophylline by 14% and increased peak theophylline levels by 15%. This interaction should be borne in mind in advising patients on the use of Tagamet HB 200. At the prescription doses of cimetidine, clinically significant pharmacokinetic interactions between cimetidine and warfarin, phenytoin, and theophylline have been reported. At prescription doses, pharmacokinetic interactions have been reported for a number of other drugs as well, such as with dihydropyridine calcium channel blockers or some short acting benzodiazepines. At the maximum recommended OTC dose level (200 mg twice a day), a pharmacokinetic study conducted in 21 normal male subjects (mean age, 38 years) showed that Tagamet HB 200, on average, increased the total AUC of triazolam by 26–28% and increased peak triazolam levels by 11–23%. Tagamet HB 200 did not alter the apparent terminal elimination half-life of triazolam.

How Supplied: Tagamet HB 200 (Cimetidine Tablets 200 mg) is available in boxes of blister packs in 6, 30, 50, & 70 tablet sizes.

Shown in Product Identification Guide, page 508

TEGRIN® DANDRUFF SHAMPOO –
EXTRA CONDITIONING

Description: Tegrin® Dandruff Shampoo contains 7% w/w Coal Tar Solution,

USP, equivalent to 0.7% w/w coal tar, in a pleasantly scented, high-foaming, cleansing shampoo base with emollients, conditioners and other formula components.

Active Ingredient: 7% w/w Coal Tar Solution, USP, Equivalent to 0.7% w/w Coal Tar.

Use: Tegrin® Dandruff Shampoo controls the flaking and itching of the scalp associated with dandruff, seborrheic dermatitis, and psoriasis.

Warnings: For external use only. Ask a doctor before use if you have psoriasis or seborrheic dermatitis that covers a large area of the body. Ask a doctor or pharmacist if you are using other forms of psoriasis therapy such as ultraviolet radiation or prescription drugs. When using this product • do not use for prolonged periods • avoid contact with eyes. If contact occurs, rinse eyes thoroughly with water. • use caution in exposing skin to sunlight after application. It may increase your tendency to sunburn for up to 24 hours after application. Stop use and ask a doctor if condition worsens or does not improve after regular use of this product as directed. Keep out of reach of children. If swallowed, get medical help or contact a Poison Control Center right away.

Directions: Shake well. Wet hair, lather, rinse, repeat. For best results use at least twice a week or as directed by a doctor.

Coal Tar is obtained in the destructive distillation of bituminous coal and is a highly effective agent for controlling the flaking and itching of the scalp associated with dandruff, seborrheic dermatitis, and psoriasis. The action of coal tar is believed to be keratolytic, antiseptic, antipruritic, and astringent. The coal tar solution used in Tegrin® Dandruff Shampoo is prepared in such a way as to reduce the itch and other irritant components found in crude coal tar without reduction in therapeutic potency.

Coal Tar Solution has been used clinically for many years as a remedy for dandruff and for scaling associated with scalp disorders such as seborrhea and psoriasis. Its mechanism of action has not been fully established, but it is believed to retard the rate of turnover of epidermal cells with regular use. A number of clinical studies have demonstrated the performance attributes of Tegrin® Dandruff Shampoo against dandruff and seborrheic dermatitis. In addition to relieving the above symptoms, Tegrin® Dandruff Shampoo, used regularly, maintains scalp and hair cleanliness and leaves the hair lustrous and manageable.

Other Information:
Store at 20°–25°C (68°–77°F)

Inactive Ingredients:
Alcohol (7.0%), Ammonium Lauryl Sulfate, Citric Acid, FD&C Blue #1, Fragrance, Glycol Stearate (and) Sodium

Continued on next page

Tegrin Extra Cond.—Cont.

Laureth Sulfate (and) Hexylene Glycol, Guar Hydroxypropyltrimonium Chloride, Hydroxypropyl Methylcellulose, Lauramide DEA, Methylparaben, Propylparaben, Sodium Lauryl Sulfate, Water.

How Supplied: Tegrin® Dandruff Shampoo is available in Extra Conditioning and Fresh Herbal formulas and supplied in 7 fl. oz. (207 ml) plastic bottles.

TEGRIN® DANDRUFF SHAMPOO-FRESH HERBAL

Description: Tegrin® Dandruff Shampoo contains 7% w/w Coal Tar Solution, USP, equivalent to 0.7% w/w coal tar, in a pleasantly scented, high-foaming, cleansing shampoo base with emollients, conditioners and other formula components.

Use: Tegrin® Dandruff Shampoo controls the flaking and itching of the scalp associated with dandruff, seborrheic dermatitis, and psoriasis.

Warnings: For external use only. Avoid contact with eyes. If contact occurs, rinse eyes thoroughly with water. If condition worsens or does not improve after regular use of this product as directed, consult a doctor. Use caution in exposing skin to sunlight after applying this product. It may increase tendency to sunburn for up to 24 hours after application. Do not use for prolonged periods without consulting a doctor. Do not use this product with other forms of psoriasis therapy, such as ultraviolet radiation or prescription drugs, unless directed by a doctor. Keep out of reach of children. In case of accidental ingestion, seek professional assistance or contact a Poison Control Center immediately.

Directions: Shake well. Wet hair. Lather, rinse, repeat. For best results use at least twice a week or as directed by a doctor.

Active Ingredient: 7% w/w Coal Tar Solution, USP, Equivalent to 0.7% w/w Coal Tar. Coal Tar is obtained in the destructive distillation of bituminous coal and is a highly effective agent for controlling the flaking and itching of the scalp associated with dandruff, seborrheic dermatitis and psoriasis. The action of coal tar is believed to be keratolytic, antiseptic, antipruritic, and astringent. The coal tar solution used in Tegrin® Dandruff Shampoo is prepared in such a way as to reduce the pitch and other irritant components found in crude coal tar without reduction in therapeutic potency.
Coal Tar Solution has been used clinically for many years as a remedy for dandruff and for scaling associated with scalp disorders such as seborrhea and psoriasis. Its mechanism of action has not been fully established, but it is believed to retard the rate of turnover of epidermal cells with regular use. A number of clinical studies have demonstrated the performance attributes of Tegrin® Dandruff Shampoo against dandruff and seborrheic dermatitis. In addition to relieving the above symptoms, Tegrin® Dandruff Shampoo, used regularly, maintains scalp and hair cleanliness and leaves the hair lustrous and manageable.

Other Information:
Store at 20°–25°C (68°–77°F)

Inactive Ingredients: Alcohol (7.0%), Citric Acid, Cocamide DEA, FD&C Blue #1, Fragrance, Glycol Stearate (and) Sodium Laureth Sulfate (and) Hexylene Glycol, Hydroxypropyl Methylcellulose, Methylparaben, Propylparaben, Sodium Lauryl Sulfate, Water.

How Supplied: Tegrin® Dandruff Shampoo is available in Extra Conditioning and Fresh Herbal formulas and supplied in 7 fl. oz. (207 ml) plastic bottles.
Shown in Product Identification Guide, page 508

TEGRIN® SKIN CREAM FOR PSORIASIS

Description: Tegrin® Skin Cream for Psoriasis contains 5% Coal Tar Solution, USP, equivalent to 0.8% Coal Tar and alcohol of 4.7%.

Indications: For relief of itching, flaking and irritation of the skin associated with psoriasis and seborrheic dermatitis.

Directions: Apply to affected areas one to four times daily or as directed by a doctor.

Warnings: For external use only. Avoid contact with eyes. If contact occurs, rinse eyes thoroughly with water. If condition worsens or does not improve after regular use of this product as directed, consult a doctor. Use caution in exposing skin to sunlight after applying this product. It may increase tendency to sunburn for up to 24 hours after application. Do not use for prolonged periods without consulting a doctor. Do not use this product with other forms of psoriasis therapy, such as ultra-violet radiation or prescription drugs, unless directed by a doctor. If the condition covers a large area of the body, consult your doctor before using this product. Keep out of reach of children. In case of accidental ingestion, seek professional assistance or contact a Poison Control Center immediately.

Active Ingredient: 5% Coal Tar Solution, USP, equivalent to 0.8% Coal Tar.

Inactive Ingredients: Acetylated Lanolin Alcohol, Alcohol (4.7%), Carbomer-934P, Ceteth-2, Ceteth-16, Cetyl Acetate, Cetyl Alcohol, D&C Red No. 28, Fragrance, Glyceryl Tribehenate, Laneth-16, Lanolin Alcohol, Laureth-23, Methyl Gluceth-20, Methylchloroisothiazolinone, Methylisothiazolinone, Mineral Oil, Octyldodecanol, Oleth-16, Petrolatum, Potassium Hydroxide, Purified Water, Steareth-16, Stearyl Alcohol, Titanium Dioxide.

How Supplied: Tegrin® Skin Cream for Psoriasis is available in a 2 oz (57g) tube.
Shown in Product Identification Guide, page 508

TUMS® Regular Antacid/Calcium Supplement Tablets
TUMS E–X® and TUMS E–X® Sugar Free Antacid/Calcium Supplement Tablets
TUMS ULTRA® Antacid/Calcium Supplement Tablets

Professional Labeling: Indicated for the symptomatic relief of hyperacidity associated with the diagnosis of peptic ulcer, gastritis, peptic esophagitis, gastric hyperacidity, and hiatal hernia.

Indications: For fast relief of acid indigestion, heartburn, sour stomach, and upset stomach associated with these symptoms.

Active Ingredient:
Tums, Calcium Carbonate 500 mg
Tums E-X, Calcium Carbonate 750 mg
Tums ULTRA, Calcium Carbonate 1000 mg

Actions: Tums provides rapid neutralization of stomach acid. Each Tums tablet has an acid-neutralizing capacity (ANC) of 10 mEq. Each Tums E-X tablet has an ANC of 15 mEq and each Tums ULTRA tablet, an ANC of 20 mEq. This high neutralization capacity makes Tums tablets an ideal antacid for management of conditions associated with hyperacidity. It effectively neutralizes free acid yet does not cause systemic alkalosis in the presence of normal renal function. A double-blind placebo-controlled clinical study demonstrated that calcium carbonate taken at a dosage of 16 Tums tablets daily for a two-week period was non-constipating/non-laxative.

Warnings: Tums: Do not take more than 15 tablets in a 24-hour period or use the maximum dosage of this product for more than 2 weeks, except under the advice and supervision of a physician. If symptoms persist for 2 weeks, stop using this product and see a physician. Keep this and all drugs out of the reach of children.
Tums E-X: Do not take more than 10 tablets in a 24-hour period or use the maximum dosage of this product for more than two weeks, except under the advice and supervision of a physician. If symptoms persist for two weeks, stop using this product and see a physician. Keep this and all drugs out of the reach of children.
Additionally, for Tums Ex Sugar Free: Phenylketonurics: Contains phenylalanine, less than 1 mg per tablet.

Supplement Facts

	Tums 2 Tablets	Tums E-X 2 Tablets	Tums E-X Sugar Free 2 Tablets	Tums Ultra 2 Tablets
Serving Size				
Amount Per Serving				
Calories	5	10	5	10
Sorbitol (g)	—	—	1	—
Sugars (g)	1	2	—	3
Calcium (mg)	400	600	600	800
% Daily Value	40	60	60	80
Sodium (mg)	—	5	—	10
% Daily Value	—	<1%	—	<1%

Tums ULTRA: Do not take more than 7 tablets in 24-hour period or use the maximum dosage of this product for more than two weeks, except under the advice and supervision of a physician. If symptoms persist for two weeks, stop using and see a physician. Keep this and all drugs out of the reach of children.

Drug Interaction Precaution: Antacids may interact with certain prescription drugs. If you are presently taking a prescription drug, do not take this product without checking with your physician or other health professional.

Dosage and Administration:
Tums: Chew 2-4 tablets as symptoms occur. Repeat hourly if symptoms return, or as directed by physician.
Tums E-X: Chew 2-4 tablets as symptoms occur. Repeat hourly if symptoms return, or as directed by a physician.
Tums ULTRA: Chew 2-3 tablets as symptoms occur. Repeat hourly if symptoms return, or as directed by a physician.

AS A DIETARY SUPPLEMENT:
Calcium Supplement Directions
Tums, Tums E-X, & Tums ULTRA:
USES: As a daily source of extra calcium. Tums is recommended by the National Osteoporosis Foundation.

IMPORTANT INFORMATION ON OSTEOPOROSIS: Research shows that certain ethnic, age and other groups are at higher risk for developing osteoporosis, including Caucasian and Asian teen and young adult women, menopausal women, older persons and those persons with a family history of fragile bones. **A balanced diet with enough calcium and regular exercise throughout life will help you to build and maintain healthy bones and may reduce your risk of developing osteoporosis.** Adequate calcium intake is important, but daily intakes above 2,000 mg are not likely to provide any additional benefit.

DIRECTIONS: Chew 2 tablets twice daily.
[See table above]

Ingredients (all variants except sugar free): Sucrose, Corn Starch, Talc, Mineral Oil, Flavors (natural and/or artificial), Sodium Polyphosphate. May also contain 1% or less of Adipic Acid, Blue 1 Lake, Yellow 6 Lake, Yellow 5 Lake, Red 40 Lake.

Ingredients (Sugar Free): Sorbitol, Acacia, Natural and Artificial Flavors, Calcium Stearate, Adipic Acid, Yellow 6 Lake, Aspartame.

How Supplied:
Tums: Peppermint flavor is available in 12-tablet rolls, 3-roll wraps, and bottles of 75, 150, and 180. **Assorted Flavors** (Cherry, Lemon, Orange, and Lime), are available in 12-tablet rolls, 3-roll wraps, and bottles of 75, 150, and 320.
Tums E-X: Wintergreen 3-roll wraps and bottles of 48, 96, and 116.
Tums E-X: Assorted Fruit, Assorted Tropical Fruit, and Assorted Berries, Fresh Blend 8 tablet rolls, 3-roll wraps, 6-roll wraps, and bottles of 48, 96, and 116. Assorted Tropical Fruit and Assorted Berries are also available in bottles of 200 tablets.
Tums EX Sugar Free: Orange Cream; bottles of 48 and 80 tablets.
Tums ULTRA: Assorted Berries, and **Spearmint** bottles of 160 tablets. **Assorted Fruit** and **Assorted Mint** bottles of 36, 72, and 86 tablets. Assorted Fruit also available in bottles of 160 tablets. **Tropical Fruit** bottles of 160 tablets.

Shown in Product Identification Guide, page 508

VIVARIN Tablets & Caplets
Alertness Aid with Caffeine
Maximum Strength

Each Tablet or Caplet Contains 200 mg. Caffeine, Equal to About Two Cups of Coffee
Take Vivarin for a safe, fast pick up anytime you feel drowsy and need to be alert. The caffeine in Vivarin is less irritating to your stomach than coffee, according to a government appointed panel of experts.

FDA APPROVED USES: Helps restore mental alertness or wakefulness when experiencing fatigue or drowsiness.

Active Ingredients: Caffeine 200 mg.

Inactive Ingredients: Tablet: Colloidal Silicon Dioxide, D&C Yellow #10 Al. Lake, Dextrose, FD&C Yellow #6 Al. Lake, Magnesium Stearate, Microcrystalline Cellulose, Starch.
Caplet: Carnauba Wax, Colloidal Silicon Dioxide, D&C Yellow #10 Al Lake, Dextrose, FD&C Yellow #6 Al Lake, Hypromellose, Magnesium Stearate, Microcrystalline Cellulose, Polyethylene Glycol, Polysorbate 80, Starch, Titanium Dioxide.

Directions: Adults and children 12 years and over: Take 1 tablet (200 mg) not more often than every 3 to 4 hours.
Warnings: The recommended dose of this product contains about as much caffeine as two cups of coffee. Limit the use of caffeine containing medications, foods, or beverages while taking this product because too much caffeine may cause nervousness, irritability, sleeplessness, and occasionally, rapid heartbeat. For occasional use only. Not intended for use as a substitute for sleep. If fatigue or drowsiness persists or continues to recur, consult a doctor. Do not give to children under 12 years of age. As with any drug, if you are pregnant or nursing a baby, seek the advice of a health professional before using this product. In case of accidental overdose, seek professional assistance or contact a poison control center immediately. Keep this and all drugs out of the reach of children.

Tamper Evident Feature: Individually sealed in foil for your protection. Do not use if foil or plastic bubble is torn or punctured.

Store at room temperature, avoid excessive heat (greater than 100°F) or humidity.

How Supplied:
Tablets: Consumer packages of 16, 40 and 80 tablets
Caplets: Consumer packages of 24 and 48 caplets

Comments or Questions? Call Toll-Free 1-800-245-1040 Weekdays.
GlaxoSmithKline Consumer Healthcare, L.P.
Pittsburgh, PA 15230. Made in U.S.A.
©1996 SmithKline Beecham
Shown in Product Identification Guide, page 508

Green Pharmaceuticals® Inc.,
1459 E. THOUSAND OAKS BLVD., #G
THOUSAND OAKS, CA 91362

Direct Inquiries and Medical Emergencies:
(800) 337 4835
mail@snorestop.com

SNORESTOP® EXTINGUISHER™
120 ORAL SPRAYS
Homeopathic Anti-snoring Medicine

Description: Uniquely formulated (U.S. Patent No. 6,491,954) to temporar-

Continued on next page

Snorestop—Cont.

ily relieve the symptoms commonly associated with non-apneic snoring. No known side effects or drug interactions.†

Important Information: This product contains no ephedrine, no pseudoephedrine, no tropane or indole alkaloids. Each substance has been highly diluted according to the *Homeopathic Pharmacopoeia of the United States:* 4X is equal to one-part-per-ten thousand, 6X is equal to one-part-per-million, and 12 X is equal to one-part-per-trillion.

Active Ingredients: Nux vomica 4X, 6X HPUS, Belladonna 6X HPUS, Ephedra vulgaris 6X HPUS, Hydrastis canadensis 6X HPUS, Kali bichromicum 6X HPUS, Teucrium marum 6X HPUS, Histaminum hydrochloricum 12X HPUS.

Mode of Action: Decongestive, anti-inflammatory, anti-histaminic and mucolytic.

Inactive Ingredients: Purified water 75%, USP Alcohol 15%, Glycerin 9.9%, Potassium sorbate 0.1%.

Directions:—Children over 5 years of age and Adults under 180 lbs.
Shake before each use. Nights 1–10, spray once under the tongue and once in the back of the throat at bedtime. When improvement is noticed, you may use *every other night* until no longer needed.
—Adults over 180 lbs. **Shake before each use.** Nights 1–10, spray once under the tongue and once in the back of the throat 30 minutes before bedtime and repeat at bedtime. When improvement is noticed, you may use *every other night* until no longer needed.

Warnings: Do not use if seal around the bottle is broken. Do not use on children under 5 years of age. This product does not treat sleep apnea. For sleep apnea, consult with a specialist. If symptoms worsen, discontinue use and consult with a licensed health care professional. As with any drug, if you are pregnant or nursing a baby, consult a health care professional before using this product. Keep this and all medications out of the reach of children.

How Supplied: .4fl oz bottle delivering 120 metered sprays (NDC 61152-196-12).
.5fl oz bottle delivering 160 metered sprays (NDC 61152-196-15).
Shown in Product Identification Guide, page 508

SNORESTOP® MAXIMUM STRENGTH CHEWABLE TABLETS
Homeopathic Anti-snoring Medicine

Description: Uniquely formulated* to temporarily relieve the symptoms commonly associated with non-apneic snoring. No known side effects or drug interactions.

*This formula has been the object of a randomized, double blind, placebo controlled independent clinical study whose positive results have been published in the peer-reviewed medical journal *Sleep and Breathing.* Vol.3. No.2. 1999.†

Important Information: This product contains no ephedrine, no pseudoephedrine, no tropane or indole alkaloids. Each substance has been highly diluted according to the *Homeopathic Pharmacopoeia of the United States*: 4X is equal to one-part-per-ten thousand, 6X is equal to one-part-per-million, and 12 X is equal to one-part-per-trillion.

Active Ingredients: Nux vomica 4X, 6X HPUS, Belladonna 6X HPUS, Ephedra vulgaris 6X HPUS, Hydrastis canadensis 6X HPUS, Kali bichromicum 6X HPUS, Teucrium marum 6X HPUS, Histaminum hydrochloricum 12X HPUS.

Mode of Action: Decongestive, anti-inflammatory, anti-histaminic and mucolytic.

Inactive Ingredients: Lactose 297 mg, magnesium stearate 3 mg.

Directions:—Children over 5 years of age and Adults under 180 lbs. Chew or suck one tablet when lying in bed. When improvement is noticed, you may start using *every other night* until no longer needed.
—Adults over 180 lbs. Chew or suck one tablet 30 minutes before bedtime and repeat at bedtime. When improvement is noticed, you may start using *every other night* until no longer needed.

Warnings: Do not use if blister seal around the tablet is broken. Do not use on children under 5 years of age. This product does not treat sleep apnea. For sleep apnea, consult with a specialist. If symptoms worsen, discontinue use and consult with a licensed health care professional. As with any drug, if you are pregnant or nursing a baby, consult a health care professional before using this product. Keep this and all medications out of the reach of children.

How Supplied: Boxes of 10 tablets (NDC 61152-195-10), 20 tablets (NDC 61152-195-20), 60 tablets (NDC 61152-195-60).
Shown in Product Identification Guide, page 508

EDUCATIONAL MATERIAL

"Snoring From A to ZZZ"
Derek LIPMAN, M.D.
The reference book for the FDA & FTC on snoring and sleep apnea
  230 pages
  Free to Physicians
  Free to Pharmacists
  $12.95 per copy to consumers

"A Randomized Double-Blind Placebo-Controlled Evaluation of the Safety and Efficacy of a Natural Over-The-Counter (OTC) Medication in the Management of Snoring"
  6 pages
  FREE
SnoreStop Maximum Strength an homeopathic drug with a clinical study.
  10 tablets
  FREE
SnoreStop The Extinguisher spray the #1 selling OTC medication for snoring
  120 doses
  Free to Physicians
  Free to Pharmacists
  $19.99 per unit to consumers

Hyland's, Inc.

See Standard Homeopathic Company

Johnson & Johnson • MERCK
Consumer Pharmaceuticals Co.
7050 CAMP HILL ROAD
FORT WASHINGTON, PA 19034

Direct Inquiries to:
Consumer Relationship Center
Fort Washington, PA 19034
(215) 273-7000

INFANTS' MYLICON® Drops
[*my 'li-con*]
Antiflatulent

Active Ingredients:
Each 0.3 mL of drops contains simethicone, 20 mg.

Uses:
Relieves the discomfort of infant gas frequently caused by air swallowing or certain formulas or foods. The defoaming action of INFANTS' MYLICON® Drops relieves flatulence by dispersing and preventing the formation of mucus-surrounded gas pockets in the gastrointestinal tract. INFANTS' MYLICON® Drops act in the stomach and intestines to change the surface tension of gas bubbles enabling them to coalesce, thereby freeing and eliminating the gas more easily by belching or passing flatus.

Directions:
• shake well before using
• all dosages may be repeated as needed, after meals and at bedtime or as directed by a physician. Do not exceed 12 doses per day.
• fill enclosed dropper to recommended dosage level and dispense liquid slowly into baby's mouth, toward the inner cheek
• dosage can also be mixed with 1 oz. cool water, infant formula or other suitable liquids

- for best results, clean dropper after each use and replace original cap.

Age (yr)	Weight (lb)	Dose
infants under 2	under 24	0.3 mL
children over 2	over 24	0.6 mL

Warnings:
Keep out of reach of children. In case of overdose get medical help or contact poison control center right away.
Other Information:
- **do not use if printed plastic overwrap or printed neck wrap is missing or broken**
- store at room temperature
- do not freeze

Inactive Ingredients: carboxymethylcellulose sodium, citric acid, D&C Red 22, D&C Red 28, flavors, maltitol, microcrystalline cellulose, purified water, sodium benzoate, sodium citrate, xanthan gum, non-staining formula contains no Red 22 or Red 28.

How Supplied:
INFANTS' MYLICON® Drops are available in bottles of 15 ml (0.5 fl oz) and 30 ml (1.0 fl oz) original pink, pleasant tasting liquid and non-staining formula. NDC 16837-630; 16837-911.

Shown in Product Identification Guide, page 509

CHILDREN'S MYLANTA® UPSET STOMACH RELIEF
CALCIUM CARBONATE/ANTACID TABLETS

Description: Children's Mylanta is a specially formulated antacid to quickly and effectively relieve the upset stomach kids sometimes experience.

Active Ingredients: Each tablet contains 400 mg of calcium carbonate.

Uses:
Relieves:
- acid indigestion
- sour stomach
- upset stomach due to these symptoms or overindulgence in food and drink

Directions:
- Find the right dose on the chart below. If possible use weight to dose; otherwise use age.
- Repeat dosing as needed.
- do not take more than 3 tablets (2–5 year old) or 6 tablets (6–11 year old) in 24 hours or use the maximum dosage for more than 2 weeks except under the advice and supervision of a doctor.

WEIGHT (LB)	AGE (YR)	TABLET
Under 24	Under 2	ask a doctor
24–47	2–5	1 tablet
48–95	6–11	2 tablets

	Regular Strength MYLANTA®	Extra Strength MYLANTA®	Purpose:
Aluminum Hydroxide (equivalent to dried gel, USP)	200 mg	400 mg	antacid
Magnesium Hydroxide	200 mg	400 mg	antacid
Simethicone	20 mg	40 mg	antigas

Acid Neutralizing Capacity:
Tablet
8 mEq

Warnings:
Ask a doctor or pharmacist before use if the child is taking a prescription drug. Antacids may interact with certain prescription drugs.
Stop use and ask a doctor if symptoms last more than 2 weeks.
Keep out of reach of children.
Other Information:
- **do not use if carton or blister is opened or broken**
- store at room temperature. Avoid excessive humidity

Inactive Ingredients: Citric acid, confectioner's sugar, cornstarch, D&C Red #27, flavors, magnesium stearate, sorbitol.

How Supplied: Children's Mylanta Upset Stomach Relief is supplied as chewable tablets in bubble gum flavor.
NDC 16837-810   Bubble Gum tablets
Shown in Product Identification Guide, page 508

REGULAR STRENGTH MYLANTA® and EXTRA STRENGTH MYLANTA®
[my-lan' ta]
Aluminum, Magnesium and Simethicone Liquid Antacid/Anti-Gas

Description: Regular Strength MYLANTA® and Extra Strength MYLANTA® are fast-acting, well-balanced, pleasant-tasting, antacid/anti-gas medications that provide consistent, effective relief of symptoms associated with heartburn, acid indigestion, sour stomach, upset stomach associated with these symptoms and relief of pressure and bloating commonly referred to as gas. Non-constipating and very low sodium. Regular Strength MYLANTA® and Extra Strength MYLANTA® contain two proven antacids, aluminum hydroxide and magnesium hydroxide, plus simethicone for gas relief.

Active Ingredients: Each 5 mL teaspoon contains:
[See table above]

Uses:
Relieves:
- heartburn
- acid indigestion
- sour stomach
- upset stomach due to these symptoms
- pressure and bloating commonly referred to as gas

Directions:
REGULAR STRENGTH MYLANTA:
- shake well
- take 2–4 teaspoonfuls between meals, at bedtime, or as directed by a doctor
- do not take more than 24 teaspoonfuls in a 24-hour period, or use the maximum dosage for more than 2 weeks
EXTRA STRENGTH MYLANTA:
- shake well
- take 2–4 teaspoonfuls between meals, at bedtime, or as directed by a doctor
- do not take more than 12 teaspoonfuls in a 24-hour period, or use the maximum dosage for more than 2 weeks

Warnings:
Ask a doctor before use if you have kidney disease.
Ask a doctor before use if you are taking a prescription drug. Antacids may interact with certain prescription drugs.
Stop use and ask a doctor if symptoms last more than 2 weeks.
Keep out of reach of children.
Other Information:
- **do not use if breakaway band on plastic cap is broken or missing**
- do not freeze

Professional Labeling

Indications: As an antacid for the symptomatic relief of hyperacidity associated with the diagnosis of peptic ulcer, gastritis, peptic esophagitis, gastric hyperacidity, or hiatal hernia. As an antiflatulent to alleviate the symptoms of gas, including post-operative gas pain.
Acid Neutralizing Capacity
Two teaspoonfuls have the following acid neutralizing capacity:

	Regular Strength MYLANTA®	Extra Strength MYLANTA®
Liquid	25.5 mEq	51.0 mEq

Warnings: Prolonged use of aluminum-containing antacids in patients with renal failure may result in or worsen dialysis osteomalacia. Elevated tissue aluminum levels contribute to the development of the dialysis encephalopathy and osteomalacia syndromes. Small amounts of aluminum are absorbed from the gastrointestinal tract and renal excretion of aluminum is impaired in renal failure. Aluminum is not well removed by dialysis because it is bound to albumin and transferrin, which do not cross dialysis membranes. As a result, aluminum is deposited in bone, and dialysis osteomalacia may develop when large amounts of aluminum are ingested orally by patients with impaired renal function. Aluminum forms insoluble complexes with phosphate in the gastrointestinal

Continued on next page

Mylanta—Cont.

tract, thus decreasing phosphate absorption. Prolonged use of aluminum-containing antacids by normophosphatemic patients may result in hypophosphatemia if phosphate intake is not adequate. In its more severe forms, hypophosphatemia can lead to anorexia, malaise, muscle weakness and osteomalacia.

Inactive Ingredients: LIQUIDS: Butylparaben, flavors, glycerin, hydroxyethyl cellulose, propylparaben, propylene glycol, purified water, sodium saccharin, and sorbitol. (Mint also contains D&C yellow #10, FD&C green #3, FD&C yellow #6 and Cherry contains FD&C red #40.)

How Supplied: Regular Strength MYLANTA® and Extra Strength MYLANTA® are available as white liquid suspensions in pleasant-tasting flavors, Original, Cherry and Mint. Liquids are supplied in bottles of 5 oz, 12 oz, and 24 oz. Also available for hospital use in liquid unit dose bottles of 1 oz and bottles of 5 oz.
Regular Strength MYLANTA®
NDC 16837-114 ORIGINAL LIQUID
NDC 16837-115 MINT LIQUID
NDC 16837-113 CHERRY LIQUID
Extra Strength MYLANTA®
NDC 16837-116 ORIGINAL LIQUID
NDC 16837-118 MINT LIQUID
NDC 16837-117 CHERRY LIQUID
Shown in Product Identification Guide, page 508

REGULAR STRENGTH MYLANTA GELCAPS and MYLANTA ULTRA TABS

[*mylan 'ta*]
Calcium Carbonate and Magnesium Hydroxide Tablets & Gelcaps
Antacid

Description: Regular Strength MYLANTA Gelcaps and MYLANTA Ultra Tabs are well balanced, pleasant tasting antacid medications that provide consistent, effective relief of symptoms associated with gastric hyperacidity. Non-constipating and very low in sodium, Regular Strength MYLANTA Gelcaps and MYLANTA Ultra Tabs contain two proven antacids, calcium carbonate and magnesium hydroxide.

Active Ingredients: Each tablet or gelcap contains:

	MYLANTA Gelcaps	MYLANTA Ultra Tabs
Calcium Carbonate	550mg	700mg
Magnesium Hydroxide	125mg	300mg

Uses: MYLANTA Gelcaps and MYLANTA Ultra Tabs
• heartburn • acid indigestion • sour stomach • upset stomach due to these symptoms • overindulgence in food and drink

Directions: Ultra tabs: • Thoroughly chew 2–4 tablets between meals, at bedtime or as directed by a doctor.
• Do not take more than 10 tablets in a 24-hour period, or use the maximum dosage for more than 2 weeks.
Gelcaps: • swallow 2–4 gelcaps as needed or as directed by a physician
• do not take more than 12 gelcaps in a 24-hour period, or use the maximum dosage for more than 2 weeks

Warnings:
Ask a doctor before use if you have kidney disease.
Ask a doctor or a pharmacist before use if you are taking a prescription drug. Antacids may interact with certain prescription drugs.
Stop use and ask a doctor if symptoms last more than 2 weeks.
Keep out of reach of children. In case of overdose get medical help or contact a poison control center right away.
Other Information: *MYLANTA Ultra Tabs*
• **do not if printed inner seal on bottle mouth or printed neck wrap is missing or broken**
• Store at room temperature in a dry place
MYLANTA Gelcaps
• **do not use if carton is opened or printed neck wrap or printed inner seal on bottle mouth is missing or broken**
• Store at room temperature, avoid high humidity and excessive heat 40°C (104°F)

Professional Labeling

Indications: MYLANTA Gelcaps and MYLANTA Ultra Tabs are also indicated as antacids for the symptomatic relief of hyperacidity associated with the diagnosis of peptic ulcer, gastritis, peptic esophagitis, heartburn and hiatal hernia.
Acid Neutralizing Capacity
Two gelcaps or chewable tablets have the following acid neutralizing capacity:

MYLANTA Gelcaps	MYLANTA U.T.
30.6mEq	48.6mEq

Inactive Ingredients: *Ultra Tabs:* Confectioner's sugar, cornstarch, flavors, magnesium stearate, sodium lauryl sulfate, sorbitol. Cherry flavor also contains D&C Red #27, citric acid, mint flavor also contains D&C yellow #10 and FD&C blue #1.
Gelcaps: Benzyl alcohol, butylparaben, castor oil, cornstarch, crospovidone, D&C Red #28, D&C Yellow #10, edetate calcium disodium, FD&C Blue #1, FD&C Red #40, gelatin, hypromellose, magnesium stearate, methylparaben, microcrystalline cellulose, propylene glycol, propylparaben, sodium lauryl sulfate, sodium propionate, titanium dioxide.

How Supplied: MYLANTA Ultra Tabs are available as a green Cool Mint Creme Chewable tablet and pink Cherry Creme chewable tablet. MYLANTA Gelcap is available as a swallowable gelcap.

MYLANTA Ultra Tabs
NDC 16837-869 Cherry Creme
NDC 16837-849 Cool Mint Creme
MYLANTA Gelcaps
NDC: 16837-850
Shown in Product Identification Guide, page 508

MYLANTA® GAS Tablets
Maximum Strength MYLANTA® GAS Tablets
MYLANTA® GAS Softgels

[*My-lan '-ta*]
Antiflatulent

Description: MYLANTA® GAS Softgels, MYLANTA® GAS, and Maximum Strength MYLANTA® GAS Tablets act in the stomach and intestines to change the surface tension of gas bubbles enabling them to coalesce, thereby freeing and eliminating the gas more easily by belching or passing flatus.

Active Ingredients: Each chewable tablet/softgel contains:

	Simethicone
MYLANTA® GAS Tablets	80 mg
Maximum Strength MYLANTA® GAS Tablets	125 mg
MYLANTA® GAS Softgels	125 mg

Uses: • Relieves bloating, pressure, and discomfort of gas which can be caused by certain foods (such as beans, bran, and broccoli) or air swallowing.

Directions:
MYLANTA® GAS Tablets
Thoroughly chew 1–2 tablets as needed after meals and at bedtime. Do not exceed six tablets per day unless directed by physician.
Maximum Strength MYLANTA® GAS Tablets
Thoroughly chew 1–2 tablets as needed after meals and at bedtime. Do not exceed 4 tablets per day unless directed by a physician.
MYLANTA® GAS Softgels
Take 1–2 softgels as needed after meals and at bedtime. Do not exceed 4 softgels per day unless directed by a physician.

Warnings: Keep out of the reach of children.
Other Information:
• Store at room temperature
• Avoid high humidity and excessive heat 40°C (104°F)

Inactive Ingredients: TABLETS: Dextrates, flavors, magnesium stearate, silicon dioxide, tribasic calcium phosphate. Cherry flavor also contains D&C Red #7 Calcium Lake.
Softgels: FD&C Blue #1, gelatin, glycerin, iron oxide black, peppermint oil, titanium dioxide.

Professional Labeling

Indications
As an antiflatulent for postoperative gas pain or for use in endoscopic examination

How Supplied: MYLANTA® GAS Tablets are available as white (mint) scored, chewable tablets identified "MYL GAS 80." Mint flavor is available in bottles of 100 tablets. Mint NDC 16837-858.

Maximum Strength MYLANTA® GAS Tablets are available as white (mint) or pink (cherry) scored, chewable tablets identified "MYL GAS 125." Mint and cherry flavors are both available in individually wrapped 24 tablet packages.

Mint NDC 16837-455

Cherry NDC 16837-861

MYLANTA® Gas Softgels are available as blue and yellow softgels identified as 'MYLANTA GAS' in individually wrapped 24 softgel packages. NDC 16837-611.

Shown in Product Identification Guide, page 509

PEPCID AC®
TABLETS, Chewable Tablets and Gelcaps

Description:
Active Ingredient: Famotidine 10 mg per tablet.

Inactive Ingredients: TABLETS: Hydroxypropyl cellulose, hypromellose, red iron oxide, magnesium stearate, microcrystalline cellulose, starch, talc, titanium dioxide.

CHEWABLE TABLETS: aspartame, cellulose acetate, flavors, hydroxypropyl cellulose, hypromellose, lactose, magnesium stearate, mannitol, microcrystalline cellulose, red ferric oxide.

GELCAPS: benzyl alcohol, black iron oxide, butylparaben, castor oil, edetate calcium disodium, FD&C red #40, gelatin, hypromellose, magnesium stearate, methylparaben, microcrystalline cellulose, pregelatinized corn starch, propylene glycol, propylparaben, sodium lauryl sulfate, sodium propionate, talc, titanium dioxide.

Product Benefits:
• **1 Tablet, Chewable Tablet or Gelcap** relieves heartburn associated with acid indigestion and sour stomach.
• prevents heartburn associated with acid indigestion and sour stomach brought on by eating or drinking certain food and beverages.

It contains famotidine, a prescription-proven medicine.

The ingredient in PEPCID AC, famotidine, has been prescribed by doctors for years to treat millions of patients safely and effectively. The active ingredient in PEPCID AC has been taken safely with many frequently prescribed medications.

Action:
It is normal for the stomach to produce acid, especially after consuming food and beverages. However, acid in the wrong place (the esophagus), or too much acid, can cause burning pain and discomfort that interfere with everyday activities.

• **Heartburn—Caused by acid in the esophagus**

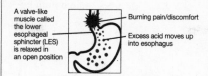

A valve-like muscle called the lower esophageal sphincter (LES) is relaxed in an open position

Burning pain/discomfort

Excess acid moves up into esophagus

In clinical studies, **PEPCID AC film-coated tablets were significantly better than placebo tablet (tablets without the medicine) in relieving and preventing heartburn. Pepcid AC chewables contain the same active ingredient.**

Percent of heartburn episodes <u>completely</u> relieved

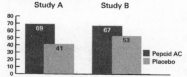

Study A Study B

Pepcid AC Placebo

Percent of patients with prevention or reduction of heartburn symptoms

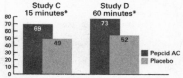

Study C 15 minutes* Study D 60 minutes*

Pepcid AC Placebo

*Time taken before eating a meal that is expected to cause symptoms.

Uses:
• **For Relief of heartburn, associated with acid indigestion, and sour stomach;**
• **For Prevention of heartburn associated with acid indigestion and sour stomach brought on by eating or drinking certain food and beverages.**

Tips for Managing Heartburn:
• Do not lie flat or bend over soon after eating.
• Do not eat late at night, or just before bedtime.
• certain foods or drinks are more likely to cause heartburn, such as rich, spicy, fatty, and fried foods, chocolate, caffeine, alcohol, and even some fruits and vegetables.
• Eat slowly and do not eat big meals.
• If you are overweight, lose weight.
• If you smoke, quit smoking.
• Raise the head of your bed.
• Wear loose fitting clothing around your stomach.

Warnings:
Allergy alert Do not use if you are allergic to famotidine or other acid reducers

Do not use:
• if you have trouble swallowing
• with other acid reducers

Stop use and ask a doctor if:
• stomach pain continues
• you need to take this product for more than 14 days

If pregnant or breast-feeding, ask a health professional before use.

Keep out of reach of children. In case of overdose, get medical help or contact a Poison Control Center right away.

Directions:
• Tablet: To relieve symptoms, swallow 1 tablet with a glass of water. Chewable Tablet: To relieve symptoms, chew one tablet thoroughly Gelcap: To relieve symptoms, swallow one gelcap with a glass of water.
• Tablet & Gelcap: To prevent symptoms, swallow one tablet or gelcap with a glass of water any time from 15 to 60 minutes before eating food or drinking beverages that cause heartburn.
• Chewable Tablet: To prevent symptoms, chew one chewable tablet before swallowing any time from 15 to 60 minutes before eating food or drinking beverages that cause heartburn.
• Do not use more than 2 tablets chewable tablets or gelcaps in 24 hours).
• Children under 12 years: ask a doctor.

Other Information:
• read the directions and warnings before use
• store at 25°–33°C (77°–86°F)
• keep the carton and package insert, they contain important information
• protect from moisture
in addition to the above the following also applies to the chewable tablet
• do not use if individual pouch is open or torn
• phenylketonurics: contains phenylalanine 1.4 mg per chewable tablet

How Supplied:
Pepcid AC Tablet is available as a rose-colored tablet identified as 'PEPCID AC'. NDC 16837-872

Pepcid AC Gelcap is available as a rose and white gelatin coated, capsule shaped tablet identified as 'PEPCID AC'. NDC 16837-856

Pepcid AC Chewable Tablet is available as a rose-colored chewable tablet identified as 'PEPCID AC'. NDC 16837-873

Shown in Product Identification Guide, page 509

PEPCID® COMPLETE
Acid Reducer + Antacid with DUAL ACTION Reduces and Neutralizes Acid

Description:

Active Ingredients: (in each chewablet tablet)	Purpose:
Famotidine 10mg	Acid Reducer
Calcium Carbonate 800 mg	Antacid
Magnesium Hydroxide 165 mg	Antacid

Inactive Ingredients:
Mint flavor: Cellulose acetate, corn starch, dextrates, flavors, hydroxypropyl cellulose, hypromellose, lactose, magnesium stearate, pregelatinized starch, red iron oxide, sodium lauryl sulfate, sugar Berry flavor: Cellulose acetate, corn starch, D&C red #7, dextrates, FD&C blue #1, FD&C red #40, flavors, hydro-

Continued on next page

In clinical studies, PEPCID COMPLETE was significantly better than placebo pills in relieving heartburn.

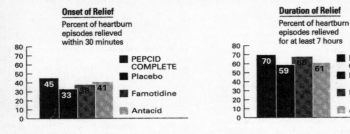

Onset of Relief
Percent of heartburn episodes relieved within 30 minutes

- ■ PEPCID COMPLETE
- □ Placebo
- ■ Famotidine
- ▨ Antacid

45, 33, 38, 41

Duration of Relief
Percent of heartburn episodes relieved for at least 7 hours

- ■ PEPCID COMPLETE
- □ Placebo
- ■ Famotidine
- ▨ Antacid

70, 59, 68, 61

Pepcid Complete—Cont.

propyl cellulose, hypromellose, lactose, magnesium stearate, pregelatinized starch, sodium lauryl sulfate, sugar

Sodium Content:
Each chewable tablet contains 0.5 mg of sodium.

Acid Neutralizing Capacity:
Each chewable tablet contains 21.7 mEq of acid neutralizing capacity.

Product Benefits: Pepcid Complete combines an acid reducer (famotidine) with antacids (calcium carbonate and magnesium hydroxide) to relieve heartburn in two different ways: Acid reducers decrease the production of new stomach acid; antacids neutralize acid that is already in the stomach. The active ingredients in PEPCID COMPLETE have been used for years to treat acid-related problems in millions of people safely and effectively.

Uses: To relieve heartburn associated with acid indigestion and sour stomach.

Action:
It is normal for the stomach to produce acid, especially after consuming food and beverages. However, acid in the stomach may move up into the wrong place (the esophagus), causing burning pain and discomfort that interfere with everyday activities.

Heartburn—Caused by acid in the esophagus

- Burning pain/discomfort in esophagus
- A valve-like muscle called the lower esophageal sphincter (LES) is relaxed in an open position
- Acid moves up from stomach

PROVEN EFFECTIVE IN CLINICAL STUDIES
[See graphic above]

Tips For Managing Heartburn
- Do not lie flat or bend over soon after eating.
- Do not eat late at night, or just before bedtime.
- Certain foods or drinks are more likely to cause heartburn, such as rich, spicy, fatty, and fried foods, chocolate, caffeine, alcohol, and even some fruits and vegetables.
- Eat slowly and do not eat big meals.
- If you are overweight, lose weight.
- If you smoke, quit smoking.
- Raise the head of your bed.

- Wear loose fitting clothing around your stomach.

Warnings:
- **Allergy alert:** Do not use if you are allergic to famotidine or other acid reducers.
- **Do not use:** if you have trouble swallowing.
- With other famotidine products or acid reducers.
- **Ask a doctor or pharmacist before use if you are** taking a prescription drug. Antacids may interact with certain prescription drugs.
- **Stop use and ask a doctor if** stomach pain continues
- You need to take this product for more than 14 days.
- **If pregnant or breast-feeding,** ask a health professional before use.
- **Keep out of reach of children.** In case of overdose, get medical help or contact a poison control center right away.

Directions:
- Adults and children 12 years and over:
  - **do not swallow tablet whole; chew completely.**
  - to relieve symptoms, **chew** 1 tablet before swallowing.
  - do not use more than 2 chewable tablets in 24 hours.
- Children under 12 years: ask a doctor.

Other Information:
- read the directions and warnings before use.
- keep the carton and package insert. They contain important information.
- store at 25°–30°C (77–86 F).
- protect from moisture.

How Supplied:
Pepcid Complete is available as a rose-colored chewable tablet identified by 'P'.
NDC 16837-888 – Mint flavor
Pepcid Complete Berry flavor
NDC 16837-291

Shown in Product Identification Guide, page 509

FACED WITH AN Rx SIDE EFFECT?
Turn to the Companion Drug Index for products that provide symptomatic relief.

Lederle Consumer Healthcare
See Wyeth Consumer Healthcare

McNeil Consumer and Specialty Pharmaceuticals
Division of McNeil-PPC, Inc.
FORT WASHINGTON, PA 19034

Direct Inquiries to:
Consumer Relationship Center
Fort Washington, PA 19034
(215) 273-7000

Maximum Strength GAS AID Softgels

Description: Each softgel of Maximum Strength GasAid contains simethicone 125 mg.

Actions: Simethicone acts in the stomach and intestines by altering the surface tension of gas bubbles enabling them to coalesce, thereby freeing and eliminating the gas more easily by belching or passing flatus.

Uses: Relieves bloating, pressure, fullness or stuffed feeling commonly referred to as gas.

Directions: Adults and children 12 years and over: take 1–2 softgels as needed after meals and at bedtime. Do not take more than 4 softgels in 24 hours unless directed by a doctor.

Warnings: Keep out of reach of children.

Other Information:
- do not use if carton or any blister unit is open or broken
- store at room temperature. Avoid high humidity and excessive heat (40°C).

Inactive Ingredients: D&C yellow #10, FD&C blue #1, FD&C red #40, gelatin, glycerin, peppermint oil, titanium dioxide.

How Supplied: Softgels in 12s, 24s, and 48s blister packaging. Each Maximum Strength GasAid softgel is oval, green in color, and imprinted with "I-G" on one side.

Shown in Product Identification Guide, page 509

IMODIUM® A–D Liquid and Caplets
(loperamide hydrochloride)

Description: Each 5 mL (teaspoon) of *IMODIUM® A-D* liquid contains

loperamide hydrochloride 1 mg. IMODIUM® A-D liquid is stable, cherry-mint flavored, and clear in color. Each caplet of IMODIUM® A-D contains 2 mg of loperamide and is scored and colored green.

Actions: IMODIUM® A-D contains a clinically proven antidiarrheal medication. Loperamide HCl acts by slowing intestinal motility and by affecting water and electrolyte movement through the bowel.

Uses: controls symptoms of diarrhea, including Travelers' Diarrhea.

Directions:
• drink plenty of clear fluids to help prevent dehydration caused by diarrhea
• find right dose on chart. If possible, use weight to dose; otherwise use age

adults and children 12 years and over	4 teaspoonfuls (1 dosage cup) or 2 caplets after the first loose stool; 2 teaspoonfuls or 1 caplet after each subsequent loose stool; but no more than 8 teaspoonfuls or 4 caplets in 24 hours
children 9–11 years (60–95 lbs)	2 teaspoonfuls (½ dosage cup) or 1 caplet after the first loose stool and 1 teaspoonful or ½ caplet after each subsequent loose stool but no more than 6 teaspoonfuls or 3 caplets in 24 hours
children 6–8 years (48–59 lbs)	2 teaspoonfuls (½ dosage cup) or 1 caplet after the first loose stool and 1 teaspoonful or ½ caplet after each subsequent loose stool but no more than 4 teaspoonfuls or 2 caplets in 24 hours
children under 6 years (up to 47 lbs)	ask a doctor

Professional Dosage Schedule for children 2–5 years old (24–47 lbs): 1 teaspoonful after first loose bowel movement, followed by 1 after each subsequent loose bowel movement. Do not exceed 3 teaspoonfuls a day.

Warnings:
Allergy alert: Do not use if you have ever had a rash or other allergic reaction to loperamide HCl
Do not use if you have bloody or black stool
Ask a doctor before use if you have
• fever • mucus in the stool • a history of liver disease
Stop use and ask a doctor if
• symptoms get worse • diarrhea lasts for more than 2 days

If pregnant or breast feeding, ask a health professional before use. **Keep out of reach of children.** In case of overdose, get medical help or contact a Poison Control Center right away.
Other Information:

Liquid:
• **do not use if carton is opened or if printed plastic neck wrap is broken or missing**
• store between 20–25°C (68–77°F)

Caplets:
• store between 20–25°C (68–77°F)
• **do not use if carton or blister unit is open or torn**

Professional Information:

Overdosage Information
Overdosage of loperamide HCl in man may result in constipation, CNS depression and nausea. A slurry of activated charcoal administered promptly after ingestion of loperamide hydrochloride can reduce the amount of drug which is absorbed. If vomiting occurs spontaneously upon ingestion, a slurry of 100 grams of activated charcoal should be administered orally as soon as fluids can be retained. If vomiting has not occurred, and CNS depression is evident, gastric lavage should be performed followed by administration of 100 gms of the activated charcoal slurry through the gastric tube. In the event of overdosage, patients should be monitored for signs of CNS depression for at least 24 hours. Children may be more sensitive to central nervous system effects than adults. If CNS depression is observed, naloxone may be administered. If responsive to naloxone, vital signs must be monitored carefully for recurrence of symptoms of drug overdose for at least 24 hours after the last dose of naloxone.

Inactive Ingredients:
Liquid: benzoic acid, citric acid, flavors, glycerin, propylene glycol, purified water, sodium benzoate, sorbitol, sucrose, contains 0.5% alcohol.
Caplets: colloidal silicon dioxide, D&C yellow no. 10, dibasic calcium phosphate, FD&C blue no. 1, magnesium stearate, microcrystalline cellulose.

How Supplied:
Liquid: Cherry-mint flavored liquid (clear) 2 fl. oz. and 4 fl. oz. tamper evident bottles with child resistant safety caps and special dosage cups.
Caplets: Green scored caplets in 6s, 12s, 18s, 24s, 48s and 72s blister packaging which is tamper evident and child resistant.

Shown in Product Identification Guide, page 509

**IMODIUM® ADVANCED
Caplets & Chewable Tablets
(loperamide HCl/simethicone)**

Description: Each easy to swallow caplet and mint-flavored chewable tablet

of Imodium® Advanced contains loperamide HCl 2 mg/simethicone 125 mg.

Actions: Imodium® Advanced combines original prescription strength Imodium® to control the symptoms of diarrhea plus simethicone to relieve bloating, pressure and cramps commonly referred to as gas. Loperamide HCl acts by slowing intestinal motility and by affecting water and electrolyte movement through the bowel. Simethicone acts in the stomach and intestines by altering the surface tension of gas bubbles enabling them to coalesce, thereby freeing and eliminating the gas more easily by belching or passing flatus.

Use: Controls symptoms of diarrhea plus bloating, pressure, and cramps commonly referred to as gas.

Directions:
• **drink plenty of clear fluids to help prevent dehydration caused by diarrhea**
• find right dose on chart. If possible, use weight to dose; otherwise use age

adults and children 12 years and over	swallow 2 caplets or chew 2 tablets after the first loose stool; 1 caplet/tablet after each subsequent loose stool; but no more than 4 caplets/tablets in 24 hours
children 9–11 years (60–95 lbs)	swallow 1 caplet or chew 1 tablet after the first loose stool; ½ caplet/tablet after each subsequent loose stool; but no more than 3 caplets/tablets in 24 hours
children 6–8 years (48–59 lbs)	swallow 1 caplet or chew 1 tablet after the first loose stool; ½ caplet/tablet after each subsequent loose stool; but no more than 2 caplets/tablets in 24 hours
children under 6 years (up to 47 lbs)	ask a doctor

Warnings:
Allergy alert: Do no use if you have ever had a rash or other reaction to loperamide HCl
Do not use if you have bloody or black stool
Ask a doctor before use if you have • fever • mucus in the stool • a history of liver disease
Ask a doctor or pharmacist before use if you are taking antibiotics
Stop use and ask a doctor if • symptoms get worse • diarrhea lasts for more than 2 days
If pregnant or breast-feeding, ask a health professional before use.

Continued on next page

Imodium Advanced—Cont.

Keep out of reach of children. In case of overdose, get medical help or contact a Poison Control Center right away.

Other Information:
Caplets:
- store between 20–25°C (68–77°F)
- protect from light
- do not use if pouch is open or torn

Chewable Tablets:
- do not use if carton is opened or if blister unit is broken or open
- store between 20–25°C (68–77°F)

Professional Information:
Overdosage Information

Overdosage of loperamide HCl in man may result in constipation, CNS depression and nausea. A slurry of activated charcoal administered promptly after ingestion of loperamide hydrochloride can reduce the amount of drug which is absorbed. If vomiting occurs spontaneously upon ingestion, a slurry of 100 grams of activated charcoal should be administered orally as soon as fluids can be retained. If vomiting has not occurred, and CNS depression is evident, gastric lavage should be performed followed by administration of 100 gms of the activated charcoal slurry through the gastric tube. In the event of overdosage, patients should be monitored for signs of CNS depression for at least 24 hours. Children may be more sensitive to central nervous system effects than adults. If CNS depression is observed, naloxone may be administered. If responsive to naloxone, vital signs must be monitored carefully for recurrence of symptoms of drug overdose for at least 24 hours after the last dose of naloxone. No treatment is necessary for the simethicone ingestion in this circumstance.

Inactive Ingredients: Caplets: acesulfame K, cellulose, dibasic calcium phosphate, flavor, sodium starch glycolate, stearic acid **Chewable Tablets:** Cellulose acetate, corn starch, D&C Yellow No. 10, dextrates, FD&C Blue No. 1, flavors, microcrystalline cellulose, polymethacrylates, saccharin sodium, sorbitol, stearic acid, sucrose, tribasic calcium phosphate.

How Supplied: Mint Chewable Tablets in 12's, 18's, 30's, and 42's blister packaging which is tamper evident and child resistant. Each Imodium® Advanced tablet is round, light green in color and has "IMODIUM" embossed on one side and "2/125" on the other side. Imodium Advanced Caplets are available in blister packs of 12's and 18's and bottles of 30's and 42's. Each Imodium® Advanced Caplet is oval, white color and has "IMO" embossed on one side and "2/125" on the other side.

Shown in Product Identification Guide, page 509

MOTRIN® IB ibuprofen Pain Reliever/ Fever Reducer Tablets, Caplets and Gelcaps

Description: Each *MOTRIN® IB Tablet, Caplet and Gelcap* contains ibuprofen 200 mg.

Uses:
Temporarily relieves minor aches and pains due to:
- headache • muscular aches • minor pain of arthritis • toothache • backache
- the common cold • menstrual cramps
Temporarily reduces fever

Directions:
- do not take more than directed

adults and children 12 years and older	• take 1 tablet, caplet, or gelcap every 4 to 6 hours while symptoms persist • if pain or fever does not respond to 1 tablet, caplet or gelcap, 2 tablets, caplets or gelcaps may be used, but do not exceed 6 tablets, caplets or gelcaps in 24 hours unless directed by a doctor • the smallest effective dose should be used
children under 12 years	• ask a doctor

Warnings:
Allergy alert: Ibuprofen may cause a severe allergic reaction which may include:
- hives • facial swelling
- asthma (wheezing) • shock

Alcohol Warning: If you consume 3 or more alcoholic drinks every day, ask your doctor whether you should take ibuprofen or other pain relievers/fever reducers. Ibuprofen may cause stomach bleeding.
Do not use if you have ever had an allergic reaction to any other pain reliever/ fever reducer.
Ask a doctor before use if you have
- stomach pain • problems or serious side effects from taking pain relievers or fever reducers.
Ask a doctor or pharmacist before use if you are
- under a doctor's care for any serious condition
- taking any other drug
- taking any other product that contains ibuprofen, or any other pain reliever/ fever reducer
When using this product give with food or milk if stomach upset occurs.
Stop use and ask a doctor if
- an allergic reaction occurs. Seek medical help right away.
- pain gets worse or lasts more than 10 days
- fever gets worse or lasts more than 3 days
- stomach pain or upset gets worse or lasts
- redness or swelling is present in the painful area

- any new symptoms appear.
If pregnant or breast-feeding, ask a health professional before use. It is especially important not to use ibuprofen during the last 3 months of pregnancy unless definitely directed to do so by a doctor because it may cause problems in the unborn child or complications during delivery.
Keep out of reach of children. In case of overdose, get medical help or contact a Poison Control Center right away.
Other Information
- **Do not use if neck wrap or foil inner seal imprinted "Safety Seal®" is broken or missing.**
- Store between 20°–25°C (68°–77°F)

Professional Information:
Overdosage Information for Adult Motrin®
IBUPROFEN

The *toxicity of ibuprofen* overdose is dependent upon the amount of drug ingested and the time elapsed since ingestion, though individual response may vary, which makes it necessary to evaluate each case individually. Although uncommon, serious toxicity and death have been reported in the medical literature with ibuprofen overdosage. The most frequently reported symptoms of ibuprofen overdose include abdominal pain, nausea, vomiting, lethargy and drowsiness. Other central nervous system symptoms include headache, tinnitus, CNS depression and seizures. Metabolic acidosis, coma, acute renal failure and apnea (primarily in very young children) may rarely occur. Cardiovascular toxicity, including hypotension, bradycardia, tachycardia and atrial fibrillation, also have been reported. The *treatment of acute ibuprofen overdose* is primarily supportive. Management of hypotension, acidosis and gastrointestinal bleeding may be necessary. In cases of acute overdose, the stomach should be emptied through ipecac-induced emesis or lavage. Emesis is most effective if initiated within 30 minutes of ingestion. Orally administered activated charcoal may help in reducing the absorption and reabsorption of ibuprofen. In children, the estimated amount of ibuprofen ingested per body weight may be helpful to predict the potential for development of toxicity although each case must be evaluated. Ingestion of less than 100 mg/kg is unlikely to produce toxicity. Children ingesting 100 to 200 mg/kg may be managed with induced emesis and a minimal observation time of four hours. Children ingesting 200 to 400 mg/kg of ibuprofen should have immediate gastric emptying and at least four hours observation in a health care facility. Children ingesting greater than 400 mg/kg require immediate medical referral, careful observation and appropriate supportive therapy. Ipecac-induced emesis is not recommended in overdoses greater than 400 mg/kg because of the risk of convulsions and the potential for aspiration of gastric contents. In adult patients the history of the dose reportedly ingested does not appear

to be predictive of toxicity. The need for referral and follow-up must be judged by the circumstances at the time of the overdose ingestion. Symptomatic adults should be admitted to a health care facility for observation.

Our Adult MOTRIN® combination products contain pseudoephedrine in addition to ibuprofen. For basic overdose information regarding pseudoephedrine, please see below. For additional emergency information, please contact your local poison control center.

PSEUDOEPHEDRINE

Symptoms from pseudoephedrine overdose consist most often of mild anxiety, tachycardia and/or mild hypertension. Symptoms usually appear within 4 to 8 hours and are transient, usually requiring no treatment.

Inactive Ingredients: Tablets and Caplets: carnauba wax, corn starch, FD&C Yellow #6, hypromellose, iron oxide, polydextrose, polyethylene glycol, silicon dioxide, stearic acid, titanium dioxide.

Gelcaps: benzyl alcohol, butylparaben, castor oil, cellulose, corn starch, edetate calcium disodium, FD&C Yellow No. 6, gelatin, hypromellose, iron oxide, methylparaben, povidone, propylparaben, silicon dioxide, sodium lauryl sulfate, sodium propionate, sodium starch glycolate, titanium dioxide.

How Supplied: Tablets: (orange, printed "MOTRIN IB" in black) in tamper evident packaging of 24, 50, 100, and 165.

Caplets: (orange, printed "MOTRIN IB" in black) in tamper evident packaging of 24, 50, 100, 165, 250, 300 and

Gelcaps: (colored orange and white, printed "MOTRIN IB" in black) in tamper evident packaging of 24, 50 and 100.

Shown in Product Identification Guide, page 511

MOTRIN® Sinus/Headache Caplets

Description: Each MOTRIN® Sinus/Headache Caplet contains ibuprofen 200 mg and pseudoephedrine HCl 30 mg.

Uses: temporarily relieves these symptoms associated with the common cold, sinusitis, and flu:
• headache • nasal congestion
• fever • minor body aches and pains

Directions:

Adults and children 12 years and older	• take 1 caplet every 4 to 6 hours while symptoms persist • If symptoms do not respond to 1 caplet, 2 caplets may be used
	• do not use more than 6 caplets in any 24-hour period unless directed by a doctor • the smallest effective dose should be used
Children under 12 years of age	Consult a doctor

Warnings:

Allergy alert: Ibuprofen may cause a severe allergic reaction which may include:
• hives • facial swelling
• asthma (wheezing) • shock

Alcohol warning: If you consume 3 or more alcoholic drinks every day, ask your doctor whether you should take ibuprofen or other pain relievers/fever reducers. Ibuprofen may cause stomach bleeding.

Do not use if you
• have ever had an allergic reaction to any other pain reliever/fever reducer
• are now taking a prescription monoamine oxidase inhibitor (MAOI) (certain drugs for depression, psychiatric or emotional conditions, or Parkinson's disease), or for 2 weeks after stopping the MAOI drug. If you do not know if your prescription drug contains an MAOI, ask a doctor or pharmacist before taking this product.

Ask a doctor before use if you have
• heart disease • high blood pressure
• thyroid disease • diabetes
• trouble urinating due to an enlarged prostate gland
• had serious side effects from taking any pain reliever/fever reducers.

Ask a doctor or pharmacist before use if you are
• taking any other product that contains ibuprofen or pseudoephedrine.
• taking any other pain reliever/fever reducer or nasal decongestant
• under a doctor's care for any continuing medical condition
• taking other drugs on a regular basis

When using this product
• do not use more than directed
• give with food or milk if stomach upset occurs

Stop use and ask a doctor if
• an allergic reaction occurs. Seek medical help right away
• you get nervous, dizzy, or sleepless
• nasal congestion lasts for more than 7 days
• symptoms continue or get worse
• new or unexpected symptoms occur
• stomach pain occurs with use of this product or even if mild symptoms persist
• fever lasts for more than 3 days

If pregnant or breast-feeding, ask a health professional before use. It is especially important not to use this product during the last 3 months of pregnancy unless definitely directed to do so by a doctor because it may cause problems in the unborn child or complications during delivery.

Keep out of reach of children. In case of overdose, get medical help or contact a Poison Control Center right away.

Other Information:
• **do not use if blister unit is broken or open**
• Store at 20–25°C (68–77°F).
• avoid excessive heat above 40°C (104°F)
• read all warnings and directions before use. Keep carton.

Professional Information:
Overdosage Information:
For overdosage information, please refer to pgs. 668–669.

Inactive Ingredients: Caplets: carnauba wax, cellulose, corn starch, FD&C Red #40, hypromellose, silicon dioxide, sodium lauryl sulfate, sodium starch glycolate, stearic acid, titanium dioxide, triacetin.

How Supplied: Caplets: (white, printed "Motrin Sinus/Headache" in red) in blister packs of 20 and 40.

Shown in Product Identification Guide, page 511

Infants' MOTRIN® ibuprofen Concentrated Drops

Children's MOTRIN® ibuprofen Oral Suspension and Chewable Tablets

Junior Strength MOTRIN® ibuprofen Caplets and Chewable Tablets

Product information for all dosages of Children's MOTRIN have been combined under this heading

Description: *Infants' MOTRIN® Concentrated Drops* are available in an alcohol-free, berry-flavored suspension and a non-staining, dye-free, berry-flavored suspension. Each 1.25 mL contains ibuprofen 50 mg. *Children's MOTRIN® Oral Suspension* is available as an alcohol-free, berry, dye-free berry, bubblegum or grape-flavored suspension. Each 5 mL (teaspoon) of *Children's MOTRIN® Oral Suspension* contains ibuprofen 100 mg. Each *Children's MOTRIN® Chewable Tablet* contains 50 mg of ibuprofen and is available as orange or grape-flavored chewable tablets. *Junior Strength MOTRIN® Chewable Tablets* and *Junior Strength MOTRIN® Caplets* contain ibuprofen 100 mg. *Junior Strength MOTRIN® Chewable Tablets* are available in orange or grape flavors. *Junior Strength MOTRIN® Caplets* are available as easy-to-swallow caplets (capsule-shaped tablet).

Uses: temporarily:
• reduces fever
• relieves minor aches and pains due to the common cold, flu, sore throat, headaches and toothaches

Directions: See Table 2: Children's Motrin Dosing Chart on pg. 672.

Warnings:
Allergy alert: Ibuprofen may cause a severe allergic reaction which may include:

Continued on next page

Motrin Infants'—Cont.

- hives • facial swelling
- asthma (wheezing) • shock

Sore throat warning: Severe or persistent sore throat or sore throat accompanied by high fever, headache, nausea, and vomiting may be serious. Consult doctor promptly. Do not use more than 2 days or administer to children under 3 years of age unless directed by doctor.

Do not use if the child has ever had an allergic reaction to any other fever reducer/pain reliever

Ask a doctor before use if the child has
- not been drinking fluids
- lost a lot of fluid due to continued vomiting or diarrhea
- stomach pain
- problems or serious side effects from taking fever reducers or pain relievers

Ask a doctor or pharmacist before use if the child
- under a doctor's care for any serious condition
- taking any other drug
- taking any other product that contains ibuprofen, or any other fever reducer/pain reliever

When using this product
- mouth or throat burning may occur; give with food or water (*Children's MOTRIN® Chewable Tablets and Junior Strength MOTRIN® Chewable Tablets* only)
- give with food or milk if stomach upset occurs

Stop use and ask a doctor if
- an allergic reaction occurs. Seek medical help right away.
- fever or pain gets worse or lasts more than 3 days
- the child does not get any relief within first day (24 hours) of treatment
- stomach pain or upset gets worse or lasts
- redness or swelling is present in the painful area
- any new symptoms appear

Keep out of reach of children. In case of overdose, get medical help or contact a Poison Control Center right away.

Other Information:

Infants', Children's and Junior Strength MOTRIN® products:
- Store at 20–25°C (68–77°F)

Infants' MOTRIN® Concentrated Drops:
- **do not use if plastic carton wrap or bottle wrap imprinted "Safety Seal®" is broken or missing.**

Children's MOTRIN® Suspension Liquid:
- **do not use if plastic carton wrap or bottle wrap imprinted "Safety Seal®" is broken or missing**

Children's MOTRIN® Chewable Tablets:
- Phenylketonurics: Contains phenylalanine 1.4 mg per tablet
- **do not use if neck wrap or foil inner seal imprinted "Safety Seal®" is broken or missing**

Junior Strength MOTRIN® Caplets and Chewable Tablets:
- phenylketonurics: contains phenylalanine 2.8 mg per tablet (tablet only)
- **do not use if neck wrap or foil inner seal imprinted "Safety Seal®" is broken or missing**

Professional Information:
Overdosage Information for all Infants', Children's & Junior Strength Motrin® Products

IBUPROFEN: The *toxicity of ibuprofen* overdose is dependent upon the amount of drug ingested and the time elapsed since ingestion, though individual response may vary, which makes it necessary to evaluate each case individually. Although uncommon, serious toxicity and death have been reported in the medical literature with ibuprofen overdosage. The most frequently reported symptoms of ibuprofen overdose include abdominal pain, nausea, vomiting, lethargy and drowsiness. Other central nervous system symptoms include headache, tinnitus, CNS depression and seizures. Metabolic acidosis, coma, acute renal failure and apnea (primarily in very young children) may rarely occur. Cardiovascular toxicity, including hypotension, bradycardia, tachycardia and atrial fibrillation, also have been reported.

The *treatment of acute ibuprofen overdose* is primarily supportive. Management of hypotension, acidosis and gastrointestinal bleeding may be necessary. In cases of acute overdose, the stomach should be emptied through ipecac-induced emesis or lavage. Emesis is most effective if initiated within 30 minutes of ingestion. Orally administered activated charcoal may help in reducing the absorption and reabsorption of ibuprofen. In children, the estimated amount of ibuprofen ingested per body weight may be helpful to predict the potential for development of toxicity although each case must be evaluated. Ingestion of less than 100 mg/kg is unlikely to produce toxicity. Children ingesting 100 to 200 mg/kg may be managed with induced emesis and a minimal observation time of four hours. Children ingesting 200 to 400 mg/kg of ibuprofen should have immediate gastric emptying and at least four hours observation in a health care facility. Children ingesting greater than 400 mg/kg require immediate medical referral, careful observation and appropriate supportive therapy. Ipecac-induced emesis is not recommended in overdoses greater than 400 mg/kg because of the risk of convulsions and the potential for aspiration of gastric contents.

In adults patients the history of the dose reportedly ingested does not appear to be predictive of toxicity. The need for referral and follow-up must be judged by the circumstances at the time of the overdose ingestion. Symptomatic adults should be admitted to a health care facility for observation.

Our Children's MOTRIN® Cold products contain pseudoephedrine in addition to ibuprofen. The following is basic overdose information regarding pseudoephedrine.

PSEUDOEPHEDRINE: Symptoms from pseudoephedrine overdose consist most often of mild anxiety, tachycardia and/or mild hypertension. Symptoms usually appear within 4 to 8 hours of ingestion and are transient, usually requiring no treatment.

For additional emergency information, please contact your local poison control center.

Inactive Ingredients: *Infants' MOTRIN® Concentrated Drops:* **Berry-Flavored:** citric acid, corn starch, FD&C Red #40, flavors, glycerin polysorbate 80, purified water, sodium benzoate, sorbitol, sucrose, xanthan gum. **Dye-Free Berry-Flavored:** artificial flavors, citric acid, corn starch, glycerin, polysorbate 80, purified water, sodium benzoate, sorbitol, sucrose, xanthan gum.

Children's MOTRIN® Oral Suspension: **Berry-Flavored:** acesulfame potassium, citric acid, corn starch, D&C Yellow #10, FD&C Red #40, glycerin, natural and artificial flavors, polysorbate 80, purified water, sodium benzoate, sucrose, xanthan gum. **Dye-Free Berry-Flavored:** acesulfame potassium, citric acid, corn starch, glycerin, natural and artificial flavors, polysorbate 80, purified water, sodium benzoate, sucrose, xanthan gum. **Bubble Gum-Flavored:** acesulfame potassium, citric acid, corn starch, FD&C Red #40, glycerin, natural and artificial flavors, polysorbate 80, purified water, sodium benzoate, sucrose, xanthan gum. **Grape-Flavored:** acesulfame potassium, citric acid, corn starch, D&C Red #33, FD&C Blue #1, FD&C Red #40, glycerin, natural and artificial flavors, polysorbate 80, purified water, sodium benzoate, sucrose, xanthan gum.

Children's MOTRIN® Chewable Tablets: **Orange-Flavored:** acesulfame K, aspartame, cellulose, citric acid, FD&C Yellow #6, flavor, fumaric acid, hydroxyethyl cellulose, hydroxypropyl methylcellulose, magnesium stearate, mannitol, povidone, sodium lauryl sulfate, sodium starch glycolate. **Grape-Flavored:** acesulfame K, aspartame, cellulose, citric acid, D&C Red #7, D&C Red #30, FD&C Blue #1, flavor, fumaric acid, hydroxyethyl cellulose, hydroxypropyl methylcellulose, magnesium stearate, mannitol, povidone, sodium lauryl sulfate, sodium starch glycolate.

Junior Strength MOTRIN® Chewable Tablets: **Orange-Flavored:** acesulfame K, aspartame, cellulose, citric acid, FD&C yellow #6, flavor, fumaric acid, hydroxyethyl cellulose, hydroxypropyl methylcellulose, magnesium stearate, mannitol, povidone, sodium lauryl sulfate, sodium starch glycolate. **Grape-Flavored:** acesulfame K, aspartame, cellulose, citric acid, D&C Red #7, D&C Red #30, FD&C Blue #1, flavor, fumaric acid, hydroxyethyl cellulose, hydroxypropyl methylcellulose, magnesium stearate, mannitol, povidone, sodium lauryl sulfate, sodium starch glycolate. **Easy-To-Swallow Caplets:** carnauba wax, cellu-

lose, corn starch, D&C Yellow #10, FD&C Yellow #6, hydroxypropyl methylcellulose, polydextrose, polyethylene glycol, propylene glycol, silicon dioxide, sodium starch glycolate, titanium dioxide, triacetin.

How Supplied: *Infants' MOTRIN® Concentrated Drops:* Berry-flavored, pink-colored liquid and Berry-Flavored, Dye-Free, white-colored liquid in ½ fl. oz. bottles.

Children's MOTRIN® Oral Suspension: Berry-flavored, pink-colored; Berry-Flavored, Dye-Free white-colored, Bubble Gum-flavored, pink-colored and Grape-flavored, purple-colored liquid in tamper evident bottles of 2 and 4 fl. oz.

Children's MOTRIN® Chewable Tablets: Orange-flavored, orange-colored and Grape-flavored, purple-colored chewable tablets in 24 count bottles.

Junior Strength MOTRIN® Chewable Tablets: Orange-flavored, orange-colored chewable tablets or Grape-flavored, purple-colored chewable tablets in 24 count bottles.

Junior Strength MOTRIN® Caplets: Easy-to-swallow caplets (capsule shaped tablets) in 24 count bottles.

Shown in Product Identification Guide, page 510

Children's MOTRIN® Cold ibuprofen/pseudoephedrine HCl Oral Suspension

Description: *Children's MOTRIN® Cold Oral Suspension* is an alcohol-free berry, dye-free berry, or grape-flavored suspension. Each 5 mL (teaspoonful) contains the pain reliever/fever reducer ibuprofen 100 mg and the nasal decongestant pseudoephedrine HCl 15 mg.

Uses: temporarily relieves these cold, sinus and flu symptoms:
• nasal and sinus congestion
• stuffy nose • headache • sore throat
• minor body aches and pains • fever

Directions: See Table 2: Children's Motrin Dosing Chart on pg. 672.

Warnings: Allergy alert: Ibuprofen may cause a severe allergic reaction which may include:
• hives • facial swelling
• asthma (wheezing) • shock

Sore throat warning: Severe or persistent sore throat or sore throat accompanied by high fever, headache, nausea, and vomiting may be serious. Consult a doctor promptly. Do not use more than 2 days or administer to children under 3 years of age unless directed by doctor.

Do not use
• if the child has ever had an allergic reaction to any other pain reliever/fever reducer and/or nasal decongestant
• in a child who is taking a prescription monoamine oxidase inhibitor [MAOI] (certain drugs for depression, psychiatric or emotional conditions, or Parkinson's disease), or for 2 weeks after

stopping the MAOI drug. If you do not know if your child's prescription drug contains an MAOI, ask a doctor or pharmacist before giving this product.

Ask a doctor before use if the child has
• not been drinking fluids
• lost a lot of fluid due to continued vomiting or diarrhea
• problems or serious side effects from taking pain relievers, fever reducers or nasal decongestants
• stomach pain
• heart disease
• high blood pressure
• thyroid disease
• diabetes

Ask a doctor or pharmacist before use if the child is
• under a doctor's care for any continuing medical condition
• taking any other drug
• taking any other product that contains ibuprofen or pseudoephedrine
• taking any other pain reliever/fever reducer and/or nasal decongestant

When using this product
• **do not exceed recommended dosage**
• give with food or milk if stomach upset occurs

Stop use and ask a doctor if
• an allergic reaction occurs. Seek medical help right away.
• the child does not get any relief within first day (24 hours) of treatment
• fever, pain or nasal congestion gets worse, or lasts for more than 3 days
• stomach pain or upset gets worse or lasts
• symptoms continue or get worse
• redness or swelling is present in the painful area
• the child gets nervous, dizzy, sleepless or sleepy
• any new symptoms appear

Keep out of reach of children. In case of overdose, get medical help or contact a Poison Control Center right away.

Other Information:
• **do not use if plastic carton wrap or bottle wrap imprinted "Safety Seal®" is broken or missing.**
• Store at 20–25°C (68–77°F)

Professional Information:
Overdosage Information
For overdosage information, please refer to pg. 670.

Inactive Ingredients: Berry Flavor: acesulfame potassium, citric acid, corn starch, D&C yellow #10, FD&C red #40, flavors, glycerin, polysorbate 80, purified water, sodium benzoate, sucrose, xanthan gum. **Dye-Free Berry Flavor:** acesulfame potassium, citric acid, corn starch, flavors, glycerin, polysorbate 80, purified water, sodium benzoate, sucrose, xanthan gum. **Grape Flavor:** acesulfame potassium, citric acid, corn starch, D&C red #33, FD&C blue #1, FD&C red #40, flavors, glycerin, polysorbate 80, purified water, sodium benzoate, sucrose, xanthan gum.

How Supplied: Berry-flavored, pink-colored, Grape-flavored, purple-colored, and Dye-Free Berry-flavored, white-colored liquid in tamper evident bottles of 4 fl. oz.

Shown in Product Identification Guide, page 510

Children's Motrin® Dosing Chart
[See table on next page]

NIZORAL® A-D KETOCONAZOLE SHAMPOO 1%

Description: *Nizoral® A-D (Ketoconazole Shampoo 1%) Anti-Dandruff Shampoo* is a light-blue liquid for topical application, containing the broad spectrum synthetic antifungal agent Ketoconazole in a concentration of 1%.

Use: Controls flaking, scaling, and itching associated with dandruff.

Directions:

Adults and children 12 years and over:	• wet hair thoroughly • apply shampoo, generously lather, rinse thoroughly. Repeat. • use every 3–4 days for up to 8 weeks or as directed by a doctor. Then use only as needed to control dandruff.
children under 12 years	• ask a doctor

Warnings:
Do Not Use
• on scalp that is broken or inflamed
• if you are allergic to ingredients in this product

When Using This Product
• avoid contact with eyes
• if product gets into eyes, rinse thoroughly with water

Stop use and ask a doctor if
• rash appears
• condition worsens or does not improve in 2–4 weeks

If pregnant or breast-feeding, ask a doctor before use.

Keep out of the reach of children.
If swallowed get medical help or contact a Poison Control Center right away.

Other Information
• store between 35° and 86°F (2° and 30°C)
• protect from light • protect from freezing

Professional Information:
Overdosage Information *Nizoral® A-D (Ketoconazole) 1% Shampoo* is intended for external use only. In the event of accidental ingestion, supportive measures should be employed. Induced emesis and gastric lavage should usually be avoided.

Inactive Ingredients: acrylic acid polymer (carbomer 1342), butylated hydroxytoluene, cocamide MEA, FD&C Blue #1, fragrance, glycol distearate, polyquaternium-7, quaternium-15, sodium chloride, sodium cocoyl sarcosinate, sodium hydroxide and/or hydrochloric acid, sodium laureth sulfate, tetrasodium EDTA, water.

Continued on next page

Table 2. Children's Motrin Dosing Chart

AGE GROUP*		0-5 mos*	6-11 mos	12-23 mos	2-3 yrs	4-5 yrs	6-8 yrs	9-10 yrs	11 yrs	Maximum doses/ 24 hrs
WEIGHT	(if possible use weight to dose; otherwise use age)	6-11 lbs	12-17 lbs	18-23 lbs	24-35 lbs	36-47 lbs	48-59 lbs	60-71 lbs	72-95 lbs	
PRODUCT FORM	INGREDIENTS Dose to be administered based on weight or age†									
Infants' Drops	Per 1.25 mL									
Infants' Motrin Concentrated Drops Berry Flavor & Dye-Free Berry Flavor	Ibuprofen 50 mg	—	1.25 mL	1.875 mL	—	—	—	—	—	4 times in 24 hrs
Children's Liquid	Per 5 mL teaspoonful (TSP)									
Children's Motrin Suspension	Ibuprofen 100 mg	—	—	—	1 TSP	1 ½ TSP	2 TSP	2 ½ TSP	3 TSP	4 times in 24 hrs
Children's Motrin Cold Suspension Liquid†	Ibuprofen 100 mg Pseudoephedrine 15 mg	—	—	—	1 TSP	1 TSP	2 TSP	2 TSP	2 TSP	4 times in 24 hrs
Children's Tablets & Caplets	Per tablet/ caplet									
Children's Motrin Chewable Tablets	Ibuprofen 50 mg	—	—	—	2 tablets	3 tablets	4 tablets	5 tablets	6 tablets	4 times in 24 hrs
Junior Strength Motrin Chewable Tablets	Ibuprofen 100 mg	—	—	—	—	—	2 tablets	2 ½ tablets	3 tablets	4 times in 24 hrs
Junior Strength Motrin Caplets	Ibuprofen 100 mg	—	—	—	—	—	2 caplets	2 ½ caplets	3 caplets	4 times in 24 hrs

†Do not give, take or chew more than directed. If needed, repeat dose every 6-8 hours; except for Children's Motrin Cold which is every 6 hours.
* Under 6 mos, call a doctor.
- Infants' Motrin Drops are more concentrated than Children's Motrin Liquids. The Infants' Concentrated Drops have been specifically designed for use only with enclosed dosing device. Do not use any other dosing device with this product.
- Children's Motrin Liquids are less concentrated than Infants' Motrin Drops. The Children's Motrin Liquids have been specifically designed for use with the enclosed measuring cup. Use only enclosed measuring cup to dose this product.
- Children's Motrin Chewable Tablets are not the same concentration as Junior Strength Motrin Chewable Tablets.
- Junior Strength Motrin Chewable Tablets contain twice as much medicine as Children's Motrin Chewable Tablets.

How Supplied: Available in 4 and 7 fl oz bottles

Shown in Product Identification Guide, page 511

**St. Joseph 81 mg Aspirin
St. Joseph 81 mg Adult Low Strength Aspirin Chewable & Enteric Coated Tablets**

Description: Each St. Joseph Adult Low Strength Aspirin tablet contains 81 mg of aspirin.

Uses:
- temporarily relieves minor aches and pains or as recommended by your doctor
- ask your doctor about other uses for St. Joseph Adult 81 mg Aspirin

Directions:
- drink a full glass of water with each dose
- **adults and children 12 years and over:**
  - take 4 to 8 tablets every 4 hours while symptoms persist
  - do not exceed 48 tablets in 24 hours or as directed by a doctor
- **children under 12:**
  - do not use unless directed by a doctor

Warnings:
Reye's syndrome: Children and teenagers should not use this drug for chicken pox or flu symptoms before a doctor is consulted about Reye's syndrome, a rare but serious illness reported to be associated with aspirin.

Allergy alert: Aspirin may cause a severe allergic reaction which may include:
- hives
- facial swelling
- asthma (wheezing)
- shock

Alcohol warning: If you consume 3 or more alcoholic drinks every day, ask your doctor whether you should take aspirin or other pain relievers/fever reducers. Aspirin may cause stomach bleeding.

Do not use
- If you have ever had an allergic reaction to any other pain reliever/fever reducer
- for at least 7 days after tonsillectomy or oral surgery unless directed by a doctor *(chewable tablet formulation only)*

Ask a doctor before use if you have
- asthma
- ulcers
- bleeding problems
- stomach problems that last or come back such as heartburn, upset stomach or pain

Ask a doctor or pharmacist before use if you are
- Taking a prescription drug for:
  - anticoagulation (blood thinning)
  - gout
  - diabetes
  - arthritis

Stop use and ask a doctor if
- allergic reaction occurs. Seek medical help right away.
- ringing in the ears or loss of hearing occurs
- pain gets worse or lasts more than 10 days

- new symptoms occur
- redness or swelling is present

If pregnant or breast-feeding, ask a health professional before use. It is especially important not to use aspirin during the last three months of pregnancy unless definitely directed to do so by a doctor because it may cause problems in the unborn child or complications during delivery.

Keep out of reach of children. In case of overdose, get medical help or contact a Poison Control Center right away.

Other Information:
- **do not use if carton is opened or neck wrap or foil inner seal imprinted with "Safety Seal®" is broken**
- store at room temperature. Avoid high humidity and excessive heat (40° C).

Inactive Ingredients: *St. Joseph 81 mg Adult Low Strength Aspirin Chewable Tablets:* corn starch, FD&C yellow #6 aluminum lake, flavor, mannitol, saccharin, silicon dioxide, stearic acid. *Enteric Coated Tablets:* cellulose, corn starch, FD&C Red #40, FD&C Yellow #6, glyceryl monostearate, iron oxide, methacrylic acid, silicon dioxide, simethicone, stearic acid, triethyl citrate.

How Supplied: *St. Joseph 81 mg Adult Low Strength Aspirin Enteric Coated Tablets:* tamper evident bottles of 36 and 108. *Enteric Coated Tablets:* tamper evident bottles of 36 and 180.

Comprehensive Prescribing Information
Description: St. Joseph Adult Low Strength Aspirin Chewable & Enteric Coated Tablets (acetylsalicylic acid) are available in 81 mg for oral administration. *St. Joseph 81 mg Adult Low Strength Aspirin Chewable Tablets* contain the following inactive ingredients: corn starch, FD&C yellow #6 aluminum lake, flavor, mannitol, saccharin, silicon dioxide, stearic acid. *St. Joseph 81 mg Adult Low Strength Aspirin Enteric Coated Tablets* contain the following inactive ingredients: cellulose, corn starch, FD&C Red #40, FD&C Yellow #6, glyceryl monostearate, iron oxide, methacrylic acid, silicon dioxide, simethicone, stearic acid, triethyl citrate. Aspirin is an odorless white, needle-like crystalline or powdery substance. When exposed to moisture, aspirin hydrolyzes into salicylic and acetic acids, and gives off a vinegary-odor. It is highly lipid soluble and slightly soluble in water.

Clinical Pharmacology:
Mechanism of Action: Aspirin is a more potent inhibitor of both prostaglandin synthesis and platelet aggregation than other salicylic acid derivatives. The differences in activity between aspirin and salicylic acid are thought to be due to the acetyl group on the aspirin molecule. This acetyl group is responsible for the inactivation of cyclo-oxygenase via acetylation.

Pharmacokinetics: Absorption: In general, immediate release aspirin is well and completely absorbed from the gastrointestinal (GI) tract. Following ab-

sorption, aspirin is hydrolyzed to salicylic acid with peak plasma levels of salicylic acid occurring within 1–2 hours of dosing (see Pharmacokinetics—Metabolism). The rate of absorption from the GI tract is dependent upon the dosage form, the presence or absence of food, gastric pH (the presence or absence of GI antacids or buffering agents), and other physiologic factors. Enteric coated aspirin products are erratically absorbed from the GI tract.

Distribution: Salicylic acid is widely distributed to all tissues and fluids in the body including the central nervous system (CNS), breast milk, and fetal tissues. The highest concentrations are found in the plasma, liver, renal cortex, heart, and lungs. The protein binding of salicylate is concentration-dependent, i.e., nonlinear. At low concentrations (100 μg/mL), approximately 90 percent of plasma salicylate is bound to albumin while at higher concentrations (>400 μg/mL), only about 75 percent is bound. The early signs of salicylic overdose (salicylism), including tinnitus (ringing in the ears), occur at plasma concentrations approximating 200 μg/mL. Severe toxic effects are associated with levels >400 μg/mL. (See Adverse Reactions and Overdosage.)

Metabolism: Aspirin is rapidly hydrolyzed in the plasma to salicylic acid such that plasma levels of aspirin are essentially undetectable 1–2 hours after dosing. Salicylic acid is primarily conjugated in the liver to form salicyluric acid, a phenolic glucuronide, and a number of minor metabolites. Salicylic acid has a plasma half-life of approximately 6 hours. Salicylate metabolism is saturable and total body clearance decreases at higher serum concentrations due to the limited ability of the liver to form both salicyluric acid and phenolic glucuronide. Following toxic doses (10–20 grams (g)), the plasma half-life may be increased to over 20 hours.

Elimination: The elimination of salicylic acid follows zero order pharmacokinetics; (i.e., the rate of drug elimination is constant in relation to plasma concentration). Renal excretion of unchanged drug depends upon urine pH. As urinary pH rises above 6.5, the renal clearance of free salicylate increases from 5 percent to >80 percent. Alkalinization of the urine is a key concept in the management of salicylate overdose. (See Overdosage.) Following therapeutic doses, approximately 10 percent is found excreted in the urine as salicylic acid, 75 percent as salicyluric acid, and 10 percent phenolic and 5 percent acyl glucuronides of salicylic acid.

Pharmacodynamics: Aspirin affects platelet aggregation by irreversibly inhibiting prostaglandin cyclo-oxygenase. The effect lasts for the life of the platelet and prevents the formation of the platelet aggregating factor thromboxane A2. Nonacetylated salicylates do not inhibit this enzyme and have no effect on plate-

Continued on next page

St. Joseph Adult—Cont.

let aggregation. At somewhat higher doses, aspirin reversibly inhibits the formation of prostaglandin I2 (prostacyclin), which is an arterial vasodilator and inhibits platelet aggregation. At higher doses, aspirin is an effective anti-inflammatory agent, partially due to inhibition of inflammatory mediators via cyclo-oxygenase inhibition in peripheral tissues. In vitro studies suggest that other mediators of inflammation may also be suppressed by aspirin administration, although the precise mechanism of action has not been elucidated. It is this nonspecific suppression of cyclo-oxygenase activity in peripheral tissues following large doses that leads to its primary side effect of gastric irritation. (See Adverse Reactions.)

Clinical Studies: Ischemic Stroke and Transient Ischemic Attack (TIA): In clinical trials of subjects with TIA's due to fibrin platelet emboli or ischemic stroke, aspirin has been shown to significantly reduce the risk of the combined endpoint of stroke or death and the combined endpoint of TIA, stroke, or death by about 13–18 percent.

Suspected Acute Myocardial Infarction (MI): In a large, multi-center study of aspirin, streptokinase, and the combination of aspirin and streptokinase in 17,187 patients with suspected acute MI, aspirin treatment produced a 23-percent reduction in the risk of vascular mortality. Aspirin was also shown to have an additional benefit in patients given a thrombolytic agent.

Prevention of Recurrent MI and Unstable Angina Pectoris: These indications are supported by the results of six large, randomized, multi-center, placebo-controlled trials of predominantly male post-MI subjects and one randomized placebo-controlled study of men with unstable angina pectoris. Aspirin therapy in MI subjects was associated with a significant reduction (about 20 percent) in the risk of the combined endpoint of subsequent death and/or nonfatal reinfarction in these patients. In aspirin-treated unstable angina patients, the event rate was reduced to 5 percent from the 10 percent rate in the placebo group.

Chronic Stable Angina Pectoris: In a randomized, multi-center, double-blind trial designed to assess the role of aspirin for prevention of MI in patients with chronic stable angina pectoris, aspirin significantly reduced the primary combined endpoint of nonfatal MI, fatal MI, and sudden death by 34 percent. The secondary endpoint for vascular events (first occurrence of MI, stroke, or vascular death) was also significantly reduced (32 percent).

Revascularization Procedures: Most patients who undergo coronary artery revascularization procedures have already had symptomatic coronary artery disease for which aspirin is indicated. Similarly, patients with lesions of the carotid bifurcation sufficient to require carotid endarterectomy are likely to have had a precedent event. Aspirin is recommended for patients who undergo revascularization procedures if there is a preexisting condition for which aspirin is already indicated.

Rheumatologic Diseases: In clinical studies in patients with rheumatoid arthritis, juvenile rheumatoid arthritis, ankylosing spondylitis and osteoarthritis, aspirin has been shown to be effective in controlling various indices of clinical disease activity.

Animal Toxicology: Ischemic Stroke and Transient Ischemic Attack (TIA): In clinical trials of subjects with TIA's due to fibrin platelet emboli or ischemic stroke, aspirin has been shown to significantly reduce the risk of the combined endpoint of stroke or death and the combined endpoint of TIA, stroke, or death by about 13–18 percent. The acute oral 50 percent lethal dose in rats is about 1.5 g/kilogram (kg) and in mice 1.1 g/kg. Renal papillary necrosis and decreased urinary concentrating ability occur in rodents chronically administered high doses. Dose-dependent gastric mucosal injury occurs in rats and humans. Mammals may develop aspirin toxicosis associated with GI symptoms, circulatory effects, and central nervous system depression. (See Overdosage.)

Indications and Usage: Vascular Indications (Ischemic Stroke, TIA, Acute MI, Prevention of Recurrent MI, Unstable Angina Pectoris, and Chronic Stable Angina Pectoris): Aspirin is indicated to: (1) Reduce the combined risk of death and nonfatal stroke in patients who have had ischemic stroke or transient ischemia of the brain due to fibrin platelet emboli, (2) reduce the risk of vascular mortality in patients with a suspected acute MI, (3) reduce the combined risk of death and nonfatal MI in patients with a previous MI or unstable angina pectoris, and (4) reduce the combined risk of MI and sudden death in patients with chronic stable angina pectoris.

Revascularization Procedures (Coronary Artery Bypass Graft (CABG), Percutaneous Transluminal Coronary Angioplasty (PTCA), and Carotid Endarterectomy): Aspirin is indicated in patients who have undergone revascularization procedures (i.e., CABG, PTCA, or carotid endarterectomy) when there is a preexisting condition for which aspirin is already indicated.

Rheumatologic Disease Indications (Rheumatoid Arthritis, Juvenile Rheumatoid Arthritis, Spondyloarthropathies, Osteoarthritis, and the Arthritis and Pleurisy of Systemic Lupus Erythematosus (SLE)): Aspirin is indicated for the relief of the signs and symptoms of rheumatoid arthritis, juvenile rheumatoid arthritis, osteoarthritis, spondyloarthropathies, and arthritis and pleurisy associated with SLE.

Contraindications: Allergy: Aspirin is contraindicated in patients with known allergy to nonsteroidal anti-inflammatory drug products in patients with the syndrome of asthma, rhinitis, and nasal polyps. Aspirin may cause severe urticaria, angioedema, or bronchospasm (asthma).

Reye's Syndrome: Aspirin should not be used in children or teenagers for viral infections, with or without fever, because of the risk of Reye's syndrome with concomitant use of aspirin in certain viral illnesses.

Warnings: Alcohol Warning: Patients who consume three or more alcoholic drinks every day should be counseled about the bleeding risks involved with chronic, heavy alcohol use while taking aspirin.

Coagulation Abnormalities: Even low doses of aspirin can inhibit platelet function leading to an increase in bleeding time. This can adversely affect patients with inherited (hemophilia) or acquired (liver disease or vitamin K deficiency) bleeding disorders.

GI Side Effects: GI side effects include stomach pain, heartburn, nausea, vomiting, and gross GI bleeding. Although minor upper GI symptoms, such as dyspepsia, are common and can occur anytime during therapy, physicians should remain alert for signs of ulceration and bleeding, even in the absence of previous GI symptoms. Physicians should inform patients about the signs and symptoms of GI side effects and what steps to take if they occur.

Peptic Ulcer Disease: Patients with a history of active peptic ulcer disease should avoid using aspirin, which can cause gastric mucosal irritation and bleeding.

Precautions:

General: Renal Failure: Avoid aspirin in patients with severe renal failure (glomerular filtration rate less than 10 mL/minute)

Hepatic Insufficiency: Avoid aspirin in patients with severe hepatic insufficiency.

Sodium Restricted Diets: Patients with sodium-retaining states, such as congestive heart failure or renal failure, should avoid sodium-containing buffered aspirin preparations because of their high sodium content.

Laboratory Tests: Aspirin has been associated with elevated hepatic enzymes, blood urea nitrogen and serum creatinine, hyperkalemia, proteinuria, and prolonged bleeding time.

Drug Interactions: Angiotensin Converting Enzyme (ACE) Inhibitors: The hyponatremic and hypotensive effects of ACE inhibitors may be diminished by the concomitant administration of aspirin due to its indirect effect on the renin-angiotensin conversion pathway.

Acetazolamide: Concurrent use of aspirin and acetazolamide can lead to high serum concentrations of acetazolamide

(and toxicity) due to competition at the renal tubule for secretion.

Anticoagulant Therapy (Heparin and Warfarin): Patients on anticoagulation therapy are at increased risk for bleeding because of drug-drug interactions and the effect on platelets. Aspirin can displace warfarin from protein binding sites, leading to prolongation of both the prothrombin time and the bleeding time. Aspirin can increase the anticoagulant activity of heparin, increasing bleeding risk.

Anticonvulsants: Salicylate can displace protein-bound phenytoin and valproic acid, leading to a decrease in the total concentration of phenytoin and an increase in serum valproic acid levels.

Beta Blockers: The hypotensive effects of beta blockers may be diminished by the concomitant administration of aspirin due to inhibition of renal prostaglandins, leading to decreased renal blood flow, and salt and fluid retention.

Diuretics: The effectiveness of diuretics in patients with underlying renal or cardiovascular disease may be diminished by the concomitant administration of aspirin due to inhibition of renal prostaglandins, leading to decreased renal blood flow and salt and fluit retention.

Methotrexate: Salicylate can inhibit renal clearance of methotrexate, leading to bone marrow toxicity, especially in the elderly or renal impaired.

Nonsteroidal Anti-Inflammatory Drugs (NSAID's): The concurrent use of aspirin with other NSAID's should be avoided because this may increase bleeding or lead to decreased renal function.

Oral Hypoglycemics: Moderate doses of aspirin may increase the effectiveness of oral hypoglycemic drugs, leading to hypoglycemia.

Uricosuric Agents (Probenecid and Sulfinpyrazone): Salicylates antagonize the uricosuric action of uricosuric agents.

Carcinogenesis, Mutagenesis, Impairment of Fertility: Administration of aspirin for 68 weeks at 0.5 percent in the feed of rats was not carcinogenic. In the Ames Salmonella assay, aspirin was not mutagenic; however, aspirin did induce chromosome aberrations in cultured human fibroblasts. Aspirin inhibits ovulation in rats. (See Pregnancy.)

Pregnancy: Pregnant women should only take aspirin if clearly needed. Because of the known effects of NSAID's on the fetal cardiovascular system (closure of the ductus arteriosus), use during the third trimester of pregnancy should be avoided. Salicylate products have also been associated with alterations in maternal and neonatal hemostasis mechanisms, decreased birth weight, and with perinatal mortality.

Labor and Delivery: Aspirin should be avoided 1 week prior to and during labor and delivery because it can result in excessive blood loss at delivery. Prolonged gestation and prolonged labor due to prostaglandin inhibition have been reported.

Nursing Mothers: Nursing mothers should avoid using aspirin because salicylate is excreted in breast milk. Use of high doses may lead to rashes, platelet abnormalities, and bleeding in nursing infants.

Pediatric Use: Pediatric dosing recommendations for juvenile rheumatoid arthritis are based on well-controlled clinical studies. An initial dose of 90–130 mg/kg/day in divided doses, with an increase as needed for anti-inflammatory efficacy (target plasma salicylate levels of 150–300 μg/mL) are effective. At high doses (i.e., plasma levels of greater than 200 μg/mL), the incidence of toxicity increases.

Adverse Reactions: Many adverse reactions due to aspirin ingestion are dose-related. The following is a list of adverse reactions that have been reported in the literature. (See Warnings.)

Body as a Whole: Fever, hypothermia, thirst.

Cardiovascular: Dysrhythmias, hypotension, tachycardia.

Central Nervous System: Agitation, cerebral edema, coma, confusion, dizziness, headache, subdural or intracranial hemorrhage, lethargy, seizures.

Fluid and Electrolyte: Dehydration, hyperkalemia, metabolic acidosis, respiratory alkalosis.

Gastrointestinal: Dyspepsia, GI bleeding, ulceration and perforation, nausea, vomiting, transient elevations of hepatic enzymes, hepatitis, Reye's Syndrome, pancreatitis.

Hematologic: Prolongation of the prothrombin time, disseminated intravascular coagulation, coagulopathy, thrombocytopenia.

Hypersensitivity: Acute anaphylaxis, angioedema, asthma, bronchospasm, laryngeal edema, urticaria.

Musculoskeletal: Rhabdomyolysis.

Metabolism: Hypoglycemia (in children), hyperglycemia.

Reproductive: Prolonged pregnancy and labor, stillbirths, lower birth weight infants, antepartum and postpartum bleeding.

Special Senses: Hearing loss, tinnitus. Patients with high frequency hearing loss may have difficulty perceiving tinnitus. In these patients, tinnitus cannot be used as a clinical indicator of salicylism.

Urogenital: Interstitial nephritis, papillary necrosis, proteinuria, renal insufficiency and failure.

Drug Abuse and Dependence: Aspirin is nonnarcotic. There is no known potential for addiction associated with the use of aspirin.

Overdosage: Salicylate toxicity may result from acute ingestion (overdose) or chronic intoxication. The early signs of salicylic overdose (salicylism), including tinnitus (ringing in the ears), occur at plasma concentrations approaching 200 μg/mL. Plasma concentrations of aspirin above 300 μg/mL are clearly toxic. Severe toxic effects are associated with

levels above 400 μg/mL (See Clinical Pharmacology.) A single lethal dose of aspirin in adults is not known with certainty but death may be expected at 30 g. For real or suspected overdose, a Poison Control Center should be contacted immediately. Careful medical management is essential.

Signs and Symptoms: In acute overdose, severe acid-base and electrolyte disturbances may occur and are complicated by hyperthermia and dehydration. Respiratory alkalosis occurs early while hyperventilation is present, but is quickly followed by metabolic acidosis.

Treatment: Treatment consists primarily of supporting vital functions, increasing salicylate elimination, and correcting the acid-base disturbance. Gastric emptying and/or lavage is recommended as soon as possible after ingestion, even if the patient has vomited spontaneously. After lavage and/or emesis, administration of activated charcoal, as a slurry, is beneficial, if less than 3 hours have passed since ingestion. Charcoal adsorption should not be employed prior to emesis and lavage. Severity of aspirin intoxication is determined by measuring the blood salicylate level. Acid-base status should be closely followed with serial blood gas and serum pH measurements. Fluid and electrolyte balance should also be maintained. In severe cases, hyperthermia and hypovolemia are the major immediate threats to life. Children should be sponged with tepid water. Replacement fluids should be administered intravenously and augmented with correction of acidosis. Plasma electrolytes and pH should be monitored to promote alkaline diuresis of salicylate if renal function is normal. Infusion of glucose may be required to control hypoglycemia. Hemodialysis and peritoneal dialysis can be performed to reduce the body drug content. In patients with renal insufficiency or in cases of life-threatening intoxication, dialysis is usually required. Exchange transfusion may be indicated in infants and young children.

Dosage and Administration: Each dose of aspirin should be taken with a full glass of water unless the patient is fluid restricted. Anti-inflammatory and analgesic dosages should be individualized. When aspirin is used in high doses, the development of tinnitus may be used as a clinical sign of elevated plasma salicylate levels except in patients with high frequency hearing loss.

Ischemic Stroke and TIA: 50–325 mg once a day. Continue therapy indefinitely

Suspected Acute MI: The initial dose of 160–162.5 mg is administered as soon as an MI is suspected. The maintenance dose of 160–162.5 mg a day is continued for 30 days post-infarction. After 30 days, consider further therapy based on dosage and administration for prevention of recurrent MI.

Continued on next page

St. Joseph Adult—Cont.

Prevention of Recurrent MI: 75–325 mg once a day. Continue therapy indefinitely. Unstable Angina Pectoris: 75–325 mg once a day. Continue therapy indefinitely. Chronic Stable Angina Pectoris: 75–325 mg once a day. Continue therapy indefinitely.
CABG: 325 mg daily starting 6 hours post-procedure. Continue therapy for 1 year post-procedure.
PTCA: The initial dose of 325 mg daily should be given 2 hours pre-surgery. Maintenance dose is 160–325 mg daily. Continue therapy indefinitely.
Carotid Endarterectomy: Doses of 80 mg once daily to 650 mg twice daily, started presurgery, are recommended. Continue therapy indefinitely.
Rheumatoid Arthritis: The initial dose is 3 g a day in divided doses. Increase as needed for anti-inflammatory efficacy with target plasma salicylate levels of 150–300 µg/mL. At high doses (i.e., plasma levels of greater than 200 µg/mL), the incidence of toxicity increases.
Juvenile Rheumatoid Arthritis: Initial dose is 90–130 mg/kg/day in divided doses. Increase as needed for anti-inflammatory efficacy with target plasma salicylate levels of 150–300 µg/mL. At high doses (i.e., plasma levels of greater than 200 µg/mL), the incidence of toxicity increases.
Spondyloarthropathies: Up to 4 g per day in divided doses.
Osteoarthritis: Up to 3 g per day in divided doses.
Arthritis and Pleurisy of SLE: The initial dose is 3 g a day in divided doses. Increase as needed for anti-inflammatory efficacy with target plasma salicylate levels of 150–300 µg/mL. At high doses (i.e., plasma levels of greater than 200 µg/mL), the incidence of toxicity increases.

How Supplied: *St. Joseph Adult Low Strength Aspirin Chewable Tablets* are round, concave, orange-flavored, orange-colored tablets that are debossed with the "SJ" logo. Available as follows:
NDC 50580-173-36 Bottle of 36 tablets
NDC Coated Tablets 50580-173-08 Bottle of 108 tablets
St Joseph Adult Low Strength Enteric Coated Tablets are round, concave, pink-coated tablets that are printed with the "St J" logo. Available as follows:
NDC 50580-126-36 Bottle of 36 tablets
NDC 50580-126-18 Bottle of 180 tablets
Store in tight container at 25 deg.C (77 deg.F); excursions permitted to 15–30 deg.C (59–86 deg.F).

SIMPLY COUGH™ LIQUID

Description: *Simply Cough™ Liquid* is Cherry Berry-flavored and contains no alcohol or aspirin. Each teaspoonful (5 mL) contains dextromethorphan HBr 5 mg.

Actions: *Simply Cough™ Liquid* is a single ingredient product that contains the cough suppressant dextromethorphan hydrobromide to provide fast, effective, temporary relief of your child's cough.

Uses: temporarily relieves cough occurring with a cold

Directions:
- find right dose on chart below. If possible, use weight to dose; otherwise use age.
- only use with enclosed measuring cup
- if needed, repeat dose every 4 hours
- do not use more than 4 times in 24 hours

AccuDose™ Chart

Weight (lb)	Age (yr)	Dose (tsp)
under 24	under 2	call a doctor
24–47	2–5	1 tsp
48–95	6–11	2 tsp

Professional Dosage Schedule: 4–11 mos (12–17 lbs): ½ teaspoonful; 12–23 mos (18–23 lbs): ¾ teaspoonful; 2–3 years (24–35 lbs) 1 teaspoonful; 4–5 yrs (36–47 lbs): 1½ teaspoonful; 6–8 yrs (48–59 lbs): 2 teaspoonsful; 9–10 yrs (60–71 lbs): 2½ teaspoonsful; 11 yrs (72–95 lbs): 3 teaspoonsful.
If needed, repeat dose every 4 to 6 hours. Do not use more than 4 times in 24 hours.

Precautions: If a rare sensitivity reaction occurs, the drug should be discontinued.

Warnings: **Do not use** in a child who is taking a prescription monoamine oxidase inhibitor (MAOI) (certain drugs for depression, psychiatric or emotional conditions, or Parkinson's disease), or for 2 weeks after stopping the MAOI drug. If you do not know if your child's prescription drug contains an MAOI, ask a doctor or pharmacist before giving this product.
Ask a doctor before use if this child has
- cough that occurs with too much phlegm (mucus)
- chronic cough that lasts or occurs with asthma

Stop use and ask a doctor if
- cough gets worse or lasts for more than 5 days, comes back or occurs with fever, rash or headache that lasts. These could be signs of a serious condition.

Keep out of reach of children.
In case of overdose, get medical help or contact a Poison Control Center right away.

Other Information:
- **do not use if carton is opened, or if neck wrap or foil inner seal imprinted with "Safety Seal®" is broken or missing**
- store at room temperature

Professional Information:
Overdosage Information:
Acute dextromethorphan overdose usually does not result in serious signs and

symptoms unless massive amounts have been ingested. Signs and symptoms of a substantial overdose may include nausea and vomiting, visual disturbances, CNS disturbances and urinary retention.

Inactive Ingredients: citric acid, corn syrup, FD&C Red #40, flavor, glycerin, purified water, sodium benzoate, sucralose

How Supplied: Red-colored-child resistant bottles of 4 fl. oz.

SIMPLY SLEEP™
Nighttime Sleep Aid

Description: *SIMPLY SLEEP™* is a non habit-forming nighttime sleep aid. Each *SIMPLY SLEEP™* Caplet contains diphenhydramine HCl 25 mg.

Actions: *SIMPLY SLEEP™* contains an antihistamine (diphenhydramine HCl) which has sedative properties.

Use: relief of occasional sleeplessness

Directions:

adults and children 12 years and over	take 2 caplets at bedtime if needed or as directed by a doctor
children under 12 years	do not use

Precautions: If a rare sensitivity reaction occurs, the drug should be discontinued.

Warnings:
Do not use
- in children under 12 years of age
Ask a doctor before use if you have
- a breathing problem such as emphysema or chronic bronchitis
- trouble urinating due to an enlarged prostate gland
- glaucoma
Ask a doctor or pharmacist before use if you are taking sedatives or tranquilizers
When using this product
- drowsiness may occur
- avoid alcoholic drinks
- do not drive a motor vehicle or operate machinery
Stop use and ask a doctor if
- sleeplessness persists continuously for more than 2 weeks. Insomnia may be a symptom of serious underlying medical illness.
If pregnant or breast-feeding, ask a health professional before use.
Keep out of reach of children. In case of overdose, get medical help or contact a Poison Control Center right away.
Other Information:
- Do not use if blister carton is opened or if blister unit is broken.
- Store at room temperature

Inactive Ingredients: carnauba wax, cellulose, croscarmellose sodium, dibasic calcium phosphate, FD&C blue #1, hydroxypropyl methylcellulose, magnesium stearate, polyethylene glycol, polysorbate 80, titanium dioxide.

How Supplied: Light blue mini-caplets embossed with "SL" on one side in blister packs of 24 and 48.

Shown in Product Identification Guide, page 511

SIMPLY STUFFY™ LIQUID

Description: *Simply Stuffy™ Liquid* is Cherry Berry-flavored and contains no alcohol or aspirin. Each teaspoonful (5 mL) contains pseudoephedrine HCL 15 mg.

Actions: *Simply Stuffy™ Liquid* is a single ingredient product that contains the decongestant pseudoephedrine hydrochloride to provide fast, effective, temporary relief of your child's nasal congestion.

Uses: temporarily relieves nasal congestion due to:
• the common cold • hay fever • upper respiratory allergies • sinusitis

Directions:
• find right dose on chart below. If possible, use weight to dose; otherwise use age.
• only use with enclosed measuring cup
• if needed, repeat dose every 4 to 6 hours
• do not use more than 4 times in 24 hours

AccuDose™ Chart

Weight (lb)	Age (yr)	Dose (tsp)
under 24	under 2	call a doctor
24–47	2–5	1 tsp
48–95	6–11	2 tsp

Professional Dosage Schedule: 4–11 mos (12–17 lbs): ½ teaspoonful; 12–23 mos (18–23 lbs): ¾ teaspoonful; 2–3 yrs (24–35 lbs) 1 teaspoonful; 4–5 yrs (36–47 lbs): 1½ teaspoonsful; 6–8 yrs (48–59 lbs): 2 teaspoonsful; 9–10 yrs (60–71 lbs): 2½ teaspoonsful; 11 yrs (72–95 lbs): 3 teaspoonsful
If needed, repeat dose every 4 to 6 hours. Do not use more than 4 times in 24 hours.

Precautions: If a rare sensitivity reaction occurs, the drug should be discontinued.

Warnings: Do not use in a child who is taking a prescription monoamine oxidase inhibitor (MAOI) (certain drugs for depression, psychiatric or emotional conditions, or Parkinson's disease), or for 2 weeks after stopping the MAOI drug. If you do not know if your child's prescription drug contains an MAOI, ask a doctor or pharmacist before giving this product.
Ask a doctor before use if this child has
• heart disease • high blood pressure
• thyroid disease • diabetes
When using this product
• do not exceed recommended dosage

Stop use and ask a doctor if
• nervousness, dizziness, or sleeplessness occur
• symptoms do not get better within 7 days or occur with a fever
Keep out of reach of children.
In case of overdose, get medical help or contact a Poison Control Center right away.
Other Information:
• do not use if carton is opened, of if neck wrap or foil inner seal imprinted with "Safety Seal®" is broken or missing
• store at room temperature
Professional Information:
Overdosage Information: Symptoms from pseudoephedrine overdose consist most often of mild anxiety, tachycardia and/or mild hypertension.
Symptoms usually appear within 4 to 8 hours of ingestion and are transient, usually requiring no treatment.

Inactive Ingredients: citric acid, corn syrup, FD&C Red #40, flavor, glycerin, purified water, sodium benzoate, sucralose

How Supplied: Red-colored-child resistant bottles of 4 fl. oz.

Regular Strength TYLENOL® acetaminophen Tablets

Extra Strength TYLENOL® acetaminophen Gelcaps, Geltabs, Caplets, Tablets

Extra Strength TYLENOL® acetaminophen Adult Liquid Pain Reliever

TYLENOL® acetaminophen Arthritis Pain Extended Relief Caplets

TYLENOL® 8 Hour Acetaminophen Extended Release Geltabs

Product information for all dosage forms of Adult TYLENOL actaminophen have been combined under this heading.

Description: *Each Regular Strength TYLENOL® Tablet* contains acetaminophen 325 mg. *Each Extra Strength TYLENOL® Gelcap, Geltab, Caplet, or Tablet* contains acetaminophen 500 mg. *Extra Strength TYLENOL® Adult Liquid* is alcohol-free and each 15 mL (1/2 fl oz or one tablespoonful) contains 500 mg acetaminophen. *Each TYLENOL® Arthritis Pain Extended Relief Caplet* and each *TYLENOL® 8 Hour Extended Release Geltab* contains acetaminophen 650 mg.

Actions: Acetaminophen is a clinically proven analgesic/antipyretic. Acetaminophen produces analgesia by elevation of the pain threshold and antipyresis through action on the hypothalamic heat-regulating center. Acetaminophen is equal to aspirin in analgesic and antipyretic effectiveness and it is unlikely to produce many of the side effects associated with aspirin and aspirin-containing

products. *Tylenol Arthritis Pain Extended Relief* and *TYLENOL 8 Hour Extended Release* uses a unique, patented, bilayer caplet. The first layer dissolves quickly to provide prompt relief while the second layer is time released to provide up to 8 hours of relief.

Uses: *Regular Strength TYLENOL® Tablets, Extra Strength TYLENOL® Gelcaps, Geltabs, Caplets, or Tablets:* temporarily relieves minor aches and pains due to:
• headache • muscular aches • backache • arthritis
• the common cold • toothache • menstrual cramps
• reduces fever
Extra Strength TYLENOL® Adult Liquid: temporarily relieves minor aches and pains due to:
• headache • muscular aches • backache • arthritis
• the common cold • toothache • menstrual cramps
reduces fever
TYLENOL® Arthritis Pain Extended Relief Caplets: temporarily relieves minor aches and pains due to:
• arthritis • the common cold • headache • toothache
• muscular aches • backache • menstrual cramps
TYLENOL® 8 Hour Extended Release Geltabs: temporarily relieves minor aches and pains due to:
• muscular aches • backache • headache • toothache • the common cold
• menstrual cramps • minor pain of arthritis

Directions: *Regular Strength TYLENOL® Tablets:*
• do not take more than directed (see overdose warning)

adults and children 12 years and over	•take 2 tablets every 4 to 6 hours as needed •do not take more than 12 tablets in 24 hours
children 6–11 years	•take 1 tablet every 4 to 6 hours as needed •do not take more than 5 in 24 hours
children under 6 years	do not use this Regular Strength product in children under 6 years of age; this will provide more than the recommended dose (overdose) of TYLENOL® and could cause serious health problems

Extra Strength TYLENOL® Gelcaps, Geltabs, Caplets, or Tablets:
• do not take more than directed (see overdose warning)

adults and children 12 years and over	•take 2 every 4 to 6 hours as needed •do not take more than 8 in 24 hours

Continued on next page

Tylenol Reg. Strength—Cont.

children under 12 years	do not use this Extra Strength product in children under 12 years of age; this will provide more than the recommended dose (overdose) of TYLENOL® and could cause serious health problems

Extra Strength TYLENOL® Adult Liquid:
- **do not take more than directed (see overdose warning)**

adults and children 12 years and over	•take 2 tablespoons (tbsp.) in dose cup provided every 4 to 6 hours as needed •do not take more than 8 tablespoons in 24 hours
children under 12 years	do not use this adult Extra Strength product in children under 12 years of age; this will provide more than the recommended dose (overdose) of TYLENOL® and could cause serious health problems

TYLENOL® Arthritis Pain Extended Relief Caplets and *TYLENOL® 8 Hour Extended Release Geltabs*
- **do not take more than directed (see overdose warning)**

adults	•take 2 every 8 hours with water •swallow whole – do not crush, chew or dissolve •do not take more than 6 in 24 hours •do not use for more than 10 days unless directed by a doctor
under 18 years of age	•ask a doctor

Precautions: If a rare sensitivity reaction occurs, the drug should be discontinued.

Warnings: *Regular Strength TYLENOL® Tablets, Extra Strength TYLENOL® Gelcaps, Geltabs, Caplets, or Tablets, Extra Strength TYLENOL® Liquid*

Alcohol warning: If you consume 3 or more alcoholic drinks every day, ask your doctor whether you should take acetaminophen or other pain relievers/ fever reducers. Acetaminophen may cause liver damage.

Do not use:
- with any other product containing acetaminophen.

Stop using and ask a doctor if:
- new symptoms occur
- redness or swelling is present
- pain gets worse or lasts for more than 10 days
- fever gets worse or lasts for more than 3 days

If pregnant or breast-feeding, ask a health professional before use.

Keep out of reach of children.

TYLENOL® Arthritis Pain Extended Relief Caplets:

Alcohol warning: If you consume 3 or more alcoholic drinks every day, ask your doctor whether you should take acetaminophen or other pain relievers/ fever reducers. Acetaminophen may cause liver damage.

Do not use
- with any other product containing acetaminophen.

Stop use and ask a doctor if
- New symptoms occur
- Redness or swelling is present
- Pain gets worse or lasts for more than 10 days

If pregnant or breast-feeding, ask a health professional before use.

Keep out of reach of children.

Overdose warning: Taking more than the recommended dose (overdose) could cause serious health problems. In case of overdose, get medical help or contact a Poison Control Center right away. Quick medical attention is critical for adults as well as for children even if you do not notice any signs or symptoms.

TYLENOL® 8 Hour Extended Release Geltabs:

Alcohol warning: If you consume 3 or more alcoholic drinks every day, ask your doctor whether you should take acetaminophen or other pain relievers/ fever reducers. Acetaminophen may cause liver damage.

Do not use
- with any other product containing acetaminophen.

Stop use and ask a doctor if
- New symptoms occur
- Redness or swelling is present
- Pain gets worse or lasts for more than 10 days

If pregnant or breast-feeding, ask a health professional before use.

Keep out of reach of children.

Overdose warning: Taking more than the recommended dose (overdose) could cause serious health problems. In case of overdose, get medical help or contact a Poison Control Center right away.

Other information

Regular Strength TYLENOL® Tablets
- **do not use if carton is opened or red neck wrap or foil inner seal imprinted with "Safety Seal®" is broken**
- store at room temperature

Extra Strength TYLENOL® Gelcaps, Geltabs, Caplets or Tablets
- **do not use if carton is opened or red neck wrap or foil inner seal imprinted with "Safety Seal®" is broken**
- store at room temperature (*tablet and caplet*)
- store at room temperature; avoid high humidity and excessive heat 40°C (104°F). (*Gelcap and Geltab*)

Extra Strength TYLENOL® Adult Liquid
- **do not use if carton is opened, or if bottle wrap or foil inner seal imprinted "Safety Seal®" is broken or missing.**
- Store at room temperature

TYLENOL® Arthritis Pain Extended Relief Caplets and *TYLENOL® 8 Hour Extended Release Geltabs*
- **do not use if carton is opened or red neck wrap or foil inner seal with "Safety Seal®" is broken**
- store at 20–25°C (68–77°F)
- avoid excessive heat at 40°C (104°F)

Professional Information:
Overdosage Information for all Adult Tylenol products
ACETAMINOPHEN: Acetaminophen in massive overdosage may cause hepatic toxicity in some patients. In adults and adolescents ($\geq$ 12 years of age), hepatic toxicity may occur following ingestion of greater than 7.5 to 10 grams over a period of 8 hours or less. Fatalities are infrequent (less than 3–4% of untreated cases) and have rarely been reported with overdoses of less than 15 grams. In children (<12 years of age), an acute overdosage of less than 150 mg/kg has not been associated with hepatic toxicity. Early symptoms following a potentially hepatotoxic overdose may include: nausea, vomiting, diaphoresis and general malaise. Clinical and laboratory evidence of hepatic toxicity may not be apparent until 48 to 72 hours postingestion. In adults and adolescents, any individual presenting with an unknown amount of acetaminophen ingested or with a questionable or unreliable history about the time of ingestion should have a plasma acetaminophen level drawn and be treated with *N*-acetylcysteine. For full prescribing information, refer to the *N*-acetylcysteine package insert. Do not await results of assays for plasma acetaminophen levels before initiating treatment with *N*-acetylcysteine. The following additional procedures are recommended: Promptly initiate gastric decontamination of the stomach. A plasma acetaminophen assay should be obtained as early as possible, but no sooner than four hours following ingestion. If an acetaminophen *extended release* product is involved, it may be appropriate to obtain an additional plasma acetaminophen level 4–6 hours following the initial acetaminophen level. If either acetaminophen level plots above the treatment line on the acetaminophen overdose nomogram, *N*-acetylcysteine treatment should be continued for a full course of therapy. Liver function studies should be obtained initially and repeated at 24-hour intervals. Serious toxicity or fatalities have been extremely infrequent following an acute acetaminophen overdose in young children, possibly because of differences in the way they metabolize acetaminophen. In children, the maximum potential amount ingested can be more easily

estimated. If more than 150 mg/kg or an unknown amount was ingested, obtain a plasma acetaminophen level as soon as possible, but no sooner than 4 hours following ingestion. If an acetaminophen *extended release* product is involved, it may be appropriate to obtain an additional plasma acetaminophen level 4–6 hours following the initial acetaminophen level. If either acetaminophen level plots above the treatment line on the acetaminophen overdose nomogram, *N*-acetylcysteine treatment should be initiated and continued for a full course of therapy. If an assay cannot be obtained and the estimated acetaminophen ingestion exceeds 150 mg/kg, dosing with *N*-acetylcysteine should be initiated and continued for a full course of therapy. For additional emergency information, call your regional poison center or call the Rocky Mountain Poison Center toll-free, (1-800-525-6115).

Our adult Tylenol® combination products contain active ingredients in addition to acetaminophen. The following is basic overdose information regarding those ingredients.

CHLORPHENIRAMINE: Chlorpheniramine toxicity should be treated as you would an antihistamine/anticholinergic overdose and is likely to be present within a few hours after acute ingestion.

DEXTROMETHORHPHAN: Acute dextromethorphan overdose usually does not result in serious signs and symptoms unless massive amounts have been ingested. Signs and symptoms of a substantial overdose may include nausea and vomiting, visual disturbances, CNS disturbances and urinary retention.

DIPHENHYDRAMINE: Diphenhydramine toxicity should be treated as you would an antihistamine/anticholinergic overdose and is likely to be present within a few hours after acute ingestion.

DOXYLAMINE: Doxylamine toxicity should be treated as you would an antihistamine/anticholinergic overdose and is likely to be present within a few hours after acute ingestion.

GUAIFENESIN: Guaifenesin should be treated as a nontoxic ingestion.

PAMABROM: Acute overexposure of diuretics is primarily associated with fluid and electrolyte loss. Fluid loss should be treated with the appropriate intravenous and/or oral fluids.

PSEUDOEPHEDRINE: Symptoms from pseudoephedrine overdose consist most often of mild anxiety, tachycardia and/or mild hypertension. Symptoms usually appear within 4 to 8 hours of ingestion and are transient, usually requiring no treatment.

For additional emergency information, please contact your local poison control center.

Alcohol Information: Chronic heavy alcohol abusers may be at increased risk of liver toxicity from excessive acetaminophen use, although reports of this event are rare. Reports usually involve cases of severe chronic alcoholics and the dosages of acetaminophen most often ex-

ceed recommended doses and often involve substantial overdose. Healthcare professionals should alert their patients who regularly consume large amounts of alcohol not to exceed recommended doses of acetaminophen.

Inactive Ingredients: *Regular Strength TYLENOL® Tablets:* cellulose, corn starch, magnesium stearate, sodium starch glycolate.

Extra Strength TYLENOL® **Tablets**: cellulose, corn starch, magnesium stearate, sodium starch glycolate. **Caplets:** cellulose, corn starch, FD&C Red #40, hypromellose, magnesium stearate, polyethylene glycol, sodium starch glycolate. **Gelcaps:** benzyl alcohol, butylparaben, castor oil, cellulose, corn starch, D&C Yellow #10, edetate calcium disodium, FD&C Blue #1, FD&C Blue #2, FD&C Red #40, gelatin, hypromellose, magnesium stearate, methylparaben, propylparaben, sodium lauryl sulfate, sodium propionate, sodium starch glycolate, titanium dioxide. **Geltabs:** benzyl alcohol, butylparaben, castor oil, cellulose, corn starch, D&C Yellow #10, edetate calcium disodium, FD&C Blue #1, FD&C Blue #2, FD&C Red #40, gelatin, hypromellose, magnesium stearate, methylparaben, propylparaben, sodium lauryl sulfate, sodium propionate, sodium starch glycolate, titanium dioxide.

Extra Strength TYLENOL® Adult Liquid: citric acid, D&C Red #33, FD&C Red #40, flavor, high fructose corn syrup, polyethylene glycol, propylene glycol, purified water, saccharin sodium, sodium benzoate, sorbitol

TYLENOL® Arthritis Pain Extended Relief Caplets: corn starch, hydroxyethyl cellulose, hypromellose, magnesium stearate, microcrystalline cellulose, povidone, powdered cellulose, pregelatinized starch, sodium starch glycolate, titanium dioxide, triacetin *TYLENOL® 8 Hour Extended Release Geltabs:* FD&C Blue #1, FD&C Blue #2, FD&C Red #40, gelatin, hydroxyethyl cellulose, hypromellose, magnesium stearate, methylparaben, povidone, propylparaben, sodium lauryl sulfate, sodium propionate, sodium starch glycolate, titanium dioxide

How Supplied: *Regular Strength TYLENOL® Tablets:* (colored white, scored, imprinted "TYLENOL" and "325")—tamper-evident bottles of 100.

Extra Strength TYLENOL® Tablets: (colored white, imprinted "TYLENOL" and "500")—tamper-evident bottles of 30, 60, 100, and 200. *Caplets* (colored white, imprinted "TYLENOL 500 mg")—vials of 10, 10 blister packs, and tamper-evident bottles of 24, 50, 100, 175, and 250. *Gelcaps* (colored yellow and red, imprinted "Tylenol 500") tamper-evident bottles of 24, 50, 100, and 225. *Geltabs* (colored yellow and red, imprinted "Tylenol 500") tamper-evident bottles of 24, 50, and 100.

Extra Strength TYLENOL® Adult Liquid: Cherry-flavored liquid (colored red)

8 fl. oz. tamper-evident bottle with child resistant safety cap and special dosage cup.

TYLENOL® Arthritis Pain Extended Relief Caplets: (colored white, engraved "TYLENOL ER") tamper-evident bottles of 24, 50, and 100, 150, 250 and 290 *TYLENOL® 8 Hour Extended Release Geltabs:* (colored white and red, imprinted "8 HOUR") tamper-evident bottles of 20, 40 and 80.

Shown in Product Identification Guide, page 512

TYLENOL® Severe Allergy Caplets

Maximum Strength TYLENOL® Allergy Sinus Night Time Caplets

Maximum Strength TYLENOL® Allergy Sinus Day Time Caplets, Gelcaps and Geltabs

Product information for all dosage forms of TYLENOL Allergy have been combined under this heading.

Description: Each *TYLENOL® Severe Allergy Caplet* contains acetaminophen 500 mg and diphenhydramine HCl 12.5 mg. Each *Maximum Strength TYLENOL® Allergy Sinus Night Time Caplet* contains acetaminophen 500 mg, diphenhydramine HCl 25 mg, and pseudoephedrine HCl 30 mg. Each *Maximum Strength TYLENOL® Allergy Sinus Day Time Caplet Gelcap and Geltab* contains acetaminophen 500 mg, chlorpheniramine maleate 2 mg, and pseudoephedrine HCl 30 mg.

Actions: *TYLENOL® Severe Allergy Caplets* contain a clinically proven analgesic-antipyretic and antihistamine. Acetaminophen produces analgesia by elevation of the pain threshold and antipyresis through action on the hypothalamic heat regulating center. Acetaminophen is equal to aspirin in analgesic and antipyretic effectiveness, and it is unlikely to produce many of the side effects associated with aspirin and aspirin-containing products.

Diphenhydramine HCl is an antihistamine which helps provide temporary relief of itchy, watery eyes, runny nose, sneezing, itching of the nose or throat due to hay fever or other respiratory allergies.

Maximum Strength TYLENOL® Allergy Sinus Night Time Caplets contain, in addition to the above ingredients, a decongestant, pseudoephedrine HCl. Pseudoephedrine is a sympathomimetic amine which provides temporary relief of nasal and sinus congestion.

Maximum Strength TYLENOL® Allergy Sinus Day Time Caplets, Gelcaps and Geltabs contain acetaminophen, pseudoephedrine HCl and the antihistamine,

Continued on next page

Tylenol Severe Allergy—Cont.

chlorpheniramine maleate. Chlorpheniramine is an antihistamine which helps provide temporary relief of runny nose, sneezing and watery and itchy eyes.

Uses: *TYLENOL® Severe Allergy:* temporarily relieves these symptoms due to hay fever or other respiratory allergies:
• itchy, watery eyes • runny nose
• sneezing • sore throat
• itching of nose or throat
Maximum Strength TYLENOL® Allergy Sinus Night Time and TYLENOL® Allergy Sinus Day Time: temporarily relieves these symptoms due to hay fever or other respiratory allergies:
• nasal congestion • sinus pressure
• sinus pain • headache
• runny nose • sneezing
• itchy, watery eyes • itchy throat

Precautions: If a rare sensitivity reaction occurs, the drug should be discontinued.

Directions: *TYLENOL® Severe Allergy:*
• **do not take more than directed (see overdose warning)**

adults and children 12 years and over	• take 2 caplets every 4 to 6 hours as needed • do not take more than 8 caplets in 24 hours
children under 12 years	• do not use this adult product in children under 12 years of age; this will provide more than the recommended dose (overdose) and could cause serious health problems.

Maximum Strength TYLENOL® Allergy Sinus Night Time:
• **do not take more than directed (see overdose warning)**

adults and children 12 years and over	• take 2 caplets every 4 to 6 hours as needed • do not take more than 8 caplets in 24 hours
children under 12 years	• do not use this adult product in children under 12 years of age; this will provide more than the recommended dose (overdose) and could cause serious health problems.

Maximum Strength TYLENOL® Allergy Sinus Day Time:
• **do not take more than directed (see overdose warning)**

adults and children 12 years and over	• take two every 4 to 6 hours as needed • do not take more than 8 caplets in 24 hours
children under 12 years	• do not use this adult product in children under 12 years of age; this will provide more than the recommended dose (overdose) and could cause serious health problems.

Warnings: Alcohol warning: If you consume 3 or more alcoholic drinks every day, ask your doctor whether your should take acetaminophen or other pain relievers/fever reducers. Acetaminophen may cause liver damage.
Sore throat warning: If sore throat is severe, persists for more than 2 days, is accompanied or followed by fever, headache, rash, nausea or vomiting, consult a doctor promptly. *(applies to TYLENOL® Severe Allergy only)*
Do not use
• if you are now taking a prescription monoamine oxidase inhibitor (MAOI) (certain drugs for depression, psychiatric or emotional conditions, or Parkinson's disease) or for 2 weeks after stopping the MAOI drug. If you do not know if your prescription drug contains an MAOI, ask a doctor or pharmacist before taking this product (does not apply to *TYLENOL® Severe Allergy*)
• with any other product containing acetaminophen
Ask a doctor or pharmacist before use if you are taking sedatives or tranquilizers
Stop use and ask a doctor if
• new symptoms occur
• redness or swelling is present
• pain gets worse or lasts for more than 7 days
• fever gets worse or lasts for more than 3 days
• you get nervous, dizzy or sleepless (does not apply to TYLENOL® Severe Allergy)
If pregnant or breast feeding, ask a health professional before use.
Keep out of reach of children. Overdose warning: Taking more than the recommended dose (overdose) could cause serious health problems. In case of overdose, get medical help or contact a Poison Control Center right away. Quick medical attention is critical for adults as well as for children even if you do not notice any signs or symptoms.
When using this product
• marked drowsiness may occur
• avoid alcoholic drinks
• alcohol, sedatives and tranquilizers may increase drowsiness

• be careful when driving a motor vehicle or operating machinery
• excitability may occur, especially in children
TYLENOL® Severe Allergy
Ask a doctor before use if you have
• glaucoma
• trouble urinating due to an enlarged prostate gland
• a breathing problem such as emphysema or chronic bronchitis
Maximum Strength TYLENOL® Allergy Sinus Night Time and Maximum Strength TYLENOL® Allergy Sinus Day Time
Ask a doctor before use if you have
• heart disease • glaucoma • diabetes
• thyroid disease • high blood pressure
• trouble urinating due to an enlarged prostate gland
• a breathing problem such as emphysema or chronic bronchitis
Other information
• **do not use if carton is opened or if blister unit is broken**
TYLENOL® Allergy Sinus Day Time Caplet and TYLENOL® Allergy Sinus Night Time Caplet:
• store at room temperature
TYLENOL® Allergy Sinus Day Time Gelcap & Geltabs
• store at room temperature; avoid high humidity and excessive heat 40°C (104°F)

Professional Information:
Overdosage Information:
For overdosage information, please refer to pgs. 678–679.

Inactive Ingredients: *TYLENOL® Severe Allergy:* **Caplets:** carnauba wax, cellulose, corn starch, D&C Yellow #10, FD&C Yellow #6, hydroxpropyl cellulose, hypromellose, iron oxide, magnesium stearate, polyethylene glycol, sodium citrate, sodium starch glycolate, titanium dioxide.
Maximum Strength TYLENOL® Allergy Sinus Night Time: **Caplets:** carnauba wax, cellulose, corn starch, D&C Yellow #10, FD&C Blue #1, hypromellose, iron oxide, magnesium stearate, polyethylene glycol, polysorbate 80, sodium citrate, sodium starch glycolate, titanium dioxide.
Maximum Strength TYLENOL® Allergy Sinus Day Time: **Caplets:** carnauba wax, cellulose, corn starch, D&C Yellow #10, FD&C Blue #1, FD&C Yellow #6, hydroxypropyl cellulose, hypromellose, iron oxide, magnesium stearate, polyethylene glycol, sodium starch glycolate, titanium dioxide. **Gelcaps and Geltabs:** benzyl alcohol, butylparaben, castor oil, cellulose, corn starch, D&C Yellow #10, FD&C Blue #1, FD&C Blue #2, gelatin, hypromellose, magnesium stearate, methylparaben, propylparaben, sodium lauryl sulfate, sodium propionate, sodium starch glycolate, titanium dioxide.

How Supplied: *TYLENOL® Severe Allergy:* **Caplets:** Yellow film-coated, imprinted with "TYLENOL Severe Allergy" on one side—blister packs of 24.
Maximum Strength TYLENOL® Allergy Sinus Night Time: **Caplets:** Light blue film-coated, imprinted with "TYLENOL A/S Night Time" on one side—blister packs of 24.

Maximum Strength TYLENOL® Allergy Sinus Day Time: **Caplets:** Yellow film-coated, imprinted with "TYLENOL Allergy Sinus" on one side—blister packs of 24.

Gelcaps and Geltabs: Green and yellow-colored, imprinted with "TYLENOL A/S"—blister packs of 24 and 48.

Shown in Product Identification Guide, page 512

**Multi-Symptom
TYLENOL® Cold Day Non-Drowsy
Caplets and Gelcaps**

**Multi-Symptom
TYLENOL® Cold Night Time
Complete
Formula Caplets**

Product information for all dosage forms of TYLENOL Cold have been combined under this heading.

Description: Each *Multi-Symptom TYLENOL® Cold Day Non-Drowsy Caplet and Gelcap* contains acetaminophen 325 mg, dextromethorphan HBr 15 mg, and pseudoephedrine HCl 30 mg. Each *Multi-Symptom TYLENOL® Cold Night Time Complete Formula Caplet* contains acetaminophen 325 mg, chlorpheniramine maleate 2 mg, dextromethorphan HBr 15 mg, and pseudoephedrine HCl 30 mg.

Actions: *Multi-Symptom TYLENOL® Cold Day Non-Drowsy* contains a clinically proven analgesic-antipyretic, a decongestant and a cough suppressant. Acetaminophen produces analgesia by elevation of the pain threshold and antipyresis through action on the hypothalamic heat regulating center. Acetaminophen is equal to aspirin in analgesic and antipyretic effectiveness and it is unlikely to produce many of the side effects associated with aspirin and aspirin-containing products. Pseudoephedrine is a sympathomimetic amine which provides temporary relief of nasal congestion. Dextromethorphan is a cough suppressant which provides temporary relief of coughs due to minor throat irritations that may occur with the common cold. *Multi-Symptom TYLENOL® Cold Night Time Complete Formula Caplets* contain, in addition to the above ingredients, an antihistamine. Chlorpheniramine is an antihistamine which helps provide temporary relief of runny nose, sneezing and watery and itchy eyes.

Uses: *Multi-Symptom TYLENOL® Cold Day Non-Drowsy:* temporarily relieves these cold symptoms:
• cough • sore throat • minor aches and pains • headaches • nasal congestion
• temporarily reduces fever
Multi-Symptom TYLENOL® Cold Night Time Complete Formula: temporarily relieves these cold symptoms:
• cough • sore throat • minor aches and pains • headache • nasal congestion
• runny nose • sneezing • watery and itchy eyes

• temporarily reduces fever

Directions: *Multi-Symptom TYLENOL® Cold Day Non-Drowsy and Multi-Symptom TYLENOL® Cold Night Time Complete Formula:*
• **do not take more than directed (see overdose warning)**

adults and children 12 years and over	• take 2 every 6 hours as needed • do not take more than 8 in 24 hours.
children under 12 years	• not intended for use in children under 12. Ask your doctor.

Precautions: If a rare sensitivity reaction occurs, the drug should be discontinued.

Warnings:
Alcohol Warning: If you consume 3 or more alcoholic drinks every day, ask your doctor whether you should take acetaminophen or other pain relievers/fever reducers. Acetaminophen may cause liver damage.
Sore throat warning: If sore throat is severe, persists for more than 2 days, is accompanied or followed by fever, headache, rash, nausea or vomiting, consult a doctor promptly.
Do not use
• if you are now taking a prescription monoamine oxidase inhibitor (MAOI) (certain drugs for depression, psychiatric or emotional conditions or Parkinson's disease), or for 2 weeks after stopping the MAOI drug. If you do not know if your prescription drug contains an MAOI, ask a doctor or pharmacist before taking this product.
• with any other product containing acetaminophen
Stop use and ask a doctor if
• new symptoms occur
• redness or swelling is present
• pain gets worse or lasts for more than 7 days
• fever gets worse or lasts for more than 3 days
• you get nervous, dizzy or sleepless
• cough lasts more than 7 days, comes back or occurs with fever, rash or headache that lasts. These could be signs of a serious condition.
If pregnant or breast-feeding, ask a health professional before use.
Keep out of reach of children.
Overdose warning: Taking more than the recommended dose (overdose) could cause serious health problems. In case of overdose, get medical help or contact a Poison Control Center right away. Quick medical attention is critical for adults as well as for children even if you don't notice any signs or symptoms.
Multi-Symptom TYLENOL® Cold Day Non-Drowsy
Ask a doctor before use if you have
• heart disease • diabetes • thyroid disease • cough that occurs with too much phlegm (mucus) • high blood pressure

• trouble urinating due to an enlarged prostate gland • chronic cough that lasts as occurs with smoking, asthma, chronic bronchitis or emphysema
When using this product
• do not exceed recommended dosage
Multi-Symptom TYLENOL® Cold Night Time Complete Formula:
Ask a doctor before use if you have
• heart disease • glaucoma • diabetes • thyroid disease • cough that occurs with too much phlegm (mucus) • high blood pressure • a breathing problem or chronic cough that lasts as occurs with smoking, asthma, chronic bronchitis or emphysema • trouble urinating due to an enlarged prostate gland
Ask a doctor or pharmacist before use if you are taking sedatives or tranquilizers
When using this product
• do not exceed recommended dosage
• drowsiness may occur • avoid alcoholic drinks • alcohol, sedatives and tranquilizers may increase drowsiness • be careful when driving a motor vehicle or operating machinery • excitability may occur, especially in children
Other information
• do not use if carton is opened or if blister unit is broken
• store at room temperature (avoid high humidity and excessive heat 40°C (104°F)—applies to TYLENOL® Cold Non-Drowsy Gelcap only)

Professional Information:
Overdosage Information
For overdosage information, please refer to pgs. 678–679.

Inactive Ingredients: *Multi-Symptom TYLENOL® Cold Day Non Drowsy Formula:* **Caplets:** carnauba wax, cellulose, corn starch, D&C Yellow #10, FD&C Blue #1, hypromellose, iron oxide, magnesium stearate, sodium starch glycolate, titanium dioxide, triacetin.
Gelcaps: benzyl alcohol, butylparaben, castor oil, cellulose, corn starch, D&C Yellow #10, edetate calcium disodium, FD&C Red #40, gelatin, hypromellose, iron oxide, magnesium stearate, methylparaben, propylparaben, sodium lauryl sulfate, sodium propionate, sodium starch glycolate, titanium dioxide.
Multi-Symptom TYLENOL® Cold Night Time Complete Formula: **Caplets:** carnauba wax, cellulose, corn starch, D&C Yellow #10, FD&C Blue #1, FD&C Yellow #6, hypromellose, iron oxide, magnesium stearate, sodium starch glycolate, titanium dioxide, triacetin.

How Supplied: *Multi-Symptom TYLENOL® Cold Day Non Drowsy* Caplets: White-colored, imprinted with "TYLENOL Cold"—blister packs of 24.
Gelcaps: Red- and tan-colored, imprinted with "TYLENOL COLD"—blister packs of 24.
Multi-Symptom TYLENOL® Cold Night Time Complete Formula Caplets: Yellow-colored, imprinted with "TYLENOL Cold"—blister packs of 24.
These products are also available in a convenience pack containing Multi-

Continued on next page

Tylenol Cold—Cont.

Symptom TYLENOL® Cold Day Non-Drowsy (pack of 12) and Multi-Symptom TYLENOL® Cold Night Time Complete Formula (pack of 12).

Shown in Product Identification Guide, page 513

Multi-Symptom TYLENOL® COLD Severe Congestion Non-Drowsy

Description: Each *Multi-Symptom TYLENOL® Cold Severe Congestion Non-Drowsy Caplet* contains acetaminophen 325 mg, dextromethorphan HBr 15 mg, guaifenesin 200 mg and pseudoephedrine HCl 30 mg.

Actions: *Multi-Symptom TYLENOL® Cold Severe Congestion Non-Drowsy Caplets* contain a clinically proven analgesic-antipyretic, decongestant, expectorant and cough suppressant. Acetaminophen produces analgesia by elevation of the pain threshold and antipyresis through action on the hypothalamic heat regulating center. Acetaminophen is equal to aspirin in analgesic and antipyretic effectiveness and is unlikely to produce many of the side effects associated with aspirin and aspirin-containing products. Pseudoephedrine is a sympathomimetic amine which provides temporary relief of nasal congestion. Guaifenesin is an expectorant which helps loosen phlegm (mucus) and thin bronchial secretions to make coughs more productive. Dextromethorphan is a cough suppressant which provides temporary relief of coughs due to minor throat irritations that may occur with the common cold.

Uses: temporarily relieves these cold symptoms:
• cough • sore throat • minor aches and pains • headaches • nasal congestion
• helps loosen phlegm (mucus) and thin bronchial secretions to make coughs more productive
• temporarily reduces fever

Directions:

adults and children 12 years and over	• take 2 caplets every 6–8 hours as needed • do not take more than 8 caplets in 24 hours
children under 12 years	• not intended for use in children under 12. Ask your doctor.

Precautions: If a rare sensitivity reaction occurs, the drug should be discontinued.

Warnings: Alcohol warning: If you consume 3 or more alcoholic drinks every day, ask your doctor whether you should take acetaminophen or other pain relievers/fever reducers. Acetaminophen may cause liver damage.

Sore throat warning: If sore throat is severe, persists for more than 2 days, is accompanied or followed by fever, headache, rash, nausea or vomiting, consult a doctor promptly.

Do not use
• if you are now taking a prescription monoamine oxidase inhibitor (MAOI) (certain drugs for depression, psychiatric or emotional conditions, or Parkinson's disease), or for 2 weeks after stopping the MAOI drug. If you do not know if your prescription drug contains an MAOI, ask a doctor or pharmacist before taking this product.
• with any other product containing acetaminophen

Ask a doctor before use if you have
• heart disease • diabetes • thyroid disease • cough that occurs with too much phlegm (mucus) • high blood pressure • trouble urinating due to an enlarged prostate gland • chronic cough that lasts as occurs with smoking, asthma, chronic bronchitis or emphysema

When using this product
• do not exceed recommended dosage

Stop use and ask a doctor if
• new symptoms occur
• redness or swelling is present
• pain gets worse or lasts for more than 7 days
• fever gets worse or lasts for more than 3 days
• you get nervous, dizzy or sleepless
• cough lasts more than 7 days, comes back or occurs with fever, rash or headache that lasts. These could be signs of a serious condition.

If pregnant or breast-feeding, ask a health professional before use.

Keep out of reach of children.

Overdose warning: Taking more than the recommended dose (overdose) could cause serious health problems. In case of overdose, get medical help or contact a Poison Control Center right away. Quick medical attention is critical for adults as well as for children even if you do not notice any signs or symptoms.

Other Information:
• do not use if carton is opened or if blister unit is broken
• Store at room temperature.

Professional Information:
Overdosage Information

For overdosage information, please refer to pgs. 678–679.

Inactive Ingredients: carnauba wax, cellulose, corn starch, D&C Yellow #10, FD&C Blue #1, FD&C Yellow #6, hypromellose, iron oxide, povidone, silicon dioxide, sodium starch glycolate, stearic acid, titanium dioxide, triacetin

How Supplied: Caplets: Buttery-tan-colored, imprinted with *"TYLENOL COLD SC"* in green ink—blister packs of 24.

Shown in Product Identification Guide, page 513

Maximum Strength TYLENOL® Flu Day Non-Drowsy Gelcaps
Maximum Strength TYLENOL® Flu NightTime Gelcaps
Maximum Strength TYLENOL® Flu NightTime Liquid

Product information for all dosage forms of TYLENOL Flu have been combined under this heading.

Description: Each *Maximum Strength TYLENOL® Flu Day Non-Drowsy Gelcap* contains acetaminophen 500 mg, dextromethorphan HBr 15 mg and pseudoephedrine HCl 30 mg. Each *Maximum Strength TYLENOL® Flu NightTime Gelcap* contains acetaminophen 500 mg, diphenhydramine HCl 25 mg and pseudoephedrine HCl 30 mg. *Maximum Strength TYLENOL® Flu NightTime Liquid:* Each 30 mL (2 tablespoonful) contains acetaminophen 1000 mg, dextromethorphan HBr 30 mg, doxylamine succinate 12.5 mg, and pseudoephedrine HCl 60 mg.

Actions: *Maximum Strength TYLENOL® Flu Day Non-Drowsy Gelcaps* contain a clinically proven analgesic-antipyretic, a decongestant and a cough suppressant. Acetaminophen produces analgesia by elevation of the pain threshold and antipyresis through action on the hypothalamic heat regulating center. Acetaminophen is equal to aspirin in analgesic and antipyretic effectiveness and it is unlikely to produce many of the side effects associated with aspirin and aspirin-containing products. Pseudoephedrine hydrochloride is a sympathomimetic amine which provides temporary relief of nasal congestion. Dextromethorphan is a cough suppressant which provides temporary relief of coughs due to minor throat irritations that may occur with the common cold.
Maximum Strength TYLENOL® Flu NightTime Gelcaps contains the same clinically proven analgesic-antipyretic and decongestant as *Maximum Strength TYLENOL Flu Day Non-Drowsy Gelcaps* along with an antihistamine. Diphenhydramine is an antihistamine which helps provide temporary relief of runny nose and sneezing. *Maximum Strength TYLENOL® Flu NightTime Liquid* contains the same clinically proven analgesic-antipyretic, decongestant and cough suppressant as *Maximum Strength TYLENOL Flu Day Non-Drowsy Gelcaps* along with an antihistamine. Doxylamine succinate is an antihistamine which helps provide temporary relief of runny nose and sneezing.

Uses: *Maximum Strength TYLENOL® Flu Day Non-Drowsy Gelcaps:* temporarily relieves these cold and flu symptoms:
• minor aches and pains • headaches
• sore throat • nasal congestion
• coughs
• temporarily reduces fever
Maximum Strength TYLENOL® Flu NightTime Gelcaps:
temporarily relieves these cold and flu symptoms:
• minor aches and pains • headaches
• sore throat • nasal congestion • runny nose • sneezing

- temporarily reduces fever

Maximum Strength TYLENOL® Flu NightTime Liquid:

temporarily relieves these cold and flu symptoms:
- body aches and headaches • coughs
- nasal congestion • sore throat • runny nose • sneezing
- temporarily reduces fever

Directions:
- do not take more than directed (see overdose warning)

Maximum Strength TYLENOL® Flu Day Non-Drowsy Gelcaps:

adults and children 12 years and over	• take 2 gelcaps every 6 hours as needed • do not take more than 8 gelcaps in 24 hours
children under 12 years	• do not use this adult product in children under 12 years of age; this will provide more than the recommended dose (overdose) and could cause serious health problems.

Maximum Strength TYLENOL® Flu NightTime Gelcaps:

adults and children 12 years and over	• take 2 gelcaps at bedtime • may repeat every 6 hours • do not take more than 8 gelcaps in 24 hours
children under 12 years	• do not use this adult product in children under 12 years of age; this will provide more than the recommended dose (overdose) and could cause serious health problems.

Maximum Strength TYLENOL® Flu NightTime Liquid:

adults and children 12 years and over	• take 2 tablespoons (tbsp) in dose cup provided every 6 hours as needed • do not take more than 8 tablespoons in 24 hours
children under 12 years	• do not use this adult product in children under 12 years of age; this will provide more than the recommended dose (overdose) and could cause serious health problems.

Precautions: If a rare sensitivity reaction occurs, the drug should be discontinued.

Warnings: Alcohol Warning: If you consume 3 or more alcoholic drinks every day, ask your doctor whether you should take acetaminophen or other pain relievers/fever reducers. Acetaminophen may cause liver damage.

Sore throat warning: If sore throat is severe, persists for more than 2 days, is accompanied or followed by fever, headache, rash, nausea or vomiting, consult a doctor promptly.

Do not use
- if you are now taking a prescription monoamine-oxidase inhibitor (MAOI) (certain drugs for depression, psychiatric or emotional conditions, or Parkinson's disease), or for 2 weeks after stopping the MAOI drug. If you do not know if your prescription drug contains an MAOI, ask a doctor or pharmacist before taking this product.
- with any other product containing acetaminophen

If pregnant or breast-feeding, ask a health professional before use.

Keep out of reach of children. Overdose warning: Taking more than the recommended dose (overdose) could cause serious health problems. In case of overdose, get medical help or contact a Poison Control Center right away. Quick medical attention is critical for adults as well as for children even if you do not notice any signs or symptoms.

Maximum Strength TYLENOL® Flu Day Non-Drowsy Gelcaps

Ask a doctor before use if you have
- heart disease • diabetes • thyroid disease • cough that occurs with too much phlegm (mucus) • high blood pressure • trouble urinating due to an enlarged prostate gland • chronic cough that lasts as occurs with smoking, asthma, chronic bronchitis or emphysema

When using this product
- do not exceed recommended dosage

Stop use and ask a doctor if
- new symptoms occur
- redness or swelling is present
- pain gets worse or lasts for more than 7 days
- fever gets worse or lasts for more than 3 days
- you get nervous, dizzy or sleepless
- cough lasts more than 7 days, comes back or occurs with fever, rash or headache that lasts. These could be signs of a serious condition.

Maximum Strength TYLENOL® Flu NightTime Gelcaps

Ask a doctor before use if you have
- heart disease • glaucoma • diabetes
- thyroid disease • high blood pressure
- trouble urinating due to an enlarged prostate gland • a breathing problem such as emphysema or chronic bronchitis

Ask a doctor or pharmacist before use if you are taking sedatives or tranquilizers

When using this product
- do not exceed recommended dosage
- marked drowsiness may occur
- avoid alcoholic drinks
- alcohol, sedatives and tranquilizers may increase drowsiness
- be careful when driving a motor vehicle or operating machinery
- excitability may occur, especially in children

Stop use and ask a doctor if
- new symptoms occur
- redness or swelling is present
- pain gets worse or lasts for more than 7 days
- fever gets worse or lasts for more than 3 days
- you get nervous, dizzy or sleepless

Maximum Strength TYLENOL® Flu NightTime Liquid

Ask a doctor before use if you have
- heart disease • glaucoma • diabetes
- thyroid disease • cough that occurs with too much phlegm (mucus)
- high blood pressure • a breathing problem such as emphysema or chronic bronchitis • trouble urinating due to an enlarged prostate gland

Ask a doctor or pharmacist before use if you are taking sedatives or tranquilizers

When using this product
- do not exceed recommended dosage
- marked drowsiness may occur
- avoid alcoholic drinks
- alcohol, sedatives and tranquilizers may increase drowsiness
- be careful when driving a motor vehicle or operating machinery
- excitability may occur, especially in children

Stop use and ask a doctor if
- new symptoms occur
- redness or swelling is present
- pain gets worse or lasts for more than 7 days
- fever gets worse or lasts for more than 3 days
- you get nervous, dizzy or sleepless
- cough lasts for more than 7 days, comes back or occurs with fever, rash or headache that lasts. These could be signs of a serious condition.

Other Information:
Maximum Strength TYLENOL® Flu Day Non-Drowsy Gelcaps and Maximum Strength TYLENOL® Flu NightTime Gelcaps:
- do not use if carton is opened or if blister unit is broken
- Store at room temperature; avoid high humidity and excessive heat 40°C (104°F)

Maximum Strength TYLENOL® Flu NightTime Liquid
- do not use if carton is opened or if bottle wrap or foil inner seal imprinted "Safety Seal®" is broken or missing
- Store at room temperature

Continued on next page

Tylenol Flu—Cont.

Professional Information:
Overdosage Information
For overdosage information, please refer to pgs. 678–679.

Inactive Ingredients: *Maximum Strength TYLENOL® Flu Day Non-Drowsy Gelcaps:* benzyl alcohol, butylparaben, castor oil, cellulose, corn starch, edetate calcium disodium, FD&C Blue #1, FD&C Red #40, gelatin, hypromellose, iron oxide, magnesium stearate, methylparaben, propylparaben, sodium lauryl sulfate, sodium propionate, sodium starch glycolate, titanium dioxide. *Maximum Strength TYLENOL® Flu NightTime Gelcaps:* benzyl alcohol, butylparaben, castor oil, cellulose, corn starch, D&C Red #28, edetate calcium disodium, FD&C Blue #1, gelatin, hypromellose, iron oxide, magnesium stearate, methylparaben, propylparaben, sodium citrate, sodium lauryl sulfate, sodium propionate, sodium starch glycolate, titanium dioxide. *Maximum Strength TYLENOL® Flu NightTime Liquid:* citric acid, corn syrup, D&C Red #33, FD&C Red #40, flavors, polyethylene glycol, propylene glycol, purified water, saccharin sodium, sodium benzoate, sorbitol.

How Supplied: *Maximum Strength TYLENOL® Flu Day Non-Drowsy* Gelcaps: Burgundy- and white-colored gelcap, imprinted with "TYLENOL FLU" in gray ink—blister packs of 24. *Maximum Strength TYLENOL® Flu NightTime:* **Gelcaps:** Blue and white-colored gelcap, imprinted with "TYLENOL FLU NT" gray ink—blister packs of 12 and 24. **Liquid:** Red-colored—bottles of 8 fl. oz with child resistant safety cap and tamper evident packaging.
Shown in Product Identification Guide, page 513

Extra Strength TYLENOL® PM
Pain Reliever/Sleep Aid Caplets, Geltabs and Gelcaps

Description: Each *Extra Strength TYLENOL® PM Caplet, Geltab* or *Gelcap* contains acetaminophen 500 mg and diphenhydramine HCl 25 mg.

Actions: *Extra Strength TYLENOL® PM Caplets, Geltabs* and *Gelcaps* contain a clinically proven analgesic-antipyretic and an antihistamine. Maximum allowable non-prescription levels of acetaminophen and diphenhydramine provide temporary relief of occasional headaches and minor aches and pains accompanying sleeplessness. Acetaminophen is equal to aspirin in analgesic and antipyretic effectiveness and it is unlikely to produce any of the side effects associated with aspirin containing products. Acetaminophen produces analgesia by elevation of the pain threshold. Diphenhydramine HCl is an antihistamine with sedative properties.

Uses: temporary relief of occasional headaches and minor aches and pains with accompanying sleeplessness.

Directions:
• do not take more than directed adults and children 12 years and over: Take 2 caplets, geltabs or gelcaps at bedtime or as directed by a doctor. children under 12 years: Do not use this adult product in children under 12 years of age; this will provide more than the recommended dose (overdose) and could cause serious health problems.

Precautions: If a rare sensitivity reaction occurs, the drug should be discontinued.

Warnings:
Alcohol Warning: If you consume 3 or more alcoholic drinks every day, ask your doctor whether you should take acetaminophen or other pain relievers/fever reducers. Acetaminophen may cause liver damage.
Do not use
• with any other product containing acetaminophen
• in children under 12 years of age
Ask a doctor before use if you have
• a breathing problem such as emphysema or chronic bronchitis
• trouble urinating due to an enlarged prostate gland
• glaucoma
When using this product
• drowsiness will occur
• avoid alcoholic drinks
• do not drive a motor vehicle or operate machinery
Stop use and ask a doctor if
• sleeplessness persists continuously for more than 2 weeks. Insomnia may be a symptom of serious underlying medical illness.
• new symptoms occur
• redness or swelling is present
• pain gets worse or lasts for more than 10 days
• fever gets worse or lasts for more than 3 days
If pregnant or breast-feeding, ask a health professional before use.
Keep out of reach of children. In case of overdose get medical help or contact a Poison Control Center right away. Quick medical attention is critical for adults as well as for children even if you do not notice any signs or symptoms.

Other information
• **do not use if carton is opened or neck wrap or foil inner seal imprinted with "Safety Seal®" is broken**
• store at room temperature

Professional Information:
Overdosage Information:
For overdosage information, please refer to pgs. 678–679.

Inactive Ingredients: Caplets: carnauba wax, cellulose, cornstarch, FD&C Blue #1, FD&C Blue #2, hydroxypropyl methylcellulose, magnesium stearate, polyethylene glycol, polysorbate 80, sodium citrate, sodium starch glycolate, titanium dioxide.
Geltabs/Gelcaps: Benzyl Alcohol, Butylparaben, Castor Oil, Cellulose, Corn Starch, D&C Red #28, Edetate Calcium Disodium, FD&C Blue #1, Gelatin, Hydroxypropyl Methylcellulose, Magnesium Stearate, Methylparaben, Propylparaben, Sodium Citrate, Sodium Lauryl Sulfate, Sodium Propionate, Sodium Starch Glycolate, Titanium Dioxide.

How Supplied: **Caplets** (colored light blue imprinted "Tylenol PM") tamper-evident bottles of 24, 50, 100, and 150 and 225.
Gelcaps (colored blue and white imprinted "TYLENOL PM") tamper-evident bottles of 24 and 50.
Geltabs (colored blue and white imprinted "TYLENOL PM") tamper-evident bottles of 24, 50, and 100 and 150.
Shown in Product Identification Guide, page 513

Maximum Strength TYLENOL® Sinus Day Non-Drowsy
Geltabs, Gelcaps and Caplets

Maximum Strength TYLENOL® Sinus Night Time Caplets

Product information for all dosage forms of TYLENOL Sinus have been combined under this heading.

Description: Each *Maximum Strength TYLENOL® Sinus Day Non-Drowsy Geltab, Gelcap,* or *Caplet* contains acetaminophen 500 mg and pseudoephedrine HCl 30 mg. Each *Maximum Strength TYLENOL® Sinus Night Time Caplet* contains acetaminophen 500 mg, doxylamine succinate 6.25 mg and pseudoephedrine HCl 30 mg.

Actions: *Maximum Strength TYLENOL® Sinus Day Non-Drowsy* contains a clinically proven analgesic-antipyretic and a decongestant. Maximum allowable non-prescription levels of acetaminophen and pseudoephedrine provide temporary relief of sinus pain and headache and congestion. Acetaminophen is equal to aspirin in analgesic and antipyretic effectiveness and it is unlikely to produce many of the side effects associated with aspirin and aspirin-containing products. Acetaminophen produces analgesia by elevation of the pain threshold and antipyresis through action on the hypothalamic heat regulating center. Pseudoephedrine hydrochloride is a sympathomimetic amine which promotes sinus cavity drainage by reducing nasopharyngeal mucosal congestion. *Maximum Strength TYLENOL® Sinus Night Time Caplets* contain, in addition to the above ingredients, an antihistamine which provides temporary relief of runny nose and itching of the nose or throat.

Uses: *Maximum Strength TYLENOL® Sinus Day Non-Drowsy:* temporarily relieves:
• sinus pain • headache • nasal and sinus congestion

Maximum Strength TYLENOL® Sinus Night Time: temporarily relieves:
• nasal congestion • sinus pressure • sinus pain • headache • runny nose • sneezing • itchy, watery eyes • itching of the nose or throat

Precautions: If a rare sensitivity reaction occurs, the drug should be discontinued.

Directions: *Maximum Strength TYLENOL® Sinus Day Non-Drowsy:*
• **do not take more than directed (see overdose warning)**

adults and children 12 years and over	• take 2 every 4–6 hours as needed • do not take more than 8 in 24 hours
children under 12 years	• do not use this adult product in children under 12 years of age; this will provide more than the recommended dose (overdose) and could cause serious health problems.

Maximum Strength TYLENOL® Sinus Night Time:
• **do not take more than directed (see overdose warning)**

adults and children 12 years and over	• take 2 caplets every 4–6 hours as needed • do not take more than 8 caplets in 24 hours
children under 12 years	• do not use this adult product in children under 12 years of age; this will provide more than the recommended dose (overdose) and could cause serious health problems.

Warnings:
Alcohol warning: If you consume 3 or more alcoholic drinks every day, ask your doctor whether you should take acetaminophen or other pain relievers/fever reducers. Acetaminophen may cause liver damage.
Do not use
• if you are now taking a prescription monamine oxidase inhibitor (MAOI) (certain drugs for depression, psychiatric or emotional conditions or Parkinson's disease), or for weeks after stopping the MAOI drug. If you do not know if your prescription drug contains an MAOI, ask a doctor or pharmacist before taking this product
• with any other product containing acetaminophen

Stop use and ask a doctor if
• new symptoms occur
• redness or swelling is present
• pains gets worse or last for more than 7 days
• fever gets worse or lasts for more than 3 days
• you get nervous, dizzy or sleepless
If pregnant or breast feeding, ask a health professional before use.
Keep out of reach of children. Overdose warning: Taking more than the recommended dose (overdose) could cause serious health problems. In case of overdose get medical help or contact a Poison Control Center right away. Quick medical attention is critical for adults as well as for children even if you do not notice any signs or symptoms.
Maximum Strength TYLENOL® Sinus Day Non-Drowsy Geltabs, Gelcaps and Caplets
Ask a doctor if you have
• heart disease • high blood pressure
• thyroid disease • diabetes
• trouble urinating due to an enlarged prostate gland
When using this product
• **do not exceed recommend dosage**
Maximum Strength TYLENOL® Sinus Night Time Caplets
Ask a doctor before use if you have
• heart disease • glaucoma • diabetes
• thyroid disease • high blood pressure
• trouble urinating due to an enlarged prostate gland • a breathing problem such as emphysema or chronic bronchitis
Ask a doctor or pharmacist before use if you are taking sedatives or tranquilizers
When using this product
• **do not exceed recommended dosage**
• marked drowsiness may occur
• avoid alcoholic drinks
• alcohol, sedatives and tranquilizers may increase drowsiness
• be careful when driving a motor vehicle or operating machinery
• excitability may occur, especially in children
Other Information
• **do not use if carton is opened or if blister unit is broken**
Maximum Strength TYLENOL® Sinus Geltabs and Gelcaps
• store at room temperature; avoid high humidity and excessive heat 40°C (104°F)
Maximum Strength TYLENOL® Sinus Caplets and Maximum Strength TYLENOL® Sinus Night Time Caplets
• store at room temperature

Professional Information:
Overdosage Information
For overdosage information, please refer to pgs. 678–679.

Inactive Ingredients: *Maximum Strength TYLENOL® Sinus Day Non-Drowsy Formula:* **Caplets:** carnauba wax, cellulose, corn starch, D&C Yellow #10, FD&C Blue #1, FD&C Red #40, hypromellose, iron oxide, magnesium stearate, polyethylene glycol, polysorbate 80, sodium starch glycolate, titanium dioxide. **Gelcaps and Geltabs:** benzyl alcohol, butylparaben, castor oil, cellulose, corn

starch, D&C Yellow #10, edetate calcium disodium, FD&C Blue #1, gelatin, hydroxypropyl methylcellulose, iron oxide, magnesium stearate, methylparaben, propylparaben, sodium lauryl sulfate, sodium propionate, sodium starch glycolate, titanium dioxide.
Maximum Strength TYLENOL® Sinus Night Time Caplets: black iron oxide, carnauba wax, cellulose, corn starch, FD&C Blue #1, FD&C Blue #2, hypromellose, propylene glycol, silicon dioxide, sodium starch glycolate, stearic acid, titanium dioxide, triacetin, yellow iron oxide.

How Supplied: *Maximum Strength TYLENOL® Sinus Day Non-Drowsy Formula:*
Caplets: Light green-colored, imprinted with "TYLENOL Sinus" in green ink—blister packs of 24 and 48.
Gelcaps: Green- and white-colored, imprinted with "TYLENOL Sinus" in dark green ink—blister packs of 24 and 48.
Geltabs: Green-colored on one side and white-colored on opposite side, imprinted with "TYLENOL Sinus" in gray ink—blister packs of 24 and 48.
Maximum Strength TYLENOL® Sinus Night Time Caplets: Green-colored, imprinted with "Tylenol Sinus NT"—blister packs of 24.
These products are also available in a convenience pack containing Maximum Strength TYLENOL® Sinus Day Non-Drowsy (pack of 12) and Maximum Strength TYLENOL® Sinus Night Time (pack of 12).

Shown in Product Identification Guide, page 513

Maximum Strength TYLENOL® Sore Throat Adult Liquid

Description: *Maximum Strength TYLENOL® Sore Throat Liquid* is available in Honey Lemon Flavor or Cherry Flavor and contains acetaminophen 1000 mg in each 30 mL (2 Tablespoonsful).

Actions: Acetaminophen is a clinically proven analgesic/antipyretic. Acetaminophen produces analgesia by elevation of the pain threshold and antipyresis through action on the hypothalamic heat regulating center. Acetaminophen is equal to aspirin in analgesic and antipyretic effectiveness and it is unlikely to produce many of the side effects associated with aspirin and aspirin-containing products.

Uses: temporarily relieves minor aches and pains due to:
• sore throat • headache • muscular aches • the common cold
• temporarily reduces fever

Directions:
• do not take more than directed (see overdose Warning)

Continued on next page

Tylenol Sore Throat Liq.—Cont.

adults and children 12 years and over	• take 2 tablespoons (tbsp) in dose cup provided every 4 to 6 hours as needed • do not take more than 8 tablespoons in 24 hours
children under 12 years	do not use this adult product in children under 12 years of age; this will provide more than the recommended dose (overdose) of TYLENOL® and could cause serious health problems.

Precautions: If a rare sensitivity reaction occurs, the drug should be discontinued.

Warnings:
Alcohol warning: If you consume 3 or more alcoholic drinks every day, ask your doctor whether you should take acetaminophen or other pain relievers/fever reducers. Acetaminophen may cause liver damage.
Sore throat warning: If sore throat is severe, persists for more than 2 days, is accompanied or followed by fever, headache, rash, nausea or vomiting, consult a doctor promptly.
Do not use
• with any other product containing acetaminophen
Stop use and ask a doctor if
• new symptoms occur
• redness or swelling is present
• pain gets worse or lasts for more than 10 days
• fever gets worse or lasts for more than 3 days
If pregnant or breast-feeding, ask a health professional before use.
Keep out of the reach of children.
Overdose Warning: Taking more than the recommended dose (overdose) could cause serious health problems. In case of overdose, get medical help or contact a Poison Control Center right away. Quick medical attention is critical for adults as well as for children even if you do not notice any signs or symptoms.
Other Information
• **Do not use if carton is opened or if bottle wrap or foil inner seal imprinted "Safety Seal®" is broken or missing**
• store at room temperature
Professional Information:
Overdosage Information
For overdosage information, please refer to pgs. 678–679.
Inactive Ingredients: *Maximum Strength TYLENOL® Sore Throat Honey-Lemon-Flavored Adult Liquid:* caramel color, citric acid, flavor, high fructose corn syrup, polyethylene glycol, propylene glycol, purified water, saccharin sodium, sodium benzoate, sorbitol

Maximum Strength TYLENOL® Sore Throat Cherry-Flavored Adult Liquid: citric acid, D&C Red # 33, FD&C Red # 40, flavor, high fructose corn syrup, polyethylene glycol, propylene glycol, purified water, saccharin sodium, sodium benzoate, sorbitol

How Supplied: Honey lemon-flavored or cherry-flavored liquid in child-resistant tamper-evident bottles of 8 fl. oz.
Shown in Product Identification Guide, page 513

Women's TYLENOL® Menstrual Relief Pain Reliever/ Diuretic Caplets

Descripton: Each *Women's Tylenol® Menstrual Relief Caplet* contains acetaminophen 500 mg and pamabrom 25 mg.

Actions: *Women's TYLENOL® Menstrual Relief Caplets* contain a clinically proven analgesic-antipyretic and a diuretic. Maximum allowable non-prescription levels of acetaminophen and pamabrom provide temporary relief of minor aches and pains due to cramps, headache, and backache and water retention, weight gain, bloating, swelling and full feeling associated with the premenstrual and menstrual periods. Acetaminophen is equal to aspirin in analgesic and antipyretic effectiveness and it is unlikely to produce many of the side effects associated with aspirin containing products. Acetaminophen produces analgesia by elevation of the pain threshold. Pamabrom is a diuretic which relieves water retention.

Uses:
• temporarily relieves minor aches and pains due to:
 • cramps • headache • backache
• temporarily relieves water-weight gain, bloating, swelling and full feeling associated with the premenstrual and menstrual periods

Directions:
• **do not take more than directed**
adults and children 12 years and over: take 2 caplets every 4 to 6 hours; do not take more than 8 caplets in 24 hours, or as directed by a doctor
children under 12 years: do not use this adult product in children under 12 years of age; this will provide more than the recommended dose (overdose) and could cause serious health problems

Precautions: If a rare sensitivity reaction occurs, the drug should be discontinued.

Warnings:
Alcohol warning: If you consume 3 or more alcoholic drinks every day, ask your doctor whether you should take acetaminophen or other pain relievers/fever reducers. Acetaminophen may cause liver damage.
Do not use
• with any other product containing acetaminophen

Stop use and ask a doctor if
• new symptoms occur
• redness or swelling is present
• pain gets worse or lasts for more than 10 days
If pregnant or breast-feeding, ask a health professional before use.
Keep out of reach of children. In case of overdose, get medical help or contact a Poison Control Center right away. Prompt medical attention is critical for adults as well as for children even if you do not notice any signs or symptoms.
Other Information
• **do not use if carton is opened, or if neck wrap or foil inner seal imprinted "Safety Seal®" is broken or missing**
• store at room temperature, avoid excessive heat 104°F (40°C)

Professional Information:
Overdosage Information
For overdosage information, please refer to pgs. 678–679.

Inactive Ingredients: cellulose, corn starch, hydroxypropyl methylcellulose, magnesium stearate, polydextrose, polyethylene glycol, sodium starch glycolate, titanium dioxide, triacetin.

How Supplied: White capsule shaped caplets with TYME printed on one side in tamper-evident bottles of 24 and 40.
Shown in Product Identification Guide, page 513

Concentrated TYLENOL® acetaminophen Infants' Drops

Children's TYLENOL® acetaminophen Suspension Liquid and Soft Chews Chewable Tablets

Junior Strength TYLENOL® acetaminophen Soft Chews Chewable Tablets

Product information for all dosages of Children's TYLENOL have been combined under this heading

Description: *Concentrated TYLENOL® Infants' Drops* are stable, alcohol-free, grape-flavored and purple in color or cherry-flavored and red in color. Each 1.6 mL contains 160 mg acetaminophen. *Concentrated TYLENOL® Infants' Drops* features the SAFE-TY-LOCK™ Bottle. The SAFE-TY-LOCK™ Bottle has a unique safety barrier inside the bottle which helps make administration easier. The integrated dropper promotes proper administration. The innovative design eliminates excess product on dropper. The star-shaped barrier inside the bottle minimizes spills and discourages pouring into a spoon. *Children's TYLENOL® Suspension Liquid* is stable, alcohol-free, cherry-flavored and red in color, or bubble gum-flavored and pink in color, or grape-flavored and purple in color. Each 5 mL (one teaspoonful) contains 160 mg acetaminophen. Each *Children's TYLENOL® Soft Chews Chewable Tablet* contains 80 mg acetaminophen in a grape, bubble gum, or fruit flavor. *Each Junior Strength TYLENOL® Soft Chews Chew-*

able Tablet contains 160 mg acetaminophen in a grape or fruit-flavored chewable tablet.

Actions: Acetaminophen is a clinically proven analgesic/antipyretic. Acetaminophen produces analgesia by elevation of the pain threshold and antipyresis through action on the hypothalamic heat-regulating center. Acetaminophen is equal to aspirin in analgesic and antipyretic effectiveness and it is unlikely to produce many of the side effects associated with aspirin and aspirin-containing products.

Uses: *Concentrated TYLENOL® Infants' Drops:* temporarily:
• reduces fever
• relieves minor aches and pains due to:
  • the common cold • flu • headaches • sore throat • immunizations • toothaches
Children's TYLENOL® Suspension Liquid and Children's TYLENOL® Soft Chews Chewable Tablets: temporarily relieves minor aches and pains due to: • the common cold • flu • headaches • sore throat • immunizations • toothaches
• temporarily reduces fever
Junior Strength TYLENOL® Soft Chews Chewable Tablets: temporarily relieves minor aches and pains due to: • the common cold • flu • headache • muscle aches • sprains • overexertion
• temporarily reduces fever

Directions: See Table 1: Children's Tylenol Dosing Chart on pgs. 691–693.

Precautions: If a rare sensitivity reaction occurs, the drug should be discontinued.

Warnings: Sore throat warning: if sore throat is severe, persists for more than 2 days, is accompanied or followed by fever, headache, rash, nausea, or vomiting, consult a doctor promptly (excluding *Junior Strength TYLENOL® Soft Chews Chewable Tablets*).

Do not use
• with any other product containing acetaminophen
When using this product
  • **do not exceed recommended dose. (see overdose warning)**
Stop use and ask a doctor if
  • new symptoms occur
  • redness or swelling is present
  • pain gets worse or lasts for more than 5 days
  • fever gets worse or lasts for more than 3 days
Keep out of the reach of children. Overdose warning: Taking more than the recommended dose (overdose) could cause serious health problems. In case of overdose, get medical help or contact a Poison Control Center right away. Quick medical attention is critical even if you do not notice any signs or symptoms.
Other Information:
Concentrated TYLENOL® Infants' Drops:
• **Do not use if plastic carton wrap or bottle wrap imprinted "Safety Seal®" is broken or missing.**

• Store at room temperature
Children's TYLENOL® Suspension Liquid:
•**Do not use if bottle wrap, or foil inner seal imprinted "Safety Seal®" is broken or missing**
• Store at room temperature
Children's TYLENOL® Soft Chews Chewable Tablets:
• phenylketonurics: fruit and grape contain phenylalanine 3 mg per tablet, bubble gum contains phenylalanine 6 mg per tablet
• **Do not use if carton is opened or if neck wrap or foil inner seal imprinted "Safety Seal®" is broken or missing.** Store at room temperature (Grape: Keep product away from direct light) *Junior Strength TYLENOL® Soft Chews Chewable Tablets:*
• Phenylketonurics: contains phenylalanine 6 mg per tablet
• **Do not use if carton is opened or if blister unit is broken**
• Store at room temperature (Grape: Keep product away from direct light)

Professional Information:
Overdosage Information for all Infants', Children's & Junior Strength Tylenol® Products
ACETAMINOPHEN: Acetaminophen in massive overdosage may cause hepatic toxicity in some patients. In adults and adolescents ($\geq$ 12 years of age), hepatic toxicity may occur following ingestion of greater than 7.5 to 10 grams over a period of 8 hours or less. Fatalities are infrequent (less than 3–4% of untreated cases) and have rarely been reported with overdoses of less than 15 grams. In children (<12 years of age), an acute overdosage of less than 150 mg/kghas not been associated with hepatic toxicity. Early symptoms following a potentially hepatotoxic overdose may include: nausea, vomiting, diaphoresis and general malaise. Clinical and laboratory evidence of hepatic toxicity may not be apparent until 48 to 72 hours postingestion. In adults and adolescents, any individual presenting with an unknown amount of acetaminophen ingested or with a questionable or unreliable history about the time of ingestion should have a plasma acetaminophen level drawn and be treated with *N*-acetylcysteine. For full prescribing information, refer to the *N*-acetylcysteine package insert. Do not await results of assays for plasma acetaminophen levels before initiating treatment with *N*-acetylcysteine. The following additional procedures are recommended: Promptly initiate gastric decontamination of the stomach. A plasma acetaminophen assay should be obtained as early as possible, but no sooner than four hours following ingestion. If an acetaminophen *extended release* product is involved, it may be appropriate to obtain an additional plasma acetaminophen level 4–6 hours following the initial acetaminophen level. If either acetaminophen level plots above the treatment line on the acetaminophen

overdose nomogram, *N*-acetylcysteine treatment should be continued for a full course of therapy. Liver function studies should be obtained initially and repeated at 24-hour intervals. Serious toxicity or fatalities have been extremely infrequent following an acute acetaminophen overdose in young children, possibly because of differences in the way they metabolize acetaminophen. In children, the maximum potential amount ingested can be more easily estimated. If more than 150 mg/kg or an unknown amount was ingested, obtain a plasma acetaminophen level as soon as possible, but no sooner than 4 hours following ingestion. If an acetaminophen *extended release* product is involved, it may be appropriate to obtain an additional plasma acetaminophen level 4–6 hours following the initial acetaminophen level. If either acetaminophen level plots above the treatment line on the acetaminophen overdose nomogram, *N*-acetylcysteine treatment should be initiated and continued for a full course of therapy. If an assay cannot be obtained and the estimated acetaminophen ingestion exceeds 150 mg/kg, dosing with *N*-acetylcysteine should be initiated and continued for a full course of therapy. For additional emergency information, call your regional poison center or call the Rocky Mountain Poison Center toll-free, (1-800-525-6115). **Our pediatric Tylenol® combination products contain active ingredients in addition to acetaminophen. The following is basic overdose information regarding those ingredients.**
CHLORPHENIRAMINE: Chlorpheniramine toxicity should be treated as you would an antihihistamine/anticholinergic overdose and is likely to be present within a few hours after acute ingestion.
DEXTROMETHORPHAN: Acute dextromethorphan overdose usually does not result in serious signs and symptoms unless massive amounts have been ingested. Signs and symptoms of a substantial overdose may include nausea and vomiting, visual disturbances, CNS disturbances and urinary retention.
DIPHENHYDRAMINE: Diphenhydramine toxicity should be treated as you would an antihihistamine/anticholinergic overdose and is likely to be present within a few hours after acute ingestion.
PSEUDOEPHEDRINE: Symptoms from pseudoephedrine overdose consist most often of mild anxiety, tachycardia and/or mild hypertension. Symptoms usually appear within 4 to 8 hours of ingestion and are transient, usually requiring no treatment.

For additional emergency information, please contact your local poison control center.

Inactive Ingredients: *Concentrated TYLENOL® Infants' Drops:* Cherry-Flavored: butylparaben, cellulose, citric acid, corn syrup, FD&C Red #40, flavors, glycerin, propylene glycol, purified water,

Continued on next page

Tylenol Infants—Cont.

sodium benzoate, sorbitol, xanthan gum. **Grape-Flavored:** butylparaben, cellulose, citric acid, corn syrup, D&C Red #33, FD&C Blue #1, flavors, glycerin, propylene glycol, purified water, sodium benzoate, sorbitol, xanthan gum. *Children's TYLENOL® Suspension Liquid:* butylparaben, cellulose, citric acid, corn syrup, flavors, glycerin, propylene glycol, purified water, sodium benzoate, sorbitol, xanthan gum. In addition to the above ingredients cherry-flavored suspension contains FD&C Red #40, bubble gum-flavored suspension contains D&C Red #33 and FD&C Red #40, and grape-flavored suspension contains D&C Red #33 and FD&C Blue #1.

Children's TYLENOL® Soft Chews Chewable Tablets: **Fruit-Flavored:** aspartame, cellulose, cellulose acetate citric acid, D&C Red #7, flavors, magnesium stearate, mannitol, povidone. **Grape-Flavored:** aspartame, cellulose, cellulose acetate, citric acid, D&C Red #7, D&C Red #30, FD&C Blue #1, flavors, magnesium stearate, mannitol, povidone. **Bubble Gum-Flavored:** aspartame, cellulose, cellulose acetate, D&C Red #7, flavors, magnesium stearate, mannitol, povidone.

Junior Strength TYLENOL® Soft Chews Chewable Tablets: **Fruit-Flavored:** aspartame, cellulose, citric acid, D&C Red #7, flavors, magnesium stearate, mannitol, povidone. **Grape-Flavored:** aspartame, cellulose, citric acid, D&C Red #7, D&C Red #30, FD&C Blue #1, flavors, magnesium stearate, mannitol, povidone.

How Supplied: *Concentrated TYLENOL® Infants' Drops:* (purple-colored grape): bottles of ½ oz (15 mL) and 1 oz (30 mL); (red-colored cherry): bottles of ½ oz and 1 oz, each with calibrated plastic dropper. *Children's TYLENOL® Suspension Liquid:* (red-colored cherry): bottles of 2 and 4 fl oz. (pink-colored bubble gum and purple-colored grape): bottles of 4 fl. oz. *Children's TYLENOL® Soft Chews Chewable Tablets:* (pink-colored fruit, purple-colored grape, pink-colored bubble gum, scored, imprinted "TY80"). Bottles of 30 and also blister packaged 60's and 96's (fruit). *Junior Strength TYLENOL® Soft Chews Chewable Tablets:* (purple-colored grape or pink-colored fruit, imprinted "TY 160") Package of 24. All packages listed above are safety sealed and use child-resistant safety caps or blisters.

Shown in Product Identification Guide, page 512

CHILDREN'S TYLENOL® Plus Allergy

Description: *Children's TYLENOL® Plus Allergy* is Bubble Gum flavored and contains no alcohol or aspirin. Each teaspoon (5 mL) contains acetaminophen 160 mg, diphenhydramine HCl 12.5 mg and pseudoephedrine HCl 15 mg.

Actions: *Children's TYLENOL® Plus Allergy* combines the analgesic-antipyretic acetaminophen with the antihistamine diphenhydramine hydrochloride and the decongestant pseudoephedrine hydrochloride to provide fast, effective, temporary relief of all your child's symptoms associated with hay fever and other respiratory allergies including sneezing, sore throat, itchy throat, itchy/watery eyes, runny nose, stuffy nose and nasal congestion. Acetaminophen is equal to aspirin in analgesic and antipyretic effectiveness and it is unlikely to produce the side effects often associated with aspirin or aspirin-containing products.

Uses: temporarily relieves these hay fever and upper respiratory allergy symptoms:
• nasal congestion • sore throat
• runny nose • sneezing
• stuffy nose • minor aches and pains
• itchy, watery eyes
• temporarily reduces fever

Directions: See Table 1: Children's Tylenol Dosing Chart on pgs. 691–693.

Precautions: If a rare sensitivity reaction occurs, the drug should be discontinued.

Warnings: Sore throat warning: If sore throat is severe, persists for more than 2 days, is accompanied or followed by fever, headache, rash, nausea or vomiting, consult a doctor promptly.

Do not use
• in a child who is taking a prescription monoamine oxidase inhibitor (MAOI) (certain drugs for depression, psychiatric, or emotional conditions, or Parkinson's disease) or for 2 weeks after stopping the MAOI drug. If you do not know if your child's prescription drug contains an MAOI, ask a doctor or pharmacist before giving this product.
• with any other product containing acetaminophen.

Ask a doctor before use if the child has
• heart disease • high blood pressure
• thyroid disease • diabetes
• glaucoma • a breathing problem such as chronic bronchitis

When using this product
• **do not exceed recommended dosage (see overdose warning)**
• marked drowsiness may occur
• excitability may occur, especially in children

Stop use and ask a doctor if
• new symptoms occur
• redness or swelling is present
• pain gets worse or lasts for more than 5 days
• fever gets worse or lasts for more than 3 days
• nervousness, dizziness or sleeplessness occurs

Keep out of reach of children.

Overdose Warning: Taking more than the recommended dose (overdose) could cause serious health problems. In case of overdose, get medical help or contact a Poison Control Center right away. Quick medical attention is critical even if you do not notice any signs or symptoms

Other Information:
• **do not use if plastic carton wrap, bottle wrap, or foil inner seal imprinted "Safety Seal®" is broken or missing.**
• store at room temperature

Professional Information:
Overdosage Information
For overdosage information, please refer to pgs. 687–688.

Inactive Ingredients: benzoic acid, citric acid, corn syrup, D&C Red #33, FD&C Red #40, flavors, polyethylene glycol, propylene glycol, purified water, sodium benzoate, sorbitol.

How Supplied: Pink-colored–child-resistant bottles of 4 fl. oz.
Shown in Product Identification Guide, page 511

Concentrated TYLENOL® Infants' Drops Plus Cold Nasal Decongestant, Fever Reducer & Pain Reliever

Concentrated TYLENOL® Infants' Drops Plus Cold & Cough Nasal Decongestant, Fever Reducer & Pain Reliever

Children's TYLENOL® Plus Cold Suspension Liquid and Chewable Tablets

Children's TYLENOL® Plus Cold & Cough Suspension Liquid and Chewable Tablets

Description: *Concentrated TYLENOL® Infants' Drops Plus Cold* are alcohol-free, aspirin-free, Bubble-Gum-flavored and red in color. Each 1.6 mL contains acetaminophen 160 mg and pseudoephedrine HCl 15 mg. *Concentrated TYLENOL® Infants' Drops Plus Cold & Cough* are alcohol-free, aspirin-free, Cherry-flavored and red in color. Each 1.6 mL contains acetaminophen 160 mg, dextromethorphan HBr 5 mg, and pseudoephedrine HCl 15 mg. *Children's TYLENOL® Plus Cold Suspension Liquid* is Grape-flavored and contains no alcohol or aspirin. Each teaspoon (5 mL) contains acetaminophen 160 mg, chlorpheniramine maleate 1 mg and pseudoephedrine HCl 15 mg. *Children's TYLENOL® Plus Cold Chewable Tablets* are Grape-flavored and each tablet contains acetaminophen 80 mg, chlorpheniramine maleate 0.5 mg and pseudoephedrine HCl 7.5 mg. *Children's TYLENOL® Plus Cold & Cough Suspension Liquid* is Cherry-flavored and contains no alcohol or aspirin. Each teaspoonful (5 mL) contains acetaminophen 160 mg, chlorpheniramine maleate 1 mg, dextromethorphan HBr 5 mg and pseudoephedrine HCl 15 mg. *Children's TYLENOL® Plus Cold & Cough Chewable Tablets* are Cherry-flavored and each tablet contains acetaminophen 80 mg, chlorpheniramine male-

ate 0.5 mg, dextromethorphan HBr 2.5 mg, and pseudoephedrine HCl 7.5 mg.

Actions: Acetaminophen is a clinically proven analgesic/antipyretic. Acetaminophen produces analgesia by elevation of the pain threshold and antipyresis through action on the hypothalamic heat-regulating center. Acetaminophen is equal to aspirin in analgesic and antipyretic effectiveness and it is unlikely to produce many of the side effects associated with aspirin and aspirin-containing products.

Pseudoephedrine hydrochloride is a sympathomimetic amine which provides temporary relief of nasal congestion. Chlorpheniramine maleate is an antihistamine that provides temporary relief of runny nose, sneezing and watery and itchy eyes.

Dextromethorphan hydrobromide is a cough suppressant which helps relieve coughs.

Uses: *Concentrated TYLENOL® Infants' Drops Plus Cold,* temporarily relieves these cold symptoms:
• minor aches and pains
• nasal congestion • headaches
• temporarily reduces fever
Concentrated TYLENOL® Infants' Drops Plus Cold & Cough, temporarily relieves these cold symptoms:
• coughs • nasal congestion
• minor aches and pains
• sore throat • headaches
• temporarily reduces fever
Children's TYLENOL® Plus Cold Suspension Liquid and *Chewable Tablets:* temporarily relieves these cold symptoms:
• nasal congestion • sore throat • runny nose • sneezing • headache • minor aches and pains
• temporarily reduces fever
Children's TYLENOL® Plus Cold & Cough Suspension Liquid and *Chewable Tablets:* temporarily relieves these cold symptoms:
• nasal congestion • sore throat • runny nose • sneezing • headache • minor aches and pains • coughs
temporarily reduces fever

Directions: See Table 1: Children's Tylenol Dosing Chart on pgs. 691–693.

Precautions: If a rare sensitivity reaction occurs, the drug should be discontinued.

Warnings: Sore throat warning: If sore throat is severe, persists for more than 2 days, is accompanied by or followed by fever, headache, rash, nausea or vomiting, consult a doctor promptly (does not apply to *Concentrated TYLENOL® Infants' Drops Plus Cold*)

Do not use
• in a child who is taking a prescription monoamine oxidase inhibitor (MAOI) (certain drugs for depression, psychiatric or emotional conditions, or Parkinson's disease), or for 2 weeks after stopping the MAOI drug. If you do not know if your child's prescription drug contains an MAOI, ask a doctor or pharmacist before giving this product.
• with any products containing acetaminophen

Keep out of reach of children.

Overdose warning: Taking more than the recommended dose (overdose) could cause serious health problems. In case of overdose, get medical help or contact a Poison Control Center right away. Quick medical attention is critical even if you do not notice any signs or symptoms.

Stop use and ask a doctor if
• new symptoms occur
• redness or swelling is present
• pain gets worse or lasts for more than 5 days
• fever gets worse or lasts for more than 3 days
• nervousness, dizziness or sleeplessness occurs
• cough lasts for more than 7 days, comes back or occurs with fever, rash or headache that lasts. These could be signs of a serious condition. (*Concentrated TYLENOL® Infants' Drops Plus Cold & Cough* and *Children's TYLENOL® Plus Cold & Cough Products* only)

Concentrated TYLENOL® Infants' Drops Plus Cold,

Ask a doctor before use if the child has
• heart disease • high blood pressure
• thyroid disease • diabetes

When using this product
• **do not exceed recommended dosage (see overdose warning)**

Concentrated TYLENOL® Infants' Drops Plus Cold & Cough

Ask a doctor before use if the child has
• heart disease • high blood pressure
• cough that occurs with too much phlegm (mucus) • thyroid disease • diabetes • chronic cough that lasts as occurs with asthma

When using this product
• **do not exceed recommended dosage (see Overdose warning)**

Children's TYLENOL® Plus Cold Suspension Liquid and Chewable Tablets

Ask a doctor before use if the child has
• heart disease • thyroid disease • glaucoma • high blood pressure • diabetes
• a breathing problem such as chronic bronchitis

When using this product
• **do not exceed recommended dosage (see overdose warning)**
• drowsiness may occur
• excitability may occur, especially in children

Children's TYLENOL® Plus Cold & Cough Suspension Liquid and Chewable Tablets

Ask a doctor before use if the child has
• heart disease • thyroid disease • glaucoma • high blood pressure • diabetes
• cough that occurs with too much phlegm (mucus) • chronic cough that lasts as occurs with asthma

When using this product
• **do not exceed recommended dosage (see overdose warning)**
• drowsiness may occur
• excitability may occur, especially in children

Other Information

Concentrated TYLENOL® Infants' Drops Plus Cold, Concentrated TYLENOL® Infants' Drops Plus Cold & Cough
• **do not use if plastic carton wrap or bottle wrap imprinted "Safety Seal®" is broken or missing**
• store at room temperature

Children's TYLENOL® Plus Cold & Cough Suspension Liquid, Children's TYLENOL® Plus Cold Suspension Liquid
• **do not use if bottle wrap or foil inner seal imprinted "Safety Seal®" is broken or missing**
• store at room temperature

Children's TYLENOL® Plus Cold Chewable Tablets
• phenylketonurics: contains phenylalanine 6 mg per tablet
• **do not use if carton is opened or if blister unit is broken**
• store at room temperature

Children's TYLENOL® Plus Cold & Cough Chewable Tablets
• phenylketonurics: contains phenylalanine 4 mg per tablet
• **do not use if carton is opened or if blister unit is broken**
• store at room temperature

Professional Information: Overdosage Information

For overdosage information, please refer to pgs. 687–688.

Inactive Ingredients: *Concentrated TYLENOL® Infants' Drops Plus Cold:* citric acid, corn syrup, FD&C Red #40, flavors, polyethylene glycol, propylene glycol, sodium benzoate, sodium saccharin.

Concentrated TYLENOL® Infants' Drops Plus Cold & Cough: acesulfame potassium, citric acid, corn syrup, FD&C Red #40, flavors, polyethylene glycol, propylene glycol, sodium benzoate.

Children's TYLENOL® Plus Cold: **Suspension Liquid:** acesulfame potassium, cellulose, citric acid, corn syrup, D&C Red #33, FD&C Blue #1, FD&C Red #40, flavors, glycerin, purified water, sodium benzoate, sorbitol, xanthan gum. **Chewable Tablets:** aspartame, basic polymethacrylate, cellulose, cellulose acetate, citric acid, D&C Red #7, FD&C Blue #1, flavors, hypromellose, magnesium stearate, mannitol.

Children's TYLENOL® Plus Cold & Cough: **Suspension Liquid:** acesulfame potassium, cellulose, citric acid, corn syrup, D&C Red #33, FD&C Red #40, flavors, glycerin, sodium benzoate, sorbitol, xanthan gum. **Chewable Tablets:** aspartame, basic polymethacrylate, cellulose, cellulose acetate, D&C Red #7, flavors, hypromellose, magnesium stearate, mannitol.

How Supplied: *Concentrated TYLENOL® Infants' Drops Plus Cold, Concentrated TYLENOL® Infants'*

Continued on next page

Tylenol Infants' Cold—Cont.

Drops Plus Cold & Cough: Red-colored drops in bottles of $1/2$ fl. oz.

Children's TYLENOL® Plus Cold: Suspension Liquid: Purple-colored-bottles of 4 fl. oz. Store at room temperature.

Chewable Tablets: Purple-colored, imprinted "TYLENOL COLD" on one side and "TC" on opposite side- blisters of 24.

Children's TYLENOL® Plus Cold & Cough: Suspension Liquid: Red-colored suspension-bottles of 4 fl. oz.

Chewable Tablets: Red-colored, imprinted TYLENOL C/C" on one side and "TC/C" on the opposite side- blisters of 24.

Shown in Product Identification Guide, page 511

Children's TYLENOL® Plus Flu

Description: *Children's TYLENOL® Plus Flu* Suspension Liquid is Bubble Gum flavored and contains no alcohol or aspirin. Each teaspoon (5 mL) contains acetaminophen 160 mg, chlorpheniramine maleate 1 mg, dextromethorphan HBr 7.5 mg and pseudoephedrine HCl 15 mg.

Actions: *Children's TYLENOL® Plus Flu* Suspension Liquid combines the analgesic-antipyretic acetaminophen with the decongestant pseudoephedrine hydrochloride, the cough suppressant dextromethorphan hydrobromide and the antihistamine chlorpheniramine maleate to provide fast, effective, temporary relief of all your child's symptoms associated with flu including fever, body aches, headache, stuffy nose, runny nose, sore throat and coughs. Acetaminophen is equal to aspirin in analgesic and antipyretic effectiveness and it is unlikely to produce the side effects often associated with aspirin or aspirin-containing products.

Uses: temporarily relieves these cold and flu symptoms:
• nasal congestion • sore throat
• runny nose • sneezing
• headache • minor aches and pains
• coughs
• temporarily reduces fever

Directions: See Table 1: Children's Tylenol Dosing Chart on pgs. 691–693.

Precautions: If a rare sensitivity reaction occurs, the drug should be discontinued.

Warnings: Sore throat warning: If sore throat is severe, persists for more than 2 days, is accompanied or followed by fever, headache, rash, nausea or vomiting, consult a doctor promptly.

Do not use
• in a child who is taking a monoamine oxidase inhibitor (MAOI) (certain drugs for depression, psychiatric or emotional conditions, or Parkinson's disease), or for 2 weeks after stopping the MAOI drug. If you do not know if

your child's prescription drug contains an MAOI, ask a doctor or pharmacist before giving this product.
• with any other product containing acetaminophen.

Ask a doctor before use if the child has
• heart disease • thyroid disease
• glaucoma • high blood pressure
• diabetes • cough that occurs with too much phlegm (mucus)
• chronic cough that lasts as occurs with asthma

When using this product
• **do not exceed recommended dosage (see overdose warning)**
• drowsiness may occur
• excitability may occur, especially in children

Stop use and ask a doctor if
• new symptoms occur
• redness or swelling is present
• pain gets worse or lasts for more than 5 days
• fever gets worse or lasts for more than 3 days
• nervousness, dizziness or sleeplessness occurs
• cough lasts more than 7 days, comes back or occurs with fever, rash or headache that lasts. These could be signs of a serious condition.

Keep out of reach of children. Overdose Warning: Taking more than the recommended dose (overdose) could cause serious health problems. In case of overdose, get medical help or contact a Poison Control Center right away. Quick medical attention is critical even if you do not notice any signs or symptoms.

Other Information:
• **do not use if bottle wrap or foil inner seal imprinted "Safety Seal®" is broken or missing**
• store at room temperature

Professional Information:
Overdosage Information
For overdosage information, please refer to pgs. 687–688.

Inactive Ingredients: acesulfame potassium, cellulose, citric acid, corn syrup, D&C Red #33, FD&C Red #40, flavors, glycerin, purified water, sodium benzoate, sorbitol, xanthan gum.

How Supplied: Pinkish-red-colored suspension liquid in bottles of 4 fl. oz.

Shown in Product Identification Guide, page 511

CHILDREN'S TYLENOL® Plus Sinus

Description: *Children's TYLENOL® Plus Sinus* Suspension Liquid is Fruit Burst-flavored and contains no alcohol or aspirin. Each teaspoon (5 mL) contains acetaminophen 160 mg and pseudoephedrine HCl 15 mg.

Actions: *Children's TYLENOL® Plus Sinus* Suspension Liquid combines the analgesic-antipyretic acetaminophen with the decongestant pseudoephedrine hydrochloride to provide fast, effective,

temporary relief of all your child's sinus symptoms including stuffy nose, sinus headache, sinus pressure, sinus pain, and nasal congestion. Acetaminophen is equal to aspirin in analgesic and antipyretic effectiveness and is unlikely to produce the side effects often associated with aspirin or aspirin-containing products.

Uses: temporarily relieves:
• sinus congestion • stuffy nose • sinus pressure • minor aches, pains and headache • temporarily reduces fever

Directions: See Table 1: Children's Tylenol Dosing Chart on pgs. 691–693.

Precautions: If a rare sensitivity reaction occurs, the drug should be discontinued.

Warnings: Do not use
• in a child who is taking a prescription monoamine oxidase inhibitor (MAOI) (certain drugs for depression, psychiatric, or emotional conditions, or Parkinson's disease), or for 2 weeks after stopping the MAOI drug. If you do not know if your child's prescription drug contains an MAOI, ask a doctor or pharmacist before giving this product.
• with any products containing acetaminophen

Ask a doctor before use if the child has
• heart disease • high blood pressure
• thyroid disease • diabetes

When using this product
• **do not exceed recommended dosage (see overdose warning)**

Stop use and ask a doctor if
• new symptoms occur
• redness or swelling is present
• pain gets worse or lasts for more than 5 days
• fever gets worse or lasts for more than 3 days
• nervousness, dizziness or sleeplessness occurs

Keep out of reach of children.

Overdose warning: Taking more than the recommended dose (overdose) could cause serious health problems. In case of overdose, get medical help or contact a Poison Control Center right away. Quick medical attention is critical even if you do not notice any signs or symptoms.

Other Information:
• **do not use if plastic carton wrap, bottle wrap, or foil inner seal imprinted "Safety Seal®" is broken or missing**
• store at room temperature

Professional Information:
Overdosage Information
For overdosage information, please refer to pgs. 687–688.

Inactive Ingredients: acesulfame potassium, cellulose, citric acid, corn syrup, D&C Red #33, FD&C Red #40, flavors, glycerin, purified water, sodium benzoate, sorbitol, xanthan gum.

How Supplied: Red-colored–child resistant bottles of 4 fl. oz.

Shown in Product Identification Guide, page 511

Children's Tylenol® Dosing Chart

[See table on pages 691 through 693]

TABLE 1
Children's Tylenol® Dosing Chart

AGE GROUP	0–3 mos	4–11 mos	12–23 mos	2–3 yrs	4–5 yrs	6–8 yrs	9–10 yrs	11 yrs	12 yrs	Maximum doses/24 hrs
WEIGHT	6–11 lbs	12–17 lbs	18–23 lbs	24–35 lbs	36–47 lbs	48–59 lbs	60–71 lbs	72–95 lbs	Over 96 lbs	
PRODUCT FORM (if possible use weight to dose; otherwise use age)	INGREDIENTS Dose to be administered based on weight or age†									

Infants' Drops — in each (0.8 mL)

PRODUCT FORM	INGREDIENTS	0–3 mos	4–11 mos	12–23 mos	2–3 yrs	4–5 yrs	6–8 yrs	9–10 yrs	11 yrs	12 yrs	Maximum doses/24 hrs
Concentrated Tylenol Infants' Drops	Acetaminophen 80 mg	(0.4 mL)*	(0.8 mL)*	(0.8 + 0.4 mL)*	(0.8 + 0.8 mL)	—	—	—	—	—	5 times in 24 hrs
Concentrated Tylenol Infants' Drops Plus Cold	Acetaminophen 80 mg Pseudoephedrine HCl 7.5 mg	(0.4 mL)*	(0.8 mL)*	(0.8 + 0.4 mL)*	(0.8 + 0.8 mL)	—	—	—	—	—	4 times in 24 hrs
Concentrated Tylenol Infants' Drops Plus Cold & Cough	Acetaminophen 80 mg Dextromethorphan HBr 2.5 mg Pseudoephedrine HCl 7.5 mg	(0.4 mL)*	(0.8 mL)*	(0.8 + 0.4 mL)*	(0.8 + 0.8 mL)	—	—	—	—	—	4 times in 24 hrs

Children's Liquids — Per 5 mL teaspoonful (TSP)

PRODUCT FORM	INGREDIENTS	0–3 mos	4–11 mos	12–23 mos	2–3 yrs	4–5 yrs	6–8 yrs	9–10 yrs	11 yrs	12 yrs	Maximum doses/24 hrs
Children's Tylenol Suspension Liquid	Acetaminophen 160 mg	—	1/2 TSP*	3/4 TSP*	1 TSP	1 1/2 TSP	2 TSP	2 1/2 TSP	3 TSP	—	5 times in 24 hrs
Children's Tylenol Plus Cold Suspension Liquid	Acetaminophen 160 mg Chlorpheniramine Maleate 1 mg Pseudoephedrine HCl 15 mg	—	1/2 TSP**	3/4 TSP**	1 TSP**	1 1/2 TSP**	2 TSP	2 1/2 TSP	3 TSP	—	4 times in 24 hrs

(Table continued on next page)

TABLE 1
Children's Tylenol® Dosing Chart *(continued)*

AGE GROUP	0–3 mos	4–11 mos	12–23 mos	2–3 yrs	4–5 yrs	6–8 yrs	9–10 yrs	11 yrs	12 yrs	Maximum doses/24 hrs
WEIGHT (if possible use weight to dose; otherwise use age)	6–11 lbs	12–17 lbs	18–23 lbs	24–35 lbs	36–47 lbs	48–59 lbs	60–71 lbs	72–95 lbs	Over 96 lbs	
PRODUCT FORM INGREDIENTS	Dose to be administered based on weight or age†									
Per 5 mL teaspoonful (TSP)										
Children's Tylenol Plus Cold & Cough Suspension Liquid — Acetaminophen 160 mg, Chlorpheniramine Maleate 1 mg, Dextromethorphan HBr 5 mg, Pseudoephedrine HCl 15 mg	—	$\frac{1}{2}$ TSP**	$\frac{3}{4}$ TSP**	1 TSP**	$1\frac{1}{2}$ TSP**	2 TSP	$2\frac{1}{2}$ TSP	3 TSP	—	4 times in 24 hrs
Children's Tylenol Plus Flu Suspension Liquid† — Acetaminophen 160 mg, Chlorpheniramine Maleate 1 mg, Dextromethorphan HBr 7.5 mg, Pseudoephedrine HCl 15 mg	—	$\frac{1}{2}$ TSP**	$\frac{3}{4}$ TSP**	1 TSP**	$1\frac{1}{2}$ TSP**	2 TSP	$2\frac{1}{2}$ TSP	3 TSP	—	4 times in 24 hrs
Children's Tylenol Plus Sinus Suspension Liquid — Acetaminophen 160 mg, Pseudoephedrine HCl 15 mg	—	$\frac{1}{2}$ TSP*	$\frac{3}{4}$ TSP*	1 TSP	$1\frac{1}{2}$ TSP	2 TSP	$2\frac{1}{2}$ TSP	3 TSP	—	4 times in 24 hrs
Children's Tylenol Plus Allergy Liquid — Acetaminophen 160 mg, Diphenhydramine HCl 12.5 mg, Pseudoephedrine HCl 15 mg	—	$\frac{1}{2}$ TSP**	$\frac{3}{4}$ TSP**	1 TSP**	$1\frac{1}{2}$ TSP**	2 TSP	$2\frac{1}{2}$ TSP	3 TSP	—	4 times in 24 hrs

Children's Liquids

Children's Tablets	Per tablet									
Children's Tylenol Soft Chews Chewable Tablets	Acetaminophen 80 mg	—	—	2 tablets	3 tablets	4 tablets	5 tablets	6 tablets	—	5 times in 24 hrs
Children's Tylenol Plus Cold Chewable Tablets	Acetaminophen 80 mg Chlorpheniramine Maleate 0.5 mg Pseudoephedrine HCl 7.5 mg	—	—	2 tablets**	3 tablets**	4 tablets	5 tablets	6 tablets	—	4 times in 24 hrs
Children's Tylenol Plus Cold & Cough Chewable Tablets	Acetaminophen 80 mg Chlorpheniramine Maleate 0.5 mg Dextromethorphan HBr 2.5 mg Pseudoephedrine HCl 7.5 mg	—	—	2 tablets**	3 tablets**	4 tablets	5 tablets	6 tablets	—	4 times in 24 hrs
Junior Strength Tylenol Soft Chews Chewable Tablets	Acetaminophen 160 mg	—	—	—	—	2 tablets	2½ tablets	3 tablets	4 tablets	5 times in 24 hrs

†All products may be dosed every 4 hours, if needed; except for Children's Tylenol Flu which is dosed every 6–8 hrs, if needed.
*Under 2 years (under 24 lbs), consult a doctor.　　　　**Under 6 years (under 48 lbs), consult a doctor.
•Infants' Tylenol Drops are more concentrated than Children's Tylenol Liquids. The Infants' Concentrated Drops have been specifically designed for use only with enclosed dropper. Do not use any other dosing device with this product.
•Children's Tylenol Liquids are less concentrated than Infants' Tylenol Concentrated Drops. The Children's Tylenol Liquids have been specifically designed for use with the enclosed measuring cup. Use only enclosed measuring cup to dose this product.
•Children's Tylenol Soft Chews Chewable Tablets are not the same concentration as Junior Strength Tylenol Soft Chews Chewable Tablets.
•Junior Strength Tylenol Soft Chews Chewable Tablets and Caplets contain twice as much medicine as Children's Tylenol Soft Chews Chewable Tablets.

Mission Pharmacal Company

10999 IH 10 WEST
SUITE 1000
SAN ANTONIO, TX 78230-1355

Direct Inquiries to:
PO Box 786099
San Antonio, TX 78278-6099
TOLL FREE: (800) 292-7364
(210) 696-8400
FAX: (210) 696-6010
For Medical Information Contact:
In Emergencies:
Mary Ann Walter
(830) 249-9822
FAX: (830) 249-1376

THERA-GESIC®
[thĕr'ə-jē-zik]
(Menthol 1%, Methyl Salicylate 15%)
TOPICAL ANALGESIC CREME

Active ingredients

	Purpose
Menthol 1%	Analgesic
Methyl Salicylate 15%	Counterirritant

Use: Temporary relief of minor aches and pains of muscles and joints associated with: Arthritis, simple backaches, strains, bruises, sprains.

Warnings:
For external use only. Use only as directed. Avoid contact with eyes or mucous membranes.
Do not use
• if skin is sensitive to oil of wintergreen (methyl salicylate)
• on wounds or damaged skin
Ask a doctor before use for children under 2 and through 12 years of age.
When using this product
• discontinue use if skin irritation develops, or redness is present
• do not swallow
• do not bandage tightly—If you intend to bandage, wrap, or cover the area where you have applied THERA-GESIC, the skin must be washed thoroughly to avoid excessive irritation
• do not use a heating pad after application of THERA-GESIC
Stop use and ask a doctor if condition worsens, or if symptoms persist for more than 7 days or clear up and occur again within a few days.
If pregnant or breast-feeding, ask a health professional before use.
Keep out of reach of children to avoid accidental poisoning. If swallowed, get medical help or contact a Poison Control Center right away.

Directions: Adults and children 12 or more years of age: Apply thin layers of creme into and around the sore or painful area, not more than 3 to 4 times daily. The number of thin layers controls the intensity of the action of THERA-GESIC. One thin layer provides a mild effect, two thin layers provide a strong effect and three thin layers provide a very strong effect. SEE WARNINGS.

Other information: Once THERA-GESIC has penetrated the skin, the area may be washed, leaving it dry, clean and fragrance-free without decreasing the effectiveness of the product.

Inactive ingredients: Carbomer 934, Dimethicone, Glycerine, Methylparaben, Propylparaben, Sodium Lauryl Sulfate, Trolamine, Water.

How Supplied:
NDC 0178-0320-03   3 oz. tube
NDC 0178-0320-05   5 oz. tube
Store at room temperature.

Novartis Consumer Health, Inc.

200 KIMBALL DRIVE
PARSIPPANY, NJ 07054-0622

Direct Product Inquiries to:
Consumer & Professional Affairs
(800) 452-0051
Fax: (800) 635-2801
Or write to above address.

DESENEX® ANTIFUNGALS

All products are Prescription Strength
Shake Powder
Liquid Spray
Spray Powder
Jock Itch Spray Powder

Indications: Cures most athlete's foot (tinea pedis), jock itch (tinea cruris) and ringworm (tinea corporis). For effective relief of the itching, burning, cracking and scaling which can accompany these conditions. Desenex powders also help keep feet dry.

Active Ingredient: *Shake Powder, Liquid Spray, Spray Powder,* and *Jock Itch Spray Powder*—Miconazole nitrate 2%.

Inactive Ingredients:
SHAKE POWDER—Corn starch, corn starch/acrylamide/sodium acrylate polymer, fragrance, talc.
LIQUID SPRAY—Polyethylene glycol 300, polysorbate 20, SD alcohol 40-B (15% w/w).
Propellant: Dimethyl ether.
SPRAY POWDER—Aloe vera gel, aluminum starch octenyl succinate, isopropyl myristate, propylene carbonate, SD alcohol 40-B (10% w/w), sorbitan monooleate, stearalkonium hectorite.
Propellant: Isobutane/propane.
JOCK ITCH SPRAY POWDER—Aloe vera gel, aluminum starch octenyl succinate, isopropyl myristate, propylene carbonate, SD alcohol 40-B (10% w/w), sorbitan monooleate, stearalkonium hectorite.
Propellant: Isobutane/propane.

Warnings: Do not use on children under 2 years of age unless directed by a doctor. For external use only. Avoid contact with the eyes. If irritation occurs, or if there is no improvement within 4 weeks (for athlete's foot or ringworm) or within 2 weeks for jock itch, discontinue use and consult a doctor. **Keep this and all drugs out of the reach of children.** In case of accidental ingestion, seek professional assistance or contact a poison control center immediately. Use only as directed. *For Spray Powders and Liquid Spray*—Avoid inhaling. Avoid contact with the eyes or other mucous membranes. Contents under pressure. Do not puncture or incinerate. Flammable mixture, do not use near fire or flame. Do not expose to heat or temperatures above 49°C (120°F). Use only as directed. Intentional misuse by deliberately concentrating and inhaling the contents can be harmful or fatal.

Directions: Clean the affected area and dry thoroughly. Apply a thin layer of the product over affected area twice daily (morning and night) or as directed by a doctor. (For Sprays: **Shake Spray can well,** and hold 4″ to 6″ from skin when applying.) For athlete's foot, pay special attention to the spaces between the toes. Wear well-fitting, ventilated shoes and change shoes and socks at least once daily. For athlete's foot or ringworm, use daily for 4 weeks. For jock itch, use daily for 2 weeks. If condition persists longer, consult a doctor. Supervise children in the use of this product. This product is not effective on the scalp or nails.

How Supplied:
Shake Powder—1.5 oz, 3 oz, 4 oz. plastic bottles.
Spray Powder—3 oz, 4 oz. cans.
Liquid Spray—3.5 oz, 4.6 oz. cans.
Store **powders/spray powders** and **liquid sprays** at room temperature, 15°–30°C (59°–86°F). See container bottom for lot number and expiration date. Spray powders: Tamper-resistant aerosol can for your protection. If clogging occurs, remove button and clean nozzle with pin.
Novartis Consumer Health, Inc.
Parsippany, NJ 07054-0622 ©2003
Shown in Product Identification Guide, page 514

EX•LAX® Chocolated Laxative Pieces

Active Ingredient: Sennosides, USP, 15mg

Use: For Relief of
• OCCASIONAL CONSTIPATION (IRREGULARITY). This product generally produces bowel movement in 6 to 12 hours.

Directions: Adults and children 12 years of age and over: chew 2 chocolated pieces once or twice daily. Children 6 to under 12 years of age: chew 1 chocolated piece once or twice daily. Children under 6 years of age: consult a doctor.

Warnings:
- as with any drug, if you are pregnant or nursing a baby, seek the advice of a health professional before using the product.

Unless directed by a doctor, do not use
- laxative products when abdominal pain, nausea, or vomiting is present.
- laxative products for a period longer than 1 week.

Consult a doctor before using a laxative if
- you have noticed a sudden change in bowel habits that persists over a period of 2 weeks.

Consult a doctor and stop using a laxative if
- rectal bleeding occurs or you fail to have a bowel movement after use because this may indicate a serious condition.

Keep this and all drugs out of the reach of children
In case of accidental overdose, seek professional assistance or contact a poison control center immediately.

Inactive Ingredients: cocoa, confectioners sugar, hydrogenated palm kernel oil, lecithin, non-fat dry milk, vanillin. Store at controlled room temperature 20–25°C (68–77°F).

How Supplied: Available in boxes of 18 ct. and 48 ct. chewable chocolated pieces.

Novartis Consumer Health, Inc.
Parsippany, NJ 07054-0622 ©2003
Shown in Product Identification Guide, page 514

EX•LAX® Laxative Pills
Regular Strength Ex•Lax® Laxative Pills
Maximum Strength Ex•Lax® Laxative Pills

Active Ingredients: *Regular Strength Ex•Lax Laxative Pills:* Sennosides, USP, 15 mg. *Maximum Relief Formula Ex•Lax Laxative Pills:* Sennosides, USP, 25 mg.

Use: For Relief of
- OCCASIONAL CONSTIPATION (IRREGULARITY). This product generally produces bowel movement in 6 to 12 hours.

Warnings:
- as with any drug, if you are pregnant or nursing a baby, seek the advice of a health professional before using this product.

Unless directed by a doctor, do not use:
- laxative products when abdominal pain, nausea, or vomiting is present.
- laxative products for a period longer than 1 week.

Consult a doctor before using a laxative if:
- you have noticed a sudden change in bowel habits that persists over a period of 2 weeks.

Consult a doctor and stop using a laxative if:
- rectal bleeding occurs or you fail to have a bowel movement after use because this may indicate a serious condition.

Keep this and all drugs out of the reach of children. In case of accidental overdose, seek professional assistance or contact a poison control center immediately.

Dosage and Administration: *Regular Strength Ex•Lax Laxative Pills, and Maximum Strength Ex•Lax Laxative Pills*—Adults and children 12 years of age and over: take 2 pills once or twice daily with a glass of water. Children 6 to under 12 years of age: take 1 pill once or twice daily with a glass of water. Children under 6 years of age: consult a doctor.

Inactive Ingredients: *Regular Strength Ex•Lax Laxative Pills*—acacia, alginic acid, carnauba wax, colloidal silicon dioxide, dibasic calcium phosphate, iron oxides, magnesium stearate, microcrystalline cellulose, sodium benzoate, sodium lauryl sulfate, starch, stearic acid, sucrose, talc, titanium dioxide. Sodium-free. *Maximum Strength Ex•Lax Laxative Pills:* acacia, alginic acid, FD&C Blue No. 1 aluminum lake, carnauba wax, colloidal silicon dioxide, dibasic calcium phosphate, magnesium stearate, microcrystalline cellulose, povidone, sodium benzoate, sodium lauryl sulfate, starch, stearic acid, sucrose, talc, titanium dioxide. Very low sodium.
Store at controlled room temperature 20–25°C (68–77°F)

How Supplied: *Regular Strength Ex•Lax Laxative Pills*—Available in boxes of 8 ct. and 30 ct. pills. *Maximum Strength Ex•Lax Laxative Pills*—Available in boxes of 24 ct., 48 ct., and 90 ct. pills.
Novartis Consumer Health, Inc.
Parsippany, NJ 07054-0622 ©2003
Shown in Product Identification Guide, page 514

Ex•Lax® Milk of Magnesia STIMULANT FREE Liquid: Laxative/Antacid, Chocolate Creme, Mint, Raspberry Creme

Indications: As a Laxative: To relieve occasional constipation (irregularity). This saline laxative product generally produces bowel movement in ½ to 6 hours.
As an Antacid: To relieve acid indigestion, sour stomach and heartburn.

Active Ingredient: Magnesium hydroxide – 400 mg per teaspoon (5 ml)

Inactive Ingredients:
Chocolate Creme: Carboxymethylcellulose sodium, flavors, glycerin, hydroxypropyl methylcellulose, microcrystalline cellulose, purified water, saccharin sodium, simethicone, sorbitol.
Mint: Carboxymethylcellulose sodium, flavor, glycerin, hydroxypropyl methylcellulose, microcrystalline cellulose, purified water, saccharin sodium, simethicone, sorbitol.
Raspberry Creme: Carboxymethylcellulose sodium, flavor, glycerin, hydroxy-

propyl methylcellulose, microcrystalline cellulose, purified water, saccharin sodium, simethicone, sorbitol.

Directions: Shake well before using.
Keep tightly closed and avoid freezing.
For Laxative Use: Adults/Children – 12 years and older: 2–4 tablespoonsful (TBSP) at bedtime or upon arising, followed by a full glass (8 oz.) of liquid.
Children: DO NOT USE DOSAGE CUP – 6–11 years: 1–2 tablespoonsful (TBSP), followed by a full glass (8 oz.) of liquid.
2–5 years: 1–3 teaspoonsful, followed by a full glass (8 oz.) of liquid.
Under 2 years: Consult a doctor.
FOR ANTACID USE: DO NOT USE DOSAGE CUP – Adults/Children - 12 years and older: 1–3 teaspoonsful with a little water, up to four times a day or as directed by a doctor.

Drug Interaction Precaution: Antacids may interact with certain prescription drugs. If you are presently taking a prescription drug, do not take this product without checking with your doctor or other health professional.

Laxative Warnings: Do not take any laxative if abdominal pain, nausea, vomiting or kidney disease are present unless directed by a doctor. If you have noticed a sudden change in bowel habits persisting for over 2 weeks, consult a doctor before using a laxative. Laxative products should not be used for a period longer than 1 week, unless directed by a doctor. Rectal bleeding or failure to have a bowel movement after use of a laxative may indicate a serious condition. Discontinue use and consult your doctor.

Antacid Warnings: Do not take more than the maximum recommended daily dosage in a 24 hour period (See Directions), or use the maximum dosage of this product for more than two weeks, or use this product if you have kidney disease, except under the advice and supervision of a doctor. May have laxative effect.

As with any drug, if you are pregnant or nursing a baby, seek the advice of a health professional before using this product. Keep this and all drugs out of the reach of children. In case of accidental overdose, seek professional assistance or contact a poison control central immediately.

How Supplied: EX•LAX MILK OF MAGNESIA is available in chocolate creme, mint and raspberry creme flavors and comes in 12 oz. (355 ml) bottles. Store at controlled room temperature 20–25°C (68–77°F).

Continued on next page

Information on Novartis Consumer Health, Inc., products appearing on these pages is effective as of November 2002.

Ex-Lax M.O.M.—Cont.

Distributed by:
NOVARTIS
Novartis Consumer Health, Inc.
Parsippany, NJ 07054-0622 ©2003
Shown in Product Identification
Guide, page 514

EX•LAX® ULTRA
Stimulant Laxative

Drug Facts:

Active Ingredient
(in each pill):   **Purpose:**
Bisacodyl 5 mg .... Stimulant laxative

Uses:
• relieves occasional constipation
• generally produces bowel movement in 6 to 12 hours

Warnings:
Ask a doctor before use if you have
• adominal pain
• nausea
• vomiting
• noticed a sudden change in bowel habits that persists over a period of 2 weeks
Ask a doctor or pharmacist before use if you are
• taking any other drug. Take this product 2 or more hours before or after other drugs. Laxatives may affect how other drugs work.
When using this product
• do not chew or crush pills
• do not take within 1 hour of taking an antacid or milk
• do not give to children under 6 years of age
• do not take if you cannot swallow without chewing
• abdominal discomfort, faintness, and cramps may occur
Stop use and ask a doctor if
• you need to use more than 1 week
• rectal bleeding or failure to have a bowel movement occur after use of a laxative.
These may be signs of a serious condition.
If pregnant or breast-feeding, ask a health care professional before use.
Keep out of reach of children. In case of overdose, get medical help or contact a Poison Control Center right away.

Directions: • take with a glass of water

adults and children 12 years of age and over	take one pill daily. If necessary, take up to a maximum of three pills in a single dose once daily.
children 6 to under 12 years of age	take one pill once daily
children under 6 years of age	ask a doctor

Other Information:
• **each pill contains:** sodium 0.1mg

• store at controlled room temperature 20–25°C (68–77°F)

Inactive Ingredients: ammonium hydroxide, butyl alcohol, colloidal silicon dioxide, croscarmellose sodium, FD&C yellow 6, iron oxide black, isopropyl alcohol, lactose, magnesium stearate, methacrylic acid, methanol, methylparaben, microcrystalline cellulose, PEG 3350, polyvinyl alcohol, propylene glycol, SD-45 alcohol, shellac, silica, sodium bicarbonate, sodium lauryl sulfate, talc, titanium dioxide, triethyl citrate.

How Supplied: Available in boxes of 24 ct. and 48 ct. cartons.
Tamper Evident Feature: Ex•Lax® Pills are sealed in blister packets. Use only if the individual seal is unbroken.
Questions? call **1-800-452-0051** 24 hours a day, 7 days a week.
Pills Non-USP (Disintegration)
Novartis Consumer Health, Inc.
Parsippany, NJ 07054-0622   ©2003
Shown in Product Identification
Guide, page 514

GAS–X® REGULAR STRENGTH
GAS–X® EXTRA STRENGTH
GAS–X® MAXIMUM STRENGTH
Antigas Softgels and Chewable Tablets

GAS–X® WITH MAALOX®
Antigas/Antacid Chewable Tablets
Antigas/Antacid Softgel

Active Ingredients:
Regular Strength—Each chewable tablet contains simethicone 80 mg.
Extra Strength—Each chewable tablet and swallowable softgel contains simethicone, 125 mg.
Maximum Strength—Each Swallowable softgel contains simethicone, 166 mg.
Gas-X with Maalox Tablets—Each extra strength chewable tablet contains simethicone 125 mg and calcium carbonate 500 mg.
Gas-X® with Maalox Softgels—Each swallowable softgel contains simethicone 62.5 mg and calcium carbonate 250 mg.

Inactive Ingredients:
Regular Strength Peppermint Creme: calcium carbonate, dextrose, flavors, maltodextrin, starch.
Regular Strength Cherry Creme: calcium carbonate, D&C Red 30 aluminum lake, dextrose, flavors, maltodextrin, propylene glycol, soy protein isolate, starch.
Extra Strength Peppermint Creme: calcium phosphate tribasic, colloidal silicon dioxide, D&C Yellow 10 aluminum lake, D&C Red 30 aluminum lake, dextrose, flavors, maltodextrin, starch.
Extra Strength Cherry Creme: calcium phosphate tribasic, colloidal silicon dioxide, D&C Red 30 aluminum lake, dextrose, flavors, maltodextrin, propylene glycol, soy protein isolate, starch.

Extra Strength Softgels: D&C Yellow 10, FD&C Blue 1, FD&C Red 40, gelatin, glycerin, peppermint oil, purified water, sorbitol, titanium dioxide.
Maximum Strength Softgels: FD&C Blue 1, FD&C Red 40, gelatin, glycerin, peppermint oil, purified water, sorbitol.
Gas-X With Maalox Wildberry Tablets: colloidal silicon dioxide, D&C Red 30, dextrose, flavors, maltodextrin, mannitol, pregelatinized starch, talc, tribasic calcium phosphate
Gas-X With Maalox Orange Tablets: colloidal silicon dioxide, dextrose, FD&C yellow 6 aluminum lake, flavors, maltodextrin, mannitol, pregelatinized starch, talc, tribasic calcium phosphate
Gas-X® With Maalox® Softgels: D&C Red 28, FD&C Blue 1 gelatin, glycerin, polyethylene glycol, polysorbate 80, silicon dioxide, sorbitol, titanium dioxide, purified water

Use:
Gas-X: For the relief of pressure and bloating commonly referred to as gas.
Gas-X with Maalox: Relief of the concurrent symptoms of gas associated with heartburn, sour stomach or acid indigestion.

Warning: **Keep out of reach of children.**

Drug Interaction Precautions: No known drug interaction.
Gax-X® with Maalox® Tablets and Softgels

Warnings:
Ask a doctor or pharmacist before use if you are now taking a prescription drug. Antacids may interact with certain prescription drugs.

Dosage and Administration: For Chewable Tablets: Adults: Chew one or two tablets as needed after meals or at bedtime. Do not exceed six Regular Strength chewable tablets or four Extra Strength chewable tablets in 24 hours except under the advice and supervision of a physician.
For Extra Strength Softgels: Adults: Swallow with water 1 or 2 softgels as needed after meals or at bedtime. Do not exceed 4 softgels in 24 hours except under the advice and supervision of a physician.
For Maximum Strength Softgels: Adults: Swallow with water one or two softgels as needed after meals or at bedtime. Do not exceed 3 softgels in 24 hours except under the advice and supervision of a physician.
For Gas-X with Maalox Tablets: Chew 1 to 2 tablets as symptoms occur or as directed by a physician. Do not take more than 4 tablets in a 24-hour period or use the maximum dosage for more than 2 weeks except under the advice and supervision of a physician.
For Gas-X® with Maalox® Softgels: Adults: Swallow with water 2 to 4 softgels as symptoms occur or as directed by a physician. Do not exceed 8 softgels in a 24 hour period or use the maximum dos-

age for more than 2 weeks except under the advice and supervision of a physician.

Professional Labeling: Gas-X may be used in the alleviation of postoperative bloating/pressure, and for use in endoscopic examination.

How Supplied:

Regular Strength Chewable tablets are available in peppermint creme and cherry creme flavored, chewable, scored tablets in boxes of 36 tablets.

Extra Strength Chewable tablets are available in peppermint creme and cherry creme flavored, chewable, scored tablets in boxes of 18 tablets.

Easy-to-swallow, tasteless/Extra Strength Softgels are available in boxes of 10 pills, 30 pills, 50 pills and 60 pills. Easy-to-swallow, tasteless/Maximum Strength Softgels are available in box of 50 pills.

Gas-X With Maalox Tablets are available in orange and wild berry flavored, chewable tablets in boxes of 8 tablets and 24 tablets

Easy-to-swallow, tasteless/Gax-X® with Maalox® Softgels are available in boxes of 24 pills and 48 pills

Shown in Product Identification Guide, page 514

LAMISIL ᴬᵀ® CREAM
Terbinafine Hydrochloride Cream 1%

Active Ingredient:	Purpose:
Terbinafine hydrochloride 1%	Antifungal

Uses:
- **cures most athlete's foot (tinea pedis)**
- **cures most jock itch (tinea cruris) and ringworm (tinea corporis)**
- **relieves itching, burning, cracking and scaling which accompany these conditions**

Warnings:

For external use only

Do not use • on nails or scalp
- in or near the mouth or the eyes
- for vaginal yeast infections

When using this product do not get into the eyes. If eye contact occurs, rinse thoroughly with water.

Stop use and ask a doctor if too much irritation occurs or gets worse.

Keep out of reach of children. If swallowed, get medical help or contact a poison control center right away.

Directions:
- adults and children 12 years and over
  - use the tip of the cap to break the seal and open the tube
  - wash the affected skin with soap and water and dry completely before applying
  - **for athlete's foot** wear well-fitting, ventilated shoes. Change shoes and socks at least once every day.
    - **between the toes only:** apply twice a day (morning and night)

for **1 week** or as directed by a doctor.

1 week between the toes

- **on the bottom or sides of the foot:** apply twice a day (morning and night) for **2 weeks** or as directed by a doctor.

2 weeks on the bottom or sides of the foot

- **for jock itch and ringworm:** apply once a day (morning **or** night) for **1 week** or as directed by a doctor.
  - wash hands after each use
- children under 12 years: ask a doctor

Other Information: • do not use if seal on tube is broken or is not visible
- store at controlled room temperature 20–25°C (68–77°F)

Inactive Ingredients: benzyl alcohol, cetyl alcohol, cetyl palmitate, isopropyl myristate, polysorbate 60, purified water, sodium hydroxide, sorbitan monostearate, stearyl alcohol.

How Supplied: Athlete's Foot — Net wt. 12g (.42 oz.) tube and 24g (.85 oz.) tube, Jock Itch — Net wt. 12g (.42 oz.) tube.

Questions? call 1-800-452-0051 24 hours a day, 7 days a week.
Novartis Consumer Health, Inc.
Parsippany, NJ 07054-0622 ©2002
Shown in Product Identification Guide, page 514

LAMISIL ᴬᵀ® ANTIFUNGAL
TERBINAFINE HYDROCHLORIDE SOLUTION 1%
CURES MOST ATHLETE'S FOOT
CURES MOST JOCK ITCH
CURES MOST RINGWORM

Active Ingredient:	Purpose:
Terbinafine Hydrochloride 1%	Antifungal

Uses:
- **Cures most athlete's foot (tinea pedis) between the toes. Effectiveness on the bottom or sides of foot is unknown.**
- **Cures most jock itch (tinea cruris) and ringworm (tinea corporis)**
- **Relieves itching, burning, cracking, and scaling which accompany these conditions**

Warnings:

For external use only:

Do not use:
- on nails or scalp
- in or near the mouth or the eyes
- for vaginal yeast infections

When using this product do not get into eyes. If contact occurs, rinse eyes thoroughly with water.

Stop use and ask a doctor if too much irritation occurs or gets worse.

Keep out of reach of children. If swallowed, get medical help or contact a poison control center right away.

Directions:
- adults and children 12 years and older
  - wash the affected skin with soap and water and dry completely before applying
  - **for athlete's foot between the toes** apply twice a day (morning and night) for 1 week or as directed by a doctor. Wear well-fitting, ventilated shoes. Change shoes and socks at least once daily.
  - **for jock itch and ringworm** apply to affected area once a day (morning **or** night) for 1 week or as directed by a doctor

1 week between the toes

  - wash hands after each use
- children under 12 years: ask a doctor

How Supplied: Bottle of 30 mL (1 fl. oz.). Solution Dropper or Spray Pump

Other Information: Store at 8°–25°C (46°–77°F).

Questions?
Call 1-800-452-0051 24 hours a day, 7 days a week.
Novartis Consumer Health, Inc.
Parsippany, NJ 07054-0622 ©2003
Shown in Product Identification Guide, page 515

MAALOX® MAX™ MAXIMUM STRENGTH
ANTACID/ANTI-GAS Liquid
Oral Suspension Antacid/Anti-Gas

Liquids
- ☐ **Lemon**
- ☐ **Cherry**
- ☐ **Mint**
- ☐ **Vanilla Crème**
- ☐ **Peaches n' Crème**
- ☐ **Wild Berry**

Composition: To provide symptomatic relief of hyperacidity plus alleviation of gas symptoms, each teaspoonful contains:
[See first table at top of next page]

Uses: For the relief of
- acid indigestion
- heartburn
- sour stomach
- upset stomach associated with these symptoms
- bloating and pressure commonly referred to as gas

Inactive Ingredients: Butylparaben, Carboxymethylcellulose Sodium, D&C Yellow #10 (Lemon Flavor only), Flavor,

Continued on next page

Information on Novartis Consumer Health, Inc., products appearing on these pages is effective as of November 2002.

Maalox Antacid—Cont.

hypromellose, Microcrystalline Cellulose, Potassium Citrate, Propylparaben, Purified Water, Saccharin Sodium, Sorbitol.

Warnings:
Ask a doctor before use if you have kidney disease.
Ask a doctor or pharmacist before use if you are taking a prescription drug. Antacids may interact with certain prescription drugs.
Stop use and ask a doctor if symptoms last for more than 2 weeks
Keep out of reach of children.

Directions
- shake well before using
- Adults/children 12 years and older: take 2 to 4 teaspoons four times a day or as directed by a physician
- do not take more than 12 teaspoonsful in 24 hours or use the maximum dosage for more than 2 weeks.
- Children under 12 years: consult a physician

To aid in establishing proper dosage schedules, the following information is provided:

MAALOX® Max™ Maximum Strength Antacid/Anti-Gas

	Per 2 Tsp. (10 mL) (Minimum Recommended Dosage)
Acid neutralizing capacity	38.8 mEq

Professional Labeling
Indications: As an antacid for symptomatic relief of hyperacidity associated with the diagnosis of peptic ulcer, gastritis, peptic esophagitis, gastric hyperacidity, or hiatal hernia. As an antiflatulent to alleviate the symptoms of gas, including postoperative gas pain.

Warnings: Prolonged use of aluminum-containing antacids in patients with renal failure may result in or worsen dialysis osteomalacia. Elevated tissue aluminum levels contribute to the development of the dialysis encephalopathy and osteomalacia syndromes. Small amounts of aluminum are absorbed from the gastrointestinal tract and renal excretion of aluminum is impaired in renal failure. Aluminum is not well removed by dialysis because it is bound to albumin and transferrin, which do not cross dialysis membranes. As a result, aluminum is deposited in bone, and dialysis osteomalacia may develop when large amounts of aluminum are ingested orally by patients with impaired renal function. Aluminum forms insoluble complexes with phosphate in the gastrointestinal tract, thus decreasing phosphate absorption. Prolonged use of aluminum-con-

taining antacids by normophosphatemic patients may result in hypophosphatemia if phosphate intake is not adequate. In its more severe forms, hypophosphatemia can lead to anorexia, malaise, muscle weakness, and osteomalacia.

Advantages: In addition to the fast acting antacid ingredients, Aluminum Hydroxide and Magnesium Hydroxide, MAALOX® Max™ Maximum Strength Antacid/Antigas contains the powerful antigas ingredient, simethicone, to provide concurrent fast relief from discomfort associated with gas.

How Supplied:
MAALOX® MAX™ MAXIMUM STRENGTH ANTACID/ANTI-GAS Liquid
Oral Suspension Antacid/Anti-Gas
Lemon is available in plastic bottles of 5 fl. oz. (148 mL), 12 fl. oz. (355 mL), and 26 fl. oz. (769 mL).
Cherry is available in plastic bottles of 12 fl. oz. (355 mL) and 26 fl. oz. (769 mL).
Mint is available in plastic bottles of 12 fl. oz. (355 mL) and 26 fl. oz. (769 mL).
Peaches n' Crème is available in Plastic Bottles of 12 fl. oz. (355 mL).
Vanilla Crème is available in Plastic Bottles of 12 fl. oz. (355 mL).
Wild Berry is available in Plastic Bottles of 12 fl. oz. (355 mL).
Novartis Consumer Health, Inc.
Parsippany, NJ 07054-0622 ©2003
Shown in Product Identification Guide, page 515

MAALOX®
Regular Strength
Liquid Antacid/Anti-Gas

Liquids
- Cooling Mint
- Smooth Cherry

Active Ingredients	Maximum Strength Maalox® Antacid/Anti-Gas Per Tsp. (5 mL)	Purpose
Aluminum Hydroxide (equivalent to dried gel, USP)	400 mg	antacid
Magnesium Hydroxide	400 mg	antacid
Simethicone	40 mg	antigas

Active Ingredients	Maalox Suspension 5 mL teaspoon	Purpose
Aluminum Hydroxide (equivalent to dried gel, USP)	200 mg	Antacid
Magnesium Hydroxide	200 mg	Antacid
Simethicone	20 mg	Antigas

[See second table above]

Uses: For the relief of
- acid indigestion
- heartburn
- sour stomach
- upset stomach associated with these symptoms
- bloating and pressure commonly referred to as gas

Inactive Ingredients: Butylparaben, Carboxymethylcellulose Sodium, Flavor, Hypromellose, Microcrystalline Cellulose, Propylparaben, Purified Water, Saccharin Sodium, Sorbitol.

	Maalox Suspension Per 2 Tsp. (10 mL) (Minimum Recommended Dosage)
Acid neutralizing capacity	19.4 mEq

Warnings:
Ask a doctor before use if you have kidney disease
Ask a doctor or pharmacist before use if you are taking a prescription drug. Antacids may interact with certain prescription drugs.
Stop use and ask a doctor if symptoms last for more than 2 weeks
Keep out of reach of children.

Directions:
- shake well before using
- Adults/children 12 years and older: take 2 to 4 teaspoons four times a day or as directed by a physician
- do not take more than 16 teaspoonsful in 24 hours or use the maximum dosage for more than 2 weeks.
- Children under 12 years: consult a physician

Professional Labeling

Indications: As an antacid for symptomatic relief of hyperacidity associated with the diagnosis of peptic ulcer, gastritis, peptic esophagitis, gastric hyperacidity, or hiatal hernia. As an antiflatulent to alleviate the symptoms of gas, including postoperative gas pain.

Warnings: Prolonged use of aluminum-containing antacids in patients with renal failure may result in or worsen dialysis osteomalacia. Elevated tissue aluminum levels contribute to the development of the dialysis encephalopathy and osteomalacia syndromes. Small amounts of aluminum are absorbed from the gastrointestinal tract and renal excretion of aluminum is impaired in renal failure. Aluminum is not well removed by dialysis because it is bound to albumin and transferrin, which do not cross dialysis membranes. As a result, aluminum is deposited in bone, and dialysis osteomalacia may develop when large amounts of aluminum are ingested orally by patients with impaired renal function. Aluminum forms insoluble complexes with phosphate in the gastrointestinal tract, thus decreasing phosphate absorption. Prolonged use of aluminum-containing antacids by normophosphatemic patients may result in hypophosphatemia if phosphate intake is not adequate. In its more severe forms, hypophosphatemia can lead to anorexia, malaise, muscle weakness, and osteomalacia.

Advantages: In addition to the fast acting antacid ingredients, Aluminum Hydroxide and Magnesium Hydroxide, MAALOX® Regular Strength Antacid/Antigas contains the powerful antigas ingredient, simethicone, to provide concurrent fast relief from discomfort associated with gas.

How Supplied:
Maalox® Cooling Mint Suspension is available in plastic bottles of 5 oz. (148 mL), 12 oz. (355 mL) and 26 oz. (769 mL)
Maalox® Smooth Cherry Suspension is available in plastic bottles of 12 oz. (355 mL)
Novartis Consumer Health, Inc.
Parsippany, NJ 07054-0622 ©2003
Shown in Product Identification Guide, page 515

Quick Dissolve
MAALOX® Regular Strength
Antacid.
Calcium Carbonate
Chewable Tablets
Assorted, Lemon and Wild Berry flavors. Quick Dissolving Tablets

MAALOX® Regular Strength

Active Ingredient:	Purpose:
(in each tablet)	
Calcium carbonate	
600 mg	Antacid

Uses: For the relief of
• acid indigestion
• heartburn

• sour stomach
• upset stomach associated with these symptoms

Warnings:
Ask a doctor or pharmacist before use if you are: presently taking a prescription drug. Antacids may interact with certain prescription drugs
Stop use and ask a doctor if symptoms last for more than 2 weeks.
Keep out of reach of children.

Directions:
• Chew 1 to 2 tablets as symptoms occur or as directed by a physician
• do not take more than 12 tablets in a 24-hour period or use the maximum dosage for more than 2 weeks except under the advice and supervision of a physician

Other Information:
• Phenylketonurics: Contains Phenylalanine, .5 mg per tablet
• store at controlled room temperature 20–25°C (68–77°F)
• keep tightly closed and dry
• Acid neutralizing capacity (per 2 tablets) is 21.6 mEq.

Inactive Ingredients: Aspartame, colloidal silicon dioxide, croscarmellose sodium, D&C Red #30 aluminum lake, D&C Yellow #10 aluminum lake, dextrose, FD&C Blue #1 aluminum lake, flavors, magnesium stearate, maltodextrin, mannitol, pregelatinized starch. May also contain: corn starch, sodium chloride.

How Supplied:
Lemon — Plastic Bottles of 45 ct. and 85 ct. Tablets.
Wild Berry — Plastic Bottles of 45 ct. Tablets.
Assorted — Plastic Bottles of 85 ct.
Questions? call 1-800-452-0051 24 hours a day, 7 days a week.
Novartis Consumer Health, Inc.
Parisppany, NJ 07054-0622 ©2003
Shown in Product Identification Guide, page 515

Quick Dissolve
MAALOX® Max™ Maximum Strength
Antacid/Antigas.
Calcium Carbonate and Simethicone
Chewable Tablets
Assorted, Lemon and Wild Berry Flavors. Quick Dissolving Tablets

Drug Facts:
MAALOX® Max™ Maximum Strength

Active Ingredients:	Purpose:
(in each tablet)	
Calcium carbonate	
1000 mg	Antacid
Simethicone 60 mg	Antigas

Uses: For the relief of
• acid indigestion
• heartburn
• sour stomach
• upset stomach associated with these symptoms
• bloating and pressure commonly referred to as gas

Warnings:
Allergy Alert: contains FD&C Yellow #5 aluminum lake (tartrazine) as a color additive
Ask a doctor or pharmacist before use if you are: presently taking a prescription drug. Antacids may interact with certain prescription drugs.
Stop use and ask a doctor if: symptoms last for more than 2 weeks.
Keep out of reach of children.

Directions:
• Chew 1 to 2 tablets as symptoms occur or as directed by a physician
• do not take more than 8 tablets in a 24-hour period or use the maximum dosage for more than 2 weeks except under the advice and supervision of a physician

Other Information:
• store at controlled room temperature 20–25°C (68–77°F)
• keep tightly closed and dry
• Acid neutralizing capacity (per 2 tablets) is 34mEq.

Inactive Ingredients: acesulfame K, colloidal silicon dioxide, croscarmellose sodium, dextrose, FD&C Red #40 aluminum lake, FD&C Yellow #5 aluminum lake, FD&C Yellow #6 aluminum lake, flavors, magnesium stearate, maltodextrin, mannitol, pregelatinized starch.

How Supplied:
Lemon — Plastic Bottles of 35 and 65 Tablets.
Wild Berry — Plastic Bottles of 35 and 65 Tablets.
Assorted — Plastic Bottles of 35, 65 and 90 Tablets.
Questions? call 1-800-452-0051 24 hours a day, 7 days a week.
Novartis Consumer Health, Inc.
Parsippany, NJ 07054-0622 ©2003
Shown in Product Identification Guide, page 515

PERDIEM®
FIBER THERAPY
Calcium Polycarbophil
Bulk Forming Laxative Caplets

Drug Facts:

Active Ingredient (in each caplet):	Purpose:
Calcium polycarbophil 625 mg equivalent to 500 mg polycarbophil	Bulk forming laxative

Uses:
• for relief of occasional constipation
• this product generally produces bowel movement in 12 to 72 hours

Warnings:
CHOKING: TAKING THIS PRODUCT WITHOUT ADEQUATE FLUID MAY CAUSE IT TO SWELL AND BLOCK

Continued on next page

Information on Novartis Consumer Health, Inc., products appearing on these pages is effective as of November 2002.

Perdiem Fiber—Cont.

YOUR THROAT OR ESOPHAGUS AND MAY CAUSE CHOKING. DO NOT TAKE THIS PRODUCT IF YOU HAVE DIFFICULTY IN SWALLOWING. IF YOU EXPERIENCE CHEST PAIN, VOMITING, OR DIFFICULTY IN SWALLOWING OR BREATHING AFTER TAKING THIS PRODUCT, SEEK IMMEDIATE MEDICAL ATTENTION.

Ask a doctor before use if you have
• abdominal pain, nausea, or vomiting
• a sudden change in bowel habits that persists over a period of 2 weeks

Ask a doctor or pharmacist before use if you are taking any other drug. Take this product 2 or more hours before or after other drugs. Laxatives may affect how other drugs work.

When using this product • do not take for more than 7 days unless directed by a doctor.
• do not take recommended dose more than 4 times in a 24 hour period unless directed by a doctor.

Stop use and ask a doctor if • rectal bleeding or failure to have bowel movement occurs after use of a laxative. These could be signs of a serious condition.

Keep out of reach of children. In case of overdose, get medical help or contact a Poison Control Center right away.

Directions:
• TAKE THIS PRODUCT (CHILD OR ADULT DOSE) WITH AT LEAST 8 OUNCES (A FULL GLASS) OF WATER OR OTHER FLUID. TAKING THIS PRODUCT WITHOUT ENOUGH LIQUID MAY CAUSE CHOKING. SEE CHOKING WARNING.
• SWALLOW CAPLET(S) WHOLE, DO NOT CRUSH, BREAK OR CHEW
• Continued use for one to three days is normally required to provide full benefit. Dosage may vary according to diet, exercise, previous laxative use or severity of constipation.

Age	Recommended dose	Daily maximum
adults & children 12 years of age and over	2 caplets once a day	Up to 4 times a day
children 6 to under 12 years of age	1 caplet once a day	Up to 4 times a day
children under 6 years of age	Consult a doctor	

Other Information:
• protect from moisture
• store at controlled room temperature 20–25°C (68–77°F)

Inactive Ingredients: caramel, carnauba wax, colloidal, silicon dioxide, crospovidone, hypromellose, microcrystalline cellulose, polyethylene glycol, povidone, stearic acid

How Supplied: Bottles of 60 caplets, NDC 0067-6026-60.

The Perdiem® Guarantee: Perdiem is guaranteed to work gently, effectively or your money back. Return product to Novartis, attention Consumer Affairs, for full refund.

Tamper Evident Feature: Protective printed inner seal beneath cap. If missing or damaged, do not use contents.

Questions? call **1-800-452-0051** 24 hours a day, 7 days a week.

Novartis Consumer Health, Inc.
Parsippany, NJ 07054-0622 ©2003
Shown in Product Identification Guide, page 515

PERDIEM® OVERNIGHT RELIEF
Sennosides, Stimulant Laxative Pills

Drug Facts:

Active Ingredient (in each pill):　　　　　**Purpose:**
Sennosides, USP, 15 mg .... Stimulant Laxative

Uses:
• relieves occasional constipation (irregularity)
• generally produces bowel movement in 6 to 12 hours

Warnings:
Do not use laxative products when abdominal pain, nausea, or vomiting are present

Ask a doctor or pharmacist before use if you
• have noticed a sudden change in bowel habits that persists over a period of 2 weeks
• are taking any other drug. Take this product 2 or more hours before or after other drugs. Laxatives may effect how other drugs work.

When using this product • do not use for a period longer than 1 week

Stop use and ask a doctor if • rectal bleeding or failure to have a bowel movement occur after use of a laxative. These may be signs of a serious condition.

If pregnant or breast-feeding, ask a health care professional before use.

Keep out of reach of children. In case of overdose, get medical help or contact a Poison Control Center right away.

Directions:
• swallow pill(s) with a glass of water
• swallow pill(s) whole, do not crush, break or chew

adults and children 12 years of age and over	take 2 pills once or twice daily
children 6 to under 12 years of age	take 1 pill once or twice daily
children under 6 years of age	consult a doctor

Other Information:
• very low sodium
• protect from moisture
• store at controlled room temperature 20–25°C (68–77°F)

Inactive Ingredients: acacia, alginic acid, black iron oxide, carnauba wax; colloidal silicon dioxide, D&C yellow #10 aluminum lake, dibasic calcium phosphate, magnesium stearate, methylparaben, microcrystalline cellulose, potassium hydroxide, povidone, pregelatinized starch, propylene glycol, propylparaben, red iron oxide, shellac, sodium benzoate, sodium lauryl sulfate, starch, stearic acid, sucrose, talc, titanium dioxide, yellow iron oxide

How Supplied: Bottles of 60 pills, NDC 0067-6025-60.

The Perdiem® Guarantee: When taken at bedtime, Perdiem® is guaranteed to work gently, effectively or your money back. Return product to Novartis, attention Consumer Affairs, for full refund.

Tamper Evident Feature: Protective printed inner seal beneath cap. If missing or damaged, do not use contents.

Questions? call **1-800-452-0051** 24 hours a day, 7 days a week.

Novartis Consumer Health, Inc.
Parsippany, NJ 07054-0622 ©2003
Shown in Product Identification Guide, page 515

TAVIST® Allergy
Antihistamine Tablets

Active Ingredient:
(in each tablet)
Clemastine fumarate, USP 1.34 mg (equivalent to 1 mg clemastine) .... Antihistamine

Uses: Temporarily reduces these symptoms of the common cold, hay fever, and other respiratory allergies:
• runny nose
• itchy, watery eyes
• sneezing
• itching of the nose or throat

Warnings:

Ask a doctor before use if you have:
• a breathing problem such as emphysema or chronic bronchitis
• glaucoma
• trouble urinating due to an enlargement of the prostate gland

Ask a doctor or pharmacist before use if you are taking sedatives or tranquilizers

When using this product
• avoid alcoholic drinks
• drowsiness may occur
• alcohol, sedatives, and tranquilizers may increase drowsiness
• be careful when driving a motor vehicle or operating machinery
• excitability may occur, especially in children

If pregnant or breast-feeding, ask a health professional before use.

Keep out of reach of children. In case of overdose, get medical help or contact a poison control center right away.

Directions:
- adults and children 12 years of age and older: take 1 tablet every 12 hours, not more than 2 tablets in 24 hours unless directed by a doctor
- children under 12 years of age: consult a doctor

Other Information:
- sodium free
- store at controlled room temperature 20–25°C (68–77°F)

Inactive Ingredients: lactose, povidone, starch, stearic acid, talc.

How Supplied: Available in 8 ct. and 16 ct. cartons.

Novartis Consumer Health, Inc.
Parsippany, NJ 07054-0622 ©2003
Shown in Product Identification Guide, page 515

TAVIST® Allergy/Sinus/Headache
Antihistamine/Nasal Decongestant/Pain Reliever/Fever Reducer Caplets*
***Capsule-shaped tablet**

Drug Facts:

Active ingredients
(in each tablet)   **Purpose:**
Acetaminophen 500 mg ... Pain reliever/ fever reducer
Clemastine fumarate 0.335 mg (equivalent to 0.25 mg clemastine) .... Antihistamine
Pseudoephedrine HCl 30 mg .... Nasal decongestant

Uses: Temporarily relieves these symptoms of hay fever or other upper respiratory allergies, and common cold:
sinus congestion and pressure, nasal congestion, headaches, itchy watery eyes, sneezing, runny nose, itching of the nose or throat, minor aches and pains, fever

Warnings:
Alcohol Warning: If you consume 3 or more alcoholic drinks daily, ask your doctor whether you should take acetaminophen or other pain relievers/fever reducers. Acetaminophen may cause liver damage.

Do not use if you are now taking a prescription monoamine oxidase inhibitor [MAOI] (certain drugs for depression, psychiatric or emotional conditions, or Parkinson's disease), or for 2 weeks after stopping the MAOI drug. If you do not know if your prescription drug contains an MAOI, ask a doctor or pharmacist before taking this product.

Ask a doctor before use if you have: heart disease, high blood pressure, thyroid disease, diabetes, glaucoma, a breathing problem such as emphysema or chronic bronchitis, trouble urinating due to an enlarged prostate gland

Ask a doctor or pharmacist before use if you are:
- taking sedatives or tranquilizers
- under a doctor's care for any continuing medical condition
- taking other drugs on a regular basis
- using another product containing acetaminophen, clemastine fumarate or pseudoephedrine HCl

When using this product • do not use more than directed:
- drowsiness may occur
- avoid alcoholic drinks
- excitability may occur, especially in children
- alcohol, sedatives, and tranquilizers may increase drowsiness
- be careful when driving a motor vehicle or operating machinery

Warnings:
Stop use and ask a doctor if
- nervousness, dizziness or sleeplessness occurs
- symptoms continue or get worse
- a fever lasts for more than 3 days
- new or unexpected symptoms occur
- nasal congestion lasts for more than 7 days

If pregnant or breast-feeding, ask a health professional before use.

Keep out of reach of children. In case of overdose, get medical help or contact a poison control center right away. Prompt medical attention is critical for adults as well as children even if you do not notice any signs or symptoms.

Directions:
- adults and children 12 years of age and over: take 2 caplets every 6 hours as needed: not more than 8 caplets in 24 hours unless directed by a doctor
- children under 12 years of age: ask a doctor

Other Information:
- store at 20–25°C (68–77°F) • **avoid excessive heat**

Inactive Ingredients: Calcium sulfate, glyceryl behenate, maltodextrin, methylcellulose, methylparaben, polyethylene glycol, silicon dioxide, sodium lauryl sulfate, starch, titanium dioxide
Questions Call **1-800-452-0051** 24 hours a day, 7 days a week.

How Supplied: Available in 24 ct. and 48 ct. caplet packages.
Novartis Consumer Health, Inc.
Parsippany, NJ 07054-0622 © 2003
Shown in Product Identification Guide, page 515

TAVIST® SINUS
Pain Reliever/Nasal Decongestant Non-Drowsy Caplets

Active Ingredients
(in each caplet):   **Purpose:**
Acetaminophen
    500 mg .... Pain reliever
Pseudoephedrine HCl
    30 mg .... Nasal decongestant

Uses: Temporarily relieves:
- nasal and sinus congestion and pressure
- sinus pain
- minor aches and pains associated with the common cold

- headache

Warnings:
Alcohol Warning If you consume 3 or more alcoholic drinks every day, ask your doctor whether you should take acetaminophen or other pain relievers/fever reducers. Acetaminophen may cause liver damage.

Do not use
- if you are now taking a prescription monoamine oxidase inhibitor (MAOI) (certain drugs for depression, psychiatric or emotional conditions, or Parkinson's disease), or for 2 weeks after stopping the MAOI drug. If you do not know if your prescription drug contains an MAOI, ask a doctor or pharmacist before taking this product.
- with any other product containing acetaminophen.

Ask a doctor before use if you have
- heart disease
- high blood pressure
- thyroid disease
- diabetes
- difficulty urinating due to an enlarged prostate gland

When using this product • do not use more than directed
Stop use and ask a doctor if
- nervousness, dizziness, or sleeplessness occurs
- symptoms do not improve for 7 days or occur with a fever
- symptoms do not improve for 10 days (pain) or for 3 days (fever). These could be signs of a serious condition.

If pregnant or breast-feeding, ask a health professional before use.

Keep out of reach of children. In case of overdose, get medical help or contact a poison control center right away. Prompt medical attention is critical for adults as well as for children even if you do not notice any signs or symptoms.

Directions:
- adults and children 12 years of age and over: take 2 caplets every 6 hours, not to exceed 8 caplets in 24 hours or as directed by a doctor
- children under 12 years of age: consult a doctor

Other information:
- each caplet contains: **sodium 3 mg**
- store at controlled room temperature 20–25°C (68–77°F)

Inactive ingredients: colloidal silicon dioxide, croscarmellose sodium, hydroxypropyl cellulose, hypromellose, lactose monohydrate, magnesium stearate, methylparaben, polydextrose powder, polyethylene glycol, pregelatinized starch, purified water, titanium dioxide, triacetin

How Supplied: Available in a 24 ct. carton.

Tamper Evident Feature: Tavist Sinus Caplets are sealed in individual caplet packages. Use only if the individual caplet seal is unbroken.

Continued on next page

Information on Novartis Consumer Health, Inc., products appearing on these pages is effective as of November 2002.

Tavist Sinus—Cont.

Questions? call **1-800-452-0051** 24 hours a day, 7 days a week.
Novartis Consumer Health, Inc.
Parsippany, NJ 07054-0622   ©2003
Shown in Product Identification Guide, page 515

TAVIST® NIGHTTIME ALLERGY
Antihistamine/Nasal Decongestant Caplets

Active Ingredients
(in each caplet):   **Purpose:**
Diphenhydramine HCl,
   USP, 25 mg .... Antihistamine
Pseudoephedrine HCl,
   USP, 60 mg .... Nasal decongestant

Uses: temporarily relieves these symptoms of the common cold, hay fever or other upper respiratory allergies:
• nasal and sinus congestion
• runny nose
• sneezing
• itchy, watery eyes
• itching of the nose or throat

Warnings:
Do not use
• if you are now taking a prescription monoamine oxidase inhibitor (MAOI) (certain drugs for depression, psychiatric or emotional conditions, or Parkinson's disease), or for 2 weeks after stopping the MAOI drug. If you do not know if your prescription drug contains an MAOI, ask a doctor or pharmacist before taking this product.
• with any other product containing diphenhydramine, even one used on skin.
Ask a doctor before use if you have
• high blood pressure
• heart disease
• glaucoma
• thyroid disease
• diabetes
• a breathing problem such as emphysema or chronic bronchitis
• trouble urinating due to an enlarged prostate gland
Ask a doctor or pharmacist before use if you are taking sedatives or tranquilizers
When using this product
• do not use more than directed
• avoid alcoholic drinks
• marked drowsiness may occur
• alcohol, sedatives, and tranquilizers may increase drowsiness
• be careful when driving a motor vehicle or operating machinery
• excitability may occur, especially in children
Stop use and ask a doctor if
• nervousness, dizziness, or sleeplessness occur
• symptoms do not improve within 7 days or occur with a fever. These could be signs of a serious condition.
If pregnant or breast-feeding, ask a health professional before use.
Keep out of reach of children. In case of overdose, get medical help or contact a poison control center right away.
Directions:
• adults and children 12 years of age and over: take 1 caplet every 4 to 6 hours; not more than 4 caplets in 24 hours or as directed by a doctor
• children under 12 years of age: consult a doctor
Other Information:
• each caplet contains: **sodium 1 mg**
• each caplet contains: **calcium 68 mg**
• store at controlled room temperature 20–25°C (68–77°F)

Inactive Ingredients: carnauba wax, dicalcium phosphate, FD&C Blue 1 aluminum lake, hypromellose, magnesium stearate, microcrystalline cellulose, polyethylene glycol, polysorbate 80, sodium starch glycolate, titanium dioxide

How Supplied: Available in a 24 ct. carton.
Tamper Evident Feature: Tavist® NightTime Allergy Caplets are sealed in individual caplet packages. Use only if the individual caplet seal is unbroken.
Questions? call **1-800-452-0051** 24 hours a day, 7 days a week.
Distributed by:
Novartis Consumer Health, Inc.,
Parsippany, NJ 07054-0622
©2003
Shown in Product Identification Guide, page 515

THERAFLU® Regular Strength
Cold & Sore Throat Night Time Hot Liquid
Pain Reliever-Fever Reducer/Antihistamine/Nasal Decongestant

THERAFLU® Regular Strength
Cold & Cough Night Time Hot Liquid
Pain Reliever-Fever Reducer/Antihistamine/Cough Suppressant/Nasal Decongestant

THERAFLU® Maximum Strength
Severe Cold & Congestion Night Time Hot Liquid
Pain Reliever-Fever Reducer/Antihistamine/Cough Suppressant/Nasal Decongestant

THERAFLU® Maximum Strength
Severe Cold & Congestion Non-Drowsy Hot Liquid
Pain Reliever-Fever Reducer/Cough Suppressant/Nasal Decongestant

THERAFLU® Maximum Strength
Flu & Sore Throat Night Time Hot Liquid
Pain Reliever-Fever Reducer/Antihistamine/Nasal Decongestant

THERAFLU® Maximum Strength
Flu & Congestion Non-Drowsy Hot Liquid
Pain Reliever-Fever Reducer/Cough Suppressant/Expectorant/Nasal Decongestant

THERAFLU® Maximum Strength
Flu & Cough Night Time Hot Liquid
Pain Reliever-Fever Reducer/Antihistamine/Cough Suppressant/Nasal Decongestant

Drug Facts:

Active Ingredients:
(in one packet of Hot Liquid or in 2 caplets)

THERAFLU® Regular Strength
Cold & Sore Throat Nighttime Hot Liquid
Acetaminophen
   650 mg ... Pain reliever/Fever reducer
Chorpheniramine Maleate
   4 mg .... Antihistamine
Pseudoephedrine HCl
   60 mg .... Nasal decongestant

THERAFLU® Regular Strength
Cold & Cough Night Time Hot Liquid
Acetaminophen
   650 mg ... Pain reliever/Fever reducer
Chorpheniramine Maleate
   4 mg .... Antihistamine
Dextromethorphan HBr
   20 mg .... Cough Suppressant
Pseudoephedrine HCl
   60 mg .... Nasal decongestant

THERAFLU® Maximum Strength
Flu & Sore Throat Night Time Hot Liquid
Acetaminophen
   1000 mg . Pain reliever/Fever reducer
Chorpheniramine Maleate
   4 mg .... Antihistamine
Pseudoephredrine HCl
   60 mg .... Nasal decongestant

THERAFLU® Maximum Strength
Flu & Congestion Non-Drowsy Citrus Flavor Hot Liquid
Acetaminophen
   1000 mg . Pain reliever/Fever reducer
Dextromethorphan HBr
   30 mg .... Cough Suppressant
Guaifensein 400 mg .... Expectorant
Pseudoephedrine HCl
   60 mg .... Nasal decongestant

THERAFLU® Maximum Strength
Flu & Cough Night Time Hot Liquid and
THERAFLU® Maximum Strength
Severe Cold & Congestion Night Time Hot Liquid (per dose/packet) & Caplets (per dose/2 caplets)
Acetaminophen
   1000 mg . Pain reliever/Fever reducer
Chorpheniramine Maleate
   4 mg .... Antihistamine
Dextromethorphan HBr
   30 mg .... Cough Suppressant
Pseudoephedrine HCl
   60 mg .... Nasal decongestant

THERAFLU® Maximum Strength
Severe Cold & Congestion Non-Drowsy Hot Liquid (per dose/packet) & Caplets (per dose/2 caplets)
Acetaminophen
   1000 mg . Pain reliever/Fever reducer
Dextromethorphan HBr
   30 mg .... Cough Suppressant
Pseudoephedrine HCl
   60 mg .... Nasal decongestant

Uses:
THERAFLU® Regular Strength
Cold & Sore Throat Night Time Hot Liquid
THERAFLU® Maximum Strength
Flu & Sore Throat Nighttime Apple Cinnamon Flavor Hot Liquid
Pain Reliever-Fever Reducer/Antihistamine/Nasal Decongestant
Temporarily relieves these symptoms:

- Headache
- Minor aches and pains
- Runny nose
- Itchy nose or throat
- Fever
- Minor sore throat pain
- Sneezing
- Nasal and sinus congestion
- Itchy, watery eyes

THERAFLU® Regular Strength Cold & Cough Night Time Hot Liquid THERAFLU® Maximum Strength Flu & Cough Night Time Hot Liquid THERAFLU® Maximum Strength Severe Cold & Congestion Night Time Hot Liquid & Caplets

Pain Reliever-Fever Reducer/Antihistamine/Cough Suppressant/Nasal Decongestant
Temporarily relieves these symptoms:
- Headache
- Minor aches and pains
- Runny nose
- Itchy nose or throat
- Fever
- Minor sore throat pain
- Sneezing
- Nasal and sinus congestion
- Itchy, watery eyes
- Cough due to minor throat and bronchial irritation

THERAFLU® Maximum Strength Severe Cold & Congestion Non-Drowsy Hot Liquid & Caplets

Pain Reliever-Fever Reducer/Cough Suppressant/Nasal Decongestant
Temporarily relieves these symptoms:
- Minor aches and pains
- Minor sore throat pain
- Nasal and sinus congestion
- Cough due to minor throat and bronchial irritation

THERAFLU® Maximum Strength Flu & Congestion Non-Drowsy Hot Liquid

Pain Reliever-Fever Reducer/Cough Suppressant/Expectorant/Nasal Decongestant
Temporarily relieves these symptoms:
- Fever
- Minor aches and pains
- Headache and sore throat
- Nasal congestion
- Chest congestion by loosening phlegm to help clear bronchial passageways

Warnings:

Alcohol Warning: If you consume 3 or more alcoholic drinks every day, ask your doctor whether you should take acetaminophen or any other pain relievers/fever reducers. Acetaminophen may cause liver damage.

Do Not Use if you are now taking a prescription monoamine oxidase inhibitor (MAOI) (certain drugs for depression, psychiatric, or emotional conditions, or Parkinson's disease), or 2 weeks after stopping MAOI drug. If you do not know if your prescription drug contains an MAOI, ask a doctor or pharmacist before taking this product.
- with any other product containing acetaminophen.

Ask a doctor before use if you have:
- heart disease
- high blood pressure
- thyroid disease
- diabetes

- glaucoma
- a breathing problem such as emphysema, asthma, or chronic bronchitis
- trouble urinating due to an enlarged prostate gland
- cough that occurs with smoking, too much phlegm (mucus) or chronic cought that lasts

For THERAFLU® Maximum Strength Severe Cold & Congestion Night Time Hot Liquid & Caplets, THERAFLU® Regular Strength Cold & Cough Night Time Hot Liquid, THERAFLU® Regular Strength Cold & Sore Throat Night Time Hot Liquid, THERAFLU® Maximum Strength Flu & Sore Throat Night Time Hot Liquid, THERAFLU® Maximum Strength Flu & Cough Night Time Hot Liquid products:

Ask a doctor or pharmacist before use if you are
- taking sedatives or tranquilizers.

When using this product:
- do not use more than directed
- avoid alcoholic drinks
- marked drowsiness may occur
- alcohol, sedatives, and tranquilizers may increase drowsiness
- be careful when driving a motor vehicle or operating machinery
- excitability may occur, especially with children

For THERAFLU® Maximum Strength Flu and Sore Throat and Regular Strength Cold & Sore Throat Night Time Hot Liquids
- drowsiness may occur

For Flu & Congestion Non-Drowsy Hot Liquid, Severe Cold & Congestion Hot Liquid Night Time and Non-Drowsy and Caplets Night Time and Non-Drowsy

When using this product:
- do not use more than directed

Stop use and ask a doctor if:
- nervousness, dizziness, or sleeplessness occurs
- symptoms do not improve for 7 days or occur with a fever
- symptoms do not improve for 10 days (pain) or for 3 days (fever)
- sore throat persists for more than 2 days, and occurs with a fever, headache, rash, nausea, or vomiting. These could be signs of a serious condition.

For Flu & Cough Night Time, Flu & Congestion Non-Drowsy, Severe Cold and Congestion (Non-Drowsy & Nighttime), Cold & Cough Night Time Hot Liquids and for Severe Cold & Congestion (Non-Drowsy & Nighttime) Caplets:
- cough persists for more than 7 days, comes back, or occurs with a fever, rash, or persistent headache.

If pregnant or breastfeeding, ask a health care professional before use.

Keep out of reach of children. In case of overdose, get medical help or contact a poison control center right away. Prompt medical attention is critical for adults as well as for children even if you do not notice any signs or symptoms.

Directions:
- take every 6 hours; do not exceed 4 packets in 24 hours or as directed by a doctor.

- adults and children 12 years of age and over: dissolve contents of one packet into 6 oz of hot water; sip while hot
- children under 12 years of age: consult a doctor
- sweeten to taste if desired.

For THERAFLU Cold and Cough and Cold and Sore Throat Night Time Hot Liquids
- take every 4–6 hours; do not exceed 4 packets in 24 hours or as directed by a doctor.
- adults and children 12 years of age and over: dissolve contents of one packet into 6 oz of hot water; sip while hot
- children under 12 years of age: consult a doctor.
- sweeten to taste if desired.

Microwave heating directions (excluding caplets):
- add contents of one package of 6 oz cool water to a microwave-safe cup and stir briskly. Microwave on high 1 ½ minutes or until hot. Do not boil water or overheat, and remember to stir liquid between reheatings.

Inactive Ingredients:

Inactive Ingredients in THERAFLU® Regular Strength Cold & Sore Throat Night Time Hot Liquid, THERAFLU® Regular Strength Cold & Cough Night Time Hot Liquid, THERAFLU® Maximum Strength Severe Cold & Congestion Nighttime Hot Liquid, THERAFLU® Maximum Strength Severe Cold & Congestion Non-Drowsy Hot Liquid: acesulfame K, aspartame, citric acid, D&C Yellow 10, flavors, maltodextrin, silicon dioxide, sodium citrate, sucrose, tribasic calcium phosphate

Inactive Ingredients in THERAFLU® Maximum Strength Flu & Cough Night Time Hot Liquid, THERAFLU® Maximum Strength Flu & Sore Throat Night Time Hot Liquid: acesulfame K, aspartame, citric acid, D&C Yellow 10, FD&C Blue 1, FD&C Red 40, flavors, maltodextrin, silicon dioxide, sodium citrate, sucrose, tribasic calcium phosphate

Inactive ingredients in THERAFLU® Maximum Strength Flu & Congestion Non-Drowsy Citrus Flavor Hot Liquid: acesulfame K, aspartame, calcium phosphate, citric acid, D&C Yellow 10, FD&C Red 40, flavors, maltodextrin, silicon dioxide, sodium citrate, sucrose

Inactive Ingredients in THERAFLU® Maximum Strength Severe Cold & Congestion Night Time Coated Caplets and THERAFLU® Maximum Strength Severe Cold & Congestion Non-Drowsy Coated Caplets: colloidal silicon dioxide, croscarmellose sodium, D&C Yellow 10 aluminum lake, FD&C Yellow 6 aluminum lake, gelatin, hydroxypropyl cellulose, hypromellose, lactose, magnesium

Continued on next page

Information on Novartis Consumer Health, Inc., products appearing on these pages is effective as of November 2002.

Theraflu—Cont.

stearate, methylparaben, polydextrose, polyethylene glycol, pregelatinized starch, titanium dioxide, triacetin.

THERAFLU® Maximum Strength Severe Cold & Congestion Night Time Coated Caplets also contains the inactive ingredient FD&C Blue 1 aluminum lake.

THERAFLU® Maximum Strength Severe Cold & Congestion Non-Drowsy Coated Caplets also contains the inactive ingredient FD&C Red 40 aluminum lake.

Other Information as follows for each product:

THERAFLU® Regular Strength Cold & Sore Throat Night Time Hot Liquid
• each packet contains: **sodium 19 mg**
• Phenylketonurics: Contains Phenylalanine 11 mg per adult dose

THERAFLU® Regular Strength Cold & Cough Night Time Hot Liquid
• each packet contains: **sodium 19 mg**
• Phenylketonurics: Contains Phenylalanine 13 mg per adult dose

THERAFLU® Maximum Strength Severe Cold & Congestion Nighttime Hot Liquid
• each packet contains: **sodium 19 mg**
• Phenylketonurics: Contains Phenylalanine 17 mg per adult dose

THERAFLU® Maximum Strength Severe Cold & Congestion Non-Drowsy Hot Liquid
• each packet contains: **sodium 19 mg**
• Phenylketonurics: Contains Phenylalanine 17 mg per adult dose

THERAFLU® Maximum Strength Flu & Sore Throat Night Time Hot Liquid
• each packet contains: **sodium 12 mg**
• Phenylketonurics: Contains Phenylalanine 22 mg per adult dose

THERAFLU® Maximum Strength Flu & Congestion Non-Drowsy Hot Liquid
• each packet contains: **sodium 15 mg**
• Phenylketonurics: Contains Phenylalanine 24 mg per adult dose

THERAFLU® Maximum Strength Flu & Cough Night Time Hot Liquid
• each packet contains: **sodium 14 mg**
• Phenylketonurics: Contains Phenylalanine 27 mg per adult dose

All products Store at Controlled room temperature 20–25°C (68–77°F)

Specific to THERAFLU® Maximum Strength Severe Cold & Congestion Night Time Coated Caplets and THERAFLU® Maximum Strength Severe Cold & Congestion Non-Drowsy Coated Caplets:

Other Information: each caplet contains: **sodium 6 mg**

How Supplied:
Hot Liquid Formulas:
powder in foil packets, 6 packets per carton

Caplet Formulas:
Caplets in blister, packs of 12's and 24's

Questions? Call **1-800-452-0051**
24 hours a day, 7 days week.
Shown in Product Identification Guide, page 516

THERAFLU® Vapor Stick
Cough Suppressant and Topical Analgesic
Non-Greasy Vapor Cream
Herbal and Menthol Scents

Active Ingredients: **Purpose:**
Camphor 4.8% .... Cough suppressant/ Topical analgesic
Menthol 2.6% .... Cough suppressant/ Topical analgesic

Uses:
on chest and throat, temporarily relieves
• cough due to a cold • cough due to minor throat and bronchial irritation
• cough to help you sleep
on muscles, temporarily relieves
• minor aches and pains

Warnings:
For external use only. Do not take by mouth or place in nostrils
Ask a doctor before use if you have
• cough that occurs with too much phlegm (mucus)
• a persistent or chronic cough such as occurs with smoking, asthma, or emphysema
When using this product, do not
• **heat • microwave**
• **add to hot water or any container where heating water. May cause splattering and result in burns.**
• use more than directed
• apply to eyes, wounds, or damaged skin • bandage tightly
Stop use and ask a doctor if
• muscle aches/pains worsen, persist for more than 7 days or come back
• cough worsens, persists for more than 7 days, comes back, or occurs with fever, rash, or persistent headache. These could be signs of a serious condition.
• too much skin irritation occurs or gets worse
If pregnant or breast-feeding, ask a health professional before use.
Keep out of reach of children. If swallowed, get medical help or contact a poison control center right away.

Directions:
• **see important warnings under "When using this product"**
• adults and children 2 years and older:
  • turn dispenser dial to the right until cream is pushed to the top
  • rub on the throat and chest (cough) or rub on sore muscles (aches/pains) in a thick layer
  • cover with a warm, dry cloth if desired
  • clothing should be loose about throat and chest to help vapors reach the nose and mouth
  • use up to 3 times daily or as directed by a doctor
  • after use, turn dial to the left so cream goes down and replace cap
• children under 2 years of age: Ask a doctor

Other Information:
• store at controlled room temperature 20–25°C (68–77°F)
• close container tightly and store away from heat

Inactive Ingredients: carbomer 940, carbomer 1342, cetyl alcohol, eucalyptus oil, fragrance, methylparaben, propylene glycol, propylparaben, purified water, sodium hydroxide
Questions? call **1-800-452-0051**
24 hours a day, 7 days a week.

How Supplied: 1.7oz stick
Novartis Consumer Health, Inc.
Parsippany, NJ 07054-0622 ©2003

TRIAMINIC® Chest Congestion Expectorant, Nasal Decongestant Citrus Flavor

Drug Facts:

Active Ingredients:
(in each 5 mL, 1 teaspoon)
Guaifenesin, USP, 50 mg .... Expectorant
Pseudoephedrine HCl, USP, 15 mg .... Nasal decongestant

Uses temporarily relieves these symptoms:
• chest congestion by loosening phlegm (mucus) to help clear bronchial passageways • nasal and sinus congestion

Warnings:
Do not use in a child who is taking a prescription monoamine oxidase inhibitor (MAOI) (certain drugs for depression, psychiatric or emotional conditions, or Parkinson's disease), or for 2 weeks after stopping the MAOI drug. If you do not know if the child's prescription drug contains an MAOI, ask a doctor or pharmacist before giving this product.
Ask a doctor before use if the child has
• heart disease • high blood pressure
• thyroid disease • diabetes • glaucoma
• cough that occurs with too much phlegm (mucus) • chronic cough that lasts or a breathing problem such as asthma or chronic bronchitis
When using this product
• do not use more than directed
Stop use and ask a doctor if
• nervousness, dizziness, or sleeplessness occur • symptoms do not improve within 7 days or occur with a fever
• cough persists for more than 7 days, comes back, or occurs with a fever, rash, or persistent headache. These could be signs of a serious condition.
Keep out of reach of children. In case of overdose, get medical help or contact a poison control center right away.

Dosage and Administration
take every 4 to 6 hours; not more than 4 doses in 24 hours or as directed by a doctor

Age	Weight	Dose
4 months to under 1 year[1]	12 to 17 lb	¼ tsp (1.25 mL)
1 to under 2 years[1]	18 to 23 lb	½ tsp (2.5 mL)

Age	Weight	Dose
2 to under 6 years	24 to 47 lb	1 tsp (5 mL)
6 to under 12 years	48 to 95 lb	2 tsp (10 mL)
12 years to adult	96+ lb	4 tsp (20 mL)

[1]The dosage for children under 2 years should be determined by the physician on the basis of the patient's weight, physical condition or other appropriate considerations. Dosages are provided as guidelines.

Other Information
• each teaspoon contains: **sodium 2 mg** • contains no aspirin • store at controlled room temperature 20–25°C (68–77°F)

Inactive Ingredients: benzoic acid, D&C Yellow 10, edetate disodium, FD&C Yellow 6, flavors, glycerin, polyethylene glycol, propylene glycol, purified water, sorbitol, sucrose

How Supplied: Bottles of 4 fl. oz. (118 mL)
Questions: call **1-800-452-0051**
For more information about Triaminic® visit our website at www.triaminic.com
Novartis Consumer Health, Inc.
Parsippany, NJ 07054-0622 ©2003
Shown in Product Identification Guide, page 516

TRIAMINIC® Cold & Allergy
Antihistamine, Nasal Decongestant-Orange Flavor
TRIAMINIC® Cold & Cough
Antihistamine, Cough Suppressant, Nasal Decongestant-Cherry Flavor
TRIAMINIC® Flu, Cough & Fever
Antihistamine, Cough Suppressant, Fever Reducer/Pain Reliever, Nasal Decongestant-Bubble Gum Flavor
TRIAMINIC® Cold & Night Time Cough
Antihistamine, Cough Suppressant, Nasal Decongestant-Grape Flavor

Drug Facts:
Active Ingredients:
(in each 5 mL, 1 teaspoon)
TRIAMINIC® Cold & Allergy
Orange Flavor
Chlorpheniramine maleate,
USP, 1 mg .... Antihistamine
Pseudoephedrine HCl,
USP, 15 mg .... Nasal decongestant
TRIAMINIC® Cold & Cough
Cherry Flavor
Chlorpheniramine maleate,
USP, 1 mg .... Antihistamine
Dextromethorphan HBr,
USP, 5 mg .... Cough suppressant
Pseudoephedrine HCl,
USP, 15 mg .... Nasal decongestant
TRIAMINIC® Flu, Cough & Fever
Bubble Gum Flavor
Acetaminophen,
USP, 160 mg .... Fever reducer/Pain reliever

Chlorpheniramine maleate,
USP, 1 mg .... Antihistamine
Dextromethorphan HBr,
USP, 7.5 mg .... Cough suppressant
Pseudoephedrine HCl,
USP, 15 mg .... Nasal decongestant
TRIAMINIC® Cold & Night Time Cough
Grape Flavor
Chlorpheniramine maleate,
USP, 1 mg .... Antihistamine
Dextromethorphan HBr,
USP, 7.5 mg .... Cough suppressant
Pseudoephedrine HCl,
USP, 15 mg .... Nasal decongestant

Uses: temporarily relieves these symptoms:
TRIAMINIC® Cold & Allergy
Antihistamine, Nasal Decongestant-Orange Flavor
• itchy, watery eyes • runny nose • itchy nose or throat • sneezing • nasal and sinus congestion
TRIAMINIC® Cold & Cough
Antihistamine, Cough Suppressant, Nasal Decongestant-Cherry Flavor
• cough due to minor throat and bronchial irritation • runny nose • nasal and sinus congestion • sneezing • itchy nose or throat • itchy, watery eyes
TRIAMINIC® Flu, Cough & Fever
Antihistamine, Cough Suppressant, Fever Reducer/Pain Reliever, Nasal Decongestant-Bubble Gum Flavor
• fever • minor aches and pains • headache and sore throat • cough due to minor throat and bronchial irritation • nasal and sinus congestion • sneezing • itchy nose or throat • itchy, watery eyes
TRIAMINIC® Cold & Night Time Cough
Antihistamine, Cough Suppressant, Nasal Decongestant-Grape Flavor
• cough due to minor throat and bronchial irritation • runny nose • nasal and sinus congestion • sneezing • itchy nose or throat • itchy, watery eyes

Warnings:
Do not use in a child who is taking a prescription monoamine oxidase inhibitor (MAOI) (certain drugs for depression, psychiatric or emotional conditions, or Parkinson's disease), or for 2 weeks after stopping the MAOI drug. If you do not know if the child's prescription drug contains an MAOI, ask a doctor or pharmacist before giving this product.
Specific to Flu, Cough & Fever: together with another product containing acetaminophen
Specific to Cold & Night Time Cough: if a child is on a sodium-restricted diet unless directed by a doctor
Ask a doctor before use if the child has
• heart disease • high blood pressure • thyroid disease • diabetes • glaucoma • cough that occurs with too much phlegm (mucus) (does not apply to Cold & Allergy) • a breathing problem such as asthma or chronic bronchitis • chronic cough that lasts (does not apply to Cold & Allergy)

Ask a doctor or pharmacist before use if the child is taking sedatives or tranquilizers.
When using this product
• do not use more than directed • excitability may occur, especially in children • marked drowsiness may occur (does not apply to Cold & Allergy) • sedatives and tranquilizers may increase drowsiness
Stop use and ask a doctor if
• nervousness, dizziness, or sleeplessness occur
• symptoms do not improve within 7 days or occur with a fever (does not apply to Flu, Cough, Fever)
• cough persists for more than 7 days, comes back, or occurs with fever, rash, or persistent headache (does not apply to Cold & Allergy)
Specific to Flu, Cough & Fever:
• symptoms do not improve within 5 days (pain) or 3 days (fever).
• sore throat persists for more than 2 days or occurs with headache, fever, rash, nausea or vomiting (does not apply to Cold & Allergy, Cold & Cough, Cold & Night Time Cough)
These could be signs of a serious condition.
Keep out of reach of children. In case of overdose, get medical help or contact a poison control center right away.
Pertains only to Flu, Cough & Fever: Prompt medical attention is critical even if you do not notice any signs or symptoms.

Dosage and Administration[1]
TRIAMINIC® Cold & Allergy
Antihistamine, Nasal Decongestant-Orange Flavor (see below Triaminic® Cold & Cough)
TRIAMINIC® Cold & Cough
Antihistamine, Cough Suppressant, Nasal Decongestant-Cherry Flavor
Take every 4 to 6 hours; not more than 4 doses in 24 hours or as directed by a doctor.
TRIAMINIC® Flu, Cough & Fever
Antihistamine, Cough Suppressant, Fever Reducer/Pain Reliever, Nasal Decongestant-Bubble Gum Flavor (see below Triaminic® Cold & Night Time Cough)
TRIAMINIC® Cold & Night Time Cough
Antihistamine, Cough Suppressant, Nasal Decongestant-Grape Flavor
Take every 6 hours; not more than 4 doses in 24 hours or as directed by a doctor.

Age	Weight	Dose
4 months to under 1 year[2]	12–17 lb	¼ tsp (1.25 mL)
1 to under 2 years[2]	18–23 lb	½ tsp (2.5 mL)

Continued on next page

Information on Novartis Consumer Health, Inc., products appearing on these pages is effective as of November 2002.

Triaminic Cold—Cont.

| 2 to under 6 years[1] | 24–47 lb | 1 tsp (5 mL) |
| 6 to under 12 years | 48–95 lb | 2 tsp (10 mL) |

[1] As with any antihistamine-containing product, use of Triaminic® Formulas containing antihistamines in children under 6 years of age should be only under the advice and supervision of a physician.

[2] The dosage for children under 2 years should be determined by the physician on the basis of patients weight, physical condition or other appropriate considerations. Dosages are provided as guidelines. Antihistamines should not be given to neonates and are contraindicated in newborns.

Other Information:

TRIAMINIC® Cold & Allergy
Antihistamine, Nasal Decongestant-Orange Flavor
• each teaspoon contains: **sodium 2 mg**
• contains no aspirin
• store at controlled room temperature 20–25°C (68–77°F).

TRIAMINIC® Cold & Cough
Antihistamine, Cough Suppressant, Nasal Decongestant-Cherry Flavor
• each teaspoon contains: **sodium 10 mg**
• contains no aspirin
• store at controlled room temperature 20–25°C (68–77°F).

TRIAMINIC® Flu, Cough & Fever
Antihistamine, Cough Suppressant, Fever Reducer/Pain Reliever, Nasal Decongestant-Bubble Gum Flavor
• each teaspoon contains: **sodium 3 mg**
• contains no aspirin
• protect from light
• store at controlled room temperature 20–25°C (68–77°F).

TRIAMINIC® Cold & Night Time Cough
Antihistamine, Cough Suppressant, Nasal Decongestant-Grape Flavor
• each teaspoon contains: **sodium 22 mg**
• contains no aspirin
• store at controlled room temperature 20–25°C (68–77°F).

Inactive Ingredients:

TRIAMINIC® Cold & Allergy
Antihistamine, Nasal Decongestant-Orange Flavor
benzoic acid, edetate disodium, FD&C Yellow 6, flavors, purified water, sorbitol, sucrose

TRIAMINIC® Cold & Cough
Antihistamine, Cough Suppressant, Nasal Decongestant-Cherry Flavor
benzoic acid, FD&C Red 40, flavors, propylene glycol, purified water, sodium chloride, sorbitol, sucrose

TRIAMINIC® Flu, Cough & Fever
Antihistamine, Cough Suppressant, Fever Reducer/Pain Reliever, Nasal Decongestant-Bubble Gum Flavor
acesulfame K, benzoic acid, citric acid, D&C Red 33, dibasic potassium phosphate, disodium edetate, FD&C Red 40, flavors, glycerin, polyethylene glycol, potassium chloride, propylene glycol, purified water, sucrose, other ingredients

TRIAMINIC® Cold & Night Time Cough
Antihistamine, Cough Suppressant, Nasal Decongestant-Grape Flavor
benzoic acid, citric acid, D&C Red 33, dibasic sodium phosphate, FD&C Blue 1, flavors, propylene glycol, purified water, sorbitol, sucrose

How Supplied:

TRIAMINIC® Cold & Cough
TRIAMINIC® Cold & Night Time Cough
Bottles of 4 fl. oz. (118 mL) and 8 fl.oz. (236 mL)
TRIAMINIC® Cold & Allergy
TRIAMINIC® Flu, Cough & Fever
Bottle of 4 fl. oz. (118 mL)
Questions: call 1-800-452-0051
For more information about Triaminic® visit our website at www.triaminic.com
Novartis Consumer Health, Inc.
Parsippany, NJ 07054-0622 ©2002
Shown in Product Identification Guide, page 516

TRIAMINIC® Cough
Cough Suppressant, Nasal Decongestant-Berry Flavor

TRIAMINIC® Cough & Congestion
Cough Suppressant, Nasal Decongestant-Orange Strawberry Flavor

TRIAMINIC® Cough & Sore Throat
Cough Suppressant, Nasal Decongestant, Pain Reliever-Fever Reducer-Grape Flavor

Drug Facts:
Active ingredients (in each 5 mL, 1 teaspoon)
TRIAMINIC® Cough
Berry Flavor
Dextromethorphan HBr, USP 5 mg .... Cough suppressant
Pseudoephedrine, HCl, USP, 15 mg .... Nasal decongestant
TRIAMINIC® Cough & Congestion
Orange Strawberry Flavor
Dextromethorphan HBr, USP, 7.5 mg .... Cough suppressant
Pseudoephedrine, HCl, USP, 15 mg .... Nasal decongestant
TRIAMINIC® Cough & Sore Throat
Grape Flavor
Acetaminophen, USP, 160 mg ..... Fever reducer, Pain reliever
Pseudoephedrine HCl, USP, 15 mg .... Nasal decongestant
Dextromethorphan HBr, USP, 7.5 mg .... Cough suppressant

Uses: Temporarily relieves these symptoms:
TRIAMINIC® Cough
Cough Suppressant, Nasal Decongestant-Berry Flavor (see Cough & Congestion)
TRIAMINIC® Cough & Congestion
Cough Suppressant, Nasal Decongestant-Orange Strawberry Flavor
• cough due to minor throat and bronchial irritation • nasal and sinus congestion

TRIAMINIC® Cough & Sore Throat
Cough Suppressant, Nasal Decongestant, Pain Reliever-Fever Reducer-Grape Flavor
• sore throat pain • minor aches and pains • cough due to minor throat and bronchial irritation • fever • nasal and sinus congestion

Warnings
Do not use in a child who is taking a prescription monoamine oxidase inhibitor (MAOI) (certain drugs for depression, psychiatric or emotional conditions, or Parkinson's disease), or for 2 weeks after stopping the MAOI drug. If you do not know if the child's prescription drug contains an MAOI, ask a doctor or pharmacist before giving this product.
Specific to Cough & Sore Throat: together with another product containing acetaminophen
Specific to Cough: if child is on a sodium-restricted diet unless directed by a doctor
Ask a doctor before use if the child has
• heart disease • high blood pressure • thyroid disease • diabetes • glaucoma • cough that occurs with too much phlegm (mucus) • chronic cough that lasts or a breathing problem such as asthma or chronic bronchitis
Ask a doctor or pharmacist before use if the child is taking sedatives or tranquilizers.
When using this product
• do not use more than directed
Stop use and ask a doctor if
• nervousness, dizziness, or sleeplessness occurs • symptoms do not improve within 7 days or occur with a fever • cough persists for more than 7 days, comes back, or occurs with fever, rash, or persistent headache. These could be signs of a serious condition.
Specific to Cough & Sore Throat:
• sore throat persists for more than 2 days, or occurs with headache, fever, rash, nausea, or vomiting. These could be signs of a serious condition. • symptoms do not improve for 5 days (pain) or 3 days (fever)
Keep out of reach of children. In case of overdose, get medical help or contact a poison control center right away. **Pertains only to cough & sore throat:** Prompt medical attention is critical even if you do not notice any signs or symptoms.

Dosage and Administration
Triaminic® Cough
Cough Suppressant, Nasal Decongestant-Berry Flavor
Take every 4 to 6 hours; not more than 4 doses in 24 hours or as directed by a doctor.
Triaminic® Cough & Congestion
Cough Suppressant, Nasal Decongestant-Orange Strawberry Flavor

Triaminic® Cough & Sore Throat
Cough Suppressant, Nasal Decongestant, Pain Reliever-Fever Reducer-Grape Flavor

Take every 6 hours; not more than 4 doses in 24 hours or as directed by a doctor.

Age	Weight	Dose
4 mos. to under 1 yr[1]	12–17 lb	¼ tsp (1.25 mL)
1 to under 2 years[1]	18–23 lb	½ tsp (2.5 mL)
2 to under 6 years	24–47 lb	1 tsp (5 mL)
6 to under 12 years	48–95 lb	2 tsp (10 mL)

[1]The dosage for children under 2 years should be determined by the physician on the basis of patients weight, physical condition or other appropriate considerations. Dosages are provided as guidelines.

Other Information
TRIAMINIC® Cough
Cough Suppressant, Nasal Decongestant-Berry Flavor
- each teaspoon contains: **sodium 20 mg**
- contains no aspirin • store at controlled room temperature 20–25°C (68–77°F)

TRIAMINIC® Cough & Congestion
Cough Suppressant, Nasal Decongestant-Orange Strawberry Flavor
- each teaspoon contains: **sodium 7 mg**
- contains no aspirin • store at controlled room temperature 20–25°C (68–77°F)

TRIAMINIC® Cough & Sore Throat
Cough Suppressant, Nasal Decongestant, Pain Reliever-Fever Reducer-Grape Flavor
- each teaspoon contains: **sodium 11 mg**
- contains no aspirin • store at controlled room temperature 20–25°C (68–77°F)

Inactive Ingredients
TRIAMINIC® Cough
Cough Suppressant, Nasal Decongestant-Berry Flavor
benzoic acid, FD&C Blue 1, FD&C Red 40, flavors, propylene glycol, purified water, sodium chloride, sorbitol, sucrose

TRIAMINIC® Cough & Congestion
Cough Suppressant, Nasal Decongestant-Orange Strawberry Flavor
benzoic acid, citric acid, dibasic sodium phosphate, edetate disodium, flavors, propylene glycol, purified water, sorbitol, sucrose

TRIAMINIC® Cough & Sore Throat
Cough Suppressant, Nasal Decongestant, Pain Reliever-Fever-Reducer-Grape Flavor
benzoic acid, D&C Red 33, dibasic sodium phosphate, edetate disodium, FD&C Blue 1, FD&C Red 40, flavors, glycerin, polyethylene glycol, propylene glycol, purified water, sucrose, tartaric acid

How Supplied:
Triaminic® Cough
Triaminic® Cough & Congestion
  Bottles of 4 fl. oz. (118 mL)
Triaminic® Cough & Sore Throat
  Bottles of 4 fl. oz. (118 mL)
Questions: call **1-800-452-0051**
For more information about Triaminic® visit our website at www.triaminic.com
Novartis Consumer Health, Inc.
Parsippany, NJ 07054-0622 ©2003
Shown in Product Identification Guide, page 516

TRIAMINIC® Softchews® Allergy
Runny Nose & Congestion—Orange Flavor
Antihistamine, Nasal Decongestant

Drug Facts:

Active Ingredients (in each tablet)
Chlorpheniramine maleate, USP, 1 mg .... Antihistamine
Pseudoephedrine HCl, USP, 15 mg .... Nasal decongestant

Uses: Temporarily relieves these symptoms:
- nasal and sinus congestion
- runny nose
- sneezing
- itchy nose or throat
- itchy, watery eyes

Warnings
Do not use in a child who is taking a prescription monoamine oxidase inhibitor (MAOI) (certain drugs for depression, psychiatric or emotional conditions, or Parkinson's disease), or for 2 weeks after stopping the MAOI drug. If you do not know if the child's prescription drug contains an MAOI, ask a doctor or pharmacist before giving this product.
Ask a doctor before use if the child has
- heart disease • high blood pressure
- thyroid disease • diabetes • glaucoma
- a breathing problem such as chronic bronchitis
Ask a doctor or pharmacist before use if the child is taking sedatives or tranquilizers.
When using this product
- do not use more than directed
- drowsiness may occur • sedatives and tranquilizers may increase drowsiness
- excitability may occur, especially in children
Stop use and ask a doctor if
- nervousness, dizziness, or sleeplessness occur symptoms do not improve within 7 days, or occur with fever, rash, or persistent headache. These could be signs of a serious condition.
Keep out of reach of children. In case of overdose, get medical help or contact a poison control center right away.

Directions
- Let Softchews® tablet dissolve in mouth or chew Softchews® tablet before swallowing, whichever is preferred
- take every 4 to 6 hours; not more than 4 doses in 24 hours or as directed by a doctor

Age	Dose
children 6 to under 12 years of age	2 tablets every 4 to 6 hours
children under 6 years of age	ask a doctor

Other Information:
- each Softchews® tablet contains: **sodium 5 mg**
- Phenylketonurics: Contains **Phenylalanine, 17.6 mg** per Softchews® tablet

Inactive Ingredients
aspartame, carnauba wax, citric acid, crospovidone, ethylcellulose, FD&C Yellow 6 aluminum lake, flavors, fractionated coconut oil, hypromellose, magnesium stearate, mannitol, microcrystalline cellulose, mono- and di-glycerides, oleic acid, polyethylene glycol, silicon dioxide, sodium bicarbonate, sodium chloride, sorbitol, starch, sucrose, triethyl citrate.

How Supplied: 18 Softchews® Tablets
Questions? call **1-800-452-0051** 24 hours a day, 7 days a week.
For more information about Triaminic® visit our website at www.triaminic.com
Novartis Consumer Health, Inc.
Parsippany, NJ 07054-0622 ©2002
Shown in Product Identification Guide, page 516

TRIAMINIC® SOFTCHEWS®
Chest Congestion
Expectorant, Nasal Decongestant

Drug Facts:

Active Ingredients (in each tablet):	Purpose:
Guaifenesin, USP, 50 mg	Expectorant
Pseudoephedrine HCl, USP, 15 mg	Nasal decongestant

Uses: temporarily relieves these symptoms:
- chest congestion by loosening phlegm (mucus) to help clear bronchial passageways
- nasal and sinus congestion

Warnings:
Do not use in a child who is taking a prescription monoamine oxidase inhibitor

Continued on next page

Triaminic Softchews—Cont.

(MAOI) (certain drugs for depression, psychiatric, or emotional conditions, or Parkinson's disease), or for 2 weeks after stopping the MAOI drug. If you do not know if the child's prescription drug contains an MAOI, ask a doctor or pharmacist before giving this product.

Ask a doctor before use if the child has
• heart disease
• high blood pressure
• thyroid disease
• diabetes
• glaucoma
• cough that occurs with too much phlegm (mucus)
• chronic cough that lasts or a breathing problem such as asthma or chronic bronchitis

When using this product • do not use more than directed

Stop use and ask a doctor if • nervousness, dizziness, or sleeplessness occur
• symptoms do not improve within 7 days or occur with a fever.
• cough persists for more than 7 days, comes back, or occurs with a fever, rash, or persistent headache. These could be signs of a serious condition.

Keep out of reach of children. In case of overdose, get medical help or contact a poison control center right away.

Directions: • Let Softchews® tablet dissolve in mouth or chew Softchews® tablet before swallowing, whichever is preferred
• take every 4 to 6 hours; not more than 4 doses in 24 hours or as directed by a doctor

children 6 to under 12 years of age	2 tablets every 4 to 6 hours
children 2 to under 6 years of age	1 tablet every 4 to 6 hours
children under 2 years of age	ask a doctor

Other Information:
• each Softchews® tablet contains: **sodium 9 mg**
• Phenylketonurics: Contains **Phenylalanine, 24.6 mg** per Softchews® tablet
• contains no aspirin • store at controlled room temperature 20–25°C (68–77°F)

Inactive Ingredients: aspartame, citric acid, corn syrup solids, crospovidone, D&C Yellow 10, dibutyl sebacate, ethylcellulose, flavors, hydroxypropyl methylcellulose, magnesium stearate, maltodextrin, mannitol, medium chain triglycerides, microcrystalline cellulose, oleic acid, polyethylene glycol, povidone, silicon dioxide, sodium bicarbonate, sodium chloride, sorbitol, starch, stearic acid, sucrose, triethyl citrate
[See table below]

How Supplied: 18 ct. Softchews® Tablets, NDC 0067-0353-18.
Questions? call **1-800-452-0051** 24 hours a day, 7 days a week.
For more information about Triaminic® visit our website at www.triaminic.com
Distributed by:
Novartis Consumer Health, Inc.
Parsippany, NJ 07054-0622 ®2003
U.S. Pat. No. 5,178,878

TRIAMINIC® Softchews® Cold & Allergy
Antihistamine, Nasal Decongestant-Orange Flavor
TRIAMINIC® Softchews® Cold& Cough
Antihistamine, Cough Suppressant, Nasal Decongestant-Cherry Flavor

Drug Facts:
Active ingredients (in each tablet)
TRIAMINIC® Softchews® Cold & Allergy-Orange Flavor
Chlorpheniramine maleate, USP, 1 mg .... Antihistamine
Pseudoephedrine, HCl, USP, 15 mg .... Nasal decongestant
TRIAMINIC® Softchews® Cold & Cough-Cherry Flavor
Pseudoephedrine HCl, USP, 15 mg .... Nasal decongestant
Dextromethorphan HBr, USP, 5 mg .... Cough suppressant
Chlorpheniramine maleate, USP, 1 mg .... Antihistamine

Uses Temporarily relieves these symptoms:
TRIAMINIC® Softchews® Cold & Allergy
Antihistamine, Nasal Decongestant-Orange Flavor
• nasal and sinus congestion • runny nose • sneezing • itchy nose or throat • itchy, watery eyes
TRIAMINIC® Softchews® Cold & Cough
Antihistamine, Cough Suppressant, Nasal Decongestant-Cherry Flavor
• cough due to minor throat and bronchial irritation • runny nose • nasal and sinus congestion • sneezing • itchy nose or throat • itchy, watery eyes

Warnings:
Do not use in a child who is taking a prescription monoamine oxidase inhibitor (MAOI) (certain drugs for depression, psychiatric or emotional conditions, or Parkinson's disease), or for 2 weeks after stopping the MAOI drug. If you do not know if the child's prescription drug contains an MAOI, ask a doctor or pharmacist before giving this product.
Ask a doctor before use if the child has
• heart disease • high blood pressure • thyroid disease • diabetes • glaucoma • a breathing problem such as asthma or chronic bronchitis
Specific to Cold & Cough: cough that occurs with too much phlegm (mucus) or chronic cough that lasts.
Ask a doctor or pharmacist before use if the child is taking sedatives or tranquilizers.
When using this product
• do not use more than directed
• marked drowsiness may occur (only applies to Softchews Cold and Cough)
• sedatives and tranquilizers may increase drowsiness • excitability may occur, especially in children
Stop use and ask a doctor if
• nervousness, dizziness, or sleeplessness occur • cough persists for more

Triaminic® Softchews® tablets provide effective, symptom-specific relief for your child.

Triaminic® Symptom-Specific Relief	Nasal Congestion	Runny Nose; Sneezing; Itchy Eyes	Dry Cough	Headache	Pain & Fever	Chest Congestion; Productive Cough
Cold & Cough	✔	✔	✔			
Cold & Allergy	✔	✔				
Cough			✔			
Cough & Sore Throat	✔		✔		✔	
Allergy Congestion	✔					
Allergy Sinus & Headache	✔			✔		
Allergy Runny Nose & Congestion	✔	✔				
Chest Congestion	✔					✔

than 7 days (not applicable to: Cold & Allergy) • symptoms do not improve within 7 days, or occur with fever, rash, or persistent headache. These could be signs of a serious condition.

Keep out of reach of children. In case of overdose, get medical help or contact a poison control center right away.

Dosage and Administration[1]:
• Let Softchews® tablet dissolve in mouth or chew Softchews® tablet before swallowing, whichever is preferred • take every 4 to 6 hours; not more than 4 doses in 24 hours or as directed by a doctor

Age	Weight	Dose
2 to under 6 years[1]	24 to 47 lb	1 tablet
6 to under 12 years	48 to 95 lb	2 tablets

[1] As with any antihistamine-containing product, use of Triaminic® Formulas containing antihistamines in children under 6 years of age should be only under the advice and supervision of a physician.

Other Information:
• each Softchews® tablet contains: **sodium 5 mg** • contains no aspirin • store at controlled room temperature 20–25°C (68–77°F)

Triaminic® Softchews® Cold & Allergy Antihistamine, Nasal Decongestant-Orange Flavor • Phenylketonurics: Contains: **Phenylalanine, 17.6 mg** per Softchews® tablet

Triaminic® Softchews® Cold & Cough Antihistamine, Cough Suppressant, Nasal Decongestant-Cherry Flavor • Phenylketonurics: Contains: **Phenylalanine, 17.6 mg** per Softchews® tablet

Inactive Ingredients:
TRIAMINIC® Softchews® Cold & Allergy
Antihistamine, Nasal Decongestant-Orange Flavor
aspartame, carnauba wax, citric acid, crospovidone, ethylcellulose, FD&C Yellow 6 aluminum lake, flavors, fractionated coconut oil, hypromellose, magnesium stearate, mannitol, microcrystalline cellulose, mono- and di-glycerides, oleic acid, polyethylene glycol, silicon dioxide, sodium bicarbonate, sodium chloride, sorbitol, starch, sucrose, triethyl citrate

TRIAMINIC® Softchews® Cold & Cough
Antihistamine, Cough Suppressant, Nasal Decongestant-Cherry Flavor
aspartame, carnauba wax, citric acid, crospovidone, D&C Red 27 aluminum lake, D&C Red 30 aluminum lake, ethylcellulose, FD&C Blue 2 aluminum lake, flavors, fractionated coconut oil, gum arabic, hypromellose, magnesium stearate, mannitol, microcrystalline cellulose, mono- and di-glycerides, oleic

acid, polyethylene glycol, sodium chloride, sorbitol, starch, triethyl citrate, povidone, silicone dioxide, sodium bicarbonate, sucrose

How Supplied: 18 Softchews® Tablets.
Questions: call **1-800-452-0051**
For more information about Triaminic® visit our website at www.triaminic.com
Novartis Consumer Health, Inc.
Parsippany, NJ 07054-0622 ©2003
Shown in Product Identification Guide, page 516

TRIAMINIC® Softchews® Cough & Sore Throat
Cough Suppressant, Nasal Decongestant, Pain Reliever-Fever Reducer-Grape Flavor

Drug Facts:
Active Ingredient: (in each tablet)
Acetaminophen, USP,
160 mg ...... Fever reducer, Pain reliever
Pseudoephedrine HCl, USP,
15 mg .... Nasal decongestant
Dextromethorphan HBr, USP,
5 mg .... Cough suppressant

Uses: Temporarily relieves these symptoms:
• fever • minor aches and pains • headache and sore throat • cough due to minor throat and bronchial irritation • nasal and sinus congestion

Warnings:
Do not use in a child who is taking a prescription monoamine oxidase inhibitor (MAOI) (certain drugs for depression, psychiatric or emotional conditions, or Parkinson's disease), or for 2 weeks after stopping the MAOI drug. If you do not know if the child's prescription drug contains an MAOI, ask a doctor or pharmacist before giving this product.
• together with another product containing acetaminophen
Ask a doctor before use if the child has
• a breathing problem such as chronic bronchitis or asthma • heart disease • high blood pressure • thyroid disease • diabetes • glaucoma • cough that occurs with too much phlegm (mucus) or chronic cough that lasts
Ask a doctor or pharmacist before use if the child is taking sedatives or tranquilizers
When using this product
• do not use more than directed
Stop use and ask a doctor if
• nervousness, dizziness, or sleeplessness occur • symptoms do not improve for 5 days (pain) or 3 days (fever) • cough persists for more than 7 days, comes back or occurs with fever, rash, or headache • sore throat persists for more than 2 days, or occurs with persistent headache, fever, rash, nausea or vomiting. These could be signs of a serious condition.
Keep out of reach of children In case of overdose, get medical help or contact a poison control center right away. Prompt medical attention is critical even if you do not notice any signs or symptoms.

Dosage and Administration
Let Softchews® tablet dissolve in mouth or chew Softchews® tablet before swallowing, whichever is preferred.
• take every 4 to 6 hours • not more than 4 doses in 24 hours.

Age	Weight	Dose
2 to under 6 years	24 to 47 lb	1 tablet
6 to under 12 years	48–97 lb	2 tablets

Other Information:
• contains no aspirin • store at controlled room temperature 20°–25°C (68°–77°F)
• each Softchews® tablet contains **sodium 8 mg**
• Phenylketonurics: Contains **Phenylalanine, 28.1 mg** per tablet

Inactive Ingredients:
aspartame, citric acid, crospovidone, D&C Red 27 aluminum lake, dextrin, ethylcellulose, FD&C Blue 1 aluminum lake, flavors, fractionated coconut oil, hypromellose, magnesium stearate, malto dextrin, mannitol, microcrystalline cellulose, oleic acid, polyethylene glycol, povidone, silicon dioxide, sodium bicarbonate, sodium chloride, sorbitol starch, sucrose, triethyl citrate

How Supplied: 18 Softchews® Tablets
Questions: call **1-800-452-0051**
For more information about Triaminic® visit our website at www.triaminic.com
Novartis Consumer Health, Inc.
Parsippany, NJ 07054-0622 ©2002
Shown in Product Identification Guide, page 516

TRIAMINIC® Vapor Patch® -Mentholated Cherry Scent
Cough Suppressant
TRIAMINIC® Vapor Patch® -Menthol Scent
Cough Suppressant

Drug Facts:
Active ingredients (in each patch)
Camphor 4.7% .... Cough suppressant
Menthol 2.6% .... Cough suppressant

Uses: Temporarily relieves cough due to:
• a cold • minor throat and bronchial irritation to help you sleep

Warnings:
For external use only
Flammable: Keep away from fire or flame

Continued on next page

Information on Novartis Consumer Health, Inc., products appearing on these pages is effective as of November 2002.

Triaminic Vapor Patch—Cont.

Ask a doctor before use if the child has
- cough that occurs with too much phlegm (mucus)
- a persistent or chronic cough such as occurs with asthma

When using this product, do not
- heat • microwave • use near an open flame
- add to hot water or any container where heating water. May cause splattering and result in burns

Additionally, do not
- apply to eyes, wounds, sensitive, irritated or damaged skin
- take by mouth or place in nostrils
- use more than directed

Stop use and ask a doctor if • cough persists for more than 7 days, comes back, or occurs with fever, rash, or persistent headache. These could be signs of a serious condition. • too much skin irritation occurs or gets worse

Keep out of reach of children. If swallowed, get medical help or contact a poison control center right away.

Directions:
- see **important warnings** under "When using this product"
- Children 2 to under 12 years of age:
  - Remove plastic backing
  - Apply patch to the throat or chest
  - If the child has sensitive skin, the patch may be applied to the same area on clothing
  - Clothing should be loose about the throat and chest to help the vapors reach the nose and mouth
  - Apply a new patch up to three times daily or as directed by a doctor
  - May use with other cough suppressant products
- Children under 2 years of age: Ask a doctor
- The patch may not adhere to some types of polyester clothing

Other Information:
- store at controlled room temperature 20–25°C (68–77°F) • protect from excessive heat

Inactive Ingredients:
TRIAMINIC® Vapor Patch®
-Mentholated Cherry Scent Cough Suppressant
acrylic ester copolymer, aloe vera gel, eucalyptus oil, glycerin, karaya, propylene glycol, purified water, wild cherry fragrance

TRIAMINIC® Vapor Patch®
-Menthol Scent Cough Suppressant
acrylic ester, copolymer, aloe vera gel, eucalyptus oil, glycerin, karaya, purified water, spirits of turpentine

How Supplied: Carton of 6 patches, ointment on a breathable cloth patch.
Questions: call **1-800-452-0051**
**For more information about Triaminic®
visit our website at www.triaminic.com**
Novartis Consumer Health, Inc.
Parsippany, NJ 07054-0622
©2003
*Shown in Product Identification
Guide, page 516*

Performance Health, Inc.
**1017 BOYD ROAD
EXPORT, PA 15632-8997**

Direct Inquiries to:
Phone - 724-733-9500
Fax - 724-733-4266
Email - PDR@Biofreeze.com

BIOFREEZE® PAIN RELIEVING GEL

Active Ingredients: Menthol 3.5% and Camphor 0.2%

Inactive Ingredients: Water, Isopropyl Alcohol, Herbal Extract (ILEX Paraguariensis), Carbomer, Triethanolamine, Silicon Dioxide, Methylparaben, FD&C Yellow #5, FD&C Blue #1

Indications: Temporary relief from minor aches and pains of muscles and joints due to arthritis, backache, strains and sprains.

Warnings: For external use only. Ask a doctor before use if you have sensitive skin. Keep away from excessive heat or open flame. Avoid contact with the eyes or mucous membranes. Do not apply to wounds or damaged skin. Do not use with other ointments, creams, sprays or liniments. Do not apply to irritated skin or if excessive irritation develops. Do not bandage. Wash hands after use. If pregnant or breast-feeding, ask a health professional before use. Keep out of reach of children. If accidentally ingested, get medical help or contact a Poison Control Center.

Directions: Adults and children 2 years of age and older: Apply to the affected areas not more than 3 to 4 times daily. Children under 2 years of age, consult physician.

How Supplied: 4 oz. tube, 3 oz. Roll-on and 5 gram packets for home use. 16 oz., 32 oz. and Gallon for professional use.

Pfizer Consumer Group, Pfizer Inc.
**201 TABOR ROAD
MORRIS PLAINS, NJ 07950**

Direct Inquiries to:
1-(800) 223-0182

For Consumer Product Information Call:
1-(800) 223-0182

CELESTIAL SEASONINGS® SOOTHERS® Herbal Throat Drops

Active Ingredients: Menthol and Pectin.

Inactive Ingredients: *HARVEST CHERRY®*—Ascorbic Acid (Vitamin C); Cherry and Elderberry Juices; Citric Acid; Corn Syrup; Natural Flavoring; Oils of Angelica Root, Anise Star, Ginger, Lemon Grass, Sage and White Thyme; Sodium Ascorbate and Sucrose. *HONEY-LEMON CHAMOMILE*—Ascorbic Acid (Vitamin C); Chamomile Flower Extract; Citric Acid; Corn Syrup; Honey; Lemon Juice; Natural Flavoring; Oils of Angelica Root, Anise Star, Ginger, Lemon Grass, Sage and White Thyme; Sodium Ascorbate; Sucrose and Tea Extract. *SUNSHINE CITRUS™*—Ascorbic Acid (Vitamin C); Beta Carotene; Citric Acid; Corn Syrup; Natural Flavoring; Oils of Angelica Root, Anise Star, Ginger, Lemon Grass, Sage and White Thyme; Orange Juice; Sodium Ascorbate, and Sucrose.

Indications: For temporary relief of occasional minor irritation, pain, sore mouth and sore throat. Provides temporary protection of irritated areas in sore mouth and sore throat.

Warnings: If sore throat is severe, persists for more than 2 days, is accompanied or followed by fever, headache, rash, nausea, or vomiting, consult a doctor promptly. If sore mouth symptoms do not improve in 7 days, see your dentist or doctor promptly. KEEP THIS AND ALL DRUGS OUT OF THE REACH OF CHILDREN.

Dosage and Administration: Adults and children 5 years and over: Dissolve 2 drops (one at a time) slowly in the mouth. May be repeated every 2 hours as needed or as directed by a dentist or doctor. Children under 5 years: Consult a dentist or doctor.

How Supplied: Celestial Seasonings Soothers Throat Drops are available in bags of 24 drops. They are available in three flavors: Harvest Cherry, Honey-Lemon Chamomile, Sunshine Citrus.
*Shown in Product Identification
Guide, page 516*

HALLS FRUIT BREEZERS™
Pectin Throat Drops

Active Ingredient (in each drop):
Pectin 7 mg
Purpose:
Oral Demulcent

Uses: temporarily relieves the following symptoms associated with sore mouth and sore throat:
- minor discomfort
- irritated areas

Warnings:
Sore throat warning: if sore throat is severe, persists for more than 2 days, is accompanied or followed by fever, headache, rash, swelling, nausea, or vomiting, consult a doctor promptly. These may be serious.

Stop use and ask a doctor if
- sore mouth does not improve in 7 days
- irritation, pain, or redness persists or worsens

Keep out of reach of children.

Directions:
- adults and children 5 years and over: dissolve 1 or 2 drops (one at a time) slowly in the mouth. Repeat as needed.
- children under 5 years: ask a doctor

Cool Berry
Inactive Ingredients: FD&C blue no. 2, FD&C red no. 40, flavors, glucose syrup, partially hydrogenated cottonseed oil sucrose, titanium dioxide, water

Tropical Chill
Inactive Ingredients: beta carotene, FD&C red no. 40, FD&C yellow no. 5 (tartrazine), FD&C yellow no. 6, flavors, glucose syrup, partially hydrogenated cottonseed oil, soy lecithin, sucrose, titanium dioxide, water

Cool Citrus Blend
Inactive Ingredients: beta carotene, flavors, glucose syrup, partially hydrogenated cottonseed oil, soy lecithin, sucrose, titanium dioxide, water

How Supplied: Halls Fruit Breezers are available in three flavors: Cool Berry, Cool Citrus Blend and Tropical Chill in bags of 25 drops and blisters of 8 (Cool Berry and Tropical Chill)
Shown in Product Identification Guide, page 517

HALLS® MENTHO–LYPTUS®
Cough Suppressant/Oral Anesthetic Drops
[Hols]

Active Ingredient: *MENTHO-LYPTUS®:* Menthol 6.5 mg per drop. *CHERRY:* Menthol 7 mg per drop. *HONEY-LEMON:* Menthol 8 mg per drop. *ICE BLUE PEPPERMINT:* Menthol 11.2 mg per drop. *SPEARMINT:* Menthol 5.6 mg per drop. *STRAWBERRY:* Menthol 3.1 mg per drop.
Purposes: Cough suppressant, Oral anesthetic

Uses: temporarily relieves: • cough due to a cold • occasional minor irritation or sore throat

Warnings:
Sore throat warning: if sore throat is severe, persists for more than 2 days, is accompanied or followed by fever, headache, rash, swelling, nausea, or vomiting, consult a doctor promptly. These may be serious.
Ask a doctor if you have • persistent or chronic cough such as occurs with smoking, asthma, or emphysema • cough accompanied by excessive phlegm (mucus)
Stop use and ask a doctor if • cough persists for more than 1 week, tends to recur, or is accompanied by fever, rash, or persistent headache. These could be signs of a serious condition. • sore mouth does not improve in 7 days • irritation, pain, or redness persists or worsens
Keep out of reach of children.

Directions: *MENTHO-LYPTUS®, CHERRY, HONEY LEMON, ICE BLUE PEPPERMINT and SPEARMINT:* • adults and children 5 years and over: dissolve 1 drop slowly in the mouth. Repeat every hour as needed. • children under 5 years: ask a doctor.
STRAWBERRY: • adults and children 5 years and over: dissolve 2 drops (one at a time) slowly in the mouth. Repeat every hour as needed. • children under 5 years: ask a doctor

Inactive Ingredients: *MENTHOLYPTUS®:* flavors, glucose syrup, sucrose. *CHERRY:* blue 2, flavors, glucose syrup, red 40, sucrose. *HONEY-LEMON:* beta carotene, flavors, glucose syrup, honey, soy lecithin, sucrose. *ICE BLUE PEPPERMINT:* blue 1, flavors, glucose syrup, sucrose. *SPEARMINT:* beta carotene, blue 1, flavors, glucose syrup, soy lecithin, sucrose. *STRAWBERRY:* flavors, glucose syrup, red 40, sucrose.

How Supplied: Halls® *Mentho-Lyptus®* Cough Suppressant Drops are available in single sticks of 9 drops each and in bags of 30. They are available in six flavors: *Regular Mentho-Lyptus®, Cherry, Honey-Lemon, Ice Blue Peppermint, Spearmint and Strawberry.* Regular Mentho-Lyptus®, Cherry, Honey-Lemon and Strawberry flavors are also available in bags of 80 drops. *Mentho-Lyptus® Cherry,* and *Strawberry* are also available in bags of 200 drops.
Shown in Product Identification Guide, page 517

HALLS® PLUS
Cough Suppressant/Oral Anesthetic Drops
[Hols]

Active Ingredients: Each drop contains Menthol 10 mg.
Purposes: Cough suppressant, Oral anesthetic

Uses: temporarily relieves: • cough due to a cold • occasional minor irritation or sore throat

Warnings: Sore throat warning: if sore throat is severe, persists for more than 2 days, is accompanied or followed by fever, headache, rash, swelling, nausea, or vomiting, consult a doctor promptly. These may be serious.
Ask a doctor before use if you have • persistent or chronic cough such as occurs with smoking, asthma, or emphysema • cough accompanied by excessive phlegm (mucus)
Stop use and ask a doctor if • cough persists for more than 1 week, tends to recur, or is accompanied by fever, rash, or persistent headache. These could be signs of a serious condition. • sore mouth does not improve in 7 days • irritation, pain, or redness persists or worsens
Keep out of reach of children.

Directions: • adults and children 5 years and over: dissolve 1 drop slowly in the mouth. Repeat every hour as needed.
• children under 5 years: ask a doctor

Inactive Ingredients: MENTHO-LYPTUS®: carrageenan, flavors, glucose syrup, glycerin, partially hydrogenated cottonseed oil, pectin, soy lecithin, sucrose. CHERRY: blue 2, carrageenan, flavors, glucose syrup, glycerin, partially hydrogenated cottonseed oil, pectin, red 40, soy lecithin, sucrose. HONEY-LEMON: beta carotene, carrageenan, flavors, glucose syrup, glycerin, honey, partially hydrogenated cottonseed oil, pectin, soy lecithin, sucrose.

How Supplied: Halls® Plus Cough Suppressant / Throat Drops are available in single sticks of 10 drops each and in bags of 25 drops. They are available in three flavors: Regular Mentho-Lyptus®, Cherry and Honey-Lemon.
Shown in Product Identification Guide, page 517

HALLS® SUGAR FREE
HALLS® SUGAR FREE SQUARES
MENTHO-LYPTUS®
Cough Suppressant/Oral Anesthetic Drops
[Hols]

Active Ingredient: Halls® Sugar Free: BLACK CHERRY and CITRUS BLEND: Menthol 5 mg per drop. MOUNTAIN MENTHOL: Menthol 5.8 mg per drop.
Halls® Sugar Free Squares: BLACK CHERRY: Menthol 5.8 mg per drop. MOUNTAIN MENTHOL: Menthol 6.8 mg per drop.
Purposes: Cough suppressant, Oral anesthetic

Uses: temporarily relieves: • cough due to a cold • occasional minor irritation or sore throat

Warnings:
Sore throat warning: if sore throat is severe, persists for more than 2 days, is accompanied or followed by fever, headache, rash, swelling, nausea, or vomiting, consult a doctor promptly. These may be serious.
Ask a doctor before use if you have • persistent or chronic cough such as occurs with smoking, asthma, or emphysema • cough accompanied by excessive phlegm (mucus)
Stop use and ask a doctor if • cough persists for more than 1 week, tends to recur, or is accompanied by fever, rash, or persistent headache. These could be signs of a serious condition. • sore mouth does not improve in 7 days • irritation, pain, or redness persists or worsens
Keep out of reach of children.

Directions: • adults and children 5 years and over: dissolve 1 drop slowly in mouth. Repeat every hour as needed.
• children under 5 years: ask a doctor

Continued on next page

Halls Sugar Free—Cont.

Additional Information:
Halls® Sugar Free:
Exchange Information*:
1 Drop = Free Exchange
10 Drops = 1 Fruit
*The dietary exchanges are based on the *Exchange Lists for Meal Planning,* Copyright ©1989 by the American Diabetes Association, Inc. and the American Dietetic Association.
Excess consumption may have a laxative effect.

Inactive Ingredients: Halls Sugar Free BLACK CHERRY: acesulfame potassium, aspartame, blue 1, carboxymethylcellulose sodium, flavors, isomalt, red 40 **Phenylketonurics: Contains 2 mg Phenylalanine Per Drop.** CITRUS BLEND: acesulfame potassium, aspartame, carboxymethylcellulose sodium, flavors, isomalt, yellow 5 (tartrazine) **Phenylketonurics: Contains 2 mg Phenylalanine Per Drop.** MOUNTAIN MENTHOL: acesulfame potassium, aspartame, carboxymethylcellulose sodium, flavors, isomalt **Phenylketonurics: Contains 2 mg Phenylalanine Per Drop.**

How Supplied: Halls® Sugar Free: Halls® Sugar Free Mentho-Lyptus® Cough Suppressant Drops are available in bags of 25 drops. They are available in three flavors: Black Cherry, Citrus Blend and Mountain Menthol. Halls® Sugar Free Squares: Halls® Sugar Free Squares Mentho-Lyptus® Cough Suppressant Drops are available in single sticks of 9 drops each. They are available in two flavors: Black Cherry and Mountain Menthol.
Shown in Product Identification Guide, page 517

HALLS DEFENSE™ MULTI-BLEND SUPPLEMENT DROPS

Supplement Facts/Ingredients:
Supplement Facts
Serving Size 1 Drop

	Amount Per Drop	% Daily Value*
Calories	15	
Sodium	10 mg	<1%*
Total Carbohydrate	4 g	1%*
Sugars	3 g	†
Vitamin C	60 mg	100%
Zinc	1.5 mg	10%
Standard Echinacea Root Extract	15 mg	†
Echinecea angustifolia and Echinecea purpurea)

* Percent Daily Value (DV) are based on a 2,000 calorie diet.

† Daily Value (DV) not established.

Other Ingredients: Sugar, Glucose Syrup, Sodium Ascorbate, Citric Acid, Cottonseed Oil, Natural Flavoring, Ascorbic Acid, Zinc Sulfate, Red 40, Blue 1, Oils of Angelica Root, Anise Star, Ginger, Lemon Grass, Sage and White Thyme.

Description: Halls Defense Vitamin C Supplement Drops help you keep going. Each drop provides 100% of the Daily Value of Vitamin C, Zinc to help support your natural resistance system*, plus Echinecea

> *** This statement has not been evaluated by the Food & Drug Administration. This product is not intended to diagnose, treat, cure, or prevent any disease.**

Indications: Dietary Supplementation

Warnings: Do not use if you have a severe systemic illness such as tuberculosis, leukosis, collagen disease, multiple sclerosis or similar condition. Do not use if you have allergies to the daisy family (Asteraceae). If you are pregnant or nursing a baby, seek the advice of a health professional before using this product. Keep out of the reach of children.

Suggested Use: As a dietary supplement, take one drop 4 times per day. Not recommended for use for more than 8 weeks consecutively.

How Supplied: Halls Defense™ Multiblend Supplement drops are available in Harvest Cherry in bags of 25 drops.
Shown in Product Identification Guide, page 516

HALLS DEFENSE™ Vitamin C Supplement Drops
[Hols]

Ingredients: *ASSORTED CITRUS*: Sugar, Glucose Syrup, Sodium Ascorbate, Citric Acid, Natural Flavoring, Ascorbic Acid, Color Added (with Soy Lecithin) and Red 40. *STRAWBERRY*: Sugar, Glucose Syrup, Sodium Ascorbate, Citric Acid, Ascorbic Acid, Natural and Artificial Flavoring, Color Added (Carmine).

Description: Halls Defense™ Vitamin C Supplement Drops are a delicious way to get 100% of the Daily Value of Vitamin C. Each drop provides 60 mg of Vitamin C (100% of the Daily Value).

Indications: Dietary Supplementation.

How Supplied: Halls Defense™ Vitamin C Supplement Drops are available in a Citrus Assortment (lemon, sweet grapefruit, orange) with all natural flavors and Strawberry in sticks of 9 drops each and in bags of 30 and 80 drops.
Shown in Product Identification Guide, page 516

TRIDENT FOR KIDS™
Sugarless Gum with Recaldent™
[Tri-dent for kids]

Ingredients: *BERRY BUBBLE GUM*: Sorbitol, Gum Base, Mannitol, Glycerin, Artificial and Natural Flavoring, Xylitol, Calcium Casein Peptone-Calcium Phosphate (Lactose-Free Milk Derivative)**, Soy Lecithin, Acetylated Monoglycerides, Sucralose, Red 40 Lake and Blue 2 Lake. **Contains a Milk-Based Ingredient.**

RECALDENT™**: A patented ingredient derived from casein, a bovine phosphoprotein found in milk. RECALDENT™ is a trademark of Bonlac Bioscience PTY Ltd.

Description: Trident For Kids™ is a dental care gum that remineralizes tooth enamel by safely delivering calcium and phosphate directly to teeth. In addition to strengthening teeth, chewing Trident for Kids™ may reduce the risk of tooth decay.

Directions: Trident For Kids™ chewed after meals provides an ideal way to deliver the benefits of Recaldent™, to help remove food particles that may adhere to teeth, and to help minimize plaque acids.

How Supplied: Trident For Kids™ with Recaldent™ is available in Berry Bubble Gum Flavor in an 8-stick pack.
Shown in Product Identification Guide, page 517

TRIDENT WHITE™
[Tri-dent White]
Sugarless Gum with Recaldent™

Ingredients: *PEPPERMINT*: Sorbitol, Gum Base, Maltitol, Mannitol, Artificial and Natural Flavoring; Less Than 2% of: Acacia, Acesulfame Potassium, Aspartame, BHT (To Maintain Freshness), Calcium Casein Peptone-Calcium Phosphate (Lactose-Free Milk Derivative)**, Candelilla Wax, Sodium Stearate and Titanium Dioxide (Color).
Contains a Milk Derived Ingredient.
Phenylketonurics: Contains Phenylalanine.

Ingredients: *WINTERGREEN*: Sorbitol, Gum Base, Maltitol, Mannitol, Artificial and Natural Flavoring; Less Than 2% of: Acacia, Acesulfame Potassium, Aspartame, BHT (To Maintain Freshness), Calcium Casein Peptone-Calcium Phosphate (Lactose-Free Milk Derivative)**, Candelilla Wax, Glycerin, Sodium Stearate, Soy Lecithin and Titanium Dioxide (Color).
Contains a Milk Derived Ingredient.
Phenylketonurics: Contains Phenylalanine.

Ingredients: *SPEARMINT*: Sorbitol, Gum Base, Maltitol, Mannitol, Artificial and Natural Flavoring; Less Than 2% of:

Acacia, Acesulfame Potassium, Aspartame, BHT (To Maintain Freshness), Calcium Casein Peptone-Calcium Phosphate (Lactose-Free Milk Derivative)**, Candelilla Wax, Sodium Stearate, Soy Lecithin and Titanium Dioxide (Color). **Contains a Milk Derived Ingredient. Phenylketonurics:** **Contains Phenylalanine.**
RECALDENT™**: A patented ingredient derived from casein, a bovine phosphoprotein found in milk. RECALDENT is a trademark of Bonlac Bioscience International PTY LTD.

Description: Trident White™ is a whitening gum that uses proprietary surfactant technology to help break up and gently remove stains from teeth. In addition to whitening teeth, chewing Trident White™ remineralizes tooth enamel by delivering calcium and phosphate beneath the tooth's surface.

Directions: When used as a part of a daily oral care regimen, Trident White helps gently remove stains caused by common beverages and food items consumed every day.

How Supplied: Trident White™ is available in Peppermint, Wintergreen and Spearmint flavors in a 12-pellet blister foil.

Shown in Product Identification Guide, page 517

Pfizer Consumer Healthcare, Pfizer Inc.

201 TABOR ROAD
MORRIS PLAINS, NJ 07950

Address Questions & Comments to:
Consumer Affairs, Pfizer Consumer Group
182 Tabor Road
Morris Plains, NJ 07950
For Medical Emergencies/Information Contact:
1-(800)-223-0182
1-800-524-2624 (Spanish)
1-(800)-378-1783 (e.p.t.)
1-(800)-337-7266 (e.p.t.-Spanish)

ACTIFED® Cold & Allergy Tablets
[ăk 'tuh-fĕd]

Drug Facts:

Active Ingredients:
(in each tablet)　　　　　**Purposes:**
Pseudoephedrine
  HCl 60 mg .... Nasal decongestant
Triprolidine
  HCl 2.5 mg .... Antihistamine

Uses:
- temporarily relieves these symptoms of hay fever or other upper respiratory allergies:
  - runny nose
  - sneezing
- itchy, watery eyes
- itching of the nose or throat
- temporarily relieves nasal congestion due to the common cold

Warnings:
Do not use if you are now taking a prescription monoamine oxidase inhibitor (MAOI) (certain drugs for depression, psychiatric, or emotional conditions, or Parkinson's disease), or for 2 weeks after stopping the MAOI drug. If you do not know if your prescription drug contains an MAOI, ask a doctor or pharmacist before taking this product.

Ask a doctor before use if you have:
- heart disease
- glaucoma
- thyroid disease
- diabetes
- high blood pressure
- trouble urinating due to an enlarged prostate gland
- a breathing problem such as emphysema or chronic bronchitis

Ask a doctor or pharmacist before use if you are taking sedatives or tranquilizers

When using this product:
- **do not use more than directed**
- drowsiness may occur
- avoid alcoholic drinks
- alcohol, sedatives, and tranquilizers may increase drowsiness
- be careful when driving a motor vehicle or operating machinery
- excitability may occur, especially in children

Stop use and ask a doctor if:
- you get nervous, dizzy, or sleepless
- symptoms do not improve within 7 days or are accompanied by fever

If pregnant or breast-feeding, ask a health professional before use.

Keep out of reach of children. In case of overdose, get medical help or contact a Poison Control Center right away.

Directions:
- take every 4 to 6 hours
- do not take more than 4 doses in 24 hours

adults and children 12 years of age and over	1 tablet
children 6 to under 12 years of age	½ tablet
children under 6 years of age	ask a doctor

Other Information:
- store at 59° to 77°F in a dry place
- protect from light

Inactive Ingredients: Flavor, hypromellose, lactose, magnesium stearate, polyethylene glycol, potato starch, povidone, sucrose, and titanium dioxide

Questions? call **1-800-223-0182**, Monday to Friday, 9 AM – 5 PM EST

How Supplied: Boxes of 12 and 24 tablets.

Shown in Product Identification Guide, page 517

ACTIFED® Cold & Sinus MS Caplets
Maximum Strength
[ak 'tuh-fed]

Drug Facts:

Active Ingredients:
(in each caplet)†　　　　　**Purposes:**
Acetaminophen
500 mg .... Pain reliever/fever reducer
Chlorpheniramine
maleate 2 mg .... Antihistamine
Pseudoephedrine
HCl 30 mg .... Nasal decongestant

†Dissolution differs from USP specification

Uses:
- temporarily relieves sinus congestion and pressure
- temporarily relieves these symptoms of hay fever:
  - itchy, watery eyes
  - sneezing
  - itching of the nose or throat
  - runny nose
- temporarily relieves these symptoms due to the common cold:
  - nasal congestion
  - headache
  - minor aches and pains
  - fever

Warnings:
Alcohol warning: If you consume 3 or more alcoholic drinks every day, ask your doctor whether you should take acetaminophen or other pain relievers/fever reducers. Acetaminophen may cause liver damage.
Do not use:
- with another product containing any of these active ingredients
- if you are now taking a prescription monoamine oxidase inhibitor (MAOI) (certain drugs for depression, psychiatric, or emotional conditions, or Parkinson's disease), or for 2 weeks after stopping the MAOI drug. If you do not know if your prescription drug contains an MAOI, ask a doctor or pharmacist before taking this product.
Ask a doctor before use if you have:
- heart disease
- glaucoma
- diabetes
- thyroid disease
- high blood pressure
- trouble urinating due to an enlarged prostate gland
- a breathing problem such as emphysema or chronic bronchitis
Ask a doctor or pharmacist before use if you are taking sedatives or tranquilizers
When using this product:
- **do not use more than directed**
- drowsiness may occur

Continued on next page

This product information was prepared in November 2002. On these and other Pfizer Consumer Healthcare Products, detailed information may be obtained by addressing Pfizer Consumer Healthcare, Pfizer, Inc., Morris Plains, NJ 07950

Actifed Cold & Sinus—Cont.

- excitability may occur, especially in children
- avoid alcoholic drinks
- alcohol, sedatives, and tranquilizers may increase drowsiness
- be careful when driving a motor vehicle or operating machinery

Stop use and ask a doctor if:
- you get nervous, dizzy, or sleepless
- new symptoms occur
- symptoms do not improve
- you need to use more than 10 days
- fever occurs and lasts more than 3 days
- redness or swelling is present

If pregnant or breast-feeding, ask a health professional before use.

Keep out of reach of children.

Overdose warning: Taking more than the recommended dose may cause liver damage. In case of overdose, get medical help or contact a Poison Control Center right away. Quick medical attention is critical for adults as well as for children even if you do not notice any signs or symptoms.

Directions:
- do not use more than directed (see overdose warning)
- adults and children 12 years of age and over: 2 caplets
- take every 6 hours while symptoms persist
- do not take more than 8 caplets in 24 hours, or as directed by a doctor
- children under 12 years of age: ask a doctor

Other Information:
- store at 59° to 77°F in a dry place

Inactive Ingredients: Calcium stearate, candelilla wax, croscarmellose sodium, crospovidone, D&C yellow no. 10 aluminum lake, FD&C yellow no. 6 aluminum lake, hypromellose, microcrystalline cellulose, polyethylene glycol, polysorbate 80, povidone, pregelatinized starch, stearic acid, and titanium dioxide.

Questions? call **1-800-223-0182**, Monday to Friday, 9AM – 5PM EST

How Supplied: Boxes of 20
Shown in Product Identification Guide, page 517

ANUSOL®
Hemorrhoidal Ointment
[ă′nū-sōl″]

Drug Facts:

Active Ingredients:	Purpose:
Mineral oil 46.6%	Skin protectant
Pramoxine HCl 1%	Pain reliever
Zinc oxide 12.5%	Skin protectant

Uses:
- temporarily relieves these local symptoms associated with hemorrhoids and other anorectal disorders:
  - pain
  - soreness
  - burning
  - itching
- temporarily forms a protective coating over inflamed tissues to help prevent drying of tissues

Warnings:
For external use only
When using this product
- do not use more than directed unless told to do so by a doctor
- do not put into the rectum by using fingers or any mechanical device or applicator

Stop use and ask a doctor if
- allergic reaction occurs
- redness, irritation, swelling, pain, or other symptoms begin or increase
- rectal bleeding occurs
- condition worsens or does not improve within 7 days

Keep out of reach of children. If swallowed, get medical help or contact a Poison Control Center right away.

Directions:
- adults: apply externally to the affected area up to 5 times daily
  - when practical, clean the affected area with mild soap and warm water and rinse thoroughly
  - gently dry by patting or blotting with toilet tissue or a soft cloth before applying
  - to use dispensing cap
    - attach it to tube, lubricate well, then gently insert part way into anus
    - squeeze tube to deliver medication
    - thoroughly cleanse dispensing cap after use
- children under 12 years of age: ask a doctor

Other Information: • store at 59° to 77°F

Inactive Ingredients: benzyl benzoate, calcium phosphate dibasic, cocoa butter, glyceryl monooleate, glyceryl monostearate, kaolin, peruvian balsam, and polyethylene wax

Questions? call **1-800-223-0182**, Monday to Friday, 9 AM - 5 PM EST

How Supplied:—1-oz (28.3g) tubes with plastic applicator.
Shown in Product Identification Guide, page 517

ANUSOL®
Hemorrhoidal Suppositories
[ă′nū-sōl″]

Drug Facts:

Active Ingredient:	Purpose:
Topical starch 51%	Skin protectant

Uses:
- temporarily relieves these local symptoms associated with hemorrhoids and other anorectal disorders:
  - itching
  - burning
  - discomfort
- temporarily forms a protective coating over inflamed tissues to help protect drying of tissue

Warnings:
For rectal use only
When using this product
- do not use more than directed unless directed by a doctor

Stop use and ask a doctor if
- rectal bleeding occurs
- condition worsens or does not improve within 7 days

If pregnant or breast-feeding, ask a health professional before use.

Keep out of reach of children. If swallowed, get medical help or contact a Poison Control Center right away.

Directions:
- see bottom panel for directions for opening suppository wrapper
- adults: insert one (1) suppository rectally up to 6 times daily or after each bowel movement by following these steps:
  - when practical, clean the affected area with mild soap and warm water and rinse thoroughly
  - gently dry by patting or blotting with toilet tissue or a soft cloth before applying
  - detach one (1) suppository from the strip of suppositories
  - remove wrapper before inserting into the rectum
- children under 12 years of age: ask a doctor

Directions for opening Suppository Wrapper:
- Detach (1) one suppository from the strip of suppositories.
- Remove wrapper before inserting into the rectum as follows: Hold suppository upright (with words "pull apart" at top) and carefully separate the plastic wrapper tabs with your fingers.

- Peel plastic slowly and evenly down both sides, exposing suppository.
- Avoid excessive handling of suppository since it is designed to melt at body temperature. If suppository seems soft, hold in plastic wrapper under cold water for 2 or 3 minutes.

Other Information:
- store at 59° to 77°F to avoid melting

Inactive Ingredients: benzyl alcohol, hydrogenated vegetable oil, and tocopheryl acetate

Questions? call **1-800-223-0182**, Monday to Friday, 9 AM - 5 PM EST

How Supplied: In boxes of 12 or 24 in plastic strips. Store at 59–77°F to avoid melting.
Shown in Product Identification Guide, page 517

ANUSOL HC-1 Hydrocortisone
Anti-Itch Ointment
[ă′nū-sōl″]

Drug Facts:

Active Ingredient:	Purpose:
Hydrocortisone acetate 1.12% (equivalent to hydrocortisone 1%)	Anti-itch

Uses:
- temporarily relieves external anal itching and itching associated with minor skin irritations and rashes

- other uses of this product should be only under the advice and supervision of a doctor

Warnings:
For external use only
Do not use
- for the treatment of diaper rash. Consult a doctor.

When using this product
- avoid contact with the eyes
- do not use more than directed unless told to do so by a doctor
- do not put into the rectum by using fingers or any mechanical device or applicator

Stop use and ask a doctor if
- condition worsens, or if symptoms persist for more than 7 days or clear up and occur again within a few days, and do not begin use of any other hydrocortisone product unless you have asked a doctor
- rectal bleeding occurs

Keep out of reach of children. If swallowed, get medical help or contact a Poison Control Center right away.

Directions:
- adults: apply externally to the affected area not more than 3 to 4 times daily
- when practical, clean the affected area with mild soap and warm water and rinse thoroughly
- gently dry by patting or blotting with toilet tissue or a soft cloth before applying
- children under 12 years of age: ask a doctor

Other Information: • store at 59° to 77° F

Inactive Ingredients: diazolidinyl urea, methylparaben, microcrystalline wax, mineral oil, propylene glycol, propylparaben, sorbitan sesquioleate, and white petrolatum

Questions? call **1-800-223-0182**, Monday to Friday, 9 AM - 5 PM EST

How Supplied: 0.7oz (19.8g) tube.
Shown in Product Identification Guide, page 517

BENADRYL® Allergy Kapseals® Capsules (also available in Ultratab™ Tablets)
[bĕ 'nă-drĭl]

Drug Facts:

Active Ingredient: **Purpose:**
(in each capsule)
Diphenhydramine HCl
   25 mg .... Antihistamine

Uses:
- temporarily relieves these symptoms due to hay fever or other upper respiratory allergies:
  - runny nose
  - sneezing
  - itchy, watery eyes
  - itching of the nose or throat
- temporarily relieves these symptoms due to the common cold:
  - runny nose
  - sneezing

Warnings:
Do not use with any other product containing diphenhydramine, including one applied topically.

Ask a doctor before use if you have:
- glaucoma
- trouble urinating due to an enlarged prostate gland
- a breathing problem such as emphysema or chronic bronchitis

Ask a doctor or pharmacist before use if you are taking sedatives or tranquilizers

When using this product:
- marked drowsiness may occur
- avoid alcoholic drinks
- alcohol, sedatives, and tranquilizers may increase drowsiness
- be careful when driving a motor vehicle or operating machinery
- excitability may occur, especially in children

If pregnant or breast-feeding, ask a health professional before use.

Keep out of reach of children. In case of overdose, get medical help or contact a Poison Control Center right away.

Directions:
- take every 4 to 6 hours
- do not take more than 6 doses in 24 hours

adults and children 12 years of age and over	25 mg to 50 mg (1 to 2 capsules)
children 6 to under 12 years of age	12.5 mg** to 25 mg (1 capsule)
children under 6 years of age	ask a doctor

**12.5 mg dosage strength is not available in this package. Do not attempt to break capsules.

Other Information:
- store at 59° to 77°F in a dry place
- protect from light

Inactive Ingredients D&C red no. 28, FD&C blue no. 1, FD&C red no. 3, FD&C red no. 40, gelatin, glyceryl monooleate, lactose, magnesium stearate, and titanium dioxide. Printed with black edible ink.

Questions? call **1-800-524-2624** (English/Spanish), weekdays, 9 AM–5 PM EST

How Supplied: Benadryl tablets are supplied in boxes of 24 and 48, bottle of 100; capsules are supplied in boxes of 24 and 48.
Shown in Product Identification Guide, page 517

BENADRYL® Dye-Free Allergy Liqui-Gels® Softgels
[bĕ 'nă-drĭl]

Drug Facts:

Active Ingredient:
(in each softgel)   **Purpose:**
Diphenhydramine
   HCl 25 mg .... Antihistamine

Uses:
- temporarily relieves these symptoms due to hay fever or other upper respiratory allergies:
  - runny nose
  - sneezing
  - itchy, watery eyes
  - itching of the nose or throat
- temporarily relieves these symptoms due to the common cold:
  - runny nose
  - sneezing

Warnings:
Do not use with any other product containing diphenhydramine, including one applied topically.

Ask a doctor before use if you have:
- glaucoma
- trouble urinating due to an enlarged prostate gland
- a breathing problem such as emphysema or chronic bronchitis

Ask a doctor or pharmacist before use if you are taking sedatives or tranquilizers

When using this product:
- marked drowsiness may occur
- avoid alcoholic drinks
- alcohol, sedatives, and tranquilizers may increase drowsiness
- be careful when driving a motor vehicle or operating machinery
- excitability may occur, especially in children

If pregnant or breast-feeding, ask a health professional before use.

Keep out of reach of children. In case of overdose, get medical help or contact a Poison Control Center right away.

Directions:
- take every 4 to 6 hours
- do not take more than 6 doses in 24 hours

adults and children 12 years of age and over	25 mg to 50 mg (1 to 2 softgels)
children 6 to under 12 years of age	12.5 mg** to 25 mg (1 softgel)
children under 6 years of age	ask a doctor

**12.5 mg dosage strength is not available in this package. Do not attempt to break softgels.

Other Information:
- store at 59° to 77°F in a dry place
- protect from heat, humidity, and light

Inactive Ingredients: Gelatin, glycerin, polyethylene glycol 400, and sorbi-

Continued on next page

This product information was prepared in November 2002. On these and other Pfizer Consumer Healthcare Products, detailed information may be obtained by addressing Pfizer Consumer Healthcare, Pfizer, Inc., Morris Plains, NJ 07950

Benadryl Dye-Free—Cont.

tol. Softgels are imprinted with edible dye-free ink.

Questions? call **1-800-524-2624** (English/Spanish), weekdays, 9 AM–5 PM EST

How Supplied: Benadryl® Dye-Free Allergy Liqui-Gels® Softgels are supplied in boxes of 24.
Liqui-Gels is a registered trademark of R.P. Scherer Corporation.

Shown in Product Identification Guide, page 517

BENADRYL® Allergy & Cold Caplets
[bĕ 'nă-drĭl]
Capsule Shaped Tablets

Drug Facts:

Active Ingredients:
(in each caplet)   **Purposes:**
Acetaminophen
  500 mg ...... Pain reliever/fever reducer
Diphenhydramine HCl
  12.5 mg .... Antihistamine
Pseudoephedrine HCl
  30 mg .... Nasal decongestant

Uses:
• temporarily relieves these symptoms of hay fever and the common cold:
  • runny nose
  • nasal congestion
  • headache
  • fever
  • sore throat
  • muscular aches
  • sneezing
  • minor aches and pains
• temporarily relieves these additional symptoms of hay fever:
  • itching of the nose or throat
  • itchy, watery eyes

Warnings:
Alcohol warning: If you consume 3 or more alcoholic drinks every day, ask your doctor whether you should take acetaminophen or other pain relievers/fever reducers. Acetaminophen may cause liver damage.
Do not use:
• with another product containing any of these active ingredients
• if you are now taking a prescription monoamine oxidase inhibitor (MAOI) (certain drugs for depression, psychiatric, or emotional conditions, or Parkinson's disease), or for 2 weeks after stopping the MAOI drug. If you do not know if your prescription drug contains an MAOI, ask a doctor or pharmacist before taking this product.
• with any other product containing diphenhydramine, including one applied topically.
Ask a doctor before use if you have:
• heart disease
• glaucoma
• thyroid disease
• diabetes
• high blood pressure
• trouble urinating due to an enlarged prostate gland
• a breathing problem such as emphysema or chronic bronchitis

Ask a doctor or pharmacist before use if you are taking sedatives or tranquilizers
When using this product:
• **do not use more than directed**
• marked drowsiness may occur
• excitability may occur, especially in children
• avoid alcoholic drinks
• alcohol, sedatives, and tranquilizers may increase drowsiness
• be careful when driving a motor vehicle or operating machinery
Stop use and ask a doctor if:
• new symptoms occur
• sore throat is severe
• you get nervous, dizzy, or sleepless
• symptoms do not get better
• you need to use more than 10 days
• redness or swelling is present
• fever occurs and lasts more than 3 days
• sore throat lasts for more than 2 days, is accompanied or followed by fever, headache, rash, swelling, nausea, or vomiting
If pregnant or breast-feeding, ask a health professional before use.
Keep out of reach of children.
Overdose warning: Taking more than the recommended dose may cause liver damage. In case of overdose, get medical help or contact a Poison Control Center right away. Quick medical attention is critical for adults as well as for children even if you do not notice any signs or symptoms.

Directions:
• do not use more than directed (see overdose warning)
• adults and children 12 years of age and over: 2 caplets
• children under 12 years of age: ask a doctor
• take every 6 hours while symptoms persist
• do not take more than 8 caplets in 24 hours or as directed by a doctor

Other Information
• store at 59° to 77°F in a dry place

Inactive Ingredients: Corn starch, croscarmellose sodium, hydroxypropyl cellulose, hypromellose, microcrystalline cellulose, polyethylene glycol, pregelatinized starch, sodium starch glycolate, stearic acid, titanium dioxide, and zinc stearate

Questions? call **1-800-524-2624** (English/Spanish), weekdays, 9 AM - 5 PM EST

How Supplied: Benadryl® Allergy & Cold caplets are supplied in boxes of 24.
Shown in Product Identification Guide, page 517

BENADRYL® Allergy & Sinus Tablets
(Formerly Benadryl Allergy/ Congestion)
[bĕ 'nă-drĭl]

Drug Facts:

Active Ingredients:
(in each tablet)   **Purposes:**
Diphenhydramine HCl
  25 mg .... Antihistamine
Pseudoephedrine HCl
  60 mg .... Nasal decongestant

Uses:
• temporarily relieves these symptoms due to hay fever or other upper respiratory allergies:
  • runny nose
  • sneezing
  • itchy, watery eyes
  • nasal congestion
  • itching of the nose or throat
• temporarily relieves these symptoms due to the common cold:
  • runny nose
  • sneezing
  • nasal congestion

Warnings:
Do not use
• if you are now taking a prescription monoamine oxidase inhibitor (MAOI) (certain drugs for depression, psychiatric, or emotional conditions, or Parkinson's disease), or for 2 weeks after stopping the MAOI drug. If you do not know if your prescription drug contains an MAOI, ask a doctor or pharmacist before taking this product.
• with any other product containing diphenhydramine, including one applied topically.
Ask a doctor before use if you have:
• heart disease
• glaucoma
• thyroid disease
• diabetes
• high blood pressure
• trouble urinating due to an enlarged prostate gland
• a breathing problem such as emphysema or chronic bronchitis
Ask a doctor or pharmacist before use if you are taking sedatives or tranquilizers
When using this product:
• **do not use more than directed**
• marked drowsiness may occur
• avoid alcoholic drinks
• alcohol, sedatives, and tranquilizers may increase drowsiness
• be careful when driving a motor vehicle or operating machinery
• excitability may occur, especially in children
Stop use and ask a doctor if:
• you get nervous, dizzy, or sleepless
• symptoms do not improve within 7 days or are accompanied by fever
If pregnant or breast-feeding, ask a health professional before use.
Keep out of reach of children. In case of overdose, get medical help or contact a Poison Control Center right away.

Directions:
• adults and children 12 years of age and over: one (1) tablet
• take every 4 to 6 hours
• do not take more than 4 tablets in 24 hours
• children under 12 years of age: ask a doctor

Other Information:
• protect from light
• store at 59° to 77°F in a dry place

Inactive Ingredients: Croscarmellose sodium, dibasic calcium phosphate dihydrate, FD&C blue no. 1 aluminum lake, hypromellose, microcrystalline cellulose, polyethylene glycol, polysorbate 80, pregelatinized starch, stearic acid, tita-

nium dioxide and zinc stearate. Printed with edible black ink.

Questions? call **1-800-524-2624** (English/Spanish), weekdays, 9 AM – 5 PM EST

How Supplied: Benadryl Allergy & Sinus Tablets are supplied in boxes of 24.

Shown in Product Identification Guide, page 517

BENADRYL® Allergy & Sinus Headache Caplets*
(also available in Gelcaps)
[bĕ 'nă-drĭl]
*Capsule Shaped Tablets

Drug Facts:

Active Ingredients:
(in each caplet)   **Purposes:**
Acetaminophen 500 mg .... Pain reliever
Diphenhydramine HCl
  12.5 mg .... Antihistamine
Pseudoephedrine HCl
  30 mg .... Nasal decongestant

Uses:
- temporarily relieves these symptoms of hay fever and the common cold:
  - runny nose
  - sneezing
  - headache
  - minor aches and pains
  - nasal congestion
- temporarily relieves these additional symptoms of hay fever:
  - itching of the nose or throat
  - itchy, watery eyes

Warnings:
Alcohol warning: If you consume 3 or more alcoholic drinks every day, ask your doctor whether you should take acetaminophen or other pain relievers/fever reducers. Acetaminophen may cause liver damage.

Do not use:
- with another product containing any of these active ingredients.
- if you are now taking a prescription monoamine oxidase inhibitor (MAOI) (certain drugs for depression, psychiatric, or emotional conditions, or Parkinson's disease), or for 2 weeks after stopping the MAOI drug. If you do not know if your prescription drug contains an MAOI, ask a doctor or pharmacist before taking this product.
- with any other product containing diphenhydramine, including one applied topically.

Ask a doctor before use if you have:
- heart disease
- glaucoma
- thyroid disease
- diabetes
- high blood pressure
- trouble urinating due to an enlarged prostate gland
- a breathing problem such as emphysema or chronic bronchitis

Ask a doctor or pharmacist before use if you are taking sedatives or tranquilizers

When using this product:
- do not use more than directed
- marked drowsiness may occur
- excitability may occur, especially in children
- avoid alcoholic drinks

- alcohol, sedatives, and tranquilizers may increase drowsiness
- be careful when driving a motor vehicle or operating machinery

Stop use and ask a doctor if:
- you get nervous, dizzy, or sleepless
- new symptoms occur
- symptoms do not get better
- you need to use more than 10 days
- fever occurs and lasts more than 3 days

If pregnant or breast-feeding, ask a health professional before use.

Keep out of reach of children.

Overdose warning: Taking more than the recommended dose may cause liver damage. In case of overdose, get medical help or contact a Poison Control Center right away. Quick medical attention is critical for adults as well as for children even if you do not notice any signs or symptoms.

Directions:
- do not use more than directed (see overdose warning)
- take every 6 hours while symptoms persist
- do not take more than 8 caplets in 24 hours or as directed by a doctor
- adults and children 12 years of age and over: 2 caplets
- children under 12 years of age: ask a doctor

Other Information
- store at 59° to 77°F in a dry place

Inactive Ingredients: (Caplets): Croscarmellose sodium, D&C yellow no. 10 aluminum lake, FD&C blue no. 1 aluminum lake, FD&C yellow no. 6 aluminum lake, hydroxypropyl cellulose, hypromellose, microcrystalline cellulose, polyethylene glycol, polysorbate 80, pregelatinized starch, sodium starch glycolate, stearic acid, titanium dioxide, and zinc stearate
(Gelcaps): Colloidal silicon dioxide, croscarmellose sodium, D&C yellow no. 10 Al lake, FD&C green no. 3 Al lake, gelatin, hypromellose, polysorbate 80, sodium lauryl sulfate, stearic acid and titanium dioxide.

Questions? call **1-800-524-2624** (English/Spanish), weekdays, 9 AM - 5 PM EST

How Supplied: Benadryl Allergy & Sinus Headache is available in boxes of 24 and 48 caplets, and boxes of 24, 48 and 72 gelcaps.

Shown in Product Identification Guide, page 518

BENADRYL® Maximum Strength Severe Allergy† & Sinus Headache Caplets*
[be' na drill]
* Capsule Shaped Tablets
† Upper Respiratory Allergies Only

Drug Facts:

Active Ingredients:
(in each caplet)   **Purposes:**
Acetaminophen
  500 mg .... Pain reliever

Diphenhydramine
  HCl 25 mg .... Antihistamine
Pseudoephedrine
  HCl 30 mg .... Nasal decongestant

Uses:
- temporarily relieves these symptoms of hay fever and the common cold:
  - runny nose
  - headache
  - sneezing
  - minor aches and pains
  - nasal congestion
- temporarily relieves these additional symptoms of hay fever:
  - itching of the nose or throat
  - itchy, watery eyes

Warnings:
Alcohol warning: If you consume 3 or more alcoholic drinks every day, ask your doctor whether you should take acetaminophen or other pain relievers/fever reducers. Acetaminophen may cause liver damage.

Do not use:
- with another product containing any of these active ingredients
- if you are now taking a prescription monoamine oxidase inhibitor (MAOI) (certain drugs for depression, psychiatric, or emotional conditions, or Parkinson's disease), or for 2 weeks after stopping the MAOI drug. If you do not know if your prescription drug contains an MAOI, ask a doctor or pharmacist before taking this product.
- with any other product containing diphenhydramine, including one applied topically.

Ask a doctor before use if you have:
- heart disease
- glaucoma
- thyroid disease
- diabetes
- high blood pressure
- trouble urinating due to an enlarged prostate gland
- a breathing problem such as emphysema or chronic bronchitis

Ask a doctor or pharmacist before use if you are taking sedatives or tranquilizers

When using this product:
- do not use more than directed
- marked drowsiness may occur
- excitability may occur, especially in children
- avoid alcoholic drinks
- alcohol, sedatives, and tranquilizers may increase drowsiness
- be careful when driving a motor vehicle or operating machinery

Stop use and ask a doctor if:
- you get nervous, dizzy, or sleepless
- new symptoms occur
- symptoms do not get better
- you need to use more than 10 days

Continued on next page

This product information was prepared in November 2002. On these and other Pfizer Consumer Healthcare Products, detailed information may be obtained by addressing Pfizer Consumer Healthcare, Pfizer, Inc., Morris Plains, NJ 07950

Benadryl Severe—Cont.

• fever occurs and lasts more than 3 days

If pregnant or breast-feeding, ask a health professional before use.

Keep out of reach of children.

Overdose warning: Taking more than the recommended dose may cause liver damage. In case of overdose, get medical help or contact a Poison Control Center right away. Quick medical attention is critical for adults as well as for children even if you do not notice any signs or symptoms.

Directions:

• do not use more than directed (see overdose warning)
• take every 6 hours while symptoms persist
• do not take more than 8 caplets in 24 hours or as directed by a doctor
• adults and children 12 years of age and over: 2 caplets
• children under 12 years of age: ask a doctor

Other Information:

• store at 59° to 77°F in a dry place

Inactive Ingredients: Carnauba wax, crospovidone, FD&C blue no. 1 aluminum lake, hypromellose, magnesium stearate, microcrystalline cellulose, polyethylene glycol, polysorbate 80, povidone, pregelatinized starch, sodium starch glycolate, stearic acid, and titanium dioxide

Questions? call **1-800-524-2624** (English/Spanish), weekdays, 9 AM – 5 PM EST

How Supplied: Available in 20 Caplets (capsule-shaped tablets).

Shown in Product Identification Guide, page 518

BENADRYL®
Allergy & Sinus FASTMELT™
Dissolving Tablets
[bĕ′nădrĭl]

Drug Facts:

Active Ingredients:
(in each tablet)   **Purposes:**
Diphenhydramine citrate
  19 mg* .... Antihistamine
Pseudoephedrine
  HCl 30 mg .... Nasal decongestant

*equivalent to 12.5 mg of diphenhydramine HCl

Uses:

• temporarily relieves these symptoms of hay fever or the common cold:
  • runny nose
  • sneezing
  • nasal congestion
• temporarily relieves these additional symptoms of hay fever:
  • itching of the nose or throat
  • itchy, watery eyes

Warnings:
Do not use:
• if you are now taking a prescription monoamine oxidase inhibitor (MAOI)

(certain drugs for depression, psychiatric, or emotional conditions, or Parkinson's disease), or for 2 weeks after stopping the MAOI drug. If you do not know if your prescription drug contains an MAOI, ask a doctor or pharmacist before taking this product.
• with any other product containing diphenhydramine, including one applied topically.

Ask a doctor before use if you have:
• heart disease
• high blood pressure
• thyroid disease
• diabetes
• glaucoma
• trouble urinating due to an enlarged prostate gland
• a breathing problem such as emphysema or chronic bronchitis

Ask a doctor or pharmacist before use if you are taking sedatives or tranquilizers

When using this product:
• **do not use more than directed**
• marked drowsiness may occur
• excitability may occur, especially in children
• avoid alcoholic drinks
• alcohol, sedatives, and tranquilizers may increase drowsiness
• be careful when driving a motor vehicle or operating machinery

Stop use and ask a doctor if:
• you get nervous, dizzy, or sleepless
• symptoms do not improve within 7 days or are accompanied by fever

If pregnant or breast-feeding, ask a health professional before use.

Keep out of reach of children. In case of overdose, get medical help or contact a Poison Control Center right away.

Directions:
• adults and children 12 years of age and over: 2 tablets
• place in mouth and allow to dissolve
• take every 4 to 6 hours
• do not take more than 8 tablets in 24 hours, or as directed by a doctor

Other Information:
• **phenylketonurics:** contains phenylalanine 4.6 mg per tablet
• store at 59° to 77°F in a dry place

Inactive Ingredients: Aspartame, citric acid, D&C red no. 7 calcium lake, ethylcellulose, flavor, lactitol, magnesium stearate, mannitol, and stearic acid

Questions? call **1-800-524-2624** (English/Spanish), weekdays, 9 AM – 5 PM EST

How Supplied: Available in boxes of 20 dissolving tablets.

Shown in Product Identification Guide, page 518

Children's BENADRYL®
Allergy
Liquid Medication
[bĕ ′nă-drĭl]
Cherry Flavored

Drug Facts:

Active Ingredient: **Purpose:**
(in each 5 mL)
Diphenhydramine
  HCl 12.5 mg .... Antihistamine

Uses:
• temporarily relieves these symptoms due to hay fever or other upper respiratory allergies:
  • runny nose
  • sneezing
  • itchy, watery eyes
  • itching of the nose or throat
• temporarily relieves these symptoms due to the common cold:
  • runny nose
  • sneezing

Warnings:
Do not use with any other product containing diphenhydramine, including one applied topically.

Ask a doctor before use if you have:
• glaucoma
• trouble urinating due to an enlarged prostate gland
• a breathing problem such as emphysema or chronic bronchitis

Ask a doctor or pharmacist before use if you are taking sedatives or tranquilizers

When using this product:
• marked drowsiness may occur
• avoid alcoholic drinks
• alcohol, sedatives, and tranquilizers may increase drowsiness
• be careful when driving a motor vehicle or operating machinery
• excitability may occur, especially in children

If pregnant or breast-feeding, ask a health professional before use.

Keep out of reach of children. In case of overdose, get medical help or contact a Poison Control Center right away.

Directions:
• take every 4 to 6 hours
• do not take more than 6 doses in 24 hours

children under 6 years of age	ask a doctor
children 6 to under 12 years of age	1 to 2 teaspoonfuls (12.5 mg to 25 mg)
adults and children 12 years of age and over	2 to 4 teaspoonfuls (25 mg to 50 mg)

Other Information:
• store at 59° to 77°F

Inactive Ingredients: Citric acid, D&C red no. 33, FD&C red no. 40, flavors, glycerin, poloxamer 407, purified water, sodium benzoate, sodium chloride, sodium citrate, and sugar

Questions? call **1-800-524-2624** (English/Spanish), weekdays, 9 AM–5 PM EST

How Supplied: Children's Benadryl Allergy Liquid Medication is supplied in 4 and 8 fluid ounce bottles.

Shown in Product Identification Guide, page 518

Children's BENADRYL® Dye-Free Allergy Liquid Medication
[bĕ 'nă-drĭl]
Bubble Gum Flavored

Drug Facts:

Active Ingredient:

(in each 5 mL)	Purpose:
Diphenhydramine HCl 12.5 mg .... Antihistamine	

Uses:
- temporarily relieves these symptoms due to hay fever or other upper respiratory allergies:
  - runny nose
  - sneezing
  - itchy, watery eyes
  - itching of the nose or throat
- temporarily relieves these symptoms due to the common cold:
  - runny nose
  - sneezing

Warnings:

Do not use with any other product containing diphenhydramine, including one applied topically.

Ask a doctor before use if you have
- glaucoma
- trouble urinating due to an enlarged prostate gland
- a breathing problem such as emphysema or chronic bronchitis

Ask a doctor or pharmacist before use if you are taking sedatives or tranquilizers

When using this product:
- marked drowsiness may occur
- avoid alcoholic drinks
- alcohol, sedatives, and tranquilizers may increase drowsiness
- be careful when driving a motor vehicle or operating machinery
- excitability may occur, especially in children

If pregnant or breast-feeding, ask a health professional before use.

Keep out of reach of children. In case of overdose, get medical help or contact a Poison Control Center right away.

Directions:
- take every 4 to 6 hours
- do not take more than 6 doses in 24 hours

children under 6 years of age	ask a doctor
children 6 to under 12 years of age	1 to 2 teaspoonfuls (12.5 mg to 25 mg)
adults and children 12 years of age and over	2 to 4 teaspoonfuls (25 mg to 50 mg)

Other Information
- store at 59° to 77°F

Inactive Ingredients: Carboxymethylcellulose sodium, citric acid, flavor, glycerin, purified water, saccharin sodium, sodium benzoate, sodium citrate, and sorbitol solution

Questions? call **1-800-524-2624** (English/Spanish), weekdays, 9 AM – 5 PM EST

How Supplied: Children's Benadryl Dye-Free Allergy Liquid Medication is supplied in 4 fl. oz. bottles.
Shown in Product Identification Guide, page 518

Children's BENADRYL® Allergy & Sinus Liquid Medication (Formerly Children's Allergy/ Congestion)
[bĕ 'nă-drĭl]
Grape Flavored

Drug Facts:

Active Ingredients:

(in each 5 mL)*	Purposes:
Diphenhydramine HCl 12.5 mg .... Antihistamine	
Pseudoephedrine HCl 30 mg .... Nasal decongestant	

*5 mL = one teaspoonful

Uses:
- temporarily relieves these symptoms due to hay fever or other upper respiratory allergies:
  - runny nose
  - sneezing
  - itchy, watery eyes
  - nasal congestion
  - itching of the nose or throat
- temporarily relieves these symptoms due to the common cold:
  - runny nose
  - sneezing
  - nasal congestion

Warnings:

Do not use
- if you are now taking a prescription monoamine oxidase inhibitor (MAOI) (certain drugs for depression, psychiatric, or emotional conditions, or Parkinson's disease), or for 2 weeks after stopping the MAOI drug. If you do not know if your prescription drug contains an MAOI, ask a doctor or pharmacist before taking this product.
- with any other product containing diphenhydramine, including one applied topically

Ask a doctor before use if you have:
- heart disease
- glaucoma
- thyroid disease
- diabetes
- high blood pressure
- trouble urinating due to an enlarged prostate gland
- a breathing problem such as emphysema or chronic bronchitis

Ask a doctor or pharmacist before use if you are taking sedatives or tranquilizers

When using this product:
- **do not use more than directed**
- marked drowsiness may occur
- avoid alcoholic drinks
- alcohol, sedatives, and tranquilizers may increase drowsiness
- be careful when driving a motor vehicle or operating machinery
- excitability may occur, especially in children

Stop use and ask a doctor if:
- you get nervous, dizzy, or sleepless
- symptoms do not improve within 7 days or are accompanied by fever

If pregnant or breast-feeding, ask a health professional before use.

Keep out of reach of children. In case of overdose, get medical help or contact a Poison Control Center right away.

Directions:
- take every 4 to 6 hours
- do not take more than 4 doses in 24 hours

children under 6 years of age	ask a doctor
children 6 to under 12 years of age	1 teaspoonful
adults and children 12 years of age and over	2 teaspoonfuls

Other Information:
- store at 59° to 77°F

Inactive Ingredients: Citric acid, FD&C blue no. 1, FD&C red no. 40, flavors, glycerin, poloxamer 407, polysorbate 20, purified water, saccharin sodium, sodium benzoate, sodium chloride, sodium citrate, and sorbitol solution

Questions? call **1-800-524-2624** (English/Spanish), weekdays, 9 AM – 5 PM EST

How Supplied: Benadryl Allergy & Sinus Liquid Medication is supplied in 4 fl. oz. bottles.
Shown in Product Identification Guide, page 518

Children's BENADRYL® Allergy Chewables
[bĕ 'nă-drĭl]
Grape Flavored

Drug Facts:

Active Ingredient:

(in each tablet)	Purpose:
Diphenhydramine HCl 12.5 mg .... Antihistamine	

Uses:
- temporarily relieves these symptoms due to hay fever or other upper respiratory allergies:
  - runny nose
  - sneezing
  - itchy, watery eyes

Continued on next page

This product information was prepared in November 2002. On these and other Pfizer Consumer Healthcare Products, detailed information may be obtained by addressing Pfizer Consumer Healthcare, Pfizer, Inc., Morris Plains, NJ 07950

Benadryl Chewables—Cont.

- itching of the nose or throat
- temporarily relieves these symptoms due to the common cold:
  - runny nose
  - sneezing

Warnings:

Do not use with any other product containing diphenhydramine, including one applied topically.

Ask a doctor before use if you have:
- glaucoma
- trouble urinating due to an enlarged prostate gland
- a breathing problem such as emphysema or chronic bronchitis

Ask a doctor or pharmacist before use if you are taking sedatives or tranquilizers

When using this product:
- marked drowsiness may occur
- avoid alcoholic drinks
- alcohol, sedatives, and tranquilizers may increase drowsiness
- be careful when driving a motor vehicle or operating machinery
- excitability may occur, especially in children

If pregnant or breast-feeding, ask a health professional before use.

Keep out of reach of children. In case of overdose, get medical help or contact a Poison Control Center right away.

Directions:

- chew tablets thoroughly before swallowing
- take every 4 to 6 hours
- do not take more than 6 doses in 24 hours

children under 6 years of age	ask a doctor
children 6 to under 12 years of age	1 to 2 tablets (12.5 mg to 25 mg)
adults and children 12 years of age and over	2 to 4 tablets (25 mg to 50 mg)

Other Information:

- **each tablet contains:** magnesium 17 mg
- **phenylketonurics:** contains phenylalanine 4.2 mg per tablet
- store at 59° to 77°F in a dry place
- protect from heat, humidity, and light

Inactive Ingredients: Aspartame, dextrates, D&C red no. 27 aluminum lake, FD&C blue no. 1 aluminum lake, flavors, magnesium stearate, magnesium trisilicate, and tartaric acid

Questions? call **1-800-524-2624** (English/Spanish), weekdays, 9 AM – 5 PM EST

How Supplied: Children's Benadryl® Allergy Chewables are supplied in boxes of 24 tablets.

Shown in Product Identification Guide, page 518

Children's BENADRYL® Allergy/Cold
FASTMELT™
Dissolving Tablets
[bĕ 'nă-drĭl]
Cherry Flavored

Drug Facts:

Active Ingredients: (in each tablet)	Purposes:
Diphenhydramine citrate 19 mg*	Antihistamine/cough suppressant
Pseudoephedrine HCl 30 mg	Nasal decongestant

*equivalent to 12.5 mg of diphenhydramine HCl

Uses:

- temporarily relieves these symptoms of hay fever or the common cold:
  - runny nose
  - sneezing
  - nasal congestion
  - cough
- temporarily relieves these additional symptoms of hay fever:
  - itching of the nose or throat
  - itchy, watery eyes

Warnings:
Do not use

- if you are now taking a prescription monoamine oxidase inhibitor (MAOI) (certain drugs for depression, psychiatric, or emotional conditions, or Parkinson's disease), or for 2 weeks after stopping the MAOI drug. If you do not know if your prescription drug contains an MAOI, ask a doctor or pharmacist before taking this product.
- with any other product containing diphenhydramine, including one applied topically.

Ask a doctor before use if you have:
- heart disease
- high blood pressure
- thyroid disease
- trouble urinating due to an enlarged prostate gland
- diabetes
- cough accompanied by excessive phlegm (mucus)
- glaucoma
- a breathing problem such as emphysema or chronic bronchitis
- persistent or chronic cough such as occurs with smoking, asthma, or emphysema

Ask a doctor or pharmacist before use if you are taking sedatives or tranquilizers

When using this product:
- **do not use more than directed**
- marked drowsiness may occur
- excitability may occur, especially in children
- avoid alcoholic drinks
- alcohol, sedatives, and tranquilizers may increase drowsiness
- be careful when driving a motor vehicle or operating machinery

Stop use and ask a doctor if:
- you get nervous, dizzy, or sleepless
- symptoms do not improve within 7 days or are accompanied by fever
- cough persists for more than 1 week, tends to recur, or is accompanied by fever, rash, or persistent headache. These could be signs of a serious condition.

If pregnant or breast-feeding, ask a health professional before use.

Keep out of reach of children. In case of overdose, get medical help or contact a Poison Control Center right away.

Directions:

- place in mouth and allow to dissolve
- take every 4 hours

adults and children 12 years of age and over	2 tablets; do not take more than 8 tablets in 24 hours or as directed by a doctor
children 6 to under 12 years of age	1 tablet; do not take more than 4 tablets in 24 hours or as directed by a doctor
children under 6 years of age	ask a doctor

Other Information:

- **phenylketonurics:** contains phenylalanine 4.6 mg per tablet
- store at 59° to 77°F in a dry place

Inactive Ingredients: Aspartame, citric acid, D&C red no. 7 calcium lake, ethylcellulose, flavor, lactitol, magnesium stearate, mannitol, and stearic acid

Questions? call **1-800-524-2624** (English/Spanish), weekdays, 9 AM - 5 PM EST

How Supplied: Available in boxes of 20 dissolving tablets.

Shown in Product Identification Guide, page 518

BENADRYL® Itch Relief Stick Extra Strength
Topical Analgesic/Skin Protectant
[bĕ 'nă-drĭl]

Drug Facts:

Active Ingredients:	Purposes:
Diphenhydramine hydrochloride 2%	Topical analgesic
Zinc acetate 0.1%	Skin protectant

Uses:

- temporarily relieves pain and itching associated with
  - insect bites
  - minor burns
  - sunburn
  - minor skin irritations
  - minor cuts
  - scrapes
  - rashes due to poison ivy, poison oak, and poison sumac
- dries the oozing and weeping of poison ivy, poison oak and poison sumac

Warnings:
For external use only

Flammable. Keep away from fire or flame.

Do not use
- more often than directed
- on chicken pox or measles
- with any other product containing diphenhydramine, even one taken by mouth

- on large areas of the body, including large areas of poison ivy, sunburn, or broken, blistered or oozing skin

When using this product
- avoid contact with eyes

Stop use and ask a doctor if
- condition worsens or does not improve within 7 days
- symptoms persist for more than 7 days or clear up and occur again within a few days

Keep out of reach of children. If swallowed, get medical help or contact a Poison Control Center right away.

Directions:
- press tip of stick on affected skin area until liquid flows, then dab sparingly
- adults and children 6 years of age and older: apply to affected area not more than 3 to 4 times daily
- children under 6 years of age: ask a doctor

Other Information:
- store at 59 to 77° F

Inactive Ingredients: alcohol 73.5% v/v, glycerin, povidone, purified water, and tromethamine

Questions? call **1-800-524-2624** (English/Spanish), Monday to Friday, 9 AM - 5 PM EST

How Supplied: Benadryl® Itch Relief Stick is available in a .47 fl. oz (14 mL) dauber.

Shown in Product Identification Guide, page 518

BENADRYL® Itch Stopping Cream Original Strength
[bĕ 'nă-drĭl]

Drug Facts
Active Ingredients: **Purpose:**
Diphenhydramine   hydrochloride 1% .... Topical analgesic
Zinc acetate 0.1% .... Skin protectant

Uses:
- temporarily relieves pain and itching associated with:
  - insect bites
  - minor burns
  - sunburn
  - minor skin irritations
  - minor cuts
  - scrapes
  - rashes due to poison ivy, poison oak, and poison sumac
- dries the oozing and weeping of poison ivy, poison oak, and poison sumac

Warnings:
For external use only
Do not use
- more often than directed
- on chicken pox or measles
- with any other product containing diphenhydramine, even one taken by mouth
- on large areas of the body, including large areas of poison ivy, sunburn, or broken, blistered or oozing skin

When using this product
- avoid contact with eyes

Stop use and ask a doctor if
- condition worsens or does not improve within 7 days
- symptoms persist for more than 7 days or clear up and occur again within a few days

Keep out of reach of children. If swallowed, get medical help or contact a Poison Control Center right away.

Directions:
- adults and children 2 years of age and older: apply to affected area not more than 3 to 4 times daily
- children under 2 years of age: ask a doctor

Other Information: • store at 59° to 77° F

Inactive Ingredients: cetyl alcohol, diazolidinyl urea, methylparaben, polyethylene glycol monostearate 1000, propylene glycol, propylparaben, and purified water

Questions? call **1-800-524-2624** (English/Spanish), Monday to Friday, 9 AM - 5 PM EST

How Supplied: Benadryl Itch Stopping Cream Original Strength is available in 1 oz (28.3 g).

Shown in Product Identification Guide, page 518

BENADRYL® Itch Stopping Cream Extra Strength
[bĕ 'nă-drĭl]

Drug Facts
Active Ingredients: **Purpose:**
Diphenhydramine   hydrochloride 2% .... Topical analgesic
Zinc acetate 0.1% .... Skin protectant

Uses:
- temporarily relieves pain and itching associated with:
  - insect bites
  - minor burns
  - sunburn
  - minor skin irritations
  - minor cuts
  - scrapes
  - rashes due to poison ivy, poison oak, and poison sumac
- dries the oozing and weeping of poison ivy, poison oak, and poison sumac

Warnings:
For external use only
Do not use
- more often than directed
- on chicken pox or measles
- with any other product containing diphenhydramine, even one taken by mouth
- on large areas of the body, including large areas of poison ivy, sunburn, or broken, blistered or oozing skin

When using this product
- avoid contact with eyes

Stop use and ask a doctor if
- condition worsens or does not improve within 7 days
- symptoms persist for more than 7 days or clear up and occur again within a few days

Keep out of reach of children. If swallowed, get medical help or contact a Poison Control Center right away.

Directions:
- adults and children 12 years of age and older: apply to affected area not more than 3 to 4 times daily
- children under 12 years of age: ask a doctor

Other Information: • store at 59° to 77° F

Inactive Ingredients: cetyl alcohol, diazolidinyl urea, methylparaben, polyethylene glycol monostearate 1000, propylene glycol, propylparaben, and purified water

Questions? call **1-800-524-2624** (English/Spanish), Monday to Friday, 9 AM - 5 PM EST

How Supplied: Benadryl Itch Stopping Cream Extra Strength is available in 1 oz (28.3 g) tubes.

Shown in Product Identification Guide, page 518

BENADRYL® Itch Stopping Gel Original Strength
[bĕ 'nă-drĭl]
Topical Analgesic Gel

Drug Facts
Active Ingredient: **Purpose:**
Diphenhydramine   hydrochloride 1% ... Topical analgesic

Uses:
- temporarily relieves pain and itching associated with:
  - insect bites
  - minor burns
  - sunburn
  - minor skin irritations
  - minor cuts
  - scrapes
  - rashes due to poison ivy, poison oak, and poison sumac

Warnings: **For external use only**
Do not use
- more often than directed
- on chicken pox or measles
- with any other product containing diphenhydramine, even one taken by mouth
- on large areas of the body, including large areas of poison ivy, sunburn, or broken, blistered or oozing skin

When using this product
- avoid contact with eyes

Stop use and ask a doctor if
- condition worsens
- symptoms persist for more than 7 days or clear up and occur again within a few days

Keep out of reach of children. If swallowed, get medical help or contact a Poison Control Center right away.

Directions:
- adults and children 6 years of age and older: apply to affected area not more than 3 to 4 times daily
- children under 6 years of age: ask a doctor

Continued on next page

This product information was prepared in November 2002. On these and other Pfizer Consumer Healthcare Products, detailed information may be obtained by addressing Pfizer Consumer Healthcare, Pfizer, Inc., Morris Plains, NJ 07950

Benadryl Itch Gel—Cont.

Other Information: • store at 59° to 77° F

Inactive Ingredients: SD alcohol 38B, camphor, citric acid, diazolidinyl urea, glycerin, hydroxypropyl methylcellulose, methylparaben, propylene glycol, propylparaben, purified water, and sodium citrate

Questions? call **1-800-524-2624** (English/Spanish), Monday to Friday, 9AM - 5 PM EST

How Supplied: Benadryl Itch Stopping Gel Original Strength is supplied in 4 fl. oz. (118mL) bottles

BENADRYL® Itch Stopping Gel Extra Strength
[bĕ 'nă-drĭl]

Drug Facts
Active Ingredient: **Purpose:**
Diphenhydramine hydrochloride 2% .... Topical analgesic

Uses:
• temporarily relieves pain and itching associated with:
  • insect bites
  • minor burns
  • sunburn
  • minor skin irritations
  • minor cuts
  • scrapes
  • rashes due to poison ivy, poison oak, and poison sumac

Warnings:
For external use only
Do not use
• more often than directed
• on chicken pox or measles
• with any other product containing diphenhydramine, even one taken by mouth
• on large areas of the body, including large areas of poison ivy, sunburn, or broken, blistered or oozing skin
When using this product
• avoid contact with eyes
Stop use and ask a doctor if
• condition worsens
• symptoms persist for more than 7 days or clear up and occur again within a few days
Keep out of reach of children. If swallowed, get medical help or contact a Poison Control Center right away.

Directions:
• adults and children 12 years of age and older: apply to affected area not more than 3 to 4 times daily
• children under 12 years of age: ask a doctor
Other Information:
• store at 59° to 77° F

Inactive Ingredients: SD alcohol 38-B, camphor, citric acid, diazolidinyl urea, glycerin, hypromellose, methylparaben, propylene glycol, propylparaben, purified water, and sodium citrate
Questions? call **1-800-524-2624** (English/Spanish), Monday to Friday, 9 AM - 5 PM EST
How Supplied: Benadryl Itch Stopping Gel Extra Strength is supplied in 4 fl. oz. (118mL) bottles

BENADRYL® Itch Stopping Spray Original Strength
[bĕ 'nă-drĭl]
Topical Analgesic/Skin Protectant

Drug Facts
Active Ingredients: **Purpose:**
Diphenhydramine hydrochloride 1% .... Topical analgesic
Zinc acetate 0.1% .... Skin protectant

Uses:
• temporarily relieves pain and itching associated with:
  • insect bites
  • minor burns
  • sunburn
  • minor skin irritations
  • minor cuts
  • scrapes
  • rashes due to poison ivy, poison oak, and poison sumac
• dries the oozing and weeping of poison ivy, poison oak, and poison sumac

Warnings:
For external use only
Flammable. Keep away from fire or flame
Do not use:
• more often than directed
• on chicken pox or measles
• with any other product containing diphenhydramine, even one taken by mouth
• on large areas of the body, including large areas of poison ivy, sunburn, or broken, blistered or oozing skin
When using this product
• avoid contact with eyes
Stop use and ask a doctor if
• condition worsens or does not improve within 7 days
• symptoms persist for more than 7 days or clear up and occur again within a few days
Keep out of reach of children. If swallowed, get medical help or contact a Poison Control Center right away.

Directions:
• adults and children 2 years of age and older: apply to affected area not more than 3 to 4 times daily
• children under 2 years of age: ask a doctor
Other Information:
• store at 59° to 77° F

Inactive Ingredients: alcohol 78% v/v, glycerin, povidone, purified water, and tris (hydroxymethyl) aminomethane
Questions? call **1-800-524-2624** (English/Spanish), Monday to Friday, 9 AM – 5 PM EST
How Supplied: Benadryl Itch Stopping Spray Original Strength is available in a 2 fl. oz. (59mL) pump spray bottle.
Shown in Product Identification Guide, page 518

BENADRYL® Itch Stopping Spray Extra Strength
[bĕ 'nă-drĭl]

Drug Facts
Active Ingredients: **Purpose:**
Diphenhydramine hydrochloride 2% .... Topical analgesic
Zinc acetate 0.1% .... Skin protectant

Uses:
• temporarily relieves pain and itching associated with:
  • insect bites
  • minor burns
  • sunburn
  • minor skin irritations
  • minor cuts
  • scrapes
  • rashes due to poison ivy, poison oak, and poison sumac
• dries the oozing and weeping of poison ivy, poison oak, and poison sumac

Warnings:
For external use only
Flammable. Keep away from fire or flame
Do not use
• more often than directed
• on chicken pox or measles
• with any other product containing diphenhydramine, even one taken by mouth
• on large areas of the body, including large areas of poison ivy, sunburn, or broken, blistered or oozing skin
When using this product
• avoid contact with eyes
Stop use and ask a doctor if
• condition worsens or does not improve within 7 days
• symptoms persist for more than 7 days or clear up and occur again within a few days
Keep out of reach of children. If swallowed, get medical help or contact a Poison Control Center right away.

Directions:
• adults and children 12 years of age and older: apply to affected area not more than 3 to 4 times daily
• children under 12 years of age: ask a doctor
Other Information: • store at 59° to 77° F

Inactive Ingredients: alcohol 78% v/v, glycerin, povidone, purified water, and tris (hydroxymethyl) aminomethane
Questions? call **1-800-524-2624** (English/Spanish), Monday to Friday, 9 AM - 5 PM EST

How Supplied: Benadryl Itch Stopping Spray Extra Strength Spray is available in a 2 fl. oz. (59mL) pump spray bottle.
Shown in Product Identification Guide, page 518

BENGAY® External Analgesic Products

Description: BENGAY products contain menthol in an alcohol base gel, combinations of methyl salicylate and menthol in cream and ointment bases, as well as a combination of methyl salicylate, menthol and camphor in a non-greasy cream base; all suitable for topical application.
In addition to the Original Formula Pain Relieving Ointment (methyl salicylate,

18.3%; menthol, 16%), BENGAY is offered as BENGAY Greaseless Pain Relieving Cream (methyl salicylate, 15%; menthol, 10%), an Arthritis Formula NonGreasy Pain Relieving Cream (methyl salicylate, 30%; menthol, 8%), an Ultra Strength NonGreasy Pain Relieving Cream (methyl salicylate 30%; menthol 10%; camphor 4%), Vanishing Scent NonGreasy Pain Relieving Gel (2.5% menthol), and S.P.A. (Site Penetrating Action) Pain Relieving Cream (10% menthol) with a fresh scent.

Action and Uses: Methyl salicylate, menthol and camphor are external analgesics which stimulate sensory receptors of warmth and/or cold. This produces a counter-irritant response which provides temporary relief of minor aches and pains of muscles and joints associated with simple backache, arthritis, strains and sprains.

Several double-blind clinical studies of BENGAY products containing mentholmethyl salicylate have shown the effectiveness of this combination in counteracting minor pain of skeletal muscle stress and arthritis.

Three studies involving a total of 102 normal subjects in which muscle soreness was experimentally induced showed statistically significant beneficial results from use of the active product vs. placebo for lowered Muscle Action Potential (spasms), greater rise in threshold of muscular pain and greater reduction in perceived muscular pain.

Six clinical studies of a total of 207 subjects suffering from minor pain due to osteoarthritis and rheumatoid arthritis showed the active product to give statistically significant beneficial results vs. placebo for greater relief of perceived pain, increased range of motion of the affected joints and increased digital dexterity. In two studies designed to measure the effect of topically applied BENGAY vs. placebo on muscular endurance, discomfort, onset of exercise pain and fatigue, 30 subjects performed a submaximal three-hour run and another 30 subjects performed a maximal treadmill run. BENGAY was found to significantly decrease the discomfort during the submaximal and maximal runs, and increase the time before onset of fatigue during the maximal run.

Applied before workouts, BENGAY relaxes tight muscles and increases circulation to make exercising more comfortable, longer.

To help reduce muscle ache and soreness after exercise, BENGAY can be applied and allowed to work before taking a shower.

Directions: Apply to affected area not more than 3 to 4 times daily.

Warnings: For external use only. Use only as directed. Do not use with a heating pad. Keep away from children to avoid accidental ingestion. Do not swallow. If swallowed, get medical help or contact a Poison Control Center immedi-

ately. Do not bandage tightly. Keep away from eyes, mucous membranes, broken or irritated skin. If skin redness or excessive irritation develops, pain lasts for more than 10 days, or with arthritis-like conditions in children under 12, do not use and call a physician.

Shown in Product Identification Guide, page 518

BENYLIN® Adult Formula Cough Suppressant
[bĕ´-nă-lĭn]

Drug Facts:

Active Ingredient: **Purpose:**
(in each 5 mL)*
Dextromethorphan
 HBr 15 mg .... Antitussive

*5 mL = one teaspoonful

Use:
• temporarily relieves cough due to minor throat and bronchial irritation due to the common cold

Warnings:
Do not use if you are now taking a prescription monoamine oxidase inhibitor (MAOI) (certain drugs for depression, psychiatric, or emotional conditions, or Parkinson's disease), or for 2 weeks after stopping the MAOI drug. If you do not know if your prescription drug contains an MAOI, ask a doctor or pharmacist before taking this product.
Ask a doctor before use if you have:
• cough accompanied by excessive phlegm (mucus)
• persistent or chronic cough such as occurs with smoking, asthma, or emphysema
Stop use and ask a doctor if:
• cough persists for more than 1 week, tends to recur, or is accompanied by fever, rash, or persistent headache. These could be signs of a serious condition.
If pregnant or breast-feeding, ask a health professional before use.
Keep out of reach of children. In case of overdose, get medical help or contact a Poison Control Center right away.

Directions:
• take every 6 to 8 hours
• do not take more than 4 doses in 24 hours

adults and children 12 years of age and over	two (2) teaspoonfuls
children 6 to under 12 years of age	one (1) teaspoonful
children 2 to under 6 years of age	one-half (1/2) teaspoonful
children under 2 years of age	ask a doctor

Other Information:
• store at 59° to 77°F

Inactive Ingredients: Caramel, citric acid, D&C red no. 33, FD&C red no. 40,

flavors, glycerin, poloxamer 407, polysorbate 20, purified water, saccharin sodium, sodium benzoate, sodium carboxymethyl cellulose, sodium citrate, and sorbitol solution

Questions? Call **1-800-223-0182,** Monday to Friday, 9 AM–5 PM EST

How Supplied: Benylin Adult Formula is supplied in 4 fl. oz. (118 mL) bottles.

Shown in Product Identification Guide, page 518

BENYLIN® Expectorant Cough Suppressant/Expectorant
[bĕ´-nă-lĭn]

Drug Facts:

Active Ingredients:
(in each 5 mL)*   **Purpose:**
Dextromethorphan HBr
 5 mg .... Antitussive
Guaifenesin 100 mg .... Expectorant

* 5 ml = one teaspoonful

Uses:
• temporarily relieves cough due to minor throat and bronchial irritation due to the common cold
• helps loosen phlegm (mucus) and thin bronchial secretions to make coughs more productive

Warnings:
Do not use if you are now taking a prescription monoamine oxidase inhibitor (MAOI) (certain drugs for depression, psychiatric or emotional conditions, or Parkinson's disease), or for 2 weeks after stopping the MAOI drug. If you do not know if your prescription drug contains an MAOI, ask a doctor or pharmacist before taking this product.
Ask a doctor before use if you have:
• cough accompanied by excessive phlegm (mucus)
• persistent or chronic cough such as occurs with smoking, asthma, chronic bronchitis, or emphysema
Stop use and ask a doctor if:
• cough persists for more than 1 week, tends to recur, or is accompanied by a fever, rash, or persistent headache. These could be signs of a serious condition.
If pregnant or breast-feeding, ask a health professional before use.
Keep out of reach of children. In case of overdose, get medical help or contact a Poison Control Center right away.

Continued on next page

This product information was prepared in November 2002. On these and other Pfizer Consumer Healthcare Products, detailed information may be obtained by addressing Pfizer Consumer Healthcare, Pfizer, Inc., Morris Plains, NJ 07950

Benylin Cough Sup/Exp—Cont.

Directions:
- take every 4 hours
- do not take more than 6 doses in 24 hours

adults and children 12 years of age and over	four (4) teaspoonfuls
children 6 to under 12 years of age	two (2) teaspoonfuls
children 2 to under 6 years of age	one (1) teaspoonful
children under 2 years of age	ask a doctor

Other Information:
- store at 59° to 77°F

Inactive Ingredients: Caramel, citric acid, D&C red no. 33, edetate disodium, FD&C red no. 40, flavors, poloxamer 407, polyethylene glycol, propyl gallate, propylene glycol, purified water, saccharin sodium, sodium benzoate, sodium chloride, sodium citrate, and sorbitol solution

Questions? Call **1-800-223-0182**, Monday to Friday, 9 AM – 5 PM EST

How Supplied: Benylin Expectorant is available in 4 fl. oz. (118 mL) bottles.
Shown in Product Identification Guide, page 518

BENYLIN® Pediatric Cough Suppressant
[bĕ '-nă-lĭn]

Drug Facts:

Active Ingredient:
(in each 5 mL)*   **Purpose:**
Dextromethorphan HBr
 7.5 mg .... Antitussive

* 5 ml = one teaspoonful

Uses:
- temporarily relieves cough due to minor throat and bronchial irritation due to the common cold

Warnings:
Do not use if you are now taking a prescription monoamine oxidase inhibitor (MAOI) (certain drugs for depression, psychiatric or emotional conditions, or Parkinson's disease), or for 2 weeks after stopping the MAOI drug. If you do not know if your prescription drug contains an MAOI, ask a doctor or pharmacist before taking this product.
Ask a doctor before use if you have:
- cough accompanied by excessive phlegm (mucus)
- persistent or chronic cough such as occurs with smoking, asthma, or emphysema
Stop use and ask a doctor if:
- cough persists for more than 1 week, tends to recur, or is accompanied by fever, rash, or persistent headache. These could be signs of a serious condition.

If pregnant or breast-feeding, ask a health professional before use.
Keep out of reach of children. In case of overdose, get medical help or contact a Poison Control Center right away.
Directions:
- take every 6 to 8 hours
- do not take more than 4 doses in 24 hours

children under 2 years of age	ask a doctor
children 2 to under 6 years of age	one (1) teaspoonful
children 6 to under 12 years of age	two (2) teaspoonfuls
adults and children 12 years of age and over	four (4) teaspoonfuls

Other Information:
- store at 59° to 77°F

Inactive Ingredients: Carboxymethyl cellulose sodium, Citric acid, D&C red no. 33, FD&C blue no. 1, flavors, glycerin, purified water, saccharin sodium, sodium benzoate, sodium chloride, sodium citrate, and sorbitol solution

Questions? Call **1-800-223-0182**, Monday to Friday, 9 AM – 5 PM EST

How Supplied: Benylin Pediatric is supplied in 4 fl. oz. (118 mL) bottles.
Shown in Product Identification Guide, page 519

BONINE®
(Meclizine hydrochloride)
Chewable Tablets

Drug Facts:

Active Ingredient
(in each tablet):   **Purpose:**
Meclizine HCl 25 mg .... Antiemetic

Uses: prevents and treats nausea, vomiting or dizziness associated with motion sickness

Warnings:
Do not use for children under 12 years of age unless directed by a doctor
Ask a doctor before use if you have
- a breathing problem such as emphysema or chronic bronchitis
- glaucoma
- trouble urinating due to an enlarged prostate gland
Ask a doctor or pharmacist before use if you are taking sedatives or tranquilizers
When using this product
- drowsiness may occur
- avoid alcoholic drinks
- alcohol, sedatives, and tranquilizers may increase drowsiness
- be careful when driving a motor vehicle or operating machinery
- do not exceed recommended dosage
If pregnant or breast-feeding, ask a health professional before use.
Keep out of reach of children. In case of overdose, get medical help or contact a Poison Control Center right away.

Directions:
- adults and children 12 years of age and over: take 1 to 2 tablets once daily or as directed by a doctor
- dosage should be taken one hour before travel starts

Other Information:
- store below 86 °F (30 °C)

Inactive Ingredients: FD&C red no. 40, lactose, magnesium stearate, purified siliceous earth, raspberry flavor, saccharin sodium, starch, and talc
Questions? call **1-800-223-0182**, Monday to Friday, 9 AM - 5 PM EST

How Supplied: BONINE® (meclizine HCl) is available in convenient packets of 8 and 16 chewable tablets of 25 mg. meclizine HCl.
Shown in Product Identification Guide, page 519

CALADRYL® Lotion
[că 'lă drĭl "]

Drug Facts:

Active Ingredients: **Purpose:**
Calamine 8% .... Skin protectant
Pramoxine HCl 1% ..... Topical analgesic

Uses:
- temporarily relieves pain and itching associated with:
  - rashes due to poison ivy, poison oak or poison sumac
  - insect bites • minor skin irritation
  - minor cuts
- dries the oozing and weeping of poison ivy, poison oak and poison sumac

Warnings:
For external use only
When using this product
- avoid contact with eyes
Stop use and ask a doctor if
- condition worsens or does not improve within 7 days
- symptoms persist for more than 7 days or clear up and occur again within a few days
Keep out of reach of children. If swallowed, get medical help or contact a Poison Control Center right away.

Directions:
- shake well before use
- adults and children 2 years of age and older: apply to affected area not more than 3 to 4 times daily
- children under 2 years of age: ask a doctor
Other Information:
- store at 59° to 77°F

Inactive Ingredients: SD alcohol 38-B, camphor, diazolidinyl urea, fragrance, glycerin, hypromellose, methylparaben, polysorbate 80, propylene glycol, propylparaben, purified water, and xanthan gum
Questions? call **1-800-223-0182**, Monday to Friday, 9 AM - 5 PM EST

How Supplied: Caladryl Lotion—6 fl. oz. (177 mL) bottles
Shown in Product Identification Guide, page 519

CALADRYL® Clear™ Lotion
[cǎ 'lǎ drǐl "]

Drug Facts

Active Ingredients: **Purpose:**
Pramoxine HCl 1% ..... Topical analgesic
Zinc acetate 0.1% .... Skin protectant

Uses:
- temporarily relieves pain and itching associated with:
  - rashes due to poison ivy, poison oak or poison sumac
  - insect bites • minor skin irritation
  - minor cuts
- dries the oozing and weeping of poison ivy, poison oak and poison sumac

Warnings:
For external use only
When using this product
- avoid contact with eyes
Stop use and ask a doctor if
- condition worsens or does not improve within 7 days
- symptoms persist for more than 7 days or clear up and occur again within a few days
Keep out of reach of children. If swallowed, get medical help or contact a Poison Control Center right away.

Directions:
- shake well before use
- adults and children 2 years of age and older: apply to affected area not more than 3 to 4 times daily
- children under 2 years of age: ask a doctor

Other Information:
- store at 59° to 77°F

Inactive Ingredients: SD alcohol 38-B, camphor, citric acid, diazolidinyl urea, fragrance, glycerin, hypromellose, methylparaben, polysorbate 40, propylene glycol, propylparaben, purified water, and sodium citrate
Questions? call   **1-800-223-0182,** Monday to Friday, 9 AM - 5 PM EST

How   Supplied: Caladryl   Clear Lotion—6 fl. oz. (177 mL) bottles
Shown in Product Identification Guide, page 519

CORTIZONE•5®
Creme

Drug Facts

Active Ingredient: **Purpose:**
Hydrocortisone 0.5% .... Anti-itch

Uses:
- temporarily relieves itching of minor skin irritations, inflammation, and rashes due to:
  - eczema
  - insect bites
  - cosmetics
  - psoriasis
  - detergents
  - soaps
  - poison ivy, oak, sumac
  - jewelry
  - seborrheic dermatitis
  - and for external anal and genital itching
- other uses of this product should be only under the advice and supervision of a doctor

Warnings:
For external use only
Do not use
- for the treatment of diaper rash. Consult a doctor.
- in the genital area if you have a vaginal discharge. Consult a doctor.
When using this product
- avoid contact with the eyes
- do not exceed the recommended daily dosage unless directed by a doctor
- do not put directly in rectum by using fingers or any mechanical device
Stop use and ask a doctor if
- rectal bleeding occurs
- condition worsens, or if symptoms persist for more than 7 days or clear up and occur again within a few days, and do not begin use of any other hydrocortisone product unless you have asked a doctor
Keep out of reach of children. If swallowed, get medical help or contact a Poison Control Center right away.

Directions:
- adults and children 2 years of age and older:
  - apply to affected area not more than 3 to 4 times daily
  - children under 2 years of age: do not use, ask a doctor
- for external anal and genital itching, adults:
  - when practical, clean the affected area with mild soap and warm water and rinse thoroughly
  - gently dry by patting or blotting with toilet tissue or a soft cloth before applying
  - apply to affected area not more than 3 to 4 times daily
  - children under 12 years of age: ask a doctor

Other Information:
- store at 15° to 30°C (59° to 86°F)

Inactive Ingredients: aloe barbadensis gel, aluminum sulfate, calcium acetate, cetearyl alcohol, glycerin, light mineral oil, maltodextrin, methylparaben, potato dextrin, propylparaben, purified water, sodium cetearyl sulfate, sodium lauryl sulfate, white petrolatum, and white wax
Questions? call **1-800-223-0182,** Monday to Friday, 9 AM - 5 PM EST

How   Supplied: CORTIZONE•5® creme: 1 oz. and 2 oz. tubes.
Shown in Product Identification Guide, page 519

CORTIZONE•5®
Ointment

Drug Facts

Active Ingredient: **Purpose:**
Hydrocortisone 0.5% .... Anti-itch

Uses:
- temporarily relieves itching of minor skin irritations, inflammation, and rashes due to:
  - eczema
  - insect bites
  - cosmetics
  - psoriasis
  - detergents
  - soaps
  - poison ivy, oak, sumac
  - jewelry
  - seborrheic dermatitis
  - and for external anal and genital itching
- other uses of this product should be only under the advice and supervision of a doctor

Warnings:
For external use only
Do not use
- for the treatment of diaper rash. Consult a doctor.
- in the genital area if you have a vaginal discharge. Consult a doctor.
When using this product
- avoid contact with the eyes
- do not exceed the recommended daily dosage unless directed by a doctor
- do not put directly in rectum by using fingers or any mechanical device
Stop use and ask a doctor if
- rectal bleeding occurs
- condition worsens, or if symptoms persist for more than 7 days or clear up and occur again within a few days, and do not begin use of any other hydrocortisone product unless you have asked a doctor
Keep out of reach of children. If swallowed, get medical help or contact a Poison Control Center right away.

Directions:
- adults and children 2 years of age and older:
  - apply to affected area not more than 3 to 4 times daily
  - children under 2 years of age: do not use, ask a doctor
- for external anal and genital itching, adults:
  - when practical, clean the affected area with mild soap and warm water and rinse thoroughly
  - gently dry by patting or blotting with toilet tissue or a soft cloth before applying
  - apply to affected area not more than 3 to 4 times daily
  - children under 12 years of age: ask a doctor

Other Information:
- store at 15° to 30°C (59° to 86°F)

Inactive Ingredients: aloe barbadensis extract and white petrolatum

Questions? call **1-800-223-0182,** Monday to Friday, 9 AM - 5 PM EST

How   Supplied: CORTIZONE•5® ointment: 1 oz. tube.
Shown in Product Identification Guide, page 519

Continued on next page

This product information was prepared in November 2002. On these and other Pfizer Consumer Healthcare Products, detailed information may be obtained by addressing Pfizer Consumer Healthcare, Pfizer, Inc., Morris Plains, NJ 07950

CORTIZONE KIDS™ CREME WITH ALOE

Drug Facts

Active Ingredient: **Purpose:**
Hydrocortisone 0.5% .... Anti-itch

Uses:
- temporarily relieves itching of minor skin irritations, inflammation, and rashes due to:
  - eczema
  - soaps
  - insect bites
  - psoriasis
  - poison ivy, oak, sumac
  - detergents
  - seborrheic dermatitis
- other uses of this product should be only under the advice and supervision of a doctor

Warnings:
For external use only
Do not use
- for the treatment of diaper rash. Consult a doctor.

When using this product
- avoid contact with the eyes

Stop use and ask a doctor if condition worsens, or if symptoms persist for more than 7 days or clear up and occur again within a few days, and do not begin use of any other hydrocortisone product unless you have asked a doctor

Keep out of reach of children. If swallowed, get medical help or contact a Poison Control Center right away.

Directions:
- children 2 years of age and older: apply to affected area not more than 3 to 4 times daily
- children under 2 years of age: do not use; ask a doctor

Other Information:
- store at 15° to 30°C (59° to 86°F)

Inactive Ingredients: aloe barbadensis gel, aluminum sulfate, calcium acetate, cetearyl alcohol, glycerin, light mineral oil, maltodextrin, methylparaben, potato dextrin, propylparaben, purified water, sodium cetearyl sulfate, sodium lauryl sulfate, white petrolatum, and white wax

Questions? call **1-800-223-0182**, Monday to Friday, 9 AM - 5 PM EST

How Supplied: CORTIZONE for KIDS™ creme: 1 oz. tubes.

Shown in Product Identification Guide, page 519

CORTIZONE•10®
Creme

Drug Facts

Active Ingredient: **Purpose:**
Hydrocortisone 1% .... Anti-itch

Uses:
- temporarily relieves itching of minor skin irritations, inflammation, and rashes due to:
  - eczema
  - insect bites
  - cosmetics
  - psoriasis
  - detergents
  - soaps
  - poison ivy, oak, sumac
  - jewelry
  - seborrheic dermatitis
  - and for external anal and genital itching
- other uses of this product should be only under the advice and supervision of a doctor

Warnings:
For external use only
Do no use
- for the treatment of diaper rash. Consult a doctor.
- in the genital area if you have a vaginal discharge. Consult a doctor.

When using this product
- avoid contact with the eyes
- do not exceed the recommended daily dosage unless directed by a doctor
- do not put directly in rectum by using fingers or any mechanical device

Stop use and ask a doctor if
- rectal bleeding occurs
- condition worsens, or if symptoms persist for more than 7 days or clear up and occur again within a few days, and do not begin use of any other hydrocortisone product unless you have asked a doctor

Keep out of reach of children. If swallowed, get medical help or contact a Poison Control Center right away.

Directions:
- adults and children 2 years of age and older:
  - apply to affected area not more than 3 to 4 times daily
  - children under 2 years of age: do not use, ask a doctor
- for external anal and genital itching, adults:
  - when practical, clean the affected area with mild soap and warm water and rinse thoroughly
  - gently dry by patting or blotting with toilet tissue or a soft cloth before applying
  - apply to affected area not more than 3 to 4 times daily
  - children under 12 years of age: ask a doctor

Other Information: • store at 15° to 30°C (59° to 86°F)

Inactive Ingredients: aloe barbadensis gel, aluminum sulfate, calcium acetate, cetearyl alcohol, glycerin, light mineral oil, maltodextrin, methylparaben, potato dextrin, propylparaben, purified water, sodium cetearyl sulfate, sodium lauryl sulfate, white petrolatum, and white wax

Questions? call **1-800-223-0182**, Monday to Friday, 9 AM - 5 PM EST

How Supplied: CORTIZONE•10® creme: .5 oz., 1 oz. and 2 oz. tubes.

CORTIZONE 10® CREME
External Anal Itch Relief

Drug Facts

Active Ingredient: **Purpose:**
Hydrocortisone 1% .... Anti-itch

Uses:
- temporarily relieves external anal itching

- other uses of this product should be only under the advice and supervision of a doctor

Warnings:
For external use only
Do not use
- for the treatment of diaper rash. Consult a doctor.

When using this product
- avoid contact with the eyes
- do not exceed the recommended daily dosage unless directed by a doctor
- do not put directly in rectum by using fingers or any mechanical device

Stop use and ask a doctor if
- rectal bleeding occurs
- condition worsens, or if symptoms persist for more than 7 days or clear up and occur again within a few days, and do not begin use of any other hydrocortisone product unless you have asked a doctor

Keep out of reach of children. If swallowed, get medical help or contact a Poison Control Center right away.

Directions:
- for external anal itching, adults:
  - when practical, clean the affected area with mild soap and warm water and rinse thoroughly
  - gently dry by patting or blotting with toilet tissue or a soft cloth before applying
  - apply to affected area not more than 3 to 4 times daily
- children under 12 years of age: ask a doctor

Other Information: • store at 15° to 30°C (59° to 86°F)

Inactive Ingredients: aloe barbadensis gel, aluminum sulfate, calcium acetate, cetearyl alcohol, glycerin, light mineral oil, maltodextrin, methylparaben, potato dextrin, propylparaben, purified water, sodium cetearyl sulfate, sodium lauryl sulfate, white petrolatum, and white wax

Questions? call **1-800-223-0182**, Monday to Friday, 9 AM - 5 PM EST

How Supplied: Cortizone•10® External Anal Itch Relief Creme: .5 oz., 1 oz. and 2 oz. tubes.

CORTIZONE•10®
Ointment

Drug Facts

Active Ingredient: **Purpose:**
Hydrocortisone 1% .... Anti-itch

Uses:
- temporarily relieves itching of minor skin irritations, inflammation, and rashes due to:
  - eczema
  - insect bites
  - cosmetics
  - psoriasis
  - detergents
  - soaps
  - poison ivy, oak, sumac
  - jewelry
  - seborrheic dermatitis
  - and for external anal and genital itching

- other uses of this product should be only under the advice and supervision of a doctor

Warnings:
For external use only
Do not use
- for the treatment of diaper rash. Consult a doctor.
- in the genital area if you have a vaginal discharge. Consult a doctor.

When using this product
- avoid contact with the eyes
- do not exceed the recommended daily dosage unless directed by a doctor
- do not put directly in rectum by using fingers or any mechanical device

Stop use and ask a doctor if
- rectal bleeding occurs
- condition worsens, or if symptoms persist for more than 7 days or clear up and occur again within a few days, and do not begin use of any other hydrocortisone product unless you have asked a doctor

Keep out of reach of children. If swallowed, get medical help or contact a Poison Control Center right away.

Directions:
- adults and children 2 years of age and older:
  - apply to affected area not more than 3 to 4 times daily
  - children under 2 years of age: do not use, ask a doctor
- for external anal and genital itching, adults:
  - when practical, clean the affected area with mild soap and warm water and rinse thoroughly
  - gently dry by patting or blotting with toilet tissue or a soft cloth before applying
  - apply to affected area not more than 3 to 4 times daily
  - children under 12 years of age: ask a doctor

Other Information:
- store at 15° to 30°C (59° to 86°F)

Inactive Ingredients: white petrolatum
Questions? call **1-800-223-0182**, Monday to Friday, 9 AM - 5 PM EST

How Supplied: CORTIZONE•10® ointment: 1 oz. and 2 oz. tubes.

CORTIZONE•10® Plus
Creme
Hydrocortisone Anti-Itch Cream

Drug Facts:

Active Ingredient: **Purpose:**
Hydrocortisone 1% .... Anti-itch

Uses:
- temporarily relieves itching of minor skin irritations, inflammation, and rashes due to:
  - eczema
  - insect bites
  - cosmetics
  - psoriasis
  - detergents
  - soaps
  - poison ivy, oak, sumac
  - jewelry
  - seborrheic dermatitis
  - and for external anal and genital itching

- other uses of this product should be only under the advice and supervision of a doctor

Warnings:
For external use only
Do not use
- for the treatment of diaper rash. Consult a doctor.
- in the genital area if you have a vaginal discharge. Consult a doctor.

When using this product
- avoid contact with the eyes
- do not exceed the recommended daily dosage unless directed by a doctor
- do not put directly in rectum by using fingers or any mechanical device

Stop use and ask a doctor if
- rectal bleeding occurs
- condition worsens, or if symptoms persist for more than 7 days or clear up and occur again within a few days, and do not begin use of any other hydrocortisone product unless you have asked a doctor

Keep out of reach of children. If swallowed, get medical help or contact a Poison Control Center right away.

Directions:
- adults and children 2 years of age and older:
  - apply to affected area not more than 3 to 4 times daily
  - children under 2 years of age: do not use, ask a doctor
- for external anal itching, adults:
  - when practical, clean the affected area with mild soap and warm water and rinse thoroughly
  - gently dry by patting or blotting with toilet tissue or a soft cloth before applying
  - children under 12 years of age: ask a doctor

Other Information: • store at 15° to 30°C (59° to 86°F)

Inactive Ingredients: aloe barbadensis gel, aluminum sulfate, calcium acetate, cetearyl alcohol, cetyl alcohol, corn oil, glycerin, isopropyl palmitate, light mineral oil, maltodextrin, methylparaben, potato dextrin, propylene glycol, propylparaben, purified water, sodium cetearyl sulfate, sodium lauryl sulfate, vitamin A palmitate, vitamin D, vitamin E, white petrolatum, and white wax

Questions? call **1-800-223-0182**, Monday to Friday, 9 AM - 5 PM EST

How Supplied: CORTIZONE•10® Plus creme: 1 oz. and 2 oz. tubes.
Shown in Product Identification Guide, page 519

CORTIZONE•10® MAXIMUM STRENGTH QUICK SHOT™ SPRAY

Drug Facts

Active Ingredient: **Purpose:**
Hydrocortisone 1% .... Anti-itch

Uses:
- temporarily relieves itching of minor skin irritations, inflammation, and rashes due to:
  - eczema
  - insect bites
  - cosmetics

- psoriasis
- detergents
- soaps
- poison ivy, oak, sumac
- jewelry
- seborrheic dermatitis
- other uses of this product should be only under the advice and supervision of a doctor

Warnings:
For external use only
Flammable - keep away from fire or flame
Do not use
- for the treatment of diaper rash. Consult a doctor.

When using this product
- avoid contact with the eyes

Stop use and ask a doctor if condition worsens, or if symptoms persist for more than 7 days or clear up and occur again within a few days, and do not begin use of any other hydrocortisone product unless you have asked a doctor

Keep out of reach of children. If swallowed, get medical help or contact a Poison Control Center right away.

Directions:
- adults and children 2 years of age and older: apply to affected area not more than 3 to 4 times daily
- children under 2 years of age: do not use; ask a doctor

Other Information:
- store at 15° to 30°C (59° to 86°F)
- store away from heat and protect from freezing

Inactive Ingredients: benzyl alcohol, propylene glycol, purified water, and SD alcohol 40-2 (60% v/v)

Questions? call **1-800-223-0182**, Monday to Friday, 9 AM - 5 PM EST

How Supplied: CORTIZONE•10® Quick Shot Spray: 1.5 oz. pump bottle
Shown in Product Identification Guide, page 519

DESITIN® CREAMY WITH ALOE and VITAMIN E
Zinc Oxide Diaper Rash Ointment

Drug Facts:

Active Ingredient: **Purpose:**
Zinc oxide 10% .... Skin protectant

Uses:
- helps treat and prevent diaper rash
- protects chafed skin due to diaper rash and helps seal out wetness

Warnings:
For external use only

Continued on next page

This product information was prepared in November 2002. On these and other Pfizer Consumer Healthcare Products, detailed information may be obtained by addressing Pfizer Consumer Healthcare, Pfizer, Inc., Morris Plains, NJ 07950

Desitin Creamy—Cont.

When using this product
• avoid contact with the eyes
Stop use and ask a doctor if:
• condition worsens or does not improve within 7 days
Keep out of reach of children. If swallowed, get medical help or contact a Poison Control Center right away.

Directions:
• change wet and soiled diapers promptly
• cleanse the diaper area
• allow to dry
• apply ointment liberally as often as necessary, with each diaper change, especially at bedtime or anytime when exposure to wet diapers may be prolonged

Other Information:
• store at 15° to 30°C (59° to 86°F)

Inactive Ingredients: aloe barbadensis gel, cyclomethicone, dimethicone, fragrance, methylparaben, microcrystalline wax, mineral oil, propylparaben, purified water, sodium borate, sorbitan sesquioleate, vitamin E, white petrolatum, and white wax

Questions? Call **1-800-223-0182**, Monday to Friday, 9 AM–5 PM EST

How Supplied: Desitin Creamy with Aloe and Vitamin E is available in 2 oz. (57g) and 4 oz. (113g) tubes.
Shown in Product Identification Guide, page 519

DESITIN® OINTMENT
Zinc Oxide Diaper Rash Ointment

Drug Facts:

Active Ingredient: **Purpose:**
Zinc oxide 40% .... Skin protectant

Uses:
• helps treat and prevent diaper rash
• protects chafed skin due to diaper rash and helps seal out wetness

Warnings:
For external use only.
When using this product
• avoid contact with the eyes
Stop use and ask a doctor if
• condition worsens or does not improve within 7 days
Keep out of reach of children. If swallowed, get medical help or contact a Poison Control Center right away.

Directions:
• change wet and soiled diapers promptly
• cleanse the diaper area
• allow to dry
• apply ointment liberally as often as necessary, with each diaper change, especially at bedtime or anytime when exposure to wet diapers may be prolonged

Other Information:
• store at 15° to 30°C (59° to 86°F)

Inactive Ingredients: BHA, cod liver oil, fragrance, lanolin, methylparaben, petrolatum, talc, and water

Questions? call **1-800-223-0182**, Monday to Friday, 9 AM - 5 PM EST

How Supplied: Desitin Ointment is available in 1 ounce (28g), 2 ounce (57g), and 4 ounce (114g) tubes, and 9 ounce (255g) and 16 ounce (454g) jars.
Shown in Product Identification Guide, page 519

---

e.p.t® PREGNANCY TEST
99% Accurate at detecting the pregnancy hormone. However, some pregnant women may not have detectable amounts of pregnancy hormone in their urine on the first day of the missed period or may have miscalculated the first day of their period

PLEASE READ INSTRUCTIONS CAREFULLY:
[See graphic below]
How to use: Remove the **e.p.t.** test stick from its foil packet just prior to use. Remove the purple cap to expose the absorbent tip. Hold the test stick by its thumb grip. Point the absorbent tip downward. Place the absorbent tip in the urine flow for just 5 seconds, or dip the absorbent tip into a clean container of urine for just 5 seconds.

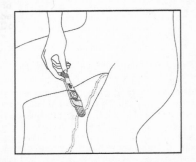

Place the test stick on a flat surface with the windows facing up for at least 3 minutes. (If you wish, replace the cap to cover the absorbent tip.) You may notice a light pink color moving across the windows.
Important: **To avoid affecting the test result, wait at least 3 minutes before lifting the stick.**

How to Read the Results:
Wait 3 minutes to read the result. A line will appear in the square window to show that the test is working properly. Be sure to read the result before 20 minutes have passed.

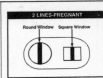

Two parallel lines, one in each window, indicate that you are **pregnant.** The lines can be different shades of pink and need not match the color in the illustration. Please see your doctor to discuss your pregnancy and the next steps. Early prenatal care is important to ensure the health of you and your baby.

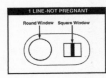

One line in the square window but none in the round window indicates that you are **not pregnant.** If your period does not start within a week, repeat the test. If you still get a negative result and your period has not started, please see your doctor.

Important: **If no line appears in the square window, the test result is invalid. Do not read the result. Call our toll-free number 1-800-378-1783 (1-800-EPT-1STEP).**

Questions? Call toll-free 1-800-378-1783

Registered nurses available 8:30 am - 5:00 pm EST weekdays, consumer specialists available until 8:00 pm, and recorded help available 24 hours, (including weekends).

Questions and Answers about e.p.t.®
When can I use e.p.t?
e.p.t can be used any time of day as soon as you miss your period and any day thereafter.

How does e.p.t work?
e.p.t detects hCG (human Chorionic Gonadotropin), a hormone present in urine only during pregnancy. **e.p.t** can detect hCG in your urine as early as the first day your period is late.

What if the lines in the round and square windows are different shades of pink? As long as 2 parallel lines appear, one in each window, the result is positive, even if the two lines are different shades of pink.

What if I think the test result is incorrect? Following the instructions carefully should yield an accurate reading. If you think the result is incorrect, or if it is

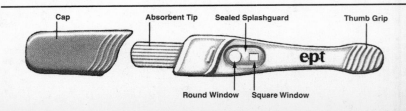

Cap · Absorbent Tip · Sealed Splashguard · Thumb Grip · ept · Round Window · Square Window

difficult to detect a line in the round window, repeat the test after 2–3 days with a new **e.p.t** stick.

Are there any factors that can affect the test result? Yes. Certain drugs which contain hCG or are used in combination with hCG (such as Humegon™, Pregnyl, Profasi, Pergonal, APL) and rare medical conditions. If you repeat the test and continue to get an unexpected result, contact your doctor.

Using **e.p.t** within 8 weeks of giving birth or having a miscarriage may cause a false positive result. The test may detect hCG still in your system from a previous pregnancy. You should ask your doctor for help in interpreting the result of your **e.p.t** test if you have recently been pregnant.

Factors which should <u>not</u> affect the test result include alcohol, analgesics (pain killers), antibiotics, birth control pills or hormone therapies containing clomiphene citrate (Clomid or Serophen). Store at room temperature 15°–30°C (59°–86°F). FOR IN-VITRO DIAGNOSTIC USE. (NOT FOR INTERNAL USE.) KEEP OUT OF THE REACH OF CHILDREN.

Please call our toll-free number 1-800-378-1783 with any questions about using e.p.t.

Shown in Product Identification Guide, page 519

LISTERINE® Antiseptic
[lĭs 'tǝrēn]

Active Ingredients: Thymol 0.064%, Eucalyptol 0.092%, Methyl Salicylate 0.060% and Menthol 0.042%.

Inactive Ingredients: Water, Alcohol 26.9%, Benzoic Acid, Poloxamer 407, Sodium Benzoate, and Caramel.

Indications: Use Listerine® Antiseptic twice daily to help:
• Prevent & Reduce Plaque
• Prevent & Reduce Gingivitis
• Fight Bad Breath
• Kill Germs Between Teeth

Actions: Listerine® Antiseptic has been shown to help prevent and reduce supragingival plaque accumulation and gingivitis when used in a conscientiously applied program of oral hygiene and regular professional care. Its effect on periodontitis has not been determined. Listerine is the only leading nonprescription mouthrinse that has received the American Dental Association's Council on Scientific Affairs Seal of Acceptance for helping to prevent and reduce plaque and gingivitis.

Directions: Rinse full strength for 30 seconds with 20 ml (²/₃ fl. ounce or 4 teaspoonfuls) morning and night. If bad breath persists, see your dentist.

Warnings: Do not administer to children under twelve years of age. **Keep this and all drugs out of the reach of**

children. Do not swallow. In case of accidental ingestion, seek professional assistance or contact a Poison Control Center immediately.

Cold weather may cloud Listerine. Its antiseptic properties are not affected. Store at 59° to 77°F.

How Supplied: Listerine® Antiseptic is supplied in 250 ml, 500 ml, 1.0 liter, 1.5 liter and 1.7 liter bottles, as well as 3 fl. oz. bottles. It is also available to professionals in 3 fl. oz. bottles and in gallons.

Shown in Product Identification Guide, page 519

COOL MINT LISTERINE® ANTISEPTIC
[lĭs 'tǝrēn]

Active Ingredients: Thymol 0.064%, Eucalyptol 0.092%, Methyl Salicylate 0.060% and Menthol 0.042%.

Inactive Ingredients: Water, Alcohol 21.6%, Sorbitol Solution, Flavoring, Poloxamer 407, Benzoic Acid, Sodium Saccharin, Sodium Benzoate, and FD&C Green No. 3.

Indications: Use Cool Mint Listerine Antiseptic twice daily to help:
• Prevent & Reduce Plaque
• Prevent & Reduce Gingivitis
• Fight Bad Breath
• Kills Germs Between teeth.

Actions: Cool Mint Listerine® Antiseptic has been shown to help prevent and reduce supragingival plaque accumulation and gingivitis when used in a conscientiously applied program of oral hygiene and regular professional care. Its effect on periodontitis has not been determined. Listerine is the only leading nonprescription mouthrinse that has received the American Dental Association's Council on Scientific Affairs Seal of Acceptance for helping to prevent and reduce plaque and gingivitis.

Directions: Rinse full strength for 30 seconds with 20 ml (²/₃ fl. ounce or 4 teaspoonfuls) morning and night. If bad breath persists, see your dentist.

Warnings: Do not administer to children under twelve years of age. **Keep this and all drugs out of the reach of children.** Do not swallow. In case of accidental ingestion, seek professional assistance or contact a Poison Control Center immediately. Cold weather may cloud Cool Mint Listerine. Its antiseptic properties are not affected. Store at 59° to 77°F.

How Supplied: Cool Mint Listerine® Antiseptic is supplied in 250 ml, 500 ml, 1.0 liter, 1.5 liter bottles and 1.7 liter bottles, as well as 3 and 58 fl. oz. bottles. It is also available to professionals in 3 fl. oz. bottles and in gallon bottles.

Shown in Product Identification Guide, page 519

FRESHBURST® LISTERINE® ANTISEPTIC
[lĭs 'tǝrēn]

Active Ingredients: Thymol 0.064%, Eucalyptol 0.092%, Methyl Salicylate 0.060% and Menthol 0.042%.

Inactive Ingredients: Water, Alcohol 21.6%, Sorbitol Solution, Flavoring, Poloxamer 407, Benzoic Acid, Sodium Saccharin, Sodium Benzoate, D&C Yellow No. 10, and FD&C Green No. 3.

Indications: Use FreshBurst Listerine Antiseptic twice daily to help:
• Prevent & Reduce Plaque
• Prevent & Reduce Gingivitis
• Fight Bad Breath
• Kill Germs Between Teeth

Actions: FreshBurst® Listerine® Antiseptic has been shown to help prevent and reduce supragingival plaque accumulation and gingivitis when used in a conscientiously applied program of oral hygiene and regular professional care. Its effect on periodontitis has not been determined. Listerine is the only leading nonprescription mouthrinse that has received the American Dental Association's Council on Scientific Affairs Seal of Acceptance for helping to prevent and reduce plaque and gingivitis.

Directions: Rinse full strength for 30 seconds with 20 ml (²/₃ fl. ounce or 4 teaspoonfuls) morning and night. If bad breath persists, see your dentist.

Warnings: Do not administer to children under twelve years of age. **Keep this and all drugs out of the reach of children.** Do not swallow. In case of accidental ingestion, seek professional assistance or contact a Poison Control Center immediately. Cold weather may cloud FreshBurst® Listerine®. Its antiseptic properties are not affected. Store at 59° to 77°F.

How Supplied: FreshBurst® Listerine® antiseptic is supplied in 250 ml, 500 ml, 1.0 liter, 1.5 liter bottles and 1.7 liter bottles, as well as 3 fl. oz. bottles. It is also available to professionals in 3 fl. oz. bottles and in gallon bottles.

Shown in Product Identification Guide, page 519

TARTAR CONTROL LISTERINE® Antiseptic
[lys'tǝrěn]

Active Ingredients: Thymol 0.064%, Eucalyptol 0.092%, Methyl Salicylate 0.060%, and Menthol 0.042.%.

Continued on next page

This product information was prepared in November 2002. On these and other Pfizer Consumer Healthcare Products, detailed information may be obtained by addressing Pfizer Consumer Healthcare, Pfizer, Inc., Morris Plains, NJ 07950

Tartar Listerine—Cont.

Inactive Ingredients: Water, Alcohol 21.6%, Sorbitol Solution, Flavoring, Poloxamer 407, Sodium Saccharin, Benzoic Acid, Zinc Chloride, Sodium Benzoate, and FD&C Blue # 1.

Indications: Use Tartar Control Listerine® Antiseptic twice daily to help:
• Prevent & Fight Tartar Build-up
• Prevent & Reduce Plaque
• Prevent & Reduce Gingivitis
• Fight Bad Breath
• Kill Germs Between Teeth

Actions: Tartar Control Listerine® Antiseptic has been shown to help prevent and reduce supragingival plaque accumulation and gingivitis when used in a conscientiously applied program of oral hygiene and regular professional care. It has also been shown to help reduce the formation of tartar above the gumline. Its effect on periodontitis has not been determined. Listerine is the only leading nonprescription mouthrinse that has received the American Dental Association's Council on Scientific Affairs Seal of Acceptance for helping to prevent and reduce plaque and gingivitis.

Directions: Rinse full strength for 30 seconds with 20ml (2/3 fluid ounce or 4 teaspoonfuls) morning and night. If bad breath persists, see your dentist.

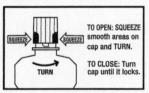

TO OPEN: SQUEEZE smooth areas on cap and TURN.

SQUEEZE ← → SQUEEZE

TURN

TO CLOSE: Turn cap until it locks.

Warnings: Do not administer to children under twelve years of age. **KEEP THIS AND ALL DRUGS OUT OF THE REACH OF CHILDREN.** Do not swallow. In case of accidental overdose, seek professional assistance or contact a Poison Control Center immediately. **Cold weather may cloud Tartar Control Listerine. Its antiseptic properties are not affected.** Store at 59° to 77°F.

How Supplied: Tartar Control. Listerine® Antiseptic is supplied in 250 ml, 500 ml, 1.0 liter and 1.5 liter bottles, as well as 3 fl. oz. bottles.
Shown in Product Identification Guide, page 519

LISTERMINT®
Alcohol-Free Mouthwash
[lĭs 'tər mĭnt]

Ingredient: Water, Glycerin, Poloxamer 335, PEG 600, Flavors, Sodium Lauryl Sulfate, Sodium Benzoate, Sodium Saccharin, Benzoic Acid, Zinc Chloride, D&C Yellow No. 10, FD&C Green No. 3.

Indications: Freshens breath; contains no fluoride.

Directions: Rinse with 30 ml (1 fl. oz.) for 30 seconds to freshen breath in the morning and after meals as needed.

Warnings: Do not swallow. Keep out of reach of children.

How Supplied: Listermint® is supplied to consumers in a 32 fl. oz. bottle and is available to professionals in 3 fl. oz. bottles and in gallons.
Shown in Product Identification Guide, page 519

LUBRIDERM® Advanced Therapy Creamy Lotion
[lū brĭ dĕrm]

Ingredients: Water, Cetyl Alcohol, Glycerin, Mineral Oil, Cyclomethicone, Propylene Glycol Dicaprylate/Dicaprate, PEG-40 Stearate, Isopropyl Isostearate, Emulsifying Wax, Lecithin, Carbomer 940, Diazolidinyl Urea, Titanium Dioxide, Sodium Benzoate, BHT, Tri(PPG-3 Myristyl Ether) Citrate, Disodium EDTA, Retinyl Palmitate, Tocopheryl Acetate, Sodium Pyruvate, Iodopropynyl Butylcarbamate, Fragrance, Sodium Hydroxide, Xanthan Gum.

Uses: Lubriderm Advanced Therapy's nourishing, rich and creamy formula helps heal extra-dry skin. Its unique combination of nutrient-enriched moisturizers penetrate dry skin leaving you with soft, smooth and comfortable skin. This non-greasy feeling lotion absorbs quickly and is non-comedogenic.

Directions: Smooth Lubriderm on hands and body every day.
For external use only.

How Supplied: Available in 6, 10, 16, and 19.6 fl. oz plastic bottles and a 3.3 fl. oz. tube.
Shown in Product Identification Guide, page 519

LUBRIDERM® Daily UV Lotion w/Sunscreen
[lū brĭ dĕrm]

Active Ingredients: Octyl Methoxycinnamate 7.5%, Octyl Salicylate 4%, Oxybenzone 3%. **Inactive Ingredients:** Purified Water, C12-15 Alkyl Benzoate, Cetearyl Alcohol (and) Ceteareth-20, Cetyl Alcohol, Glyceryl Monostearate, Propylene Glycol, Petrolatum, Diazolidinyl Urea, Triethanolamine, Disodium EDTA, Xanthan Gum, Acrylates/C10-30 Alkyl Acrylate Crosspolymer, Tocopheryl Acetate, Iodopropynyl Butylcarbamate, Fragrance, Carbomer.

Actions and Uses: Lubriderm Daily UV Lotion's unique formula combines light, daily moisturization with dermatologist-recommended SPF 15 sun protection. This non-greasy feeling lotion

moisturizes dry skin and helps protect against the damaging rays of the sun.

Directions: Apply liberally as often as necessary. Children under 6 months of age: consult a doctor.

Warnings: For external use only. Avoid contact with the eyes. If contact occurs, rinse eyes thoroughly with water. Discontinue use if signs of irritation or rash appear. If irritation or rash persists, consult a doctor. Keep out of reach of children. In case of accidental ingestion, seek professional assistance or contact a Poison Control Center immediately. Store between 59°–77°F.

How Supplied: Available in 6, 10, 16 fl. oz plastic bottles and a 3.3 fl. oz. tube.
Shown in Product Identification Guide, page 519

LUBRIDERM®
Seriously Sensitive® Lotion
[lū brĭ dĕrm]

Ingredients: Water, Butylene Glycol, Mineral Oil, Petrolatum, Glycerin, Cetyl Alcohol, Propylene Glycol Dicaprylate/ Dicaprate, PEG-40 Stearate, C11-13 Isoparaffin, Glyceryl Stearate, Tri (PPG-3 Myristyl Ether) Citrate, Emulsifying Wax, Dimethicone, DMDM Hydantoin, Methylparaben, Carbomer 940, Ethylparaben, Propylparaben, Titanium Dioxide, Disodium EDTA, Sodium Hydroxide, Butylparaben, Xanthan Gum.

Uses: Lubriderm Seriously Sensitive Lotion's unique combination of emollients provides sensitive dry skin with the moisture it needs while helping to create a protective layer. It is non-comedogenic, 100% lanolin free, fragrance free, and dye free so its appropriate for skin that is sensitive to these ingredients. It is nongreasy feeling and absorbs quickly.

Directions: Smooth on hands and body everyday. Particularly effective when used after showering or bathing. For external use only.

How Supplied: Available in 1, 6, 10, and 16 fl. oz. plastic bottles and 3.3 fl. oz. tube.
Shown in Product Identification Guide, page 519

LUBRIDERM®
Skin Firming Body Lotion
[lū brĭ dĕrm]

Ingredients: Water, isostearic acid, stearic acid, steareth-21, sodium lactate, PPG 12/SMDI copolymer, lactic acid, steareth-2, magnesium aluminum silicate, cetyl alcohol, imidurea, fragrance, potassium sorbate, xanthan gum.

Uses: Lubriderm Skin Firming Body Lotion, with its unique dual action formula of Alpha Hydroxy Acid and moisturizers, will improve the firmness and appearance of your skin. This advanced non-greasy feeling lotion has been shown in a clinical study to help increase skin firmness in just 8 weeks, leaving improved skin texture and healthy-looking skin.

Directions: Apply liberally twice daily. Gently massage lotion all over body. Rub in a circular motion to stimulate circulation and promote firming in problem areas like legs, thighs and arms. Daily use of sun protection (such as Lubriderm Daily UV) is advisable when using this product.

How Supplied: Available in 10 fl. oz. plastic bottles.

Shown in Product Identification Guide, page 520

LUBRIDERM®
Skin Therapy Moisturizing Lotion
[lū brĭ dĕrm]

Ingredients: Scented—Water, Mineral Oil, Petrolatum, Sorbitol Solution, Stearic Acid, Lanolin, Lanolin Alcohol, Cetyl Alcohol, Glyceryl Stearate/PEG-100 Stearate, Triethanolamine, Dimethicone, Propylene Glycol, Microcrystalline Wax, Tri(PPG-3 Myristyl Ether) Citrate, Disodium EDTA, Methylparaben, Ethylparaben, Propylparaben, Fragrance, Xanthan Gum, Butylparaben, Methyldibromo Glutaronitrile.

Fragrance Free—Contains Water, Mineral Oil, Petrolatum, Sorbitol Solution, Stearic Acid, Lanolin, Lanolin Alcohol, Cetyl Alcohol, Glyceryl Stearate/PEG-100 Stearate, Triethanolamine, Dimethicone, Propylene Glycol, Microcrystalline Wax, Tri(PPG-3 Myristyl Ether) Citrate, Disodium EDTA, Methylparaben, Ethylparaben, Propylparaben, Xanthan Gum, Butylparaben, Methyldibromo Glutaronitrile.

Uses: Lubriderm provides the essential moisturizing elements that contribute to healthy skin. Its unique combination of emollients penetrate dry skin to effectively moisturize without leaving a greasy feel. Lubriderm helps heal and protect skin from dryness, absorbs rapidly for a clean, natural feel and is non-comedogenic so it won't clog pores.

Directions: Smooth on hands and body every day. Particularly effective when used after showering or bathing. For external use only.

How Supplied:
Scented: Available in 6, 10, 16 and 19.6 oz fl. oz. plastic bottles.
Fragrance Free: Available in 6, 10 and 16 fl. oz. plastic bottles and 3.3 fl. oz. tube.

Shown in Product Identification Guide, page 520

NEOSPORIN® Ointment
[nē "uh-spō' rŭn]

Drug Facts:

Active Ingredients: **Purpose:**
(in each gram):
Bacitracin
  400 units .... First aid antibiotic
Neomycin
  3.5 mg .... First aid antibiotic
Polymyxin B
  5,000 units .... First aid antibiotic

Use: first aid to help prevent infection in minor:
• cuts
• scrapes
• burns

Warnings:
For external use only
Do not use if you are allergic to any of the ingredients
Ask a doctor before use if you have
• deep or puncture wounds
• animal bites
• serious burns
When using this product
• do not use in the eyes
• do not apply over large areas of the body
Stop use and ask a doctor if
• you need to use more than 1 week
• condition persists or gets worse
• rash or other allergic reaction develops
Keep out of reach of children. If swallowed, get medical help or contact a Poison Control Center right away.

Directions:
• clean the affected area
• apply a small amount of this product (an amount equal to the surface area of the tip of a finger) on the area 1 to 3 times daily
• may be covered with a sterile bandage

Other Information: • store at 59° to 77°F

Inactive Ingredients: cocoa butter, cottonseed oil, olive oil, sodium pyruvate, tocopheryl acetate, and white petrolatum

Questions? call **1-800-223-0182**, Monday to Friday, 9 AM - 5 PM EST

How Supplied: Tubes, ¹/₂ oz (14.2 g), 1 oz (28.3 g), ¹/₃₂ oz (0.9 g) foil packets packed 10 per box (Neo To Go™) or 144 per box.

Shown in Product Identification Guide, page 520

NEOSPORIN® + PAIN RELIEF MAXIMUM STRENGTH Cream
[nē "uh-spō'rŭn]

Drug Facts:

Active Ingredients: **Purpose:**
(in each gram):
Neomycin 3.5 mg ..... First aid antibiotic
Polymyxin B
  10,000 units .... First aid antibiotic
Pramoxine HCl 10 mg ...... Pain reliever

Uses: first aid to help prevent infection and for temporary relief of pain or discomfort in minor:

• cuts
• scrapes
• burns

Warnings:
For external use only
Do not use if you are allergic to any of the ingredients
Ask a doctor before use if you have
• deep or puncture wounds
• animal bites
• serious burns
When using this product
• do not use in the eyes
• do not apply over large areas of the body
Stop use and ask a doctor if
• you need to use more than 1 week
• condition persists or gets worse
• symptoms persist for more than 1 week or clear up and occur again within a few days
• rash or other allergic reaction develops
Keep out of reach of children. If swallowed, get medical help or contact a Poison Control Center right away.

Directions:
• adults and children 2 years of age and older:
  • clean the affected area
  • apply a small amount of this product (an amount equal to the surface area of the tip of a finger) on the area 1 to 3 times daily
  • may be covered with a sterile bandage
• children under 2 years of age: ask a doctor

Other information: • store at 59° to 77°F

Inactive Ingredient: emulsifying wax, methylparaben, mineral oil, propylene glycol, purified water, and white petrolatum

Questions? call **1-800-223-0182**, Monday to Friday, 9 AM - 5 PM EST

How Supplied: ½ oz (14.2 g) tubes.
Shown in Product Identification Guide, page 520

NEOSPORIN® + PAIN RELIEF MAXIMUM STRENGTH Ointment
[nē "uh-spō 'rŭn]

Drug Facts:

Active Ingredients: **Purpose:**
(in each gram):
Bacitracin
  500 units .... First aid antibiotic
Neomycin 3.5 mg ..... First aid antibiotic

Continued on next page

This product information was prepared in November 2002. On these and other Pfizer Consumer Healthcare Products, detailed information may be obtained by addressing Pfizer Consumer Healthcare, Pfizer, Inc., Morris Plains, NJ 07950

Neosporin Plus Ointment—Cont.

Polymyxin B
  10,000 units .... First aid antibiotic
Pramoxine HCl 10 mg ...... Pain reliever

Uses: first aid to help prevent infection and for temporary relief of pain or discomfort in minor:
• cuts
• scrapes
• burns

Warnings:
For external use only
Do not use if you are allergic to any of the ingredients
Ask a doctor before use if you have
• deep or puncture wounds
• animal bites
• serious burns
When using this product
• do not use in the eyes
• do not apply over large areas of the body
Stop use and ask a doctor if
• you need to use more than 1 week
• condition persists or gets worse
• symptoms persist for more than 1 week or clear up and occur again within a few days
• rash or other allergic reaction develops
Keep out of reach of children. If swallowed, get medical help or contact a Poison Control Center right away.

Directions:
• adults and children 2 years of age and older:
  • clean the affected area
  • apply a small amount of this product (an amount equal to the surface area of the tip of a finger) on the area 1 to 3 times daily
  • may be covered with a sterile bandage
• children under 2 years of age: ask a doctor

Other Information: • store at 59° to 77°F

Inactive Ingredient: white petrolatum
Questions? call **1-800-223-0182**, Monday to Friday, 9 AM - 5 PM EST

How Supplied: $^{1}/_{2}$ oz (14.2 g) and 1 oz (28.3 g) tubes.

Shown in Product Identification Guide, page 520

NIX® Creme Rinse
Permethrin
Lice Treatment
[nĭks]

Each Fluid Ounce Contains: Active Ingredient: permethrin 280 mg (1%). Also contains: balsam canada, cetyl alcohol, citric acid, FD&C Yellow No. 6, fragrance, hydrolyzed animal protein, hydroxyethylcellulose, polyoxyethylene 10 cetyl ether, propylene glycol, stearalkonium chloride, water, isopropyl alcohol 5.6 g (20%), methylparaben 56 mg (0.2%), and propylparaben 22 mg (0.08%).

Product Benefits: Nix Creme Rinse kills lice and their unhatched eggs with usually only one application. Nix protects against head lice reinfestation for 14 days. The creme rinse formula leaves hair manageable and easy to comb.

Indications: For the treatment of head lice.

Directions for Use: Nix Creme Rinse should be used after hair has been washed with your regular shampoo, rinsed with water and towel dried. A sufficient amount should be applied to saturate hair and scalp (especially behind the ears and on the nape of the neck). Leave on hair for 10 minutes but no longer. Rinse with water. A single application is usually sufficient. If live lice are observed seven days or more after the first application of this product, a second treatment should be given. For proper head lice management, remove nits with the nit comb provided.

Head lice live on the scalp and lay small white eggs (nits) on the hair shaft close to the scalp. The nits are most easily found on the nape of the neck or behind the ears. All personal headgear, scarfs, coats, and bed linen should be disinfected by machine washing in hot water and drying, using the hot cycle of a dryer for at least 20 minutes. Personal articles of clothing or bedding that cannot be washed may be dry-cleaned, sealed in a plastic bag for a period of about 2 weeks, or sprayed with a product specifically designed for this purpose. Personal combs and brushes may be disinfected by soaking in hot water (above 130°F) for 5 to 10 minutes. Thorough vacuuming of rooms inhabited by infected patients is recommended.
Shake well before using.

Warnings: For external use only. Keep out of eyes when rinsing hair. Adults and children: Close eyes and do not open eyes until product is rinsed out. If product gets into the eyes, immediately flush with water. Do not use near the eyes or permit contact with mucous membranes, such as inside the nose, mouth, or vagina, as irritation may occur. Children: Also protect children's eyes with a washcloth, towel, or other suitable material or method. This product should not be used on children less than 2 months of age. Itching, redness, or swelling of the scalp may occur. If skin irritation persists or infection is present or develops, discontinue use and consult a doctor. Consult a doctor if infestation of eyebrows or eyelashes occurs. This product may cause breathing difficulty or an asthmatic episode in susceptible persons. As with any drug, if you are pregnant or nursing a baby, seek the advice of a health professional before using this product. Keep this and all drugs out of the reach of children. In case of accidental ingestion, seek professional assistance or contact a Poison Control Center immediately.

Professional Labeling:
Indications: For the treatment of head lice. For prophylactic use during head lice epidemics.

Warnings: For external use only. Keep out of eyes when rinsing hair. Adults and children: Close eyes and do not open eyes until product is rinsed out. If product gets into the eyes, immediately flush with water. Do not use near the eyes or permit contact with mucous membranes, such as inside the nose, mouth, or vagina, as irritation may occur. Children: Also protect children's eyes with a washcloth, towel, or other suitable material or method. This product should not be used on pediatric patients less than 2 months of age. Itching, redness, or swelling of the scalp may occur. If skin irritation persists or infection is present or develops, discontinue use and consult a doctor. Consult a doctor if infestation of eyebrows or eyelashes occurs. This product may cause breathing difficulty or an asthmatic episode in susceptible persons. As with any drug, if you are pregnant or nursing a baby, seek the advice of a health professional before using this product. Keep this and all drugs out of the reach of children. In case of accidental ingestion, seek professional assistance or contact a Poison Control Center immediately.

Dosage and Administration
Treatment
Nix Creme Rinse should be used after hair has been washed with patient's regular shampoo, rinsed with water and towel dried. A sufficient amount should be applied to saturate hair and scalp (especially behind the ears and on the nape of the neck). Leave on hair for 10 minutes but no longer. Rinse with water. A single application is usually sufficient. If live lice are observed seven days or more after the first application of this product a second treatment should be given. For proper head lice management, remove nits with the nit comb provided.

Head lice live on the scalp and lay small white eggs (nits) on the hair shaft close to the scalp. The nits are most easily found on the nape of the neck or behind the ears. All personal headgear, scarfs, coats, and bed linen should be disinfected by machine washing in hot water and drying, using the hot cycle of a dryer for a least 20 minutes. Personal articles of clothing or bedding that cannot be washed may be dry-cleaned, sealed in a plastic bag for a period of about 2 weeks, or sprayed with a product specifically designed for this purpose. Personal combs and brushes may be disinfected by soaking in hot water (above 130°F) for 5 to 10 minutes. Thorough vacuuming of rooms inhabited by infected patients is recommended.

Prophylaxis
Prophylactic use of Nix Creme Rinse is only recommended for individuals exposed to head lice epidemics in which at least 20% of the population at an institution are infested and for immediate household members of infested individuals. Casual use is strongly discouraged. The method of application of Nix Creme Rinse for prophylaxis is identical to that described above for treatment of a lice

infestation except nit removal is not required.

Directions for Use
One application of Nix Creme Rinse has been shown to protect greater than 95% of patients against reinfestation for at least two weeks. In epidemic settings, a second prophylactic application is recommended two weeks after the first because the life cycle of a head louse is approximately four weeks.

How Supplied: Bottles of 2 fl. oz. (59 mL) with nit removal comb and Family Pack of 2 bottles, 2 fl. oz. (59 mL) each, with two nit removal combs. Store at 15° to 25°C (59° to 77°F).
Shown in Product Identification Guide, page 520

NIX® LICE CONTROL SPRAY
For Bedding and Furniture

NOT FOR USE IN HUMANS

Directions for Use: It is a violation of Federal law to use this product in a manner inconsistent with its labeling.

FOR USE IN NON-FOOD AREA OF HOMES
Indoor Application: Surface Spraying: To kill lice, spray in an inconspicuous area to test for possible staining or discoloration. Inspect again after drying, then proceed to spray entire area to be treated. Spray from a distance of 8 to 10 inches. Treat only those garments and parts of bedding, including mattresses and furniture that cannot be either laundered or dry cleaned. Allow all treated articles to dry thoroughly before use.
Do not use in food/feed areas of food/feed handling establishments, restaurants or other areas where food/feed is commercially prepared or processed. Do not use in serving areas while food is exposed or facility is in operation. Serving areas are areas where prepared foods are served such as dining rooms, but excluding areas where foods may be prepared or held.
In the home, cover all food handling surfaces, cover or remove all food and cooking utensils or wash thoroughly after treatment.
Do not apply to classrooms while in use. Not for use in Federally Inspected Meat and Poultry Plants.
Storage and Disposal: Do not contaminate water, food or feed by storing or disposal.
Pesticide Storage and Spill Procedures: Keep from freezing. Store upright at room temperature. Avoid exposure to extreme temperatures. In case of spill or leakage, soak up with an absorbent material such as sand, sawdust, earth, fuller's earth, etc. Dispose of with chemical waste.
Pesticide Disposal: Pesticide or rinse water that cannot be used according to label instructions must be disposed of at or by an approved waste disposal facility.

Container Disposal: Do not reuse empty container. Wrap container and put in trash collection.

READ ENTIRE LABEL BEFORE EACH USE.

Observe all precautionary statements and follow directions for use carefully.

Environmental Hazards: This product is extremely toxic to fish and aquatic organisms. Do not apply directly to any body of water. Do not contaminate water when disposing of equipment washwater. This pesticide is toxic to honey bees and other beneficial pollinators exposed to an application. Do not apply when bees are actively visiting blooming plants (vegetables, flowers, fruit/ornamental trees) Do not allow this product to come in direct contact with bee hives at any time.

QUESTIONS OR COMMENTS:
Call Toll Free 1-888-542-3546
Shown in Product Identification Guide, page 520

POLYSPORIN® Ointment
[pŏl 'ē-spō 'rŭn]

Drug Facts
Active Ingredients
(in each gram): **Purpose**
Bacitracin
500 units .... First aid antibiotic
Polymyxin B
10,000 units .... First aid antibiotic

Use: first aid to help prevent infection in minor:
• cuts
• scrapes
• burns

Warnings:
For external use only
Do not use if you are allergic to any of the ingredients
Ask a doctor before use if you have
• deep or puncture wounds
• animal bites
• serious burns
When using this product
• do not use in the eyes
• do not apply over large areas of the body
Stop use and ask a doctor if
• you need to use more than one week
• condition persists or gets worse
• rash or other allergic reaction develops
Keep out of reach of children. If swallowed, get medical help or contact a Poison Control Center right away.

Directions:
• clean the affected area
• apply a small amount of this product (an amount equal to the surface area of the tip of a finger) on the area 1 to 3 times daily
• may be covered with a sterile bandage
Other Information: • store at 15° to 25°C (59° to 77°F)

Inactive Ingredient: white petrolatum base

Questions?
call **1-800-223-0182**, Monday to Friday, 9 AM - 5 PM EST

How Supplied: Tubes, $1/2$ oz (14.2 g), 1 oz (28.3 g); $1/32$ oz (0.9 g) foil packets packed in cartons of 144.
Shown in Product Identification Guide, page 520

POLYSPORIN® Powder
[pŏl 'ē-spō 'rŭn]

Drug Facts
Active Ingredients
(in each gram): **Purpose**
Bacitracin
500 units .... First aid antibiotic
Polymyxin B
10,000 units .... First aid antibiotic

Use: first aid to help prevent infection in minor:
• cuts
• scrapes
• burns

Warnings:
For external use only
Do not use if you are allergic to any of the ingredients
Ask a doctor before use if you have
• deep or puncture wounds
• animal bites
• serious burns
When using this product
• do not use in the eyes
• do not apply over large areas of the body
Stop use and ask a doctor if
• you need to use more than one week
• condition persists or gets worse
• rash or other allergic reaction develops
Keep out of reach of children. If swallowed, get medical help or contact a Poison Control Center right away.

Directions:
• clean the affected area
• apply a light dusting of the powder on the area 1 to 3 times daily
• may be covered with a sterile bandage

Other Information:
• store at 15° to 25°C (59° to 77°F)
• do not refrigerate

Inactive Ingredient: lactose base

Questions? call **1-800-223-0182**, Monday to Friday, 9 AM – 5 PM EST

How Supplied: 0.35 oz (10 g) shaker-vial.
Shown in Product Identification Guide, page 520

Continued on next page

This product information was prepared in November 2002. On these and other Pfizer Consumer Healthcare Products, detailed information may be obtained by addressing Pfizer Consumer Healthcare, Pfizer, Inc., Morris Plains, NJ 07950

ROLAIDS® Antacid Tablets
Original Peppermint, Spearmint, and Cherry

Drug Facts:

Active ingredients
(in each tablet): **Purpose:**
Calcium carbonate 550 mg Antacid
Magnesium hydroxide 110 mg Antacid

Uses: relieves: • heartburn • sour stomach • acid indigestion • upset stomach due to these symptoms

Warnings:
Ask a doctor or pharmacist before use if you are
• presently taking a prescription drug. Antacids may interact with certain prescription drugs.
• do not take more than 12 tablets in a 24-hour period, or use the maximum dosage for more than 2 weeks, except under the advice and supervision of a physician.
Keep out of reach of children.

Directions
• chew 2 to 4 tablets, hourly if needed

Other Information:
• each tablet contains: calcium 220 mg and magnesium 45 mg
• store at 59° to 77°F in a dry place

Inactive ingredients: Peppermint and Spearmint Flavors: dextrose, flavoring, magnesium stearate, polyethylene glycol, pregelatinized starch and sucrose
Cherry Flavor: dextrose, flavoring, magnesium stearate, polyethylene glycol, pregelatinized starch, D&C red no. 27 aluminum lake, and sucrose

Actions: Rolaids® provides rapid neutralization of stomach acid. Each tablet has an acid-neutralizing capacity of 14.7 mEq and the ability to maintain the pH of stomach contents at 3.5 or greater for a significant period of time.

Dosage and Administration: Chew 2 to 4 tablets as symptoms occur. Repeat hourly if symptoms return, or as directed by a physician.

How Supplied: Rolaids® is available in 12-tablet rolls, 3-packs containing three 12-tablet rolls and in bottles containing 150 or 300 tablets.
Shown in Product Identification Guide, page 520

EXTRA STRENGTH ROLAIDS®
Antacid Tablets
Freshmint, Fruit, Cool Strawberry, and Tropical Punch Flavors

Drug Facts:

Active Ingredients:
(in each tablet): **Purpose:**
Calcium carbonate 675 mg Antacid
Magnesium hydroxide 135 mg Antacid

Uses: relieves: • heartburn • sour stomach • acid indigestion • upset stomach due to these symptoms

Warnings: Ask a doctor or pharmacist before use if you are
• presently taking a prescription drug. Antacids may interact with certain prescription drugs.
• do not take more than 10 tablets in a 24-hour period, or use the maximum dosage for more than 2 weeks, except under the advice and supervision of a physician.
Keep out of reach of children.

Directions:
• chew 2 to 4 tablets, hourly if needed

Other Information:
• each tablet contains: calcium 271 mg and magnesium 56 mg
• store at 59° to 77° F in a dry place

Inactive Ingredients: Freshmint Flavor: dextrose, flavoring, magnesium stearate, polyethylene glycol, pregelatinized starch and sucrose
Fruit Flavor: dextrose, flavoring, magnesium stearate, polyethylene glycol, pregelatinized starch, sucrose and FD&C yellow no. 5 aluminum lake (tartrazine)
Cool Strawberry and Tropical Punch: carmine, dextrose, flavoring, magnesium stearate, polyethylene glycol, pregelatinized starch and sucrose

Actions: Extra Strength Rolaids® provides rapid neutralization of stomach acid. Each tablet has an acid-neutralizing capacity of 18.2 mEq and the ability to maintain the pH of stomach contents at 3.5 or greater for a significant period of time.

Dosage and Administration: Chew 2 to 4 tablets as symptoms occur. Repeat hourly if symptoms return, or as directed by a physician.

How Supplied: Extra Strength Rolaids® is available in 10-tablet rolls, 3-packs containing three 10-tablet rolls and in bottles containing 100 tablets.
Shown in Product Identification Guide, page 520

SINUTAB® Non-Drying
Liquid Caps
[sîn 'ū tăb]

Drug Facts:

Active Ingredients: **Purposes:**
(in each liquid cap)
Guaifenesin
200 mg .... Expectorant
Pseudoephedrine
HCl 30 mg .... Nasal decongestant

Uses:
• temporarily relieves nasal congestion associated with sinusitis
• helps loosen phlegm (mucus) and thin bronchial secretions to drain bronchial passageways of bothersome mucus and make coughs more productive

Warnings:
Do not use if you are now taking a prescription monoamine oxidase inhibitor (MAOI) (certain drugs for depression, psychiatric, or emotional conditions, or

Parkinson's disease), or for 2 weeks after stopping the MAOI drug. If you do not know if your prescription drug contains an MAOI, ask a doctor or pharmacist before taking this product.
Ask a doctor before use if you have:
• heart disease
• high blood pressure
• thyroid disease
• diabetes
• trouble urinating due to an enlarged prostate gland
• persistent or chronic cough such as occurs with smoking, asthma, chronic bronchitis, or emphysema
• cough occurs with too much phlegm (mucus)
When using this product:
• do not use more than directed
Stop use and ask a doctor if:
• you get nervous, dizzy, or sleepless
• symptoms do not improve within 7 days or are accompanied by fever
• cough persists for more than 1 week, tends to recur, or is accompanied by a fever, rash, or persistent headache. These could be signs of a serious condition.
If pregnant or breast-feeding, ask a health professional before use.
Keep out of reach of children. In case of overdose, get medical help or contact a Poison Control Center right away.

Directions:
• adults and children 12 years of age and over: 2 liquid caps
• children under 12 years of age: ask a doctor
• take every 4 hours
• do not take more than 8 liquid caps in 24 hours

Other Information:
• store at 59° to 77° F
• protect from heat, humidity, and light

Inactive Ingredients: FD&C blue no. 1, gelatin, glycerin, polyethylene glycol 400, povidone, propylene glycol, and sorbitol. Printed with edible white ink.

Questions? Call **1-800-223-0182,** Monday to Friday, 9 AM–5 PM EST

How Supplied: Sinutab® Non-Drying supplied in a box of 24 liquid caps.
Shown in Product Identification Guide, page 520

SINUTAB® Sinus Allergy
Medication, Maximum Strength Formula,
Caplets
[sîn 'ū tăb]

Drug Facts:

Active Ingredients:
(in each caplet)+ **Purposes:**
Acetaminophen 500 mg .... Pain reliever
Chlorpheniramine maleate
2 mg .... Antihistamine
Pseudoephedrine HCl
30 mg .... Nasal decongestant

+Dissolution differs from USP specification

Uses: Temporarily relieves these symptoms of hay fever or other upper respiratory allergies:

- runny nose
- sneezing
- itchy, watery eyes
- itching of the nose or throat
- headache
- minor aches and pains
- nasal congestion

Warnings:
Alcohol warning: If you consume 3 or more alcoholic drinks every day, ask your doctor whether you should take acetaminophen or other pain relievers/fever reducers. Acetaminophen may cause liver damage.
Do not use:
- with another product containing any of these active ingredients
- if you are now taking a prescription monoamine oxidase inhibitor (MAOI) (certain drugs for depression, psychiatric, or emotional conditions, or Parkinson's disease), or for 2 weeks after stopping the MAOI drug. If you do not know if your prescription drug contains an MAOI, ask a doctor or pharmacist before taking this product.

Ask a doctor before use if you have:
- glaucoma
- high blood pressure
- heart disease
- thyroid disease
- diabetes
- trouble urinating due to an enlarged prostate gland
- a breathing problem such as emphysema or chronic bronchitis

Ask a doctor or pharmacist before use if you are taking sedatives or tranquilizers
When using this product:
- do not use more than directed
- drowsiness may occur
- excitability may occur, especially in children
- avoid alcoholic drinks
- alcohol, sedatives, and tranquilizers may increase drowsiness
- be careful when driving a motor vehicle or operating machinery

Stop use and ask a doctor if:
- you get nervous, dizzy, or sleepless
- new symptoms occur
- symptoms do not get better
- you need to use more than 10 days
- fever occurs and lasts more than 3 days

If pregnant or breast-feeding, ask a health professional before use.
Keep out of reach of children.
Overdose warning: Taking more than the recommended dose may cause liver damage. In case of overdose, get medical help or contact a Poison Control Center right away. Quick medical attention is critical for adults as well as for children even if you do not notice any signs or symptoms.

Directions:
- do not use more than directed (see overdose warning)
- adults and children 12 years of age and over: 2 caplets
- children under 12 years of age: ask a doctor
- take every 6 hours while symptoms persist
- do not take more than 8 caplets in 24 hours or as directed by a doctor

Other Information:
- store at 59° to 77°F in a dry place

Inactive Ingredients: Calcium stearate, candelilla wax, croscarmellose sodium, crospovidone, D&C yellow no. 10 aluminum lake, FD&C yellow no. 6 aluminum lake, hypromellose, microcrystalline cellulose, polyethylene glycol, polysorbate 80, povidone, pregelatinized starch, stearic acid, and titanium dioxide
Questions? call **1-800-223-0182**, Monday to Friday, 9 AM – 5 PM EST
How Supplied: Sinutab® Sinus Allergy Medication, Maximum Strength Formula Caplets are supplied in child-resistant blister packs in boxes of 24 tablets or caplets.
Shown in Product Identification Guide, page 520

SINUTAB® Sinus Medication, Maximum Strength Without Drowsiness Formula, Caplets (also available in Tablets)
[sîn 'ū tăb]

Drug Facts:

Active Ingredients:
(in each caplet)   **Purposes:**
Acetaminophen 500 mg ... Pain reliever
Pseudoephedrine
  HCl 30 mg .... Nasal decongestant
Uses:
- temporarily relieves nasal congestion associated with sinusitis
- temporarily relieves headache, minor aches, and pains

Warnings:
Alcohol warning: If you consume 3 or more alcoholic drinks every day, ask your doctor whether you should take acetaminophen or other pain relievers/fever reducers. Acetaminophen may cause liver damage.
Do not use:
- with another product containing any of these active ingredients
- if you are now taking a prescription monoamine oxidase inhibitor (MAOI) (certain drugs for depression, psychiatric, or emotional conditions, or Parkinson's disease), or for 2 weeks after stopping the MAOI drug. If you do not know if your prescription drug contains an MAOI, ask a doctor or pharmacist before taking this product.

Ask a doctor before use if you have:
- heart disease
- high blood pressure
- thyroid disease
- diabetes
- trouble urinating due to an enlarged prostate gland

When using this product:
- do not use more than directed
Stop use and ask a doctor if:
- you get nervous, dizzy, or sleepless
- new symptoms occur
- symptoms do not get better
- you need to use more than 10 days
- fever occurs and lasts more than 3 days

If pregnant or breast-feeding, ask a health professional before use.
Keep out of reach of children.
Overdose warning: Taking more than the recommended dose may cause liver

damage. In case of overdose, get medical help or contact a Poison Control Center right away. Quick medical attention is critical for adults as well as for children even if you do not notice any signs or symptoms.

Directions:
- do not use more than directed (see overdose warning)
- adults and children 12 years of age and over: 2 caplets
- children under 12 years of age: ask a doctor
- take every 6 hours while symptoms persist
- do not take more than 8 caplets in 24 hours or as directed by a doctor

Other Information:
- store at 59° to 77°F in a dry place

Inactive Ingredients: Calcium stearate, candelilla wax, croscarmellose sodium, crospovidone, FD&C yellow no. 6 aluminum lake, hypromellose, microcrystalline cellulose, polyethylene glycol, polysorbate 80, povidone, pregelatinized starch, stearic acid, and titanium dioxide
Questions? call **1-800-223-0182**, Monday to Friday, 9 AM – 5 PM EST
How Supplied: Sinutab® Sinus Medication, Maximum Strength Without Drowsiness Formula, Caplets and Tablets are supplied in child-resistant blister packs in boxes of 24 tablets or caplets.
Shown in Product Identification Guide, page 520

SUDAFED® Non-Drowsy 12 Hour Nasal Decongestant Tablets
[sū 'duh-fĕd]
*Capsule-shaped Tablets

Drug Facts:

Active Ingredient:
(in each tablet)   **Purpose:**
Pseudoephedrine
  HCl 120 mg .... Nasal decongestant
Uses:
- temporarily relieves nasal congestion due to the common cold, hay fever or other upper respiratory allergies, and nasal congestion associated with sinusitis
- temporarily relieves sinus congestion and pressure

Warnings:
Do not use if you are now taking a prescription monoamine oxidase inhibitor (MAOI) (certain drugs for depression,

Continued on next page

This product information was prepared in November 2002. On these and other Pfizer Consumer Healthcare Products, detailed information may be obtained by addressing Pfizer Consumer Healthcare, Pfizer, Inc., Morris Plains, NJ 07950

Sudafed 12 Hour—Cont.

psychiatric, or emotional conditions, or Parkinson's disease), or for 2 weeks after stopping the MAOI drug. If you do not know if your prescription drug contains an MAOI, ask a doctor or pharmacist before taking this product.

Ask a doctor before use if you have:
- heart disease
- high blood pressure
- thyroid disease
- diabetes
- trouble urinating due to an enlarged prostate gland

When using this product:
- do not use more than directed

Stop use and ask a doctor if:
- you get nervous, dizzy, or sleepless
- symptoms do not improve within 7 days or are accompanied by fever

If pregnant or breast-feeding, ask a health professional before use.

Keep out of reach of children. In case of overdose, get medical help or contact a Poison Control Center right away.

Directions:
- adults and children 12 years of age and over: one tablet every 12 hours not to exceed two tablets in 24 hours
- children under 12 years of age: use of product not recommended

Other Information:
- store at 59° to 77°F in a dry place
- protect from light

Inactive Ingredients: hypromellose, magnesium stearate, microcrystalline cellulose, polyethylene glycol, povidone, and titanium dioxide. May also contain: candelilla wax or carnauba wax. Printed with edible blue ink.

Questions? call **1-800-524-2624** (English/Spanish), weekdays, 9 AM–5 PM EST

How Supplied: Boxes of 10 and 20.
Shown in Product Identification Guide, page 521

SUDAFED® Non-Drowsy 24 Hour Nasal Decongestant Tablets
[sū 'duh-fĕd]

Drug Facts:

Active Ingredient:
(in each tablet)   **Purpose:**
Pseudoephedrine HCl 240 mg .... Nasal decongestant

Uses:
- temporarily relieves nasal congestion due to the common cold, hay fever or other upper respiratory allergies, and nasal congestion associated with sinusitis
- reduces swelling of nasal passages
- relieves sinus pressure

Warnings:
Do not use if you are now taking a prescription monoamine oxidase inhibitor (MAOI) (certain drugs for depression, psychiatric, or emotional conditions, or Parkinson's disease), or for 2 weeks after stopping the MAOI drug. If you do not

know if your prescription drug contains an MAOI, ask a doctor or pharmacist before taking this product.

Ask a doctor before use if you have:
- heart disease
- high blood pressure
- thyroid disease
- trouble urinating due to an enlarged prostate gland
- diabetes
- had obstruction or narrowing of the bowel. Rarely, tablets of this kind may cause bowel obstruction (blockage), usually in people with severe narrowing of the bowel (esophagus, stomach or intestine).

When using this product:
- do not use more than directed

Stop use and ask a doctor if:
- you get nervous, dizzy, or sleepless
- symptoms do not improve within 7 days or are accompanied by fever
- you experience persistent abdominal pain or vomiting

If pregnant or breast-feeding, ask a health professional before use.

Keep out of reach of children. In case of overdose, get medical help or contact a Poison Control Center right away.

Directions:
- adults and children 12 years of age and over: **swallow one** whole tablet with fluid every 24 hours
- **do not exceed one tablet in 24 hours**
- **do not divide, crush, chew or dissolve the tablet**
- the tablet does not completely dissolve and may be seen in the stool (this is normal)
- not for use in children under 12 years of age

Other Information:
- store at 59° to 77°F in a dry place

Inactive Ingredients: Cellulose, cellulose acetate, hydroxypropyl cellulose, hypromellose, magnesium stearate, polyethylene glycol, polysorbate 80, povidone, sodium chloride, and titanium dioxide

Questions? call **1-800-524-2624** (English/Spanish), weekdays, 9 AM – 5 PM EST

How Supplied: Box of 5 tablets and 10 tablets. **BLISTER PACKAGED FOR YOUR PROTECTION. DO NOT USE IF INDIVIDUAL SEALS ARE BROKEN.**
Shown in Product Identification Guide, page 521

SUDAFED® Non-drowsy Cold & Cough Liquid Caps
[sū 'duh-fĕd]

Drug Facts:

Active Ingredients: **Purposes:**
(in each liquid cap)
Acetaminophen 250 mg ..... Pain reliever/fever reducer
Dextromethorphan HBr 10 mg .... Cough suppressant
Guaifenesin 100 mg .... Expectorant
Pseudoephedrine HCl 30 mg .... Nasal decongestant

Uses:
- temporarily relieves these symptoms due to the common cold:
  - nasal congestion
  - headache
  - minor aches and pains
  - muscular aches
  - fever
  - sore throat
  - cough
- helps loosen phlegm (mucus) and thin bronchial secretions to drain bronchial tubes and make coughs more productive

Warnings:
Alcohol warning: If you consume 3 or more alcoholic drinks every day, ask your doctor whether you should take acetaminophen or other pain relievers/fever reducers. Acetaminophen may cause liver damage.

Do not use:
- with another product containing any of these active ingredients
- if you are now taking a prescription monoamine oxidase inhibitor (MAOI) (certain drugs for depression, psychiatric, or emotional conditions, or Parkinson's disease), or for 2 weeks after stopping the MAOI drug. If you do not know if your prescription drug contains an MAOI, ask a doctor or pharmacist before taking this product.

Ask a doctor before use if you have:
- heart disease
- thyroid disease
- diabetes
- high blood pressure
- trouble urinating due to an enlarged prostate gland
- cough accompanied by excessive phlegm (mucus)
- persistent or chronic cough such as occurs with smoking, asthma, chronic bronchitis, or emphysema

When using this product:
- do not use more than directed

Stop use and ask a doctor if:
- new symptoms occur
- redness or swelling is present
- symptoms do not improve
- sore throat is severe
- you get nervous, dizzy, or sleepless
- fever gets worse or lasts more than 3 days
- sore throat lasts for more than 2 days, is accompanied or followed by fever, headache, rash, swelling, nausea, or vomiting
- you need to use more than 10 days
- cough persists for more than 7 days, tends to recur, or is accompanied by rash or persistent headache. These could be signs of a serious condition.

If pregnant or breast-feeding, ask a health professional before use.

Keep out of reach of children.

Overdose warning: Taking more than the recommended dose may cause liver damage. In case of overdose, get medical help or contact a Poison Control Center right away. Quick medical attention is critical for adults as well as for children even if you do not notice any signs or symptoms.

Directions:
- do not use more than directed (see overdose warning)

- adults and children 12 years of age and over: 2 liquid caps
- take every 4 hours while symptoms persist
- do not take more than 8 liquid caps in 24 hours, or as directed by a doctor
- children under 12 years of age: ask a doctor

Other Information:
- store at 59° to 77°F in a dry place
- protect from heat, humidity, and light

Inactive Ingredients: D&C yellow no. 10, FD&C red no. 40, gelatin, glycerin, mannitol, polyethylene glycol 400, povidone, propylene glycol, and sorbitol. Printed with edible white ink.

Questions? call **1-800-524-2624** (English/Spanish), weekdays, 9 AM – 5 PM EST

How Supplied: Boxes of 10 and 20.
Shown in Product Identification Guide, page 520

SUDAFED® Non-Drowsy Nasal Decongestant 30-mg Tablets
[sū 'duh-fĕd]

Drug Facts:

Active Ingredient:
(in each tablet)   **Purpose:**
Pseudoephedrine HCl
 30 mg .... Nasal decongestant

Uses:
- temporarily relieves nasal congestion due to the common cold, hay fever or other upper respiratory allergies, and nasal congestion associated with sinusitis
- temporarily relieves sinus congestion and pressure

Warnings:
Do not use if you are now taking a prescription monoamine oxidase inhibitor (MAOI) (certain drugs for depression, psychiatric, or emotional conditions, or Parkinson's disease), or for 2 weeks after stopping the MAOI drug. If you do not know if your prescription drug contains an MAOI, ask a doctor or pharmacist before taking this product.
Ask a doctor before use if you have:
- heart disease
- high blood pressure
- thyroid disease
- diabetes
- trouble urinating due to an enlarged prostate gland

When using this product:
- **do not use more than directed**
Stop use and ask a doctor if:
- you get nervous, dizzy, or sleepless
- symptoms do not improve within 7 days or are accompanied by fever
If pregnant or breast-feeding, ask a health professional before use.
Keep out of reach of children. In case of overdose, get medical help or contact a Poison Control Center right away.

Directions:
- take every 4 to 6 hours
- do not take more than 4 doses in 24 hours

adults and children 12 years of age and over	2 tablets
children 6 to under 12 years of age	1 tablet
children under 6 years of age	ask a doctor

Other Information:
- store at 59° to 77°F in a dry place

Inactive Ingredients: Acacia, candelilla wax, corn starch, FD&C red no. 40 aluminum lake, FD&C yellow no. 6 aluminum lake, hydroxypropyl methylcellulose, lactose, magnesium stearate, pharmaceutical glaze, poloxamer 407, polyethylene glycol, polyethylene oxide, polysorbate 60, povidone, sodium benzoate, sodium lauryl sulfate, stearic acid, sucrose, and titanium dioxide. Printed with edible black ink.

Questions? call **1-800-524-2624** (English/Spanish), weekdays, 9 AM – 5 PM EST

How Supplied: Boxes of 24, 48 and 96.
Shown in Product Identification Guide, page 521

SUDAFED® NON-DROWSY NON-DRYING SINUS, LIQUID CAPS
[sū 'duh-fĕd]

Drug Facts:

Active Ingredients: **Purposes:**
(in each liquid cap)
Guaifenesin 200 mg .... Expectorant
Pseudoephedrine
 HCl 30 mg .... Nasal decongestant

Uses:
- temporarily relieves nasal congestion associated with sinusitis
- promotes nasal and/or sinus drainage
- temporarily relieves sinus congestion and pressure
- helps loosen phlegm (mucus) and thin bronchial secretions to rid the bronchial passageways of bothersome mucus and make coughs more productive

Warnings:
Do not use if you are now taking a prescription monoamine oxidase inhibitor (MAOI) (certain drugs for depression, psychiatric, or emotional conditions, or Parkinson's disease), or for 2 weeks after stopping the MAOI drug. If you do not know if your prescription drug contains an MAOI, ask a doctor or pharmacist before taking this product.
Ask a doctor before use if you have:
- heart disease
- high blood pressure
- thyroid disease
- diabetes
- trouble urinating due to an enlarged prostate gland
- cough that occurs with too much phlegm (mucus)
- persistent or chronic cough such as occurs with smoking, asthma, chronic bronchitis, or emphysema

When using this product:
- **do not use more than directed**
Stop use and ask a doctor if:
- you get nervous, dizzy, or sleepless
- symptoms do not improve within 7 days or are accompanied by fever
- cough persists for more than 1 week, tends to recur, or is accompanied by a fever, rash, or persistent headache. These could be signs of a serious condition.
If pregnant or breast-feeding, ask a health professional before use.
Keep out of reach of children. In case of overdose, get medical help or contact a Poison Control Center right away.

Directions:
- adults and children 12 years of age and over: swallow 2 liquid caps
- take every 4 hours
- do not exceed 8 liquid caps in 24 hours
- children under 12 years of age: ask a doctor

Other Information:
- store at 59° to 77°F
- protect from heat, humidity, and light

Inactive Ingredients: FD&C blue no. 1, gelatin, glycerin, polyethylene glycol 400, povidone, propylene glycol, and sorbitol. Printed with edible white ink.

Questions? call **1-800-524-2624** (English/Spanish), weekdays, 9 AM - 5 PM EST

How Supplied: Sudafed Non-Drying Sinus is supplied in boxes of 24 liquid caps.
Shown in Product Identification Guide, page 521

SUDAFED® Non-drowsy Severe Cold Caplets (Formerly Sudafed Severe Cold Formula)
[sū 'duh-fĕd]

Drug Facts:

Active Ingredients: **Purpose:**
(in each caplet)
Acetaminophen
 500 mg ...... Pain reliever/fever reducer
Dextromethorphan HBr
 15 mg .... Antitussive
Pseudoephedrine HCl
 30 mg .... Nasal decongestant

Uses:
- temporarily relieves these symptoms due to the common cold:
  - nasal congestion
  - headache
  - minor aches and pains

Continued on next page

This product information was prepared in November 2002. On these and other Pfizer Consumer Healthcare Products, detailed information may be obtained by addressing Pfizer Consumer Healthcare, Pfizer, Inc., Morris Plains, NJ 07950

Sudafed Severe Cold—Cont.

- muscular aches
- cough
- sore throat
- fever

Warnings:
Alcohol warning: If you consume 3 or more alcoholic drinks every day, ask your doctor whether you should take acetaminophen or other pain relievers/ fever reducers. Acetaminophen may cause liver damage.
Do not use:
- with another product containing any of these active ingredients
- if you are now taking a prescription monoamine oxidase inhibitor (MAOI) (certain drugs for depression, psychiatric, or emotional conditions, or Parkinson's disease), or for 2 weeks after stopping the MAOI drug. If you do not know if your prescription drug contains an MAOI, ask a doctor or pharmacist before taking this product.

Ask a doctor before use if you have:
- heart disease
- thyroid disease
- diabetes
- high blood pressure
- trouble urinating due to an enlarged prostate gland
- cough accompanied by excessive phlegm (mucus)
- persistent or chronic cough as occurs with smoking, asthma, or emphysema

When using this product:
- **do not use more than directed**
Stop use and ask a doctor if:
- new symptoms occur
- sore throat is severe
- you get nervous, dizzy, or sleepless
- symptoms do not get better
- you need to use more than 10 days
- redness or swelling is present
- fever gets worse or lasts more than 3 days
- cough persists for more than 7 days, tends to recur, or is accompanied by rash, or persistent headache. These could be signs of a serious condition.
- sore throat lasts for more than 2 days, is accompanied or followed by fever, headache, rash, swelling, nausea, or vomiting

If pregnant or breast-feeding, ask a health professional before use.
Keep out of reach of children.
Overdose warning: Taking more than the recommended dose may cause liver damage. In case of overdose, get medical help or contact a Poison Control Center right away. Quick medical attention is critical for adults as well as for children even if you do not notice any signs or symptoms.

Directions:
- do not use more than directed (see overdose warning)
- adults and children 12 years of age and over: 2 caplets
- children under 12 years of age: ask a doctor
- take every 6 hours while symptoms persist
- do not take more than 8 caplets in 24 hours or as directed by a doctor

Other Information:
- store at 59° to 77°F in a dry place

Inactive Ingredients: candelilla wax, crospovidone, hypromellose, magnesium stearate, microcrystalline cellulose poloxamer 407, polyethylene glycol, polyethylene oxide, povidone, pregelatinized starch, silicon dioxide, sodium lauryl sulfate, stearic acid, and titanium dioxide

Questions? call toll free **1-800-524-2624,** Monday to Friday, 9 AM – 5 PM EST

How Supplied: Boxes of 12 and 24 caplets; boxes of 12 tablets.
Shown in Product Identification Guide, page 521

SUDAFED® Sinus & Allergy Tablets
(Formerly Sudafed Cold & Allergy)
[sū 'duh-fĕd]

Drug Facts:

Active Ingredients: **Purposes:**
(in each tablet)
Chlorpheniramine maleate
     4 mg .... Antihistamine
Pseudoephedrine HCl
     60 mg .... Nasal decongestant

Uses:
- temporarily relieves these symptoms due to hay fever (allergic rhinitis) or other upper respiratory allergies:
  - runny nose
  - sneezing
  - itchy, watery eyes
  - nasal congestion
  - itching of the nose or throat
- temporarily relieves these symptoms due to the common cold:
  - runny nose
  - sneezing
  - nasal congestion

Warnings:
Do not use if you are now taking a prescription monoamine oxidase inhibitor (MAOI) (certain drugs for depression, psychiatric, or emotional conditions, or Parkinson's disease), or for 2 weeks after stopping the MAOI drug. If you do not know if your prescription drug contains an MAOI, ask a doctor or pharmacist before taking this product.

Ask a doctor before use if you have:
- high blood pressure
- thyroid disease
- heart disease
- glaucoma
- diabetes
- trouble urinating due to an enlarged prostate gland
- a breathing problem such as emphysema or chronic bronchitis

Ask a doctor or pharmacist before use if you are taking sedatives or tranquilizers
When using this product:
- **do not use more than directed**
- drowsiness may occur
- excitability may occur, especially in children
- avoid alcoholic drinks
- alcohol, sedatives, and tranquilizers may increase drowsiness
- be careful when driving a motor vehicle or operating machinery
Stop use and ask a doctor if:
- you get nervous, dizzy, or sleepless
- symptoms do not improve within 7 days or are accompanied by fever

If pregnant or breast-feeding, ask a health professional before use.
Keep out of reach of children. In case of overdose, get medical help or contact a Poison Control Center right away.

Directions:
- take every 4 to 6 hours
- do not take more than 4 doses in 24 hours

adults and children 12 years of age and over	1 tablet
children 6 to under 12 years of age	½ tablet
children under 6 years of age	ask a doctor

Other Information:
- store at 59° to 77°F in a dry place

Inactive Ingredients: Lactose, magnesium stearate, potato starch, and povidone

Questions? call **1-800-524-2624** (English/Spanish), weekdays, 9 AM–5 PM EST

How Supplied: Boxes of 24 tablets.
Shown in Product Identification Guide, page 520

SUDAFED® NON-DROWSY SINUS & COLD
(Formerly Sudafed Cold & Sinus)
Liquid Caps
[sū 'duh-fed]

Drug Facts:

Active Ingredients: **Purposes:**
(in each liquid cap)
Acetaminophen
     325 mg .... Pain reliever/fever reducer
Pseudoephedrine HCl
     30 mg .... Nasal decongestant

Uses:
- temporarily relieves these symptoms due to the common cold:
  - nasal congestion
  - headache
  - minor aches and pains
  - muscular aches
  - sore throat
  - fever
- temporarily restores freer breathing through the nose
- temporarily relieves sinus congestion and pressure

Warnings:
Alcohol warning: If you consume 3 or more alcoholic drinks every day, ask your doctor whether you should take acetaminophen or other pain relievers/ fever reducers. Acetaminophen may cause liver damage.
Do not use:
- with another product containing any of these active ingredients.
- if you are now taking a prescription monoamine oxidase inhibitor (MAOI) (certain drugs for depression, psychiatric, or emotional conditions, or Parkinson's disease), or for 2 weeks after stopping the MAOI drug. If you do not know if your prescription drug contains an MAOI, ask a doctor or pharmacist before taking this product.

Ask a doctor before use if you have:
- heart disease
- thyroid disease
- diabetes
- high blood pressure
- trouble urinating due to an enlarged prostate gland

When using this product:
- **do not use more than directed**

Stop use and ask a doctor if:
- redness or swelling is present
- you get nervous, dizzy, or sleepless
- new symptoms occur
- you need to use more than 10 days
- symptoms do not improve
- fever gets worse or lasts more than 3 days
- sore throat is severe
- sore throat lasts for more than 2 days, is accompanied or followed by fever, headache, rash, swelling, nausea, or vomiting

If pregnant or breast-feeding, ask a health professional before use.

Keep out of reach of children.

Overdose warning: Taking more than the recommended dose may cause liver damage. In case of overdose, get medical help or contact a Poison Control Center right away. Quick medical attention is critical for adults as well as for children even if you do not notice any signs or symptoms.

Directions:
- do not use more than directed (see overdose warning)
- adults and children 12 years of age and over: 2 liquid caps
- take every 4 to 6 hours while symptoms persist
- do not take more than 8 liquid caps in 24 hours, or as directed by a doctor
- children under 12 years of age: ask a doctor

Other Information:
- **each liquid cap contains:** sodium 16 mg
- store at 59° to 77°F
- protect from heat, humidity, and light

Inactive Ingredients: FD&C blue no. 1, FD&C red no. 40, gelatin, glycerin, polyethylene glycol, povidone, sodium acetate, and sorbitol. Printed with edible white ink.

Questions? call **1-800-524-2624** (English/Spanish), weekdays, 9 AM – 5 PM EST

How Supplied: Boxes of 10 and 20 liquid caps.

Shown in Product Identification Guide, page 521

SUDAFED® Non-drowsy Sinus Headache Caplets and Tablets (Formerly Sudafed Sinus)
[sū 'duh-fĕd]

Drug Facts:

Active Ingredients:
(in each caplet)   **Purposes:**
Acetaminophen 500 mg .... Pain reliever
Pseudoephedrine
  HCl 30 mg .... Nasal decongestant

Uses:
- temporarily relieves nasal congestion associated with sinusitis
- temporarily relieves headache, minor aches, and pains

Warnings:

Alcohol warning: If you consume 3 or more alcoholic drinks every day, ask your doctor whether you should take acetaminophen or other pain relievers/fever reducers. Acetaminophen may cause liver damage.

Do not use:
- with another product containing any of these active ingredients.
- if you are now taking a prescription monoamine oxidase inhibitor (MAOI) (certain drugs for depression, psychiatric, or emotional conditions, or Parkinson's disease), or for 2 weeks after stopping the MAOI drug. If you do not know if your prescription drug contains an MAOI, ask a doctor or pharmacist before taking this product.

Ask a doctor before use if you have:
- heart disease
- thyroid disease
- diabetes
- high blood pressure
- trouble urinating due to an enlarged prostate gland

When using this product:
- **do not use more than directed**

Stop use and ask a doctor if:
- you get nervous, dizzy, or sleepless
- new symptoms occur
- symptoms do not get better
- you need to use more than 10 days
- fever occurs and lasts for more than 3 days

If pregnant or breast-feeding, ask a health professional before use.

Keep out of reach of children.

Overdose warning: Taking more than the recommended dose may cause liver damage. In case of overdose, get medical help or contact a Poison Control Center right away. Quick medical attention is critical for adults as well as for children even if you do not notice any signs or symptoms.

Directions:
- do not use more than directed (see overdose warning)
- children under 12 years of age: ask a doctor
- adults and children 12 years of age and over: 2 caplets every 6 hours while symptoms persist
- do not take more than 8 caplets in 24 hours or as directed by a doctor

Other Information:
- store at 59° to 77°F in a dry place

Inactive Ingredients: calcium stearate, candelilla wax, croscarmellose sodium, crospovidone, FD&C yellow no. 6 aluminum lake, hypromellose, microcrystalline cellulose, polyethylene glycol, polysorbate 80, povidone, pregelatinized starch, stearic acid and titanium dioxide.

Questions? call **1-800-524-2624** (English/Spanish), weekdays, 9 AM–5 PM EST

How Supplied: Boxes of 24 and 48 caplets; boxes of 24 tablets.

Shown in Product Identification Guide, page 521

SUDAFED® SINUS NIGHTTIME
[sū' duh-fĕd]

Drug Facts:

Active Ingredients:
(in each tablet)   **Purposes:**
Pseudoephedrine HCl
  60 mg .... Nasal decongestant
Triprolidine HCl
  2.5 mg .... Antihistamine

Uses:
- temporarily relieves these symptoms of hay fever or other upper respiratory allergies:
  - runny nose
  - sneezing
  - nasal and sinus congestion
  - itchy, watery eyes
  - itching of the nose or throat
- temporarily relieves nasal and sinus congestion due to the common cold or associated with sinusitis

Warnings:

Do not use if you are now taking a prescription monoamine oxidase inhibitor (MAOI) (certain drugs for depression, psychiatric, or emotional conditions, or Parkinson's disease), or for 2 weeks after stopping the MAOI drug. If you do not know if your prescription drug contains an MAOI, ask a doctor or pharmacist before taking this product.

Ask a doctor before use if you have:
- high blood pressure
- heart disease
- thyroid disease
- diabetes
- glaucoma
- trouble urinating due to an enlarged prostate gland
- a breathing problem such as emphysema or chronic bronchitis

Ask a doctor or pharmacist before use if you are taking sedatives or tranquilizers

When using this product
- **do not use more than directed**
- drowsiness may occur
- avoid alcoholic drinks
- alcohol, sedatives, and tranquilizers may increase drowsiness
- be careful when driving a motor vehicle or operating machinery
- excitability may occur, especially in children

Stop use and ask a doctor if
- you get nervous, dizzy, or sleepless
- symptoms do not improve within 7 days or are accompanied by fever

If pregnant or breast-feeding, ask a health professional before use.

Keep out of reach of children. In case of overdose, get medical help or contact a Poison Control Center right away.

Continued on next page

This product information was prepared in November 2002. On these and other Pfizer Consumer Healthcare Products, detailed information may be obtained by addressing Pfizer Consumer Healthcare, Pfizer, Inc., Morris Plains, NJ 07950

Sudafed Nighttime—Cont.

Directions:
- take every 4 to 6 hours
- do not take more than 4 doses in 24 hours

adults and children 12 years of age and over	1 tablet
children 6 to under 12 years of age	1/2 tablet
children under 6 years of age	ask a doctor

Other Information:
- store at 59° to 77°F in a dry place
- protect from light

Inactive Ingredients: Flavor, hypromellose, lactose, magnesium stearate, polyethylene glycol, potato starch, povidone, sucrose, and titanium dioxide

Questions? call **1-800-524-2624** (English/Spanish), weekdays, 9 AM–5 PM EST

How Supplied: Boxes of 12 tablets.
Shown in Product Identification Guide, page 521

SUDAFED® Sinus Nighttime Plus Pain Relief
[sū'duh - fēd]

Drug Facts:

Active Ingredients:
(in each caplet)   **Purposes:**
Acetaminophen
  500 mg .... Pain reliever
Diphenhydramine HCl
  25 mg .... Antihistamine
Pseudoephedrine HCl
  30 mg .... Nasal decongestant

Uses:
- temporarily relieves these symptoms of hay fever, the common cold or other upper respiratory allergies:
  - runny nose
  - sneezing
  - nasal and sinus congestion
  - headache
  - minor aches and pains
- temporarily relieves these additional symptoms of hay fever or other upper respiratory allergies:
  - itching of the nose or throat
  - itchy, watery eyes
- temporarily relieves nasal and sinus congestion associated with sinusitis

Warnings:
Alcohol warning: If you consume 3 or more alcoholic drinks every day, ask your doctor whether you should take acetaminophen or other pain relievers/fever reducers. Acetaminophen may cause liver damage.
Do not use:
- with another product containing any of these active ingredients
- if you are now taking a prescription monoamine oxidase inhibitor (MAOI) (certain drugs for depression, psychi-

atric, or emotional conditions, or Parkinson's disease), or for 2 weeks after stopping the MAOI drug. If you do not know if your prescription drug contains an MAOI, ask a doctor or pharmacist before taking this product.
- with any other product containing diphenhydramine, including one applied topically

Ask a doctor before use if you have:
- heart disease
- glaucoma
- thyroid disease
- diabetes
- high blood pressure
- trouble urinating due to an enlarged prostate gland
- a breathing problem such as emphysema or chronic bronchitis

Ask a doctor or pharmacist before use if you are taking sedatives or tranquilizers
When using this product:
- **do not use more than directed**
- marked drowsiness may occur
- avoid alcoholic drinks
- alcohol, sedatives, and tranquilizers may increase drowsiness
- excitability may occur, especially in children
- be careful when driving a motor vehicle or operating machinery
Stop use and ask a doctor if:
- you get nervous, dizzy, or sleepless
- new symptoms occur
- fever occurs and lasts more than 3 days
- symptoms do not get better
- you need to use more than 10 days
If pregnant or breast-feeding, ask a health professional before use.
Keep out of reach of children.
Overdose warning: Taking more than the recommended dose may cause liver damage. In case of overdose, get medical help or contact a Poison Control Center right away. Quick medical attention is critical for adults as well as for children even if you do not notice any signs or symptoms.

Directions:
- do not use more than directed (see overdose warning)
- take every 6 hours while symptoms persist
- do not take more than 8 caplets in 24 hours or as directed by a doctor
- adults and children 12 years of age and over: 2 caplets
- children under 12 years of age: ask a doctor

Other Information:
- store at 59° to 77°F in a dry place

Inactive Ingredients: Carnauba wax, crospovidone, FD&C blue no. 1 aluminum lake, hypromellose, magnesium stearate, microcrystalline cellulose, polyethylene glycol, polysorbate 80, povidone, pregelatinized starch, sodium starch glycolate, stearic acid, and titanium dioxide

Questions? call **1-800-524-2624** (English/Spanish), weekdays, 9 AM – 5 PM EST

How Supplied: Boxes of 20 caplets. Capsule shaped tablets.
Shown in Product Identification Guide, page 521

CHILDREN'S SUDAFED®
Non-Drowsy Cold & Cough Liquid
[sū 'duh-fĕd]

Drug Facts:

Active Ingredients: **Purposes:**
(in each 5 mL*)
Dextromethorphan HBr
  5 mg .... Antitussive
Pseudoephedrine HCl
  15 mg .... Nasal decongestant

---
*5 mL = one teaspoonful

Uses:
- temporarily relieves nasal congestion due to the common cold
- temporarily quiets cough due to minor throat and bronchial irritation occurring with a cold or inhaled irritants

Warnings:
Do not use if you are now taking a prescription monoamine oxidase inhibitor (MAOI) (certain drugs for depression, psychiatric, or emotional conditions, or Parkinson's disease), or for 2 weeks after stopping the MAOI drug. If you do not know if your prescription drug contains an MAOI, ask a doctor or pharmacist before taking this product.
Ask a doctor before use if you have:
- heart disease
- thyroid disease
- diabetes
- high blood pressure
- trouble urinating due to an enlarged prostate gland
- cough accompanied by excessive phlegm (mucus)
- persistent or chronic cough such as occurs with smoking, asthma, or emphysema
When using this product:
- **do not use more than directed**
Stop use and ask a doctor if:
- you get nervous, dizzy, or sleepless
- symptoms do not improve within 7 days or are accompanied by fever
- cough persists for more than 1 week, tends to recur, or is accompanied by fever, rash, or persistent headache. These could be signs of a serious condition.
If pregnant or breast-feeding, ask a health professional before use.
Keep out of reach of children. In case of overdose, get medical help or contact a Poison Control Center right away.

Directions:
- take every 4 hours
- do not take more than 4 doses in 24 hours, or as directed by a doctor

children under 2 years of age	ask a doctor
children 2 to under 6 years of age	one (1) teaspoonful
children 6 to under 12 years of age	two (2) teaspoonfuls
adults and children 12 years of age and over	four (4) teaspoonfuls

Other Information:
- store at 59° to 77°F

Inactive Ingredients: Carboxymethylcellulose sodium, citric acid, D&C red

no. 33, FD&C red no. 40, flavors, glycerin, poloxamer 407, polyethylene glycol 1450, purified water, saccharin sodium, sodium benzoate, sodium chloride, sodium citrate, and sorbitol solution

Questions? call **1-800-524-2624** (English/Spanish), weekdays, 9 AM–5 PM EST

How Supplied: Sudafed Children's Cold and Cough Non-Drowsy Liquid is supplied in 4 fl. oz. bottles.
Shown in Product Identification Guide, page 521

CHILDREN'S SUDAFED®
Non-drowsy Nasal Decongestant Chewables
[sū ' duh-fĕd]

Drug Facts:

Active Ingredient:

(in each tablet)	Purpose:
Pseudoephedrine HCl 15 mg	Nasal decongestant

Uses:
- temporarily relieves nasal congestion due to the common cold, hay fever or other upper respiratory allergies, and nasal congestion associated with sinusitis
- temporarily relieves sinus congestion and pressure
- promotes nasal and/or sinus drainage

Warnings:
Do not use if you are now taking a prescription monoamine oxidase inhibitor (MAOI) (certain drugs for depression, psychiatric, or emotional conditions, or Parkinson's disease), or for 2 weeks after stopping the MAOI drug. If you do not know if your prescription drug contains an MAOI, ask a doctor or pharmacist before taking this product.
Ask a doctor before use if you have:
- heart disease
- high blood pressure
- thyroid disease
- diabetes
- trouble urinating due to an enlarged prostate gland
When using this product:
- **do not use more than directed**
Stop use and ask a doctor if:
- you get nervous, dizzy, or sleepless
- symptoms do not improve within 7 days or are accompanied by fever
If pregnant or breast-feeding, ask a health professional before use.
Keep out of reach of children. In case of overdose, get medical help or contact a Poison Control Center right away.

Directions:
- take every 4 to 6 hours
- do not take more than 4 doses in 24 hours

children under 2 years of age	ask a doctor
children 2 to under 6 years of age	one (1) chewable tablet
children 6 to under 12 years of age	two (2) chewable tablets
adults and children 12 years of age and over	four (4) chewable tablets

Other Information:
- **phenylketonurics:** contains phenylalanine 0.78 mg per tablet
- store at 59° to 77°F in a dry place
- protect from light

Inactive Ingredients: Ascorbic acid, aspartame, carnauba wax, citric acid, crospovidone, FD&C yellow no. 6 aluminum lake, flavors, hypromellose, magnesium stearate, mannitol, microcrystalline cellulose, sodium chloride, and tartaric acid

Questions? call **1-800-524-2624** (English/Spanish), weekdays, 9 AM – 5 PM EST

How Supplied: Box of 24 chewable tablets.
Shown in Product Identification Guide, page 521

CHILDREN'S SUDAFED®
NON-DROWSY NASAL DECONGESTANT LIQUID
[sū 'duh-fĕd]

Drug Facts:

Active Ingredient:

(in each 5 mL*)	Purpose:
Pseudoephedrine HCl 15 mg	Nasal decongestant

*5 mL = one teaspoonful

Uses:
- temporarily relieves nasal congestion due to the common cold, hay fever or other upper respiratory allergies, and nasal congestion associated with sinusitis
- temporarily relieves sinus congestion and pressure
- promotes nasal and/or sinus drainage

Warnings:
Do not use if you are now taking a prescription monoamine oxidase inhibitor (MAOI) (certain drugs for depression, psychiatric, or emotional conditions, or Parkinson's disease), or for 2 weeks after stopping the MAOI drug. If you do not know if your prescription drug contains an MAOI, ask a doctor or pharmacist before taking this product.
Ask a doctor before use if you have:
- heart disease
- high blood pressure
- thyroid disease
- diabetes
- trouble urinating due to an enlarged prostate gland
When using this product:
- **do not use more than directed**
Stop use and ask a doctor if:
- you get nervous, dizzy, or sleepless
- symptoms do not improve within 7 days or are accompanied by fever
If pregnant or breast-feeding, ask a health professional before use.
Keep out of reach of children. In case of overdose, get medical help or contact a Poison Control Center right away.

Directions:
- take every 4 to 6 hours
- do not take more than 4 doses in 24 hours

children under 2 years of age	ask a doctor
children 2 to under 6 years of age	one (1) teaspoonful
children 6 to under 12 years of age	two (2) teaspoonfuls
adults and children 12 years of age and over	four (4) teaspoonfuls

Other Information:
- store at 59° to 77°F

Inactive Ingredients: Citric acid, edetate disodium, FD&C red no. 40, FD&C blue no. 1, flavors, glycerin, poloxamer 407, polyethylene glycol 1450, povidone K-90, purified water, saccharin sodium, sodium benzoate, sodium citrate, and sorbitol solution

Questions? Call **1-800-524-2624** (English/Spanish), weekdays, 9 AM – 5 PM EST

How Supplied: Sudafed Children's Nasal Decongestant is supplied in 4 fl. oz. bottles
Shown in Product Identification Guide, page 521

TUCKS®
Hemorrhoidal Pads
[tŭks]

Drug Facts:

Active Ingredient:	Purpose:
Witch hazel 50%	Hemorrhoidal pad

Use: temporarily relieves these external symptoms associated with hemorrhoids:
- itching
- burning
- irritation

Warnings:
For external use only
When using this product
- do not exceed the recommended daily dosage unless directed by a doctor
- do not put directly in rectum by using fingers or any mechanical device
Stop use and ask a doctor if
- condition worsens or does not improve within 7 days
- rectal bleeding occurs
Keep out of reach of children. If swallowed, get medical help or contact a Poison Control Center right away.

Continued on next page

This product information was prepared in November 2002. On these and other Pfizer Consumer Healthcare Products, detailed information may be obtained by addressing Pfizer Consumer Healthcare, Pfizer, Inc., Morris Plains, NJ 07950

Tucks—Cont.

Directions:
- as a hemorrhoidal treatment for adults:
  - when practical, clean the affected area with mild soap and warm water and rinse thoroughly
  - gently dry by patting or blotting with toilet tissue or a soft cloth before applying
  - gently apply to the affected area by patting and then discard tissue
  - can be used up to six times daily or after each bowel movement
- children under 12 years of age: ask a doctor

Other Information: • store at 59° to 77°F

Inactive Ingredients: water, glycerin, alcohol, propylene glycol, sodium citrate, diazolidinyl urea, citric acid, methylparaben, and propylparaben

Questions? call **1-800-223-0182**, Monday to Friday, 9 AM – 5 PM EST

How Supplied: Jars of 40 and 100 pads. Also available TUCKS® individual foil-wrapped towelettes.
Shown in Product Identification Guide, page 521

MAXIMUM STRENGTH UNISOM SLEEPGELS®
Nighttime Sleep Aid

Drug Facts

Active Ingredient
(in each softgel): **Purpose:**
Diphenhydramine HCl
  50 mg .... Nighttime sleep-aid

Use:
- helps to reduce difficulty falling asleep

Warnings:
Do not use
- for children under 12 years of age
- with any other product containing diphenhydramine, including one applied topically
Ask a doctor before use if you have
- a breathing problem such as emphysema or chronic bronchitis
- glaucoma
- trouble urinating due to an enlarged prostate gland
Ask a doctor or pharmacist before use if you are taking sedatives or tranquilizers
When using this product avoid alcoholic drinks
Stop use and ask a doctor if sleeplessness persists continuously for more than 2 weeks. Insomnia may be a symptom of serious underlying medical illness.
If pregnant or breast-feeding, ask a health professional before use.
Keep out of reach of children. In case of overdose, get medical help or contact a Poison Control Center right away.

Directions:
- adults and children 12 years of age and over: 1 softgel (50 mg) at bedtime if needed, or as directed by a doctor

Other information:
- store at 59° to 86°F (15° to 30°C)

Inactive ingredients: FD&C blue no. 1, gelatin, glycerin, polyethylene glycol, polyvinyl acetate phthalate, propylene glycol, purified water, sorbitol, and titanium dioxide

Questions? call **1-800-223-0182**, Monday to Friday, 9 AM – 5 PM EST

How Supplied: Boxes of 16 liquid filled softgels in child resistant blisters and boxes of 8 with non-child resistant packaging. Also in a 32 count easy to open child resistant bottle.
Store between 15° and 30°C (59° and 86°F)
Shown in Product Identification Guide, page 521

UNISOM® SleepTabs™
[yu 'na-som]
Nighttime Sleep Aid
(doxylamine succinate)

Drug Facts

Active Ingredient: **Purpose:**
(in each tablet)
Doxylamine succinate
  25 mg .... Nighttime sleep-aid

Use:
- helps to reduce difficulty in falling asleep

Warnings:
Ask a doctor before use if you have
- a breathing problem such as asthma, emphysema or chronic bronchitis
- glaucoma
- trouble urinating due to an enlarged prostate gland
Ask a doctor or pharmacist before use if you are taking any other drugs
When using this product
- avoid alcoholic beverages
- take only at bedtime
Stop use and ask a doctor if sleeplessness persists continuously for more than two weeks. Insomnia may be a symptom of serious underlying medical illness.
If pregnant or breast-feeding, ask a health professional before use.
Keep out of reach of children. In case of overdose, get medical help or contact a Poison Control Center right away.

Directions:
- adults: take one tablet 30 minutes before going to bed; take once daily or as directed by a doctor
- do not give to children under 12 years of age

Other information:
- store at 59° to 86°F (15° to 30°C)

Inactive ingredients: dibasic calcium phosphate, FD&C blue no. 1 aluminum lake, magnesium stearate, microcrystalline cellulose, and sodium starch glycolate

Questions?
call **1-800-223-0182**, Monday to Friday, 9 AM - 5 PM EST

How Supplied: Boxes of 8, 32 and 48 tablets in child resistant packaging. Boxes of 16 tablets in non-child resistant packaging.
Shown in Product Identification Guide, page 522

VISINE® ORIGINAL
Tetrahydrozoline Hydrochloride/Redness Reliever Eye Drops

Description: Visine Original is a redness reliever eye drop that gives fast relief of redness of the eye due to minor eye irritation caused by conditions such as smoke, dust, other airborne pollutants and swimming.
Visine Original is a sterile, isotonic, buffered ophthalmic solution containing tetrahydrozoline hydrochloride. The effectiveness of Visine in relieving conjunctival hyperemia has been demonstrated by numerous clinicals, including several double-blind studies, involving more than 2,000 subjects suffering from acute or chronic hyperemia induced by a variety of conditions. Visine was found to be efficacious in providing relief from conjunctival hyperemia.

Active Ingredient: **Purpose:**
Tetrahydrozoline
  HCl 0.05% .... Redness reliever

Use:
- for the relief of redness of the eye due to minor eye irritations

Warnings:
Ask a doctor before use if you have narrow angle glaucoma
When using this product
- pupils may become enlarged temporarily
- overuse may cause more eye redness
- remove contact lenses before using
- do not use if this solution changes color or becomes cloudy
- do not touch tip of container to any surface to avoid contamination
- replace cap after each use
Stop use and ask a doctor if
- you feel eye pain
- changes in vision occur
- redness or irritation of the eye lasts
- condition worsens or lasts more than 72 hours
If pregnant or breast-feeding, ask a health professional before use.
Keep out of reach of children. If swallowed, get medical help or contact a Poison Control Center right away.

Directions:
- put 1 to 2 drops in the affected eye(s) up to 4 times daily
- children under 6 years of age: ask a doctor

Other Information:
- store at 15° to 30°C (59° to 86°F)

Inactive Ingredients: benzalkonium chloride, boric acid, edetate disodium, purified water, sodium borate, and sodium chloride
Questions? call **1-800-223-0182**, Monday to Friday, 9 AM – 5 PM EST

Caution: Do not use if Visine-imprinted neckband on bottle is broken or missing.

How Supplied: In 0.5 fl. oz. and 1.0 fl. oz. plastic dispenser bottle and 0.5 fl. oz. plastic bottle with eye dropper.
Shown in Product Identification Guide, page 522

VISINE-A®
ANTIHISTAMINE & REDNESS RELIEVER EYE DROPS

Drug Facts:

Active Ingredients:	Purpose:
Naphazoline hydrochloride 0.025%	Redness reliever
Pheniramine maleate 0.3%	Antihistamine

Uses: Temporarily relieves itchy, red eyes due to:
- pollen
- ragweed
- grass
- animal hair and dander

Warnings:
Do not use
- if you are sensitive to any ingredient in this product

Ask a doctor before use if you have:
- heart disease
- high blood pressure
- narrow angle glaucoma
- trouble urinating due to an enlarged prostate gland

When using this product:
- pupils may become enlarged temporarily
- do not touch tip of container to any surface to avoid contamination
- replace cap after each use
- remove contact lenses before using
- do not use if this solution changes color or becomes cloudy
- overuse may cause more eye redness

Stop use and ask a doctor if:
- you feel eye pain
- changes in vision occur
- redness or irritation of the eye lasts
- condition worsens or lasts more than 72 hours

Keep out of reach of children. If swallowed, get medical help or contact a Poison Control Center right away. Accidental swallowing by infants and children may lead to coma and marked reduction in body temperature.

Directions:
- adults and children 6 years of age and over: put 1 or 2 drops in the affected eye(s) up to 4 times a day
- children under 6 years of age: consult a doctor

Other Information:
- some users may experience a brief tingling sensation
- store between 15° and 25°C (59° and 77°F)

Inactive Ingredients: boric acid and sodium borate buffer system preserved with benzalkonium chloride (0.01%) and edetate disodium (0.1%), sodium hydroxide and/or hydrochloric acid (to adjust pH), and purified water

Questions? call **1-800-223-0182**, Monday to Friday, 9 AM – 5 PM EST

Caution: Do not use if Visine imprinted neckband on bottle is broken or missing.

How Supplied: In 0.5 fl. oz. plastic dispenser bottle.
Shown in Product Identification Guide, page 522

VISINE A.C.®
Astringent/Redness Reliever Eye Drops

Drug Facts:

Active Ingredients:	Purposes:
Tetrahydrozoline HCl 0.05%	Redness reliever
Zinc sulfate 0.25%	Astringent

Use:
- for temporary relief of discomfort and redness of the eye due to minor eye irritations

Warnings:
Ask a doctor before use if you have narrow angle glaucoma
When using this product:
- pupils may become enlarged temporarily
- overuse may cause more eye redness
- remove contact lenses before using
- do not use if this solution changes color or becomes cloudy
- do not touch tip of container to any surface to avoid contamination
- replace cap after each use

Stop use and ask a doctor if:
- you feel eye pain
- changes in vision occur
- redness or irritation of the eye lasts
- condition worsens or lasts more than 72 hours

If pregnant or breast-feeding, ask a health professional before use.
Keep out of reach of children. If swallowed, get medical help or contact a Poison Control Center right away.

Directions:
- put 1 to 2 drops in the affected eye(s) up to 4 times daily
- children under 6 years of age: ask a doctor

Other information:
- some users may experience a brief tingling sensation
- store at 15° to 30°C (59° to 86°F)

Inactive Ingredients: benzalkonium chloride, boric acid, edetate disodium, purified water, sodium chloride, and sodium citrate

Questions? call **1-800-223-0182**, Monday to Friday, 9 AM – 5 PM EST

Caution: Do not use if Visine-imprinted neckband on bottle is broken or missing.

How Supplied: In 0.5 fl. oz. and 1.0 fl. oz. plastic dispenser bottle.
Shown in Product Identification Guide, page 522

ADVANCED RELIEF VISINE®
Lubricant/Redness Reliever Eye Drops

Drug Facts:

Active Ingredients:	Purposes:
Dextran 70 0.1%	Lubricant
Polyethylene glycol 400 1%	Lubricant
Povidone 1%	Lubricant
Tetrahydrozoline HCl 0.05%	Redness reliever

Uses:
- for the relief of redness of the eye due to minor eye irritations
- for use as a protectant against further irritation or to relieve dryness of the eye

Warnings:
Ask a doctor before use if you have narrow angle glaucoma
When using this product:
- pupils may become enlarged temporarily
- overuse may cause more eye redness
- remove contact lenses before using
- do not use if this solution changes color or becomes cloudy
- do not touch tip of container to any surface to avoid contamination
- replace cap after each use

Stop use and ask a doctor if:
- you feel eye pain
- changes in vision occur
- redness or irritation of the eye lasts
- condition worsens or lasts more than 72 hours

If pregnant or breast-feeding, ask a health professional before use.
Keep out of reach of children. If swallowed, get medical help or contact a Poison Control Center right away.

Directions:
- put 1 or 2 drops in the affected eye(s) up to 4 times daily
- children under 6 years of age: ask a doctor

Other Information:
- store at 15° to 30°C (59° to 86°F)

Inactive Ingredients: benzalkonium chloride, boric acid, edetate disodium, purified water, sodium borate, and sodium chloride

Questions? call **1-800-223-0182**, Monday to Friday, 9 AM – 5 PM EST

Caution: Do not use if Visine-imprinted neckband on bottle is broken or missing.

How Supplied: In 0.5 fl. oz. and 1.0 fl. oz. plastic dispenser bottle.
Shown in Product Identification Guide, page 522

Continued on next page

This product information was prepared in November 2002. On these and other Pfizer Consumer Healthcare Products, detailed information may be obtained by addressing Pfizer Consumer Healthcare, Pfizer, Inc., Morris Plains, NJ 07950

VISINE L.R.®
Redness Reliever Eye Drops

Drug Facts:

Active Ingredient: **Purpose:**
Oxymetazoline HCl
0.025% .... Redness reliever

Use:
- for the relief of redness of the eye due to minor eye irritations

Warnings:
Ask a doctor before use if you have narrow angle glaucoma
When using this product:
- overuse may cause more eye redness
- remove contact lenses before using
- do not use if this solution changes color or becomes cloudy
- do not touch tip of container to any surface to avoid contamination
- replace cap after each use
Stop use and ask a doctor if:
- you feel eye pain
- changes in vision occur
- redness or irritation of the eye lasts
- condition worsens or lasts more than 72 hours
If pregnant or breast-feeding, ask a health professional before use.
Keep out of reach of children. If swallowed, get medical help or contact a Poison Control Center right away.

Directions:
- adults and children 6 years of age and over: put 1 or 2 drops in the affected eye(s)
- this may be repeated as needed every 6 hours or as directed by a doctor
- children under 6 years of age: ask a doctor

Other Information:
- store at 15° to 30°C (59° to 86°F)

Inactive Ingredients: benzalkonium chloride, boric acid, edetate disodium, purified water, sodium borate, and sodium chloride

Questions? call **1-800-223-0182**, Monday to Friday, 9 AM – 5 PM EST

Caution: Do not use if Visine-imprinted neckband on bottle is broken or missing.

How Supplied: In 0.5 fl. oz. and 1 fl. oz. plastic dispenser bottle.
Shown in Product Identification Guide, page 522

VISINE TEARS®
Lubricant Eye Drops

Description: Visine Tears® Lubricant Eye Drops cools and comforts your dry, scratchy, irritated eyes, and helps them feel their best. It relieves the dryness caused by computer use, reading, wind, heat and air conditioning, while it protects your eyes from further irritation. Visine Tears is safe to use as often as needed.

Active Ingredients: **Purpose:**
Glycerin 0.2% .... Lubricant
Hypromellose 0.2% .... Lubricant
Polyethylene glycol 400 1% ... Lubricant

Uses:
- for the temporary relief of burning and irritation due to dryness of the eye
- for protection against further irritation

Warnings:
When using this product
- remove contact lenses before using
- do not use if this solution changes color or becomes cloudy
- do not touch tip of container to any surface to avoid contamination
- replace cap after each use
Stop use and ask a doctor if:
- you feel eye pain
- changes in vision occur
- redness or irritation of the eye lasts
- condition worsens or lasts more than 72 hours
If pregnant or breast-feeding, ask a health professional before use.
Keep out of reach of children. If swallowed, get medical help or contact a Poison Control Center right away.

Directions:
- put 1 or 2 drops in the affected eye(s) as needed
- children under 6 years of age: ask a doctor

Other information:
- store at 15° to 30°C (59° to 86°F)

Inactive Ingredients: ascorbic acid, benzalkonium chloride, boric acid, dextrose, disodium phosphate, glycine, magnesium chloride, potassium chloride, purified water, sodium borate, sodium chloride, sodium citrate, and sodium lactate

Questions? call **1-800-223-0182**, Monday to Friday, 9 AM – 5 PM EST

Caution: Do not use if Visine-imprinted neckband on bottle is broken or missing.

How Supplied: In 0.5 fl. oz. and 1 fl. oz. plastic dispenser bottle.
Shown in Product Identification Guide, page 522

VISINE TEARS®
Preservative Free, Single-Use Containers
Lubricant Eye Drops

Drug Facts:

Active Ingredients: **Purpose:**
Glycerin 0.2% .... Lubricant
Hypromellose 0.2% .... Lubricant
Polyethylene glycol 400 1% ... Lubricant

Uses:
- for the temporary relief of burning and irritation due to dryness of the eye
- for protection against further irritation

Warnings:
When using this product
- remove contact lenses before using
- do not use if this solution changes color or becomes cloudy
- do not touch tip of container to any surface to avoid contamination
- do not reuse; once opened, discard
Stop use and ask a doctor if:
- you feel eye pain
- changes in vision occur
- redness or irritation of the eye lasts
- condition worsens or lasts more than 72 hours
If pregnant or breast-feeding, ask a health professional before use.
Keep out of reach of children. If swallowed, get medical help or contact a Poison Control Center right away.

Directions:
- put 1 or 2 drops in the affected eye(s) as needed
- children under 6 years of age: ask a doctor

Other Information:
- store at 15° to 30°C (59° to 86°F)

Inactive Ingredients: ascorbic acid, dextrose, disodium phosphate, glycine, magnesium chloride, potassium chloride, purified water, sodium chloride, sodium citrate, sodium lactate, and sodium phosphate

Questions? call **1-800-223-0182**, Monday to Friday, 9 AM - 5 PM EST

Caution: Use only if unit dose container is intact.

How Supplied: 1 box contains 28 single-use containers, 0.01 fl. oz. (0.4 mL) each
Shown in Product Identification Guide, page 522

MAXIMUM STRENGTH WART–OFF®
SALICYLIC ACID • WART REMOVER
Liquid

Drug Facts:

Active Ingredient: **Purpose:**
Salicylic acid 17% w/w .... Wart remover

Uses: For the removal of common warts and plantar warts on the bottom of the foot. The common wart is easily recognized by the rough "cauliflower-like" appearance of the surface. The plantar wart is recognized by its location only on the bottom of the foot, its tenderness, and the interruption of the footprint pattern.

Warnings:
For external use only.
Extremely flammable: Keep away from fire or flame
Do not use:
- on irritated skin, on any area that is infected or reddened, if you are a diabetic, or if you have poor blood circulation
- on moles, birthmarks, warts with hair growing from them, genital warts, or warts on the face or mucous membranes
When using this product:
- if product gets into the eye, flush with water for 15 minutes
- avoid inhaling vapors
- cap bottle tightly and store at room temperature away from heat
Stop use and ask a doctor if
- discomfort persists
Keep out of reach of children. If swallowed, get medical help or contact a Poison Control Center right away.

Directions:
- wash affected area
- dry area thoroughly
- apply one drop at a time with applicator to sufficiently cover each wart
- let dry
- repeat this procedure once or twice daily as needed (until wart is removed) for up to 12 weeks

Other Information:
- store at 15° to 30°C (59° to 86°F)

Inactive Ingredients:
Alcohol 26.3% w/w, *t*-butyl alcohol, denatonium benzoate, flexible collodion, and propylene glycol dipelargonate.

Questions? Call **1-800-723-7529,** Monday to Friday, 9 AM – 5 PM EST

How Supplied: 0.45 fluid ounce (13.3mL) bottle.

ZANTAC® 75
Ranitidine Tablets 75 mg
Acid Reducer
[*zan ' tak*]

Drug Facts:

Active Ingredient:
(in each tablet)　　　　　　　　**Purpose:**
Ranitidine 75 mg
(as ranitidine
hydrochloride 84 mg) .... Acid reducer

Uses:
- relieves heartburn associated with acid indigestion and sour stomach
- prevents heartburn associated with acid indigestion and sour stomach brought on by certain foods and beverages

Warnings:
Allergy alert: Do not use if you are allergic to ranitidine or other acid reducers
Do not use:
- if you have trouble swallowing
- with other acid reducers
Stop use and ask a doctor if:
- stomach pain continues
- you need to take this product for more than 14 days
If pregnant or breast-feeding, ask a health professional before use.
Keep out of reach of children. In case of overdose, get medical help or contact a Poison Control Center right away.

Directions:
- adults and children 12 years and over:
  - to **relieve** symptoms, swallow 1 tablet with a glass of water
  - to **prevent** symptoms, swallow 1 tablet with a glass of water **30 to 60 minutes before** eating food or drinking beverages that cause heartburn
  - can be used up to twice daily (up to 2 tablets in 24 hours)
- children under 12 years: ask a doctor

Other Information:
- do not use if foil under bottle cap or individual blister unit is open or torn
- store at 20°–25°C (68°–77°F)
- avoid excessive heat or humidity
- this product is sodium and sugar free

Inactive Ingredients: Hydroxypropyl methylcellulose, magnesium stearate, microcrystalline cellulose, synthetic red iron oxide, titanium dioxide, triacetin

Read the Label: Read the directions, consumer information leaflet and warnings before use. Keep the carton. It contains important information.

Questions? call **1-800-223-0182.** Information is available 24 hours a day, 7 days a week.

How Supplied: Zantac 75 is available in convenient blister packs in boxes of 4, 10, 20 and 30 tablets, and in bottles of 60, 80 and 110 count.
Shown in Product Identification Guide, page 522

Pharmacia Consumer Healthcare
PEAPACK, NJ 07977

For Medical and Pharmaceutical Information, Including Emergencies:
(269) 833-8244
(800) 253-8600 ext. 3-8244

DRAMAMINE® Original Formula Tablets
DRAMAMINE® Chewable Formula Tablets
Antiemetic

Description: DRAMAMINE Original Formula Tablets and DRAMAMINE Chewable Formula Tablets contain dimenhydrinate, which is the chlorotheophylline salt of the antihistaminic agent diphenhydramine.

Active Ingredient: Dimenhydrinate 50 mg per tablet.

Indications: For prevention and treatment of the symptoms associated with motion sickness including nausea, vomiting, and dizziness

Directions: To prevent motion sickness, the first dose should be taken ½ to 1 hour before starting activity. To prevent or treat motion sickness, use the following dosing.
Adults and children 12 years and over: 1 to 2 tablets every 4–6 hours; not more than 8 tablets in 24 hours, or as directed by a doctor
Children 6 to under 12 years: ½ to 1 tablet every 6–8 hours: not more than 3 tablets in 24 hours, or as directed by a doctor
Children 2 to under 6 years: ¼ to ½ tablet every 6–8 hours; not more than 1 ½ tablets in 24 hours, or as directed by a doctor

Warnings:
Do not use in children under 2 years of age unless directed by a doctor.
Ask a doctor before use if you have
- a breathing problem such as emphysema or chronic bronchitis • glaucoma • difficulty in urination due to enlargement of the prostate gland

Ask a doctor or pharmacist before use if you are taking sedatives or tranquilizers
When using these products
- marked drowsiness may occur • avoid alcoholic drinks • alcohol, sedatives, and tranquilizers may increase drowsiness • be careful when driving a motor vehicle or operating machinery
If pregnant or breast-feeding, ask a health professional before use.
Keep out of reach of children.
In case of overdose, get medical help or contact a Poison Control Center right away.

Other Information:
Chewable Formula Tablets: Phenylketonurics: contains **phenylalanine** 1.5 mg per tablet. Also contains FD&C yellow No. 5 (tartrazine) as a color additive

Inactive Ingredients: DRAMAMINE Original Formula Tablets: colloidal silicon dioxide, croscarmellose sodium, lactose, magnesium stearate, microcrystalline cellulose
DRAMAMINE Chewable Formula Tablets: aspartame, citric acid, FD&C yellow no. 5, FD&C yellow no. 6, flavor, magnesium stearate, methacrylic acid copolymer, sorbitol

How Supplied: Original Formula Tablets: scored, white tablets, available in 12 ct. vials, 36 ct. and 100 ct. packages
Chewable Formula Tablets: scored, orange tablets, available in 8 ct. and 24 ct. packages
Store at room temperature

DRAMAMINE® Less Drowsy Formula Tablets
Antiemetic

Description: DRAMAMINE Less Drowsy Formula contains meclizine hydrochloride.
Active Ingredient: Meclizine hydrochloride 25 mg per tablet

Indications: for prevention and treatment of the symptoms associated with motion sickness including nausea, vomiting, and dizziness

Directions: To prevent motion sickness, the first dose should be taken 1 hour before starting activity. To prevent or treat motion sickness, use the following dosing.
Adults and children 12 years and over: 1 to 2 tablets once daily, or as directed by a doctor

Warnings:
Do not use in children under 12 years of age unless directed by a doctor.
Ask a doctor before use if you have:
- a breathing problem such as emphysema or chronic bronchitis • glaucoma • difficulty in urination due to enlargement of the prostate gland
Ask a doctor or pharmacist before use if you are taking sedatives or tranquilizers

Continued on next page

Dramamine Less Drowsy—Cont.

When using these products:
• drowsiness may occur • avoid alcoholic drinks • alcohol, sedatives, and tranquilizers may increase drowsiness • be careful when driving a motor vehicle or operating machinery
If pregnant or breast-feeding, ask a health professional before use.
Keep out of reach of children.
In case of overdose, get medical help or contact a Poison Control Center right away.

Inactive Ingredients: Colloidal silicon dioxide, corn starch, D&C yellow no. 10 (aluminum lake), lactose, magnesium stearate, microcrystalline cellulose

How Supplied: Yellow tablets in 8 ct. vials
Store at controlled room temperature 20°–25°C (68°–77°F)

EMETROL®
(Phosphorated Carbohydrate Solution)
For the relief of nausea associated with upset stomach

Description: EMETROL is an oral solution containing balanced amounts of dextrose (glucose) and levulose (fructose) and phosphoric acid with controlled hydrogen ion concentration. Available in original lemon-mint or cherry flavor. EMETROL quickly relieves nausea by local action on the wall of the hyperactive G.I. tract.

Active Ingredients: Each 5 mL teaspoonful contains dextrose (glucose), 1.87 g; levulose (fructose), 1.87 g; and phosphoric acid, 21.5 mg.

Indications: For the relief of nausea due to upset stomach from intestinal flu and food or drink indiscretions. For other conditions, take only as directed by your physician.

Directions:

Usual Adult Dose: One or two tablespoonfuls (1 tbsp equals 3 tsps). Repeat every 15 minutes until distress subsides.

Usual Children's Dose (2 to 12 years): One or two teaspoonfuls. Repeat dose every 15 minutes until distress subsides.

Important: For maximum effectiveness never dilute EMETROL or drink fluids of any kind immediately before or after taking a dose.

Caution: Not to be taken for more than one hour (5 doses) without consulting a physician. If nausea continues or recurs frequently, consult a physician promptly as it may be a sign of a serious condition.

Warnings: This product contains fructose and should not be taken by persons with hereditary fructose intolerance (HFI).

As with any drug, if you are pregnant or nursing a baby, seek the advice of a health professional before using this product.
This product contains sugar and should not be taken by diabetics except under the advice and supervision of a physician.
Keep this and all medications out of the reach of children.
In case of accidental overdose, contact a Poison Control Center or physician immediately.

Inactive Ingredients: glycerin, methylparaben, purified water; D&C Yellow No. 10 and natural lemon-mint flavor in lemon-mint Emetrol; FD&C Red No. 40 and artificial cherry flavor in cherry Emetrol.

How Supplied: Yellow, Lemon-Mint: Bottles of 4 & 8 fluid ounces.
Red, Cherry: Bottles of 4 & 8 fluid ounces.

KAOPECTATE® Anti-Diarrheal, CHILDREN'S KAOPECTATE® Anti-Diarrheal

Description: KAOPECTATE®, is a pleasant testing oral suspension for use in the control of diarrhea. Each 15 mL of **KAOPECTATE® Anti-Diarrheal** contains bismuth subsalicylate 262 mg, contributing 130 mg total salicylates. **KAOPECTATE® Anti-Diarrheal** is low sodium, with each 15 mL tablespoonful containing 10 mg sodium. Each 5 mL of **CHILDREN'S KAOPECTATE® Anti-Diarrheal** contains bismuth subsalicylate 87 mg, contributing 43.4 mg total salicylates. **CHILDREN'S KAOPECTATE® Anti-Diarrheal** is low sodium, with each 5 mL tablespoonful containing 3.3 mg sodium

Active Ingredient: Bismuth subsalicylate.

Indication: Anti-diarrheal. Controls diarrhea within 24 hours.

Warnings: Reye's syndrome: children and teenagers who have or are recovering from chicken pox, flu symptoms, or flu should NOT use this product. If nausea, vomiting, or fever occur, consult a doctor because these symptoms could be an early sign of Reye's syndrome, a rare but serious illness.
This product contains salicylate. If taken with aspirin and ringing in the ears occurs, stop using.
Do not use • if you are allergic to salicylates (including aspirin) unless directed by a doctor • for more than 2 days in the presence of fever, or in children under 3 years of age unless directed by a doctor
Ask a doctor before use if you are
• taking a prescription drug for anticoagulation (thinning of the blood), diabetes, gout or arthritis unless directed by a doctor

If pregnant or breast-feeding, ask a health professional before use. **Keep out of reach of children.** In case of overdose, get medical help or contact a Poison Control Center right away.

Directions: KAOPECTATE® Anti-Diarrheal, CHILDREN'S KAOPECTATE® Anti-Diarrheal • shake well before each use • for accurate dosing, use convenient pre-measured dose cup • repeat dose every 1/2 hour to 1 hour as needed, to a maximum of 8 doses in a 24-hour period • drink plenty of clear fluids to help prevent dehydration which may accompany diarrhea • this medication may cause a temporary and harmless darkening of the tongue or stool

Dosing Chart—Regular Strength, Children's KAOPECTATE®

Age	Dose
adults and children 12 years and over	30 mL or 2 tablespoonfuls
9 to 11 years	15 mL or 1 tablespoonful
6 to 8 years	10 mL or 2 teaspoonfuls
3 to 5 years	5 mL or 1 teaspoonful
under 3 years	ask a doctor

Inactive Ingredients:
KAOPECTATE® Anti-Diarrheal — Peppermint: caramel, carboxymethylcellulose sodium, FD&C red no. 40, flavor, microcrystalline cellulose, purified water, sodium salicylate, sorbic acid, sucrose, titanium dioxide, xanthan gum
KAOPECTATE® Anti-Diarrheal Regular Flavor (vanilla): caramel, carboxymethylcellulose sodium, flavor, microcrystalline cellulose, purified water, sodium salicylate, sorbic acid, sucrose, titanium dioxide, xanthan gum
CHILDREN'S KAOPECTATE® Anti-Diarrheal (cherry): caramel, carboxymethylcellulose sodium, FD&C red no. 40, flavor, microcrystalline cellulose, purified water, sodium salicylate, sorbic acid, sucrose, titanium dioxide, xanthan gum
How Supplied: KAOPECTATE® Anti-Diarrheal 262 mg Peppermint and **262 mg Regular Flavor (vanilla):** available in 8 and 12 oz bottles; **CHILDREN'S KAOPECTATE® Anti-Diarrheal (cherry):** available in 6 oz bottles. Store at room temperature 20° to 25C (68° to 77°F). Avoid excessive heat.
Do not use if inner seal is broken or missing.

EXTRA STRENGTH KAOPECTATE® Anti-Diarrheal

Description: EXTRA STRENGTH KAOPECTATE® is a pleasant testing oral suspension for use in the control of diarrhea. Each 15 mL of **EXTRA**

STRENGTH KAOPECTATE® Anti-Diarrheal contains bismuth subsalicylate 525 mg, contributing 236 mg total salicylates. **EXTRA STRENGTH KAOPECTATE®** is low sodium. Each 15 mL tablespoonful contains **sodium 11 mg.**:

Active Ingredient: Bismuth subsalicylate.

Indication: Anti-diarrheal. Controls diarrhea within 24 hours.

Warnings: Reye's syndrome: children and teenagers who have or are recovering from chicken pox, flu symptoms, or flu should NOT use this product. If nausea, vomiting, or fever occur, consult a doctor because these symptoms could be an early sign of Reye's syndrome, a rare but serious illness.
This product contains salicylate. If taken with aspirin and ringing in the ears occurs, stop using.
Do not use • if you are allergic to salicylates (including aspirin) unless directed by a doctor • for more than 2 days in the presence of fever, or in children under 3 years of age unless directed by a doctor
Ask a doctor before use if you are • taking a prescription drug for anticoagulation (thinning of the blood), diabetes, gout or arthritis unless directed by a doctor
If pregnant or breast-feeding, ask a health professional before use. **Keep out of reach of children.** In case of overdose, get medical help or contact a Poison Control Center right away.

Directions: EXTRA STRENGTH KAOPECTATE® Anti-Diarrheal
• **shake well** immediately before each use • for accurate dosing, use convenient pre-measured dose cup • repeat dose every hour as needed, to a maximum of 4 doses in a 24-hour period • drink plenty of clear fluids to help prevent dehydration which may accompany diarrhea • this medication may cause a temporary and harmless darkening of the tongue or stool

Dosing Chart—Extra Strength KAOPECTATE®

Age	Dose
adults and children 12 years and over	30 mL or 2 tablespoonfuls
9 to 11 years	15 mL or 1 tablespoonful
6 to 8 years	10 mL or 2 teaspoonfuls
3 to 5 years	5 mL or 1 teaspoonful
under 3 years	ask a doctor

Inactive Ingredients: caramel, carboxymethylcellulose sodium, FD&C red no. 40, flavor, microcrystalline cellulose, purified water, sodium salicylate, sorbic acid, sucrose, titanium dioxide, xanthan gum, salicylate, sorbic acid, sucrose, titanium dioxide, xanthan gum

How Supplied: EXTRA STRENGTH KAOPECTATE® Anti-Diarrheal **525 mg - Peppermint:** available in 8 oz bottles. Store at room temperature 20° to 25C (68° to 77°F). Avoid excessive heat. **Do not use if inner seal is broken or missing.**

NASALCROM® Nasal Spray
Nasal Allergy Symptom Controller

Description: NASALCROM Nasal Spray contains a liquid formulation of cromolyn sodium that stabilizes mast cells that release histamine. NASALCROM is neither an antihistamine nor a decongestant nor a corticosteroid. In addition to treating nasal allergy symptoms, it decreases the allergic reaction by reducing the release of histamine, the trigger of allergy symptoms, from mast cells. NASALCROM has no known drug interactions and is safe to use with medications including other allergy medications.

Active Ingredient: (per spray) Cromolyn sodium 5.2mg

Indications: To prevent and relieve nasal symptoms of hay fever and other nasal allergies:
• runny/itchy nose • sneezing • allergic stuffy nose

Directions:
• parent or care provider must supervise the use of this product by young children. Adults and children 2 years and older:
• spray once into each nostril. Repeat 3–4 times a day (every 4–6 hours). If needed, may be used up to 6 times a day.
• use every day while in contact with the cause of your allergies (pollen, molds, pets, and dust)
• to **prevent** nasal allergy symptoms, use before contact with the cause of your allergies. For best results, start using up to one week before contact.
• if desired, you can use this product with other medications, including other allergy medications.
• children under 2 years: Do not use unless directed by a doctor

Warnings:
Do not use • if you are allergic to any of the ingredients
Ask a doctor before use if you have • fever • discolored nasal discharge • sinus pain • wheezing
When using this product • it may take several days of use to notice an effect. Your best effect may not be seen for 1 to 2 weeks • brief stinging or sneezing may occur right after use • do not use to treat sinus infection, asthma, or cold symptoms • do not share this bottle with anyone else as this may spread germs

Stop use and ask a doctor if
• shortness of breath, wheezing, or chest tightness occurs • hives or swelling of the mouth or throat occurs • your symptoms worsen • you have new symptoms • your symptoms do not begin to improve within two weeks
• you need to use more than 12 weeks
If pregnant or breast feeding ask a health professional before use.
Keep out of reach of children. If swallowed, get medical help or contact a Poison Control Center right away.

Inactive Ingredients: benzalkonium chloride, edetate disodium, purified water

How Supplied: NASALCROM Nasal Spray is available in 13mL (100 metered sprays) and 26mL (200 metered sprays) sizes
Store between 20°–25°C (68°–77°F). Keep away from light.

PEDIACARE® Multisymptom Cold Liquid
PEDIACARE® Multisymptom Cold Chewable
PEDIACARE® NightRest Cough-Cold Liquid
PEDIACARE® Cold & Allergy Liquid
PEDIACARE® Long-Acting Cough Plus Cold Liquid
PEDIACARE® Long-Acting Cough Plus Cold Chewable
PEDIACARE® Infants' Drops Decongestant
PEDIACARE® Infants' Drops Decongestant Plus Cough

Description: PEDIACARE products are available in eight different formulas, allowing you to select the ideal product to temporarily relieve your patient's symptoms. **PEDIACARE® Multisymptom Cold Liquid** and **PEDIACARE® Multisymptom Cold Chewable** contain an antihistamine, chlorpheniramine maleate, a nasal decongestant, pseudoephedrine HCl, and a cough suppressant, dextromethorphan hydrobromide, to provide temporary relief of nasal congestion, runny nose, sneezing and coughing due to the common cold, hay fever or other upper respiratory allergies. **PEDIACARE® NightRest Cough-Cold Liquid** contains a decongestant, pseudoephedrine hydrochloride, an antihistamine, chlorpheniramine maleate, and a cough suppressant, dextromethorphan hydrobromide, to provide temporary relief of coughs, nasal congestion, runny nose and sneezing due to the common cold, hayfever or other upper respiratory allergies. **PEDIACARE® Cold & Allergy Liquid** contains a decongestant, pseudoephedrine hydrochloride, and an antihistamine, chlorpheniramine maleate, to provide temporary relief of nasal congestion, runny nose and sneezing due to the common cold, hayfever or other

Continued on next page

Pediacare—Cont.

respiratory allergies. **PEDIACARE® Long-Acting Cough Plus Cold Liquid** and **PEDIACARE® Long-Acting Cough Plus Cold Chewable** contain a decongestant, pseudoephedrine hydrochloride, and a cough suppressant, dextromethorphan hydrobromide, to provide temporary relief of nasal congestion and coughing due to the common cold, hayfever or other respiratory allergies. **PEDIACARE® Infants' Drops Decongestant** contains a decongestant, pseudoephedrine hydrochloride, to provide temporary relief of nasal congestion due to the common cold, hay fever or other upper respiratory allergies. **PEDIACARE® Infants' Drops Decongestant Plus Cough** contains a decongestant, pseudoephedrine hydrochloride, and a cough suppressant, dextromethorphan hydrobromide, to provide temporary relief of nasal congestion and coughing due to common cold, hay fever or other upper respiratory allergies.

Active Ingredients: Each 5 mL of **PEDIACARE® Multisymptom Cold Liquid** contains pseudoephedrine hydrochloride 15 mg, chlorpheniramine maleate 1 mg and dextromethorphan hydrobromide 5 mg. Each chewable tablet of **PEDIACARE® Multisymptom Cold Chewable** contains pseudoephedrine hydrochloride 15mg, chlorpheniramine maleate 1mg and dextromethorphan hydrobromide 5 mg. Each 0.8 mL oral dropper of **PEDIACARE® Infants' Drops Decongestant** contains pseudoephedrine hydrochloride 7.5 mg. Each 0.8 mL of **PEDIACARE® Infants' Drops Decongestant Plus Cough** contains pseudoephedrine hydrochloride 7.5 mg and dextromethorphan hydrobromide 2.5 mg. Each 5 mL of **PEDIACARE® NightRest Cough-Cold Liquid** contains pseudoephedrine hydrochloride 15 mg, chlorpheniramine maleate 1 mg and dextromethorphan hydrobromide 7.5 mg. Each 5mL of **PEDIACARE® Cold & Allergy Liquid** contains pseudoephedrine hydrochloride 15mg and chlorpheniramine maleate 1mg. Each 5mL of **PEDIACARE® Long-Acting Cough Plus Cold Liquid** contains pseudoephedrine hydrochloride 15mg and dextromethorphan hydrobromide 7.5mg. Each chewable tablet of **PEDIACARE® Long-Acting Cough Plus Cold Chewable** contains pseudoephedrine hydrochloride 15mg and dextromethorphan hydrobromide 7.5mg. **PEDIACARE® Multisymptom Cold Liquid** and **NightRest Cough-Cold Liquid** are cherry flavored, alcohol free and red in color. **PEDIACARE® Cold & Allergy Liquid** is bubblegum flavored, alcohol free and pink in color. **PEDIACARE® Long-Acting Cough Plus Cold Liquid** is grape flavored, alcohol free and purple in color. **PEDIACARE® Multisymptom Cold Chewable tablets** are cherry flavored, pink in color with PC3 imprinting.

PEDIACARE® Long-Acting Cough Plus Cold Chewable tablets are grape flavored, purple in color with PC2 imprinting. **PEDIACARE® Infants' Drops Decongestant** is fruit flavored, alcohol free and red in color. **PEDIACARE® Infants' Drops Decongestant Plus Cough** is cherry flavored, alcohol free and clear, non-staining in color.

Professional Dosage: A calibrated dosage cup is provided for accurate dosing of the **PEDIACARE** Liquid formulas. A calibrated oral dropper is provided for accurate dosing of **PEDIACARE® Infants' Drops.** All doses of **PEDIACARE® Multisymptom Cold, Cold & Allergy Liquid,** as well as **PEDIACARE® Infants' Drops** may be repeated every 4–6 hours, not to exceed 4 doses in 24 hours. **PEDIACARE® Night-Rest Liquid** and **Long-Acting Cough Plus Cold Liquid** may be repeated every 6–8 hrs, not to exceed 4 doses in 24 hours.

[See table at top of next page]

Warnings: Keep this and all medication out of the reach of children. In case of accidental overdosage, contact a physician or poison control center immediately.

The following information appears on the appropriate package labels:

PEDIACARE® Multisymptom Cold Liquid, Night Rest Cough-Cold Liquid, Cold & Allergy Liquid and **PEDIACARE® Multisymptom Cold Chewable:** Do not exceed recommended dosage. If nervousness, dizziness or sleeplessness occur, discontinue use and consult a doctor. If symptoms do not improve within 7 days or are accompanied by fever, consult a doctor. A persistent cough may be a sign of a serious condition. If cough persists for more than one week, tends to recur or is accompanied by fever, rash, or persistent headache, consult a doctor. Do not give this product for persistent or chronic cough such as occurs with asthma or if cough is accompanied by excessive phlegm (mucus) unless directed by a doctor. May cause excitability especially in children. May cause drowsiness. Sedatives and tranquilizers may increase the drowsiness effect. Do not give this product to children who are taking sedatives or tranquilizers without first consulting the child's doctor. Do not give this product to children who have a breathing problem such as chronic bronchitis, or who have glaucoma, heart disease, high blood pressure, thyroid disease or diabetes, without first consulting the child's doctor.

PEDIACARE® Long-Acting Cough Plus Cold Liquid and **PEDIACARE® Long-Acting Cough Plus Cold Chewable:** Do not exceed recommended dosage. If nervousness, dizziness, or sleeplessness occur, discontinue use and consult a doctor. If symptoms do not improve within 7 days or are accompanied by fever, consult a doctor. A persistent cough may be a sign of a serious condition. If cough persists for more than one week, tends to

recur or is accompanied by fever, rash, or persistent headache, consult a doctor. Do not give this product for persistent or chronic cough such as occurs with asthma or if cough is accompanied by excessive phlegm (mucus) unless directed by a doctor. Do not give this product to a child who has heart disease, high blood pressure, thyroid disease or diabetes unless directed by a doctor. Take by mouth only.

PEDIACARE® Infants' Drops Decongestant: Do not exceed the recommended dosage. If nervousness, dizziness or sleeplessness occur, discontinue use and consult a doctor. If symptoms do not improve within 7 days or are accompanied by fever, consult a physician. Do not give this product to a child who has heart disease, high blood pressure, thyroid disease or diabetes unless directed by a doctor. Take by mouth only. Not for nasal use.

PEDIACARE® Infants' Drops Decongestant Plus Cough: Do not exceed recommended dosage. If nervousness, dizziness, or sleeplessness occur, discontinue use and consult a doctor. If symptoms do not improve within 7 days or are accompanied by fever, consult a doctor. A persistent cough may be a sign of a serious condition. If cough persists for more than one week, tends to recur or is accompanied by fever, rash, or persistent headache, consult a doctor. Do not give this product for persistent or chronic cough such as occurs with asthma or if cough is accompanied by excessive phlegm (mucus) unless directed by a doctor. Do not give this product to a child who has heart disease, high blood pressure, thyroid disease or diabetes unless directed by a doctor. Take by mouth only. Not for nasal use.

Drug Interaction Precaution: Do not give this product to a child who is taking a prescription monoamine oxidase inhibitor (MAOI) (certain drugs for depression, psychiatric or emotional conditions), or for 2 weeks after stopping the MAOI drug. If you are uncertain whether your child's prescription drug contains an MAOI, consult a health professional before giving this product.

Overdosage: Acute dextromethorphan overdose usually does not result in serious signs and symptoms unless massive amounts have been ingested. Signs and symptoms of a substantial overdose may include nausea and vomiting, visual disturbances, CNS disturbances, and urinary retention. Symptoms from pseudoephedrine overdose consist most often of mild anxiety, tachycardia and/or mild hypertension. Symptoms usually appear within 4 to 8 hours of ingestion and are transient, usually requiring no treatment. Chlorpheniramine toxicity should be treated as you would an antihistamine/anticholinergic overdose and is likely to be present within a few hours after acute ingestion.

Inactive Ingredients: PEDIACARE® Multisymptom Cold Liquid: citric

Age Group	0–3 mos	4–11 mos	12–23 mos	2–3 yrs	4–5 yrs	6–8 yrs	9–10 yrs	11 yrs	Dosage
Weight (lbs)	6–11 lbs	12–17 lbs	18–23 lbs	24–35 lbs	36–47 lbs	48–59 lbs	60–71 lbs	72–95 lbs	
PEDIACARE® Infants' Drops Decongestant*	$1/_2$ dropper (0.4 mL)	1 dropper (0.8 mL)	$1^1/_2$ droppers (1.2 mL)	2 droppers (1.6 mL)					q4–6h
PEDIACARE® Infants' Drops Decongestant Plus Cough*	$1/_2$ dropper (0.4 mL)	1 dropper (0.8 mL)	$1^1/_2$ droppers (1.2 mL)	2 droppers (1.6 mL)					q4–6h
PEDIACARE® Long-Acting Cough Plus Cold Liquid*			$1/_2$ tsp	1 tsp	$1^1/_2$ tsp	2 tsp	$2^1/_2$ tsp	3 tsp	q6–8h
PEDIACARE® Multisymptom Cold Liquid**				1 tsp	$1^1/_2$ tsp	2 tsp	$2^1/_2$ tsp	3 tsp	q4–6h
PEDIACARE® NightRest Liquid**				1 tsp	$1^1/_2$ tsp	2 tsp	$2^1/_2$ tsp	3 tsp	q6–8h
PEDIACARE® Cold & Allergy Liquid**				1 tsp	$1^1/_2$tsp	2 tsp	$2^1/_2$ tsp	3 tsp	q4–6h
PEDIACARE® Long-Acting Cough Plus Cold Chewable*				1 tablet	1 tablet	2 tablets	2 tablets	3 tablets	q6–8h
PEDIACARE® Multisymptom Cold Chewable**				1 tablet	1 tablet	2 tablets	2 tablets	3 tablets	q4–6h

*Administer to children under 2 years only on the advice of a physician.
**Administer to children under 6 years only on the advice of a physician.

acid, corn syrup, FD&C red no. 40, flavors, glycerin, propylene glycol, purified water, sodium benzoate, sodium carboxymethylcellulose, sorbitol.
PEDIACARE® Multisymptom Cold Chewable: aspartame, carnauba wax, citric acid, colloidal silicon dioxide, crospovidone, D&C red no. 27 aluminum lake, ethylcellulose, flavors, hydroxypropyl methylcellulose, magnesium stearate, mannitol, microcrystalline cellulose, mono & diglycerides, povidone, silcon dioxide, sucrose
PEDIACARE® NightRest Cough-Cold: citric acid, corn syrup, FD&C red no. 40, flavors, glycerin, propylene glycol, purified water, sodium benzoate, sodium carboxymethylcellulose, sorbitol.
PEDIACARE® Cold & Allergy Liquid: citric acid, corn syrup, FD&C red no. 40, flavors, glycerin, propylene glycol, purified water, sodium benzoate, sodium carboxymethylcellulose, sorbitol.
PEDIACARE® Long-Acting Cough Plus Cold Liquid: citric acid, corn syrup, FD&C blue no. 1, FD&C red no. 40, flavors, glycerin, propylene glycol, purified water, sodium benzoate, sodium carboxymethylcellulose, sorbitol.
PEDIACARE® Long-Acting Cough Plus Cold Chewable: aspartame, citric acid, colloidal silicon dioxide, crospovidone, D&C red no. 27 aluminum lake, ethylcellulose, FD&C blue no. 1 aluminum lake, flavor, magnesium stearate, mannitol, microcrystalline cellulose, povidone, sucrose
PEDIACARE® Infants' Drops Decongestant: benzoic acid, citric acid, FD&C red no. 40, flavors, glycerin, polyethylene glycol, purified water, sodium benzoate, sorbitol, sucrose.
PEDIACARE® Infants' Drops Decongestant Plus Cough: citric acid, flavors, glycerin, purified water, sodium benzoate, sorbitol.
How Supplied: PEDIACARE® **Multisymptom Cold Liquid,** Night-Rest Cough-Cold Liquid, **Cold & Allergy** (color pink), and **Long-Acting Cough Plus Cold** (color purple)-bottles of 4 fl. oz. (120 mL) with child-resistant safety cap and calibrated dosage cup. **Multisymptom Cold Chewable Tablets** (color pink, imprinted PC3), and **Long-Acting Cough Plus Cold Chewable Tablets** (color purple, imprinted PC2)-individually sealed blister packaging in boxes of 18. **PEDIACARE® Infants' Drops Decongestant** (color red) and **PEDIACARE® Infants' Drops Decongestant Plus Cough** (clear)—bottles of $1/_2$ fl. oz. (15 mL) with calibrated dropper.

Store bottled product in original outer carton until depleted.

MEN'S ROGAINE® EXTRA STRENGTH
(5% Minoxidil Topical Solution)
Hair Regrowth Treatment

Description: Men's ROGAINE Extra Strength is a colorless solution for use only on the scalp to help regrow hair in men.

Active Ingredient: Minoxidil 5% w/v

Indication: Hair regrowth treatment for men

Directions: Apply 1 mL (twice a day, every day, directly onto the scalp) in the hair loss area. Using more or using more often will not improve results.

Warnings:
For external use only
Flammable: Keep away from fire or flame
Do not use if:
• you are a woman
• you have no family history of hair loss
• your hair loss is sudden and/or patchy
• you do not know the reason for your hair loss

Continued on next page

Rogaine Extra Strength—Cont.

- you are under 18 years of age. Do not use on babies and children.
- scalp irritation or redness occurs
- you are using other medicines on the scalp

Ask a doctor before use if you have heart disease

When using this product:

- do not apply on other parts of the body
- avoid contact with the eyes. In case of accidental contact, rinse eyes with large amounts of cool tap water.
- some people have experienced changes in hair color and/or texture
- it takes time to regrow hair. Results may occur at 2 months with twice a day usage. For some men, you may need to use this product for at least 4 months before you see results.
- the amount of hair regrowth is different for each person. This product will not work for all men.

Stop use and ask a doctor if:

- chest pain, rapid heartbeat, faintness, or dizziness occurs
- sudden, unexplained weight gain occurs
- your hands or feet swell
- scalp irritation occurs, and continues or worsens
- unwanted facial hair growth occurs
- you do not see hair regrowth in 4 months

May be harmful if used when pregnant or breast-feeding.

Keep out of reach of children. If swallowed, get medical help or contact a Poison Control Center right away.

Inactive Ingredients: Alcohol (30% v/v), propylene glycol (50% v/v), and purified water.

How Supplied: Men's ROGAINE Extra Strength is available in packs of one, three, or four 60 mL bottles. (One 60 mL bottle is a one-month supply.) Store at controlled room temperature 20° to 25°C (68° to 77°F)

Women's ROGAINE®
(2% Minoxidil Topical Solution)
Hair Regrowth Treatment

Description: ROGAINE is a colorless liquid medication for use on the scalp to help regrow hair.

Active Ingredient: Minoxidil 2% w/v

Indication: Hair regrowth treatment.

Directions: Apply one mL (twice a day, every day, directly onto the scalp) in the hair loss area. Using more or using more often will not improve results.

Warnings:
For external use only
Flammable: Keep away from fire or flame
Do not use if

- you have no family history of hair loss
- your hair loss is sudden and/or patchy
- hair loss is associated with childbirth
- you do not know the reason for your hair loss
- you are under 18 years of age. Do not use on babies and children.

- scalp irritation or redness occurs
- you use other medicines on the scalp

Ask a doctor before use if you have heart disease

When using this product

- do not apply on other parts of the body
- avoid contact with the eyes. In case of accidental contact, rinse eyes with large amounts of cool tap water.
- some people have experienced changes in hair color and/or texture
- it takes time to regrow hair. You may need to use this product 2 times a day for at least 4 months before you see results.
- the amount of hair regrowth is different for each person. This product will not work for everyone

Stop use and ask a doctor if

- chest pain, rapid heartbeat, faintness, or dizziness occurs
- sudden, unexplained weight gain occurs
- your hands or feet swell
- redness or irritation occurs
- unwanted facial hair growth occurs
- you do not see hair regrowth in 4 months

If pregnant or breast-feeding ask a health professional before use.

Keep out of reach of children. If swallowed, get medical help or contact a Poison Control Center right away.

Side Effects:

The most common side effects are itching and other skin irritations of the treated area of the scalp. If scalp irritation continues, stop use and see a doctor.

Although unwanted facial hair growth has been reported on the face and on other parts of the body, such reports have been infrequent. The unwanted hair growth may be caused by the transfer of ROGAINE to areas other than the scalp, or by absorption into the circulatory system of low levels of the active ingredient, or by a medical condition not related to the use of ROGAINE. If you experience unwanted hair growth, discontinue using ROGAINE and see your doctor for recommendations about appropriate treatment. After stopping use of ROGAINE, the unwanted hair, if caused by the use of ROGAINE, should go away over time.

Inactive Ingredients: Alcohol (60% v/v), propylene glycol (20% v/v), and purified water.

How Supplied: Women's ROGAINE is available in packs of one, three, or four 60 mL bottles. (One 60 mL bottle is a one-month supply.) Store at Controlled Room Temperature 20° to 25°C (68° to 77°F).

**IF YOU SUSPECT
AN INTERACTION...**
The 1,800-page
PDR Companion Guide™ can help.
Use the order form
in the front of this book.

The Procter & Gamble Company
P. O. BOX 599
CINCINNATI, OH 45201

Direct Inquiries to:
Consumer Relations
(800) 832–3064
For Medical Emergencies:
Call Collect: (513) 636-5107

HEAD & SHOULDERS CLASSIC CLEAN DANDRUFF SHAMPOO

Head & Shoulders Classic Clean Dandruff Shampoo for normal/oily hair offers effective control of persistent dandruff and beautiful hair from a pleasant-to-use formula. Double-blind, expert-graded testing have proven that it reduces dandruff very effectively. It is also gentle enough to use every day for clean, manageable hair.

The formula ingredients below are for Classic Clean version. Head & Shoulders is also available in a Classic Clean 2-in-1 version for increased manageability and hair damage prevention. The key formula difference is increased dimethicone conditioner and substitution of Polyquaternium-10 polymer instead of Guar Hydroxypropyltrimonium Chloride.

Drug Facts

Active Ingredient: **Purpose:**
Pyrithione zinc 1%   Anti-dandruff

Uses: helps prevent recurrence of flaking and itching associated with dandruff

Warnings:
For external use only
When using this product

- avoid contact with eyes. If contact occurs, rinse eyes thoroughly with water.

Stop use and ask a doctor if

- condition worsens or does not improve after regular use of this product as directed.

Keep this and all drugs out of reach of children. If swallowed, get medical help or contact a Poison Control Center right away.

Directions:

- for maximum dandruff control, use every time you shampoo.
- wet hair.
- massage onto scalp
- rinse.
- repeat if desired.
- for best results use <u>at least</u> twice a week or as directed by a doctor.

Inactive Ingredients: Water, Ammonium laureth sulfate, Ammonium lauryl sulfate, Glycol distearate, Dimethicone, Cetyl alcohol, Cocamide MEA, Fragrance, Sodium chloride, Guar hydroxypropyltrimonium chloride, Hydrogenated polydecene, Sodium citrate, Sodium benzoate, Trimethylolpropane tricaprylate/tricaprate, Citric acid, Benzyl alcohol, Methylchloroisothiazolinone,

Methylisothiazolinone, Ext. D&C violet no. 2, FD&C blue no. 1, Ammonium xylenesulfonate

How Supplied: Head & Shoulders Classic Clean Dandruff Shampoo is available in 2.0 FL, 6.8 FL OZ, 13.5 FL OZ, 25.4 FL OZ, 33.9 FL OZ unbreakable plastic bottles.

Questions [or comments]? 1-800-723-9569

HEAD & SHOULDERS DRY SCALP CARE DANDRUFF SHAMPOO

Head & Shoulders Dry Scalp Care Dandruff Shampoo offers effective control of persistent dandruff and beautiful hair from a pleasant-to-use formula. Double-blind, expert-graded testing have proven that it reduces dandruff very effectively. It is also gentle enough to use every day for clean, manageable hair.

The formula ingredients below are for Dry Scalp version. Head & Shoulders is also available in a conditioning Smooth & Silky 2-in-1 version whose primary formula difference is a lower level of the moisturizing and protective conditioning ingredient Dimethicone and substitution of Polyquarternium-10 polymer for a portion of the Guar Hydroxypropyltrimonium Chloride.

Drug Facts

Active Ingredient: **Purpose:**
Pyrithione zinc 1% Anti-dandruff

Uses: Helps prevent recurrence of flaking and itching associated with dandruff

Warnings:
For external use only
When using this product
• avoid contact with eyes. If contact occurs, rinse eyes thoroughly with water.
Stop use and ask a doctor if
• condition worsens or does not improve after regular use of this product as directed.
Keep this and all drugs out of reach of children. If swallowed, get medical help or contact a Poison Control Center right away.

Directions:
• for maximum dandruff control, use every time you shampoo.
• wet hair.
• massage onto scalp.
• rinse.
• repeat if desired.
• for best results use at least twice a week or as directed by a doctor.

Inactive Ingredients: Water, Ammonium laureth sulfate, Ammonium lauryl sulfate, Dimethicone, Glycol distearate, Cetyl alcohol, Cocamide MEA, Fragrance, Sodium chloride, Polyquaternium-10, Hydrogenated polydecene, Sodium citrate, Sodium benzoate, Trimethylolpropane tricaprylate/tricaprate, Citric acid, Benzyl alcohol, Methylchloroisothiazolinone, Methylisothiazolinone, Ext. D&C violet no. 2, FD&C blue no. 1, Ammonium xylenesulfonate

How Supplied: Head & Shoulders Dry Scalp Care Dandruff Shampoo is available in 6.8 FL OZ, 13.5 FL OZ, 25.4 FL OZ, 33.9 FL OZ unbreakable plastic bottles.

Questions [or comments]? 1-800-723-9569

HEAD & SHOULDERS® INTENSIVE TREATMENT DANDRUFF AND SEBORRHEIC DERMATITIS SHAMPOO

Head & Shoulders Intensive Treatment Dandruff and Seborrheic Dermatitis Shampoo offers effective control of persistent dandruff and beautiful hair from a pleasant-to-use formula. Double-blind, expert-graded testing have proven that it reduces dandruff very effectively. It is also gentle enough to use every day for clean, manageable hair.

Drug Facts
Active Ingredient: **Purpose:**
Selenium Sulfide 1% Anti-dandruff
Anti-seborrheic dermatitis

Uses: Helps stop itching, flaking, scaling, irritation and redness associated with dandruff and seborrheic dermatitis.

Warnings:
For external use only
Ask a doctor before use if you have a condition that covers a large portion of the body.
When using this product
• avoid contact with eyes. If contact occurs, rinse eyes thoroughly with water.
Stop use and ask a doctor if
• condition worsens or does not improve after regular use of this product as directed.
Keep this and all drugs out of reach of children. If swallowed, get medical help or contact a Poison Control Center right away.

Directions:
• wet hair.
• massage onto scalp
• rinse thoroughly
• for best results use at least twice a week or as directed by a doctor.
• caution: if used on bleached, tinted, grey, or permed hair, rinse for 5 minutes
• for maximum dandruff control, use every time you shampoo

Inactive Ingredients: Water, Ammonium laureth sulfate, Ammonium lauryl sulfate, Glycol distearate, Cocamide MEA, Fragrance, Dimethicone, Tricetylmonium chloride, Ammonium xylenesulfonate, Cetyl alcohol, DMDM hydantoin, Sodium chloride, Stearyl alcohol, Hydroxypropyl methylcellulose, FD&C red no. 4

How Supplied: Head & Shoulders Intensive Treatment Dandruff and Seborrheic Dermatitis Shampoo is available in 13.5 FL OZ unbreakable plastic bottles.

Questions [or comments]? 1-800-723-9569

METAMUCIL® FIBER LAXATIVE
[met uh-mū sil]
(psyllium husk)
Also see **Metamucil Dietary Fiber Supplement** *in Dietary Supplement Section*

Description: Metamucil contains psyllium husk (from the plant *Plantago ovata*), a bulk forming, natural therapeutic fiber for restoring and maintaining regularity when recommended by a physician. Metamucil contains no chemical stimulants and does not disrupt normal bowel function. Each dose of Metamucil powder and Metamucil Fiber Wafers contains approximately 3.4 grams of psyllium husk (or 2.4 grams of soluble fiber). Inactive ingredients, sodium, calcium, potassium, calories, carbohydrate, dietary fiber, and phenylalanine content are shown in the following table for all versions and flavors. Metamucil Smooth Texture Sugar-Free Regular Flavor and Metamucil capsules contains no sugar and no artificial sweeteners; Metamucil Smooth Texture Sugar-Free Orange Flavor contains aspartame (phenylalanine content per dose is 25 mg). Metamucil powdered products and Metamucil capsules are gluten-free. Metamucil Fiber Wafers contain gluten: Apple Crisp contains 0.7g/dose, Cinnamon Spice contains 0.5g/dose. Each two-wafer dose contains 5 grams of fat.

Actions: The active ingredient in Metamucil is psyllium husk, a natural fiber which promotes elimination due to its bulking effect in the colon. This bulking effect is due to both the water-holding capacity of undigested fiber and the increased bacterial mass following partial fiber digestion. These actions result in enlargement of the lumen of the colon, and softer stool, thereby decreasing intraluminal pressure and straining, and speeding colonic transit in constipated patients.

Indications: Metamucil is indicated for the treatment of occasional constipation, and when recommended by a physician, for chronic constipation and constipation associated with irritable bowel syndrome, diverticulosis, hemorrhoids, convalescence, senility and pregnancy. Pregnancy: Category B. If considering use of Metamucil as part of a cholesterol-lowering program, see **Metamucil Dietary Fiber Supplement** in Dietary Supplement Section.

Drug Facts

Active Ingredient:
(in each DOSE) **Purpose:**
Psyllium husk
approximately 3.4 g ..... Fiber therapy
for regularity

For Metamucil capsules each dose of 5 capsules contains approximately 2.6 gm of psyllium husk.

Continued on next page

Metamucil—Cont.

Uses:
- effective in treating occasional constipation and restoring regularity

Warnings:

Choking: Taking this product without adequate fluid may cause it to swell and block your throat or esophagus and may cause choking. Do not take this product if you have difficulty in swallowing. If you experience chest pain, vomiting, or difficulty in swallowing or breathing after taking this product, seek immediate medical attention.

Ask a doctor before use if you have:
- a sudden change in bowel habits persisting for 2 weeks
- abdominal pain, nausea or vomiting

Adults 12 yrs. & older	Powders: 1 dose in 8 oz of liquid. Capsules: 5 capsules with 8 oz of liquid (swallow one capsule at a time). Wafers: 1 dose with 8 oz of liquid. Take at the first sign of irregularity; can be taken up to 3 times daily. Generally produces effect in 12 – 72 hours.
6 – 11 yrs.	Powders: ½ adult dose in 8 oz of liquid. Wafers: 1 wafer with 8 oz of liquid. Can be taken up to 3 times daily. Capsules: consider use of powder or wafer products
Under 6 yrs.	consult a doctor

When using this product:
- may cause allergic reaction in people sensitive to inhaled or ingested psyllium

Stop use and ask a doctor if:
- constipation lasts more than 7 days
- rectal bleeding occurs

These may be signs of a serious condition.

Keep out of reach of children. In case of overdose, get medical help or contact a Poison Control Center right away.

Directions: For Powders: Put one dose into an empty glass. Fill glass with at least 8 oz of water or your favorite beverage. Stir briskly and drink promptly. If mixture thickens, add more liquid and

Metamucil Fiber Laxative/Dietary Fiber Supplement

Versions/Flavors	Ingredients (alphabetical order)	Sodium mg/ dose	Calcium mg/ dose	Potassium mg/ dose	Calories kcal/ dose	Total Carbohydrate g/dose	Dietary Fiber/ (Soluble) g/dose	Dosage (Weight in gms)	How Supplied
Smooth Texture Orange Flavor Metamucil Powder	Citric Acid, FD&C Yellow #6, Natural and Artificial Flavor, Psyllium Husk, Sucrose	5	7	30	45	12	3 (2.4)	1 rounded tablespoon ~12g	Canisters: Doses: 48, 72, 114; Cartons: 30 single-dose packets.
Smooth Texture Sugar-Free Orange Flavor Metamucil Powder	Aspartame, Citric Acid, FD&C Yellow #6, Maltodextrin, Natural and Artificial Flavor, Psyllium Husk	5	7	30	20	5	3 (2.4)	1 rounded teaspoon ~5.8g	Canisters: Doses: 30, 48, 72 114, 180; Cartons: 30 single-dose packets.
Smooth Texture Sugar-Free Regular Flavor Metamucil Powder	Citric Acid, Maltodextrin, Psyllium Husk	4	7	30	20	5	3 (2.4)	1 rounded teaspoon ~5.4g	Canisters: Doses: 48, 72 114.
Original Texture Regular Flavor Metamucil Powder	Psyllium Husk, Sucrose	3	6	30	25	7	3 (2.4)	1 rounded teaspoon ~7g	Canisters: Doses: 48, 72 114.
Original Texture Orange Flavor Metamucil Powder	Citric Acid, FD&C Yellow #6, Natural and Artificial Flavor, Psyllium Husk, Sucrose	5	6	30	40	11	3 (2.4)	1 rounded tablespoon ~11g	Canisters: Doses: 48,72 114.
Metamucil Capsules	Caramel color, FD&C Blue No. 1 Aluminum Lake, FD&C Red No. 40 Aluminum Lake, FD&C Yellow No. 6 Aluminum Lake, gelatin, polysorbate 80, psyllium husk	0	5	0	10	3	3 (2.4)	6 capsules 3.2g	Bottles: 100 ct 160 ct

Fiber Laxative
Wafers

Apple Crisp (1) Metamucil Wafers		20	14	60	120	17	6	2 wafers 24 g	Cartons: 12 doses
Cinnamon Spice (2) Metamucil Wafers		20	14	60	120	17	6	2 wafers 24 g	Cartons: 12 doses

(1) ascorbic acid, brown sugar, cinnamon, corn oil, corn starch, fructose, lecithin, molasses, natural and artificial flavors, oat hull fiber, psyllium husk, sodium bicarbonate, sucrose, water, wheat flour
(2) ascorbic acid, cinnamon, corn oil, corn starch, fructose, lecithin, molasses, natural and artificial flavors, nutmeg, oat hull fiber, oats, psyllium husk, sodium bicarbonate, sucrose, water, wheat flour

stir. Mix this product (child or adult dose) with at least 8 ounces (a full glass) of water or other fluid. For capsules: Take product with 8 oz of liquid (swallow 1 capsule at a time) up to 3 times daily. Take this product with at least 8 oz (a full glass) of liquid. For Wafers: Take this product (child or adult dose) with at least 8 ounces (a full glass) of liquid. Taking these products without enough liquid may cause choking. See choking warning.
[See table at top of previous page]
Laxatives, including bulk fibers, may affect how well other medicines work. If you are taking a prescription medicine by mouth, take this product at least 2 hours before or 2 hours after the prescribed medicine. As your body adjusts to increased fiber intake, you may experience changes in bowel habits or minor bloating. **New Users:** Start with 1 dose per day; gradually increase to 3 doses per day as necessary.

Other Information:
- **Each product contains:** sodium (See table for amount/dose)
- **PHENYLKETONURICS: Smooth Texture Sugar Free Orange product contains phenylalanine** 25 mg per dose
- Each product contains a 100% natural, therapeutic fiber

Inactive Ingredients: See table
Notice to Health Care Professionals: To minimize the potential for allergic reaction, health care professionals who frequently dispense powdered psyllium products should avoid inhaling airborne dust while dispensing these products.
Handling and Dispensing: To minimize generating airborne dust, spoon product from the canister into a glass according to label directions.

How Supplied: Powder: canisters and cartons of single-dose packets. Capsules: 100 and 160 count bottles. Wafers: cartons of single dose packets. (See table) [See table at bottom of previous page]
Questions? 1-800-983-4237
Shown in Product Identification Guide, page 522

**PEPTO-BISMOL®
ORIGINAL LIQUID,
MAXIMUM STRENGTH LIQUID,
ORIGINAL AND CHERRY FLAVOR
CHEWABLE TABLETS
AND EASY-TO-SWALLOW CAPLETS
For upset stomach, indigestion, heartburn, nausea and diarrhea.**

Multi-symptom Pepto-Bismol® contains bismuth subsalicylate and is the only leading OTC stomach remedy clinically proven effective for both upper and lower GI symptoms. It has been clinically proven in double-blind placebo-controlled trials for relief of upset stomach symptoms and diarrhea.

**Active Ingredient: (per tablespoon/ per tablet/per caplet)
Original Liquid/Tablets/Caplets**
Bismuth subsalicylate 262 mg
Maximum Strength Liquid
Bismuth subsalicylate 525 mg

Inactive Ingredients:
[Original Liquid] benzoic acid, flavor, magnesium aluminum silicate, methylcellulose, red 22, red 28, saccharin sodium, salicylic acid, sodium salicylate, sorbic acid, water
[Maximum Strength Liquid] benzoic acid, flavor, magnesium aluminum silicate, methylcellulose, red 22, red 28, saccharin sodium, salicylic acid, sodium salicylate, sorbic acid, water
[Original Tablets] calcium carbonate, flavor, magnesium stearate, mannitol, povidone, red 27 aluminum lake, saccharin sodium, talc
[Cherry Tablets] adipic acid, calcium carbonate, flavor, magnesium stearate, mannitol, povidone, red 27 aluminum lake, red 40 aluminum lake, saccharin sodium, talc
[Caplets] calcium carbonate, magnesium stearate, mannitol, microcrystalline cellulose, polysorbate 80, povidone, red 27 aluminum lake, silicon dioxide, sodium starch glycolate.

Other Information:
Sodium Content
Original Liquid – each Tbsp contains: sodium 6 mg • low sodium
Maximum Strength Liquid - each Tbsp contains: sodium 6 mg • low sodium
Chewable Tablets – each Original or Cherry Flavor Tablet contains: sodium less than 1 mg • very low sodium
Caplets – each Caplet contains: sodium 2 mg • low sodium
Salicylate Content
Original Liquid – each Tbsp contains: salicylate 130 mg
Maximum Strength Liquid – each Tbsp contains: salicylate 236 mg
Chewable Tablets – each tablet contains: [original] salicylate 102 mg [cherry] salicylate 99 mg
Caplets – each caplet contains: salicylate 99 mg
All Forms are sugar free.

Indications:
- relieves upset stomach symptoms (i.e., indigestion, heartburn, nausea and fullness caused by over-indulgence in food and drink) without constipating; and,
- controls diarrhea (including Travelers' Diarrhea).

Actions: For upset stomach symptoms, the active ingredient is believed to work via a topical effect on the stomach mucosa. For diarrhea, it is believed to work by several mechanisms in the gastrointestinal tract, including: 1) normalizing fluid movement via an antisecretory mechanism, 2) binding bacterial toxins and 3) antimicrobial activity.

Warnings:
Do not use
- for children and teenagers who have or are recovering from chicken pox or flu. If nausea or vomiting occurs, ask a doctor because this could be an early sign of Reye Syndrome, a rare but serious illness.
- if you are allergic to salicylates including aspirin
Ask a doctor if you are taking medicines for
- anticoagulation (thinning the blood)
- diabetes • gout

Stop use and ask a doctor if
- taken with other salicylates such as aspirin and ringing in the ears occurs
- diarrhea occurs with a fever or lasts more than 2 days
- other symptoms last more than 2 weeks
If pregnant or breast feeding, ask a health professional before use.
Keep out of reach of children.
Notes: May cause a temporary and harmless darkening of the tongue or stool. Stool darkening should not be confused with melena.
While no lead is intentionally added to Pepto-Bismol, this product contains certain ingredients that are mined from the ground and thus contain small amounts of naturally occurring lead. For example, bismuth, contained in the active ingredient of Pepto-Bismol, is mined and therefore contains some naturally occurring lead. The small amounts of naturally occurring lead in Pepto-Bismol are low in comparison to average daily lead exposure; this is for the information of healthcare professionals. Pepto-Bismol is indicated for treatment of acute upset stomach symptoms and diarrhea. It is not intended for chronic use.

Overdosage: In case of overdose, patients are advised to contact a physician or Poison Control Center. Emesis induced by ipecac syrup is indicated in large ingestions provided ipecac can be administered within one hour of ingestion. Activated charcoal should be administered after gastric emptying. Patients should be evaluated for signs and symptoms of salicylate toxicity.

Directions:
Pepto-Bismol® Original Liquid, Original & Cherry Flavor Chewable Tablets, and Caplets
[Original Liquid]
- shake well before using
- for easy dosing, use dose cup
[Original Tablet, Cherry Tablets]
- chew or dissolve in mouth
[Caplets]
- swallow with water, do not chew

AGE	DOSAGE
adults & children 12 yrs & older	2 Tbsp. or 30 ml, 2 tablets or 2 caplets
children 9 to under 12 yrs	1 Tbsp or 15 ml, 1 tablet or 1 caplet
children 6 to under 9 yrs	2 tsp or 10 ml, 2/3 tablet or 2/3 caplet
children 3 to under 6 yrs	1 tsp or 5 ml, 1/3 tablet or 1/3 caplet
children under 3 yrs	ask a doctor

- repeat every ½ to 1 hour as needed
- not more than 8 doses in 24 hours

Continued on next page

Pepto-Bismol Original—Cont.

Pepto-Bismol® Maximum Strength Liquid
- shake well before using
- for easy dosing, use dose cup

AGE	DOSAGE
adults & children 12 yrs & older	2 Tbsp. or 30 ml
children 9 to under 12 yrs	1 Tbsp or 15 ml
children 6 to under 9 yrs	2 tsp or 10 ml
children 3 to under 6 yrs	1 tsp or 5 ml
children under 3 yrs	ask a doctor

- repeat every hour as needed
- not more than 4 doses in 24 hours

How Supplied: Pepto-Bismol® Original and Maximum Strength Liquids are pink. Pepto-Bismol® Original Liquid is available in: 4, 8, 12 and 16 fl oz bottles. Pepto-Bismol® Maximum Strength Liquid is available in: 4, 8 and 12 fl oz bottles. Pepto-Bismol® Original and Cherry Flavor Tablets are pink, round, chewable tablets imprinted with a debossed triangle and "Pepto-Bismol" on one side. Tablets are available in: boxes of 30 and 48. Pepto-Bismol® Caplets are pink and imprinted with "Pepto-Bismol" on one side. Caplets are available in bottles of 24 and 40.
- avoid excessive heat (over 104°F or 40°C)
- protect liquids from freezing

Questions: 1-800-717-3786
www.pepto-bismol.com
Shown in Product Identification Guide, page 522

THERMACARE®
[thərm' ă-kār]
Therapeutic Heat Wraps with Air-Activated Heat Discs

Uses:
Back/Hip Wrap: Provides temporary relief of minor muscular back aches and pains associated with overexertion, strains and sprains.
Neck to Arm Wrap: Provides temporary relief of minor muscular and joint aches and pains associated with overexertion, strains, sprains and arthritis.
Menstrual Patch: Provides temporary relief of minor menstrual cramp pain.

Warnings:
Skin warning This product has the potential to cause skin irritation or burns. Do not use ThermaCare in the same location for more than 8 hours in any 24 hour period.
Ingestion warning Each heat disc contains iron (~2 grams) which can be harmful if ingested. If ingested, rinse mouth with water and call a Poison Control Center right away. If heat disc contents come in contact with your skin or eyes, rinse right away with water.
Flammability warning To avoid the risk of fire, do not microwave or attempt to reheat this product.

Do not use:
- if the material covering the heat discs is damaged or torn
- with medicated lotions, creams or ointments
- on skin that is damaged or broken
- on areas of bruising or swelling that have occurred within 48 hours
- on people unable to remove the product on their own, including children and infants
- on areas of the body where heat cannot be felt
- if you are bedridden or prone to skin ulcers
- with other forms of therapeutic heat, including electric heating pads

Ask a doctor before use if you:
- are pregnant
- have diabetes
- have poor blood circulation
- have rheumatoid arthritis

When using this product:
- it is normal to experience slight skin redness after removing the wrap. If your skin is still red after a few hours, stop using ThermaCare until the redness goes away completely. To reduce the risk of prolonged redness in the future, we recommend you:
  (a) wear ThermaCare for a shorter period of time
  (b) wear looser clothing over ThermaCare
  (c) wear ThermaCare over a thin layer of clothing instead of directly against your skin
- periodically check your skin:
  (a) if you know your skin is sensitive to heat
  (b) if you feel your tolerance to heat has decreased over the years
  (c) when lying down or leaning against the product
  (d) when wearing a tight fitting belt or waistband over the product
- if you know your skin is sensitive to heat, consider wearing ThermaCare during the day to gain experience with the level of heat before deciding to use ThermaCare during sleep

Stop use and ask a doctor if:
- after 7 days of product use (4 days for menstrual product) the pain you are treating gets worse or remains unchanged. This could be a sign of a more serious condition
- you experience any discomfort, swelling, rash or other changes in your skin that persist where the wrap is worn

Keep out of reach of children and pets.

Directions: Tear open the pouch when ready to use. It may take up to 30 minutes for ThermaCare to reach its therapeutic temperature. For maximum effectiveness, we recommend you wear ThermaCare for the full 8 hours. Do not use for more than 8 hours in any 24 hour period OR for more than 7 days in a row (4 days in a row for menstrual product).

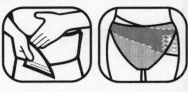

Place on pain area on lower back or hip with darker discs toward skin. Attach firmly.

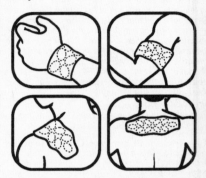

Peel away paper to reveal adhesive side. Place on pain area with adhesive side toward skin. Attach firmly.

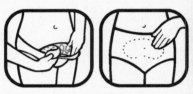

Peel away paper to reveal adhesive side. Place on pain area with adhesive side toward panties. Attach firmly.

How Supplied:
Back/Hip Wrap: Available in trial size of 1 L/XL or in boxes of 2 S/M or L/XL wraps.
Neck to Arm: Available in boxes of 3 wraps.
Menstrual: Available in boxes of 3 patches.
Shown in Product Identification Guide, page 522

VICKS® 44® COUGH
RELIEF
Dextromethorphan HBr/
Cough Suppressant
Alcohol 5%

- Maximum Strength
- Non-Drowsy
- For Adults & Children

Drug Facts:

Active Ingredient:
(per 15 ml tablespoon)   **Purpose:**
Dextromethorphan HBr
  30 mg .... Cough suppressant

Uses: Temporarily relieves cough due to minor throat and bronchial irritation associated with a cold

Warnings:

Do not use if you are now taking a prescription monoamine oxidase inhibitor (MAOI) (certain drugs for depression, psychiatric or emotional conditions, or Parkinson's disease), or for 2 weeks after stopping the MAOI drug. If you do not know if your prescription drug contains an MAOI, ask a doctor or pharmacist before taking this product.

Ask a doctor before use if you have:
- cough that occurs with too much phlegm (mucus)
- persistent or chronic cough such as occurs with smoking, asthma, or emphysema

Stop use and ask a doctor if:
- cough lasts more than 7 days, comes back, or occurs with fever, rash, or headache that lasts. These could be signs of a serious condition.

If pregnant or breast feeding, ask a health professional before use.

Keep out of reach of children. In case of overdose, get medical help or contact a Poison Control Center right away.

Directions:
- use teaspoon (tsp), tablespoon (TBSP) or dose cup
- do not exceed 4 doses per 24 hours

Under 6 yrs.	ask a doctor
6–11 yrs.	1½ tsp (7½ ml) every 6-8 hours
12 yrs. & older	1 TBSP (15 ml) every 6-8 hours

Other Information:
- **each tablespoon contains** sodium 31 mg
- store at room temperature

Inactive Ingredients: Alcohol, FD&C blue no.1, FD&C red 40, carboxymethylcellulose sodium, citric acid, flavor, high fructose corn syrup, polyethylene oxide, polyoxyl 40 stearate, propylene glycol, purified water, saccharin sodium, sodium benzoate, sodium citrate.

How Supplied: Available in 4 FL OZ (118 ml) 6 FL OZ (177 ml) plastic bottle. A calibrated dose cup accompanies each bottle.

TAMPER EVIDENT: Do not use if imprinted shrinkband is missing or broken.

Questions? 1-800-342-6844

Dist. by Procter & Gamble, Cincinnati, OH 45202.

US Pat 5,458,879   42434792

Shown in Product Identification Guide, page 522

VICKS® 44D®
COUGH & HEAD CONGESTION RELIEF
Cough Suppressant/
Nasal Decongestant
Alcohol 5%
- Maximum Strength
- Non-Drowsy
- For Adults & Children

Drug Facts:

Active Ingredients:
(per 15 ml tablespoon)   Purpose:
Dextromethorphan HBr
   30 mg .... Cough suppressant

Pseudoephedrine HCl
   60 mg .... Nasal decongestant

Uses: Temporarily relieves these cold symptoms
- cough
- nasal congestion

Warnings:
Failure to follow these warnings could result in serious consequences.

Do not use if you are now taking a prescription monoamine oxidase inhibitor (MAOI) (certain drugs for depression, psychiatric or emotional conditions, or Parkinson's disease), or for 2 weeks after stopping the MAOI drug. If you do not know if your prescription drug contains an MAOI, ask a doctor or pharmacist before taking this product.

Ask a doctor before use if you have:
- heart disease
- cough that lasts or is chronic such as occurs with smoking, asthma, or emphysema
- thyroid disease
- diabetes
- high blood pressure
- cough that occurs with too much phlegm (mucus)
- trouble urinating due to enlarged prostate gland

When using this product do not take more than directed.

Stop use and ask a doctor if:
- symptoms do not get better within 7 days or are accompanied by fever.
- you get nervous, dizzy or sleepless
- cough lasts more than 7 days, comes back, or occurs with fever, rash, or headache that lasts. These could be signs of a serious condition.

If pregnant or breast-feeding, ask a health professional before use.

Keep out of reach of children. In case of overdose, get medical help or contact a Poison Control Center right away.

Directions:
- use teaspoon (tsp), tablespoon (TBSP) or dose cup
- do not exceed 4 doses in a 24 hour period

Under 6 yrs.	ask a doctor
6–11 yrs.	1½ tsp (7½ ml) every 6 hours
12 yrs. & older	1 TBSP (15 ml) every 6 hours

Other Information:
- **each tablespoonful contains** sodium 31 mg
- store at room temperature

Inactive Ingredients: Alcohol, FD&C blue no. 1, carboxymethylcellulose sodium, citric acid, flavor, high fructose corn syrup, polyethylene oxide, polyoxyl 40 stearate, propylene glycol, purified water, FD&C red no. 40, saccharin sodium, sodium benzoate, sodium citrate.

How Supplied: Available in 1 FL OZ (30 ml) 4 FL OZ (118 ml) 6 FL OZ (177 ml) and 8 FL OZ (236 ml) plastic bottles. A calibrated dose cup accompanies each bottle.

TAMPER EVIDENT: Do not use if imprinted shrinkband is missing or broken.

Question? 1-800-342-6844

Dist. by Procter & Gamble, Cincinnati OH 45202.

US Pat 5,458,879   42434796

Shown in Product Identification Guide, page 522

VICKS® 44E®
Cough & Chest Congestion Relief
Cough Suppressant/Expectorant
Alcohol 5%
- Non-Drowsy
- For Adults & Children

Drug Facts:

Active Ingredients:
(per 15 ml tablespoon)   Purpose:
Dextromethorphan HBr
   20 mg .... Cough suppressant
Guaifenesin
   200 mg .... Expectorant

Uses:
- temporarily relieves cough due to the common cold
- helps loosen phlegm and thin bronchial secretions to rid the bronchial passageways of bothersome mucus

Warnings:
Do not use
- if you are now taking a prescription monoamine oxidase inhibitor (MAOI) (certain drugs for depression, psychiatric or emotional conditions, or Parkinson's disease), or for 2 weeks after stopping the MAOI drug. If you do not know if your prescription drug contains an MAOI, ask a doctor or pharmacist before taking this product.

Ask a doctor before use if you have:
- a sodium restricted diet
- persistent or chronic cough such as occurs with smoking, asthma, chronic bronchitis or emphysema
- cough that occurs with too much phlegm (mucus)

Stop use and ask a doctor if:
- cough lasts more than 7 days, comes back, or occurs with fever, rash, or headache that lasts. These could be signs of a serious condition.

If pregnant or breast-feeding, ask a health professional before use.

Keep out of reach of children. In case of overdose, get medical help or contact a Poison Control Center right away.

Directions:
- use teaspoon (tsp), tablespoon (TBSP) or dose cup
- do not exceed 6 doses per 24 hours

Under 6 yrs.	ask a doctor
6–11 yrs.	1½ tsp (7½ ml) every 4 hours
12 yrs. & older.	1 TBSP (15 ml) every 4 hours

Other Information:
- **each tablespoon contains** sodium 31 mg
- store at room temperature

Inactive Ingredients: Alcohol, FD&C blue 1, carboxymethylcellulose sodium, citric acid, flavor, high fructose corn syrup, polyethylene oxide, polyoxyl 40 stearate, propylene glycol, purified water, FD&C red no. 40, saccharin sodium, sodium benzoate, sodium citrate.

Continued on next page

Vicks 44E—Cont.

How Supplied: Available in 4 FL OZ (118 ml) 6 FL OZ (177 ml) and 8 FL OZ (236 ml) plastic bottles. A calibrated dose cup accompanies each bottle.
TAMPER EVIDENT: Do not use if imprinted shrinkband is missing or broken.
Questions? 1-800-342-6844
Dist. by Procter & Gamble, Cincinnati OH 45202.
US Pat 5,458,879   42434800
Shown in Product Identification Guide, page 522

VICKS® 44M®
COUGH, COLD & FLU RELIEF
Cough Suppressant/Nasal Decongestant/Antihistamine/ Pain Reliever–Fever Reducer
Alcohol 10%

Maximum strength cough formula
Drug Facts:

Active Ingredients:
(per 5 ml teaspoon)   Purpose:
Acetaminophen
  162.5 mg ... Pain reliever/fever reducer
Chlorpheniramine maleate
  1 mg .... Antihistamine
Dextromethorphan HBr
  7.5 mg .... Cough suppressant
Pseudoephedrine HCl
  15 mg .... Nasal decongestant

Uses: Temporarily relieves cough/cold/flu symptoms
• cough
• sneezing
• headache
• muscular aches
• sore throat
• fever
• runny nose
• nasal congestion

Warnings:
Failure to follow these warnings could result in serious consequences.
Alcohol warning If you consume 3 or more alcoholic drinks every day, ask your doctor whether you should take acetaminophen or other pain relievers/fever reducers. Acetaminophen may cause liver damage.
Sore throat warning If sore throat is severe, persists more than two days, is accompanied or followed by a fever, headache, rash, nausea or vomiting, consult a doctor promptly.
Do not use with other medicines containing acetaminophen if you are now taking a prescription monoamine oxidase inhibitor (MAOI) (certain drugs for depression, psychiatric or emotional conditions, or Parkinson's disease), or for 2 weeks after stopping the MAOI drug. If you do not know if your prescription drug contains an MAOI, ask a doctor or pharmacist before taking this product.
Ask a doctor before use if you have:
• heart disease
• breathing problems or chronic cough such as occurs with smoking, asthma, chronic bronchitis or emphysema

• thyroid disease
• diabetes
• glaucoma
• high blood pressure
• cough that occurs with too much phlegm (mucus)
• trouble urinating due to enlarged prostate gland
Ask a doctor or pharmacist before use if you are taking sedatives or tranquilizers.

When using this product:
• **do not use more than directed**
• excitability may occur, especially in children
• drowsiness may occur
• avoid alcoholic drinks
• be careful when driving a motor vehicle or operating machinery
• alcohol, sedatives, and tranquilizers may increase drowsiness

Stop use and ask a doctor if:
• you get nervous, dizzy or sleepless
• fever gets worse or lasts more than 3 days
• new symptoms occur
• redness or swelling is present
• symptoms do not get better within 7 days or are accompanied by fever
• cough lasts more than 7 days, comes back, or occurs with fever, rash, or headache that lasts.
These could be signs of a serious condition.
If pregnant or breast-feeding, ask a health professional before use.
Keep out of reach of children.
Overdose Warning: Taking more than recommended dose can cause serious health problems. In case of overdose, get medical help or contact a Poison Control Center right away. Quick medical attention is critical for adults as well as for children even if you do not notice any signs or symptoms.

Directions:
• take only as recommended—see **Overdose Warning**
• use teaspoon or dose cup
• do not exceed 4 doses per 24 hours
• children 12 and under: ask a doctor.
• 12 yrs. & older: take 4 teaspoons (20 ml) every 6 hours.

Other Information:
• **each teaspoon contains** sodium 8 mg
• store at room temperature

Inactive Ingredients: Alcohol, FD&C blue 1, carboxymethylcellulose sodium, citric acid, flavor, high fructose corn syrup, polyethylene glycol, polyethylene oxide, propylene glycol, purified water, FD&C red 40, saccharin sodium, sodium citrate.

How Supplied: Available in 4 FL OZ (118 ml) 6 FL OZ (177 ml) and 8 FL OZ (236 ml) plastic bottles. A calibrated dose cup accompanies each bottle.
TAMPER EVIDENT: Do not use if imprinted shrinkband is missing or broken. Not recommended for children.
Questions? 1-800-342-6844
Dist. by Procter & Gamble, Cincinnati OH 45202.
US Pat 5,458,879   42434741
Shown in Product Identification Guide, page 522

CHILDREN'S VICKS® NYQUIL® COLD/COUGH RELIEF
Antihistamine/Nasal Decongestant/ Cough Suppressant

Children's NyQuil was specially formulated with three effective ingredients to relieve nighttime cough, nasal congestion, and runny nose so children can rest. Children's NyQuil® is alcohol free and analgesic free and has a pleasant cherry flavor.

Drug Facts:

Active Ingredients: Purpose:
(per tablespoon, 15 ml)
Chlorpheniramine maleate
  2 mg .... Antihistamine
Dextromethorphan HBr
  15 mg .... Cough suppressant
Pseudoephedrine HCl
  30 mg .... Nasal decongestant

Uses: Temporarily relieves cold symptoms:
• cough due to minor throat and bronchial irritation
• sneezing
• runny nose
• nasal congestion

Warnings:
Failure to follow these warnings could result in serious consequences.

Do not use
• if you are now taking a prescription monoamine oxidase inhibitor (MAOI) (certain drugs for depression, psychiatric or emotional conditions, or Parkinson's disease), or for 2 weeks after stopping the MAOI durg. If you do not know if your prescription drug contains an MAOI, ask a doctor or pharmacist before taking this product.

Ask a doctor before use if you have:
• heart disease
• a breathing problem or chronic cough that lasts or as occurs with smoking, asthma, chronic bronchitis or emphysema
• thyroid disease
• diabetes
• glaucoma
• high blood pressure
• cough that occurs with too much phlegm (mucus)
• a sodium-restricted diet
• trouble urinating due to enlarged prostate gland
Ask a doctor or pharmacist before use if you are taking sedatives or tranquilizers.

When using this product:
• **do not use more than directed**
• excitability may occur, especially in children
• drowsiness may occur
• avoid alcoholic drinks
• be careful when driving a motor vehicle or operating machinery
• alcohol, sedatives, and tranquilizers may increase drowsiness

Stop use and ask a doctor if:
• you get nervous, dizzy or sleepless
• symptoms do not get better within 7 days or accompanied by a fever

- cough lasts more than 7 days, comes back, or occurs with fever, rash, or headache that lasts.
  These could be signs of a serious condition.

If pregnant or breast-feeding, ask a health professional before use.

Keep out of reach of children. In case of overdose, get medical help or contact a Poison Control Center right away. Quick medical attention is critical for adults as well as for children even if you do not notice any signs or symptoms.

Directions:
- use tablespoon (TBSP) or dose cup
- do not exceed 4 doses per 24 hours
  under 6 yrs. .... ask a doctor
  6–11 yrs. .... 1 TBSP or 15 ml every 6 hours
  12 yrs. & older .... 2 TBSP or 30 ml every 6 hours

Other Information:
- **each tablespoon contains** sodium 71 mg
- store at room temperature

Inactive Ingredients: Citric acid, flavor, potassium sorbate, propylene glycol, purified water, FD&C red 40, sodium citrate, sucrose.

How Supplied: Available in 4 FL OZ (118 ml) plastic bottles with child-resistant, tamper-evident cap and a calibrated medicine cup.

Questions? 1-800-362-1683
Exp. Date: See Bottom.   42434744
Dist. by Procter & Gamble, Cincinnati OH 45202.

Shown in Product Identification Guide, page 523

VICKS® Cough Drops
Menthol Cough Suppressant/
Oral Anesthetic
Menthol and Cherry Flavors

CONSUMER INFORMATION: Vicks Cough Drops provide fast and effective relief. Each drop contains effective medicine to suppress your impulse to cough as it dissolves into a soothing syrup to relieve your sore throat.

Drug Facts:

Active Ingredient:
Menthol:

Active Ingredient:	**Purpose:**
(per drop)	

Menthol 3.3 mg ...... Cough suppressant/ oral anesthetic

Cherry:

Active Ingredient:	**Purpose:**
(per drop)	

Menthol 1.7 mg ...... Cough suppressant/ oral anesthetic

Uses: Temporarily relieves:
- sore throat
- coughs due to colds or inhaled irritants

Warnings:
Ask a doctor before use if you have:
- cough associated with excessive phlegm (mucus)
- persistent or chronic cough such as those caused by asthma, emphysema, or smoking

- a severe sore throat accompanied by difficulty in breathing or that lasts more than 2 days
- a sore throat accompanied or followed by fever, headache, rash, swelling, nausea or vomiting

Stop use and ask a doctor if:
- you need to use more than 7 days
- cough lasts more than 7 days, comes back, or occurs with fever, rash, or headache that lasts. These could be the signs of a serious condition.

If pregnant or breast-feeding, ask a health professional before use.

Keep out of reach of children.

Directions:
- under 5 yrs.: ask a doctor (menthol)
- adults & children 5 yrs & older: allow 2 drops to dissolve slowly in mouth (cherry)
- adults & children 5 yrs & older: allow 3 drops to dissolve slowly in mouth
Cough: may be repeated every hour.
Sore Throat: may be repeated every 2 hours.

Other Information:
- store at room temperature

Inactive Ingredients:
Menthol: Ascorbic acid, caramel, corn syrup, eucalyptus oil, sucrose.
Cherry: Ascorbic acid, citric acid, corn syrup, eucalyptus oil, FD&C blue 1, flavor, FD&C red 40, sucrose.

How Supplied: Vicks® Cough Drops are available in boxes of 20 triangular drops. Each red or green drop is debossed with "V."

Questions? 1-800-707-1709
Made in Mexico by Procter & Gamble Manufactura S. de R.I. de C.V. Dist. by Procter & Gamble
Cincinnati OH 45202
50144381

VICKS® DAYQUIL® LIQUID
VICKS® DAYQUIL® LIQUICAPS®
Multi-Symptom Cold/Flu Relief
Nasal Decongestant/
Pain Reliever/Cough
Suppressant/Fever Reducer
Non-drowsy

Drug Facts:

Active Ingredients:

LIQUID:

Active Ingredients:	**Purpose:**
(per 15 ml tablespoon)	

Acetaminophen
  325 mg ...... Pain reliever/fever reducer
Dextromethorphan HBr
  10 mg .... Cough suppressant
Pseudoephedrine HCl
  30 mg .... Nasal decongestant

LIQUICAP®:

Active Ingredients:	**Purpose:**
(per softgel)	

Acetaminophen
  250 mg ...... Pain reliever/fever reducer
Dextromethorphan HBr
  10 mg .... Cough suppressant

Pseudoephedrine HCl
  30 mg .... Nasal decongestant

Uses: Temporarily relieves common cold/flu symptoms:
- nasal congestion
- cough due to minor throat and bronchial irritation
- sore throat
- headache
- minor aches and pains
- muscular aches
- fever

Warnings:
Failure to follow these warnings could result in serious consequences.
Alcohol warning: If you consume 3 or more alcoholic drinks every day, ask your doctor whether you should take acetaminophen or other pain relievers/fever reducers. Acetaminophen may cause liver damage.
Sore throat warning: If sore throat is severe, persists more than 2 days, is accompanied by fever, nausea, rash or vomiting, consult a doctor promptly.
Do not use • with other medicines containing acetaminophen • if you are now taking a prescription monoamine oxidase inhibitor (MAOI) (certain drugs for depression, psychiatric or emotional conditions, or Parkinson's disease), or for 2 weeks after stopping the MAOI drug. If you do not know if your prescription drug contains an MAOI, ask a doctor or pharmacist before taking this product.
Ask a doctor before use if you have:
- heart disease
- thyroid disease
- diabetes
- persistent or chronic cough such as occurs with smoking, asthma, or emphysema
- high blood pressure
- cough that occurs with too much phlegm (mucus)
- trouble urinating due to enlarged prostate gland
- sodium-restricted diet (Specific to DayQuil Liquid only)
When using this product:
- **do not use more than directed**
Stop use and ask a doctor if:
- you get nervous, dizzy or sleepless
- fever gets worse or lasts more than 3 days
- new symptoms occur
- symptoms do not get better within 7 days
- redness or swelling is present
- symptoms do not get better within 7 days (adults) or 5 days (children)
- cough lasts more than 7 days, comes back, or occurs with fever, rash, or headache that lasts. These could be the signs of a serious condition.
If pregnant or breast-feeding, ask a health professional before use.
Keep out of reach of children. Overdose warning: Taking more than the recommended dose can cause serious health problems. In case of overdose, get medical help or contact a Poison Control Center right away. Quick medical attention is critical for adults as well as for children even if you do not notice any signs or symptoms.

Continued on next page

Vicks DayQuil—Cont.

Directions:
- take only as recommended – see Overdose warning

LIQUID:
- use tablespoon (TBSP) or dose cup
- do not exceed 4 doses per 24 hours
  under 6 yrs. .... ask a doctor
  6–11 yrs. .... 1 TBSP or 15 ml
  every 4 hours
  12 yrs. & older .... 2 TBSP or 30 ml
  every 4 hours
- If taking NyQuil® and DayQuil, limit total to 4 doses per 24 hours.

LIQUICAP:
- take only as recommended – see **Overdose Warning**
- do not exceed 4 doses per 24 hours
  under 6 yrs. .... ask a doctor
  6–11 yrs. .... 1 softgel with water
  every 4 hours
  12 yrs. & older .. 2 softgels with water
  every 4 hours
- If taking NyQuil® and DayQuil, limit total to 4 doses per 24 hours.

Other Information:
LIQUID:
- **each tablespoon contains** sodium 71 mg
- store at room temperature
LIQUICAP:
- store at room temperature

Inactive Ingredients:
LIQUID: Citric acid, FD&C yellow 6, flavor, glycerin, polyethylene glycol, propylene glycol, purified water, saccharin sodium, sodium citrate, sucrose.
LIQUICAP: FD&C red 40, FD&C yellow 6, gelatin, glycerin, polyethylene glycol, povidone, propylene glycol, purified water, sorbitol special.

How Supplied: Available in: **LIQUID** 6 FL OZ (177 ml) and 10 FL OZ (295 ml) plastic bottles with child-resistant, tamper-evident cap and a calibrated medicine cup.
LIQUICAP: in 2-count, 12-count and 36-count child-resistant packages and 20-nonchild-resistant packages. Each softgel is imprinted: "DayQuil."
LIQUID:
TAMPER EVIDENT: Do not use if imprinted shrinkband is missing or broken.
LIQUICAP, 12- and 36-count:
TAMPER EVIDENT: This package is safety sealed and child resistant. Use only if blisters are intact. If difficult to open, use scissors.
LIQUICAP, 20-count:
This Package for households without young children.
TAMPER EVIDENT: Use only if blisters are intact. If difficult to open, use scissors.

Questions? 1-800-251-3374
Made in Canada
Dist. by Procter & Gamble
Cincinnati OH 45202
42435018

Shown in Product Identification Guide, page 522

VICKS® NYQUIL® COUGH
Antihistamine
Cough Suppressant
All Night Cough Relief
Cherry Flavor

alcohol 10%

Drug Facts:

Active Ingredients: **Purpose:**
(per 15 ml tablespoon)
Dextromethorphan HBr
  15 mg .... Cough suppressant
Doxylamine succinate
  6.25 mg .... Antihistamine

Uses:
Temporarily relieves cold symptoms
- cough
- runny nose and sneezing

Warnings:
Do not use if you are now taking a prescription monoamine oxidase inhibitor (MAOI) (certain drugs for depression, psychiatric or emotional conditions, or Parkinson's disease), or for 2 weeks after stopping the MAOI drug. If you do not know if your prescription drug contains an MAOI, ask a doctor or pharmacist before taking this product.
Ask a doctor before use if you have:
- asthma
- emphysema
- breathing problems
- excessive phlegm (mucus)
- glaucoma
- chronic bronchitis
- persistent or chronic cough
- cough associated with smoking
- trouble urinating due to enlarged prostate gland
Ask a doctor or pharmacist before use if you are:
taking sedatives or tranquilizers.
When using this product:
- **do not use more than directed**
- marked drowsiness may occur
- avoid alcoholic drinks
- excitability may occur, especially in children
- be careful when driving a motor vehicle or operating machinery
- alcohol, sedatives, and tranquilizers may increase drowsiness
Stop use and ask a doctor if:
- cough lasts more than 7 days, comes back, or occurs with fever, rash, or headache that lasts.
These could be signs of a serious condition.
If pregnant or breast-feeding, ask a health professional before use.
Keep out of reach of children. In case of overdose, get medical help or contact a Poison Control Center right away.

Directions: [1 oz bottle] use tablespoon (TBSP)
Use tablespoon (TBSP) or dose cup
- do not exceed 4 doses per 24 hours
Under 12 yrs. .... ask a doctor
12 yrs. and older .... 2 TBSP or 30 ml
every 6 hours
[6 & 10 oz bottle, twin, quad pack]
- if taking NyQuil and DayQuil®, limit total to 4 doses per day.
Other Information:
- **each tablespoon contains** sodium 17 mg
- store at room temperature

Inactive Ingredients: Alcohol, F&C blue no. 1, citric acid, flavor, high fructose corn syrup, polyethylene glycol, propylene glycol, purified water, FD&C red no. 40, saccharin sodium, sodium citrate

How Supplied: Available in 1 FL OZ (30 ml) 6 FL OZ (177 ml), 10 FL OZ (295 ml) plastic bottles with child-resistant, tamper-evident cap and calibrated Medicine cup.
TAMPER EVIDENT: Do not use if imprinted shrinkband is missing or broken.
Questions? 1-800-362-1683
Dist. by Procter & Gamble,
Cincinnati OH 45202. 42437885
Shown in Product Identification Guide, page 523

VICKS® NYQUIL® LIQUICAPS®
VICKS® NYQUIL® LIQUID
(Original and Cherry)
Multi-Symptom Cold/Flu Relief
Antihistamine/Cough
Suppressant/Pain Reliever/
Nasal Decongestant/
Fever Reducer

Liquid (Original and Cherry)—alcohol 10%

Drug Facts:

Active Ingredients:
LiquiCaps®:
Active Ingredients: **Purpose:**
(per softgel)
Acetaminophen
  250 mg ...... Pain reliever/fever reducer
Dextromethorphan HBr
  10 mg .... Cough suppressant
Doxylamine succinate
  6.25 mg .... Antihistamine
Pseudoephedrine HCl
  30 mg .... Nasal decongestant
Liquid (Original and Cherry):
Active Ingredients: **Purpose:**
(per 15 ml tablespoon)
Acetaminophen
  500 mg ...... Pain reliever/fever reducer
Dextromethorphan HBr
  15 mg .... Cough suppressant
Doxylamine succinate
  6.25 mg .... Antihistamine
Pseudoephedrine HCl
  30 mg .... Nasal decongestant

Uses:
LiquiCaps®:
Temporarily relieves these common cold/flu symptoms:
- nasal congestion
- cough due to minor throat & bronchial irritation
- sore throat
- headache
- minor aches and pains
- muscular aches
- fever
- runny nose and sneezing
Liquid (Original and Cherry):
Temporarily relieves these common cold/flu symptoms:
- minor aches and pains
- headache
- muscular aches

- sore throat
- fever
- runny nose and sneezing
- nasal congestion
- cough due to minor throat and bronchial irritation

Warnings:
Failure to follow these warnings could result in serious consequences.
Alcohol warning If you consume 3 or more alcoholic drinks every day, ask your doctor whether you should take acetaminophen or other pain relievers/fever reducers. Acetaminophen may cause liver damage.
Sore throat warning If sore throat is severe, persists more than 2 days, is accompanied or followed by fever, rash, nausea, or vomiting, consult a doctor promptly.
Do not use • with other medications containing acetaminophen • if you are now taking a prescription monoamine oxidase inhibitor (MAOI) (certain drugs for depression, psychiatric or emotional conditions, or Parkinson's disease), or for 2 weeks after stopping the MAOI drug. If you do not know if your prescription drug contains an MAOI, ask a doctor or pharmacist before taking this product.
Ask a doctor before use if you have:
- heart disease
- a breathing problem or chronic cough such as occurs with smoking, asthma, chronic bronchitis, or emphysema
- thyroid disease
- diabetes
- glaucoma
- high blood pressure
- cough that occurs with too much phlegm (mucus)
- chronic bronchitis

Ask a doctor or pharmacist before use if you are taking sedatives or tranquilizers.
When using this product
- **do not use more than directed**
- excitability may occur, especially in children
- marked drowsiness may occur
- avoid alcoholic drinks
- be careful when driving a motor vehicle or operating machinery
- alcohol, sedatives, and tranquilizers may increase drowsiness

Stop use and ask a doctor if:
- symptoms do not get better within 7 days or are accompanied by fever.
- you get nervous, dizzy or sleepless
- fever gets worse or lasts more than 3 days
- new symptoms occur
- swelling or redness is present.
- cough lasts more than 7 days, comes back, or occurs with fever, rash, or headache that lasts. These could be signs of a serious condition.

If pregnant or breast-feeding, ask a health professional before use.
Keep out of reach of children.
Overdose warning: Taking more than the recommended dose can cause serious health problems. In case of overdose, get medical help or contact a Poison Control Center right away. Quick medical attention is critical for adults as well as for children even if you do not notice any signs or symptoms.

Directions:
LiquiCaps®:
- take only as recommended – see **Overdose warning**
- children under 12 yrs.: ask a doctor.
- do not exceed 4 doses per 24 hours
- 12 yrs and older . . . . 2 softgels with water every 4 hours
- If taking NyQuil and DayQuil®, limit total to 4 doses per 24 hours.

Liquid (Original and cherry):

AGE	DOSAGE
take only as recommended – see **Overdose warning**	
use tablespoon (TBSP) or dose cup	
do not exceed 4 doses per 24 hours	
children under 12	ask a doctor
adults and children 12 years and over	2 TBSP (30 ml) every 6 hours

If taking NyQuil and DayQuil®, limit total to 4 doses per 24 hours.

Other Information:
LiquiCaps®:
- store at room temperature
Liquid (Original and Cherry):
- **each tablespoon contains** sodium 17 mg
- store at room temperature

Inactive Ingredients:
LiquiCaps®: FD&C Blue no. 1, gelatin, glycerin, polyethylene glycol, povidone, propylene glycol, purified water, sorbitol special, D&C Yellow no. 10.
Liquid (Original): Alcohol, citric acid, flavor, FD&C Green no. 3, high fructose corn syrup, polyethylene glycol, propylene glycol, purified water, saccharin sodium, sodium citrate, yellow 6, D&C Yellow 10.
Liquid (Cherry): Alcohol, FD&C Blue 1, citric acid, flavor, high fructose corn syrup, polyethylene glycol, propylene glycol, purified water, FD&C Red 40, saccharin sodium, sodium citrate.

How Supplied:
LiquiCaps®: Available in 2-count 12- and 36-count child-resistant blister packages and 20-count non-child resistant blister packages. Each softgel is imprinted: "NyQuil".
Liquid: Available in 1 FL OZ (30 ml) 6 and 10 FL OZ (177 ml and 295 ml, respectively) 16 FL OZ (473 ml) plastic bottles with child-resistant, tamper-evident cap and calibrated medicine cup.
LiquiCaps®: 12- and 36-ct
TAMPER EVIDENT: This package is safety sealed and child resistant. Use only if blisters are intact. If difficult to open, use scissors.
LiquiCaps, 20-count:
This package for households without young children.
TAMPER EVIDENT: Use only if blisters are intact. If difficult to open, use scissors.

Liquid (Original and cherry):
TAMPER EVIDENT: Do not use if imprinted shrinkband is missing or broken.
Questions? 1-800-362-1683
Liqui Caps®:
Made in Canada
Dist. by Procter & Gamble,
Cincinnati OH 45202.
©2001   42435017
Liquid (Original): Dist. by Procter & Gamble
Cincinnati OH 45202   42434786
Liquid (Cherry): Dist. by Procter & Gamble
Cincinnati OH 45202   42434789
Shown in Product Identification Guide, page 523

PEDIATRIC VICKS® 44e®
Cough & Chest Congestion Relief
Cough suppressant/Expectorant

- Non-drowsy
- Alcohol-free
- Aspirin-free

Drug Facts:

Active Ingredients:
(per 15 ml tablespoon)   **Purpose:**
Dextromethorphan
   HBr 10 mg .... Cough suppressant
Guaifenesin 100mg .... Expectorant

Uses:
- temporarily relieves cough due to the common cold
- helps loosen phlegm and thin bronchial secretions to rid bronchial passageways of bothersome mucus

Warnings:
Do not use
- if you are now taking a prescription monoamine oxidase inhibitor (MAOI) (certain drugs for depression, psychiatric or emotional conditions, or Parkinson's disease), or for 2 weeks after stopping the MAOI drug. If you do not know if your prescription drug contains an MAOI, ask a doctor or pharmacist before taking this product.

Ask a doctor before use if you have:
- a sodium restricted diet
- cough that occurs with too much phlegm (mucus)
- persistent or chronic cough such as occurs with smoking, asthma, chronic bronchitis or emphysema

Stop use and ask a doctor if:
- cough lasts more than 7 days, comes back, or occurs with fever, rash, or headache that lasts. These could be signs of a serious condition.

If pregnant or breast-feeding, ask a health professional before use.
Keep out of reach of children. In case of overdose, get medical help or contact a Poison Control Center right away.

Directions:
- use tablespoon (TBSP) or dose cup
- do not exceed 6 doses per 24 hours
  Under 2 yrs. .... ask a doctor
  2–5 yrs. .... ½ TBSP (7½ ml) every 4 hours
  6–11 yrs. .... 1 TBSP (15 ml) every 4 hours

Continued on next page

Vicks Pediatric 44e—Cont.

12 yrs.&
older .... 2 TBSP (30 ml)
every 4 hours

Other Information:
- **each tablespoon contains** sodium 30 mg
- store at room temperature

Inactive Ingredients: Carboxymethylcellulose sodium, citric acid, FD&C red no. 40, flavor, high fructose corn syrup, polyethylene oxide, polyoxyl 40 stearate, propylene glycol, purified water, saccharin sodium, sodium benzoate, sodium citrate.

How Supplied: 4 FL OZ (118 ml) plastic bottles. A calibrated dose cup accompanies each bottle.

TAMPER EVIDENT: Do not use if imprinted shrinkband is missing or broken.
***Questions?* 1-800-342-6844**
Dist. by Procter & Gamble, Cincinnati OH 45202.
US Pat 5,458,879   42434802
Shown in Product Identification Guide, page 522

PEDIATRIC VICKS® 44m®
Cough & Cold Relief
Cough Suppressant/Nasal Decongestant/Antihistamine

- Alcohol-free
- Aspirin-free

Drug Facts:

Active Ingredients:
(per 15 ml tablespoon)   Purpose:
Chlorpheniramine maleate
2 mg .... Antihistamine
Dextromethorphan HBr
15 mg .... Cough suppressant
Pseudoephedrine HCl
30 mg .... Nasal decongestant

Uses: Temporarily relieves cough/cold symptoms
- cough
- sneezing
- runny nose
- nasal congestion

Warnings:
Failure to follow these warnings could result in serious consequences.
Do not use:
- if you are now taking a prescription monoamine oxidase inhibitor (MAOI) (certain drugs for depression, psychiatric or emotional conditions, or Parkinson's disease), or for 2 weeks after stopping the MAOI drug. If you do not know if your prescription drug contains an MAOI, ask a doctor or pharmacist before taking this product.

Ask a doctor before use if you have:
- heart disease
- a sodium restricted diet
- a breathing problem or chronic cough that lasts or occurs with smoking, asthma, chronic bronchitis or emphysema
- thyroid disease
- diabetes
- glaucoma

- high blood pressure
- cough that occurs with too much phlegm (mucus)
- trouble urinating due to enlarged prostate gland

Ask a doctor or pharmicist before use if you are taking sedatives or tranquilizers.

When using this product:
- **do not use more than directed**
- excitability may occur, especially in children
- drowsiness may occur
- avoid alcoholic drinks
- be careful when driving a motor vehicle or operating machinery
- alcohol, sedatives, and tranquilizers may increase drowsiness

Stop use and ask a doctor if:
- you get nervous, dizzy or sleepless
- symptoms do not get better within 7 days or are accompanied by a fever.
- cough last more than 7 days, comes back, or occurs with fever, rash, or headache that lasts
These could be signs of a serious condition.

If pregnant or breast-feeding, ask a health professional before use.

Keep out of reach of children. In case of overdose, get medical help or contact a Poison Control Center right away.

Directions:
- use tablespoon (TBSP) or dose cup
- do not exceed 4 doses per 24 hours
Under 6 yrs. .... ask a doctor
6–11 yrs. .... 1 TBSP or 15 ml every 6 hours
12 yrs. & older .... 2 TBSP or 30 ml every 6 hours

Other Information:
- **each tablespoon contains** sodium 30 mg
- store at room temperature

Inactive Ingredients: Carboxymethylcellulose sodium, citric acid, FD&C red 40, flavor, high fructose corn syrup, polyethylene oxide, polyoxyl 40 stearate, propylene glycol, purified water, saccharin sodium, sodium benzoate, sodium citrate.

How Supplied: 4 FL OZ (118 ml) plastic bottles. A calibrated dose cup accompanies each bottle.

TAMPER EVIDENT: Do not use if imprinted shrinkband is missing or broken.
***Questions?* 1-800-342-6844**
Dist. by Procter & Gamble, Cincinnati OH 45202.
US Pat 5,458,879   42434743
Shown in Product Identification Guide, page 522

VICKS® SINEX® [NASAL SPRAY]
[Ultra Fine Mist] for Sinus Relief
[sī 'něx]
Phenylephrine HCl Nasal Decongestant

Drug Facts:

Active Ingredients: Purpose:
Phenylephrine
HCl 0.5% .... Nasal decongestant

Uses: Temporarily relieves sinus/nasal congestion due to
- colds
- hay fever
- upper respiratory allergies
- sinusitis

Warnings:
Ask a doctor before use if you have:
- heart disease
- thyroid disease
- diabetes
- high blood pressure
- trouble urinating due to enlarged prostate gland

When using this product:
- **do not exceed recommended dosage**
- use of this container by more than one person may cause infection
- temporary burning, stinging, sneezing, or increased nasal discharge may occur
- frequent or prolonged use may cause nasal congestion to recur or worsen

Stop use and ask a doctor if:
- symptoms persist for more than 3 days

If pregnant or breast-feeding, ask a health professional before use.

Keep out of reach of children. In case of accidental ingestion, get medical help or contact a poison control center right away.

Directions:
Nasal Spray:
- under 12 yrs. ask a doctor
- adults & children 12 yrs. & older: 2 or 3 sprays in each nostril without tilting your head, not more often than every 4 hours.

Ultra Fine Mist: Remove protective cap. Before using for the first time, prime the pump by firmly depressing its rim several times. Hold container with thumb at base and nozzle between first and second fingers. Without tilting your head, insert nozzle into nostril. Fully depress rim with a firm, even stroke and inhale deeply.
- under 12 yrs.: ask a doctor
- adults & children 12 yrs. & older: 2 or 3 sprays in each nostril, not more often than every 4 hours.

Other Information:
- store at room temperature

Inactive Ingredients: Benzalkonium chloride, camphor, chlorhexidine gluconate, citric acid, disodium EDTA, eucalyptol, menthol, purified water, tyloxapol.

How Supplied: Available in $1/2$ FL OZ (14.7 ml) plastic squeeze bottle and $1/2$ FL OZ (14.7 ml) measured dose Ultra Fine mist pump. Note: This container is properly filled when approximately half full. Air space equal to one half of volume is necessary to propel the fine spray.

TAMPER EVIDENT:

Do not use if imprinted shrinkband is missing or broken.
Questions? 1-800-873-8276
Nasal Spray 42436771
Ultra Fine Mist 42436765
Dist. by Procter & Gamble
Cincinnati OH 45202

VICKS® SINEX®
[sĭ 'nĕx]
12-HOUR [Nasal Spray]
[Ultra Fine Mist] for Sinus Relief
Oxymetazoline HCl
Nasal Decongestant

Drug Facts:

Active Ingredients:	Purpose:
Oxymetazoline HCl 0.05%	Nasal decongestant

Uses: Temporarily relieves sinus/nasal congestion due to
- colds
- hay fever
- upper respiratory allergies
- sinusitis

Warnings:
Ask a doctor before use if you have:
- heart disease
- thyroid disease
- diabetes
- high blood pressure
- trouble urinating due to enlarged prostate gland

When using this product:
- **do not exceed recommended dosage**
- temporary burning, stinging, sneezing, or increased nasal discharge may occur
- frequent or prolonged use may cause nasal congestion to recur or worsen
- use of this container by more than one person may cause infection

Stop use and ask a doctor if:
- symptoms persist for more than 3 days

If pregnant or breast-feeding, ask a health professional before use.

Keep out of reach of children. In case of accidental ingestion, get medical help or contact a poison control center right away.

Directions:
Nasal Spray:
- under 6 yrs: ask a doctor
- adults & children 6 yrs. & older (with adult supervision): 2 or 3 sprays in each nostril without tilting your head, not more often than every 10 to 12 hours. Do not exceed 2 doses in 24 hours.

Ultra Fine Mist: Remove protective cap. Before using for the first time, prime the pump by firmly depressing its rim several times. Hold container with thumb at base and nozzle between first and second fingers. Without tilting your head, insert nozzle into nostril. Fully depress rim with a firm, even stroke and inhale deeply.
- under 6 yrs.: ask a doctor
- adults & children 6 yrs. & older (with adult supervision): 2 or 3 sprays in each nostril, not more often than every 10 to 12 hours. Do not exceed 2 doses in 24 hours.

Other Information:
- store at room temperature

Inactive Ingredients: Benzalkonium chloride, camphor, chlorhexidine gluconate, disodium EDTA, eucalyptol, menthol, potassium phosphate, purified water, sodium chloride, sodium phosphate, tyloxapol.

How Supplied: Available in ½ FL OZ (14.7 ml) plastic squeeze bottle and ½ FL OZ (14.7 ml) measured-dose Ultra Fine mist pump.
TAMPER EVIDENT: Do not use if imprinted shrinkband is missing or broken.
Nasal Spray 42436768
Ultra Fine Mist 42436763
Questions? 1-800-873-8276
Dist. by
Procter & Gamble,
Cincinnati OH 45202

VICKS® VAPOR INHALER
Levmetamfetamine/Nasal Decongestant

Drug Facts:

Active Ingredients:	Purpose:
(per inhaler) Levmetamfetamine 50 mg	Nasal decongestant

Uses: Temporarily relieves nasal congestion due to:
- a cold
- hay fever or other upper respiratory allergies
- sinusitis

Warnings:
When using this product:
- **do not exceed recommended dosage**
- temporary burning, stinging, sneezing, or increased nasal discharge may occur
- frequent or prolonged use may cause nasal congestion to recur or worsen
- do not use for more than 7 days
- do not use container by more than one person as it may spread infection
- use only as directed

Stop use and ask a doctor if:
- symptoms persist

If pregnant or breast-feeding, ask a health professional before use.

Keep out of reach of children. If swallowed, get medical help or contact a poison control center right away.

Directions:
The product delivers in each 800 ml air 0.04 to 0.15 mg of levmetamfetamine.
- do not use more often than every 2 hours
- under 6 yrs.: ask a doctor
- 6–11 yrs.: with adult supervision, 1 inhalation in each nostril.
- 12 yrs. & older: 2 inhalation in each nostril.

Other Information:
- store at room temperature
- keep inhaler tightly closed.
- This inhaler is effective for a minimum of 3 months after first use.

Inactive Ingredients: Bornyl acetate, camphor, lavender oil, menthol.

How Supplied: Available as a cylindrical plastic nasal inhaler.
Net weight: 0.007 OZ (198 mg).
TAMPER EVIDENT: Use only if imprinted wrap is intact.
Questions? 1-800-873-8276
Dist. by Procter & Gamble, Cincinnati OH 45202. ©2001 42438038

VICKS® VAPORUB®
VICKS® VAPORUB® CREAM
(greaseless)
[vā 'pō-rub]
Nasal Decongestant/Cough Suppressant/Topical Analgesic

Drug Facts:

Active Ingredients:
Vicks® VapoRub®:

Active Ingredients:	Purpose:
Camphor 4.8%	Cough suppressant, nasal decongestant & topical analgesic
Eucalyptus oil 1.2%	Cough suppressant & nasal decongestant
Menthol 2.6%	Cough suppressant, nasal decongestant & topical analgesic

Vicks® VapoRub® Cream:

Active Ingredients:	Purpose:
Camphor 5.2%	Cough suppressant, nasal decongestant & topical analgesic
Eucalyptus oil 1.2%	Cough suppressant & nasal decongestant
Menthol 2.8%	Cough suppressant, nasal decongestant & topical analgesic

Uses: • On chest & throat temporarily relieves cough and nasal congestion due to the common cold
- on aching muscles temporarily relieves minor aches & pains

Warnings:
Failure to follow these warnings could result in serious consequences.
For external use only; avoid contact with eyes.
Do not use:
- by mouth
- with tight bandages
- in nostrils
- on wounds or damaged skin

Ask a doctor before use if you have:
- cough that occurs with too much phlegm (mucus)
- persistent or chronic cough such as occurs with smoking, asthma or emphysema

When using this product do not:
- heat
- microwave
- use near an open flame
- add to hot water or any container where heating water. May cause splattering and result in burns.

Stop use and ask a doctor if:
- muscle aches/pains persist more than 7 days or come back
- cough lasts more than 7 days, comes back, or occurs with fever, rash, or headache that lasts.
These could be signs of a serious condition.

If pregnant or breast-feeding, ask a health professional before use.

Keep out of reach of children. In case of accidental ingestion, get medical help or contact a Poison Control Center right away.

Directions: • **See important warnings under "When using this product"**

Continued on next page

Vicks VapoRub—Cont.

- under 2 yrs.: ask a doctor
- adults and children 2 yrs. & older: Rub a thick layer on chest & throat or rub on sore aching muscles. If desired, cover with a soft cloth but keep clothing loose. Repeat up to three times per 24 hours or as directed by a doctor.

Other Information:
- store at room temperature

Inactive Ingredients:
Vicks® VapoRub®: Cedarleaf oil, nutmeg oil, special petrolatum, thymol, turpentine oil
Vicks® VapoRub® Cream: Carbomer 954, cedarleaf oil, cetyl alcohol, cetyl palmitate, cyclomethicone copolyol, dimethicone copolyol, dimethicone, EDTA, glycerin, imidazolidinyl urea, isopropyl palmitate, methylparaben, nutmeg oil, peg-100 stearate, propylparaben, purified water, sodium hydroxide, stearic acid, stearyl alcohol, thymol, titanium dioxide, turpentine oil

How Supplied:
Vicks VapoRub®: Available in 1.76 oz (50 g) 3.53 oz (100 g) and 6 oz (170 g) plastic jars 0.45 oz (12 g) tin.
Vicks® VapoRub® Cream: Available in 2 oz (60 g) tube ¹/₆ oz pouch.
Questions? 1-800-873-8276
www.vicks.com
Vicks® VapoRub® 50142932
Vicks® VapoRub® Cream 50117758
US Pat. 5,322,689
Made in Mexico by Procter & Gamble
Manufactura, S. de R.L. de C.V.
Dist. by Procter & Gamble,
Cincinnati OH 45202

VICKS® VAPOSTEAM®
[vā 'pō "stēm]
Liquid Medication for Hot Steam Vaporizers. Camphor/Cough Suppressant

Drug Facts:

Active Ingredient: **Purpose:** Camphor 6.2% .... Cough suppressant

Uses: Temporarily relieves cough associated with a cold.

Warnings:
Failure to follow these warnings could result in serious consequences.
For external use only
Flammable Keep away from fire or flame. Cap container tightly and store at room temperature away from heat.
Ask a doctor before use if you have:
- a persistent or chronic cough
- cough associated with smoking
- emphysema
- excessive phlegm (mucus)
- asthma
When using this product do not
- heat
- microwave
- use near an open flame
- take by mouth
- direct steam from the vaporizer too close to the face

- add to hot water or any container where heating water except when adding to cold water only in a hot steam vaporizer. May cause splattering and result in burns.
Stop use and ask a doctor if:
- cough lasts more than 7 days, comes back, or occurs with fever, rash, or headache that lasts.
These could be signs of a serious condition.
Keep out of reach of children. In case of eye exposure (flush eyes with water); or in case of accidental ingestion; seek medical help or contact a Poison Control Center right away.

Directions:
see important warnings under "When using this product"
- under 2 yrs.: ask a doctor
- adults & children 2 yrs. & older: use 1 tablespoon of solution for each quart of water or 1½ teaspoonsful of solution for each pint of water
- add solution directly to cold water only in a hot steam vaporizer
- follow manufacturer's directions for using vaporizer. Breathe in medicated vapors. May be repeated up to 3 times a day.

Inactive Ingredients: Alcohol 78%, cedarleaf oil, eucalyptus oil, laureth-7, menthol, nutmeg oil, poloxamer 124, silicone.

How Supplied: Available in 4 FL OZ (118 ml) and 8 FL OZ (235 ml) bottles.
Questions? 1-800-873-8276
Made in Mexico by Procter & Gamble
Manufactura S. de R.L. de C.V.
Dist. by Procter & Gamble
Cincinnati OH 45202
50144018

EDUCATIONAL MATERIAL

The Procter & Gamble Company offers to health care professionals a variety of journal reprints and patient education materials. For this information, please call **1-800-832-3064** or write:
Scientific Communications
The Procter & Gamble Company
P.O. Box 599
Cincinnati, OH 45201
Information is also available by visiting www.pg.com. Select the brand of interest from the *Product Help* section. Each brand site offers a *Contact Us* page in case of additional questions.

**IF YOU SUSPECT
AN INTERACTION. . .**
The 1,800-page
PDR Companion Guide™ can help.
Use the order form
in the front of this book.

The Purdue Frederick Company
ONE STAMFORD FORUM
STAMFORD, CT 06901-3431

For Medical Information Contact:
Medical Department
(888) 726–7535

**BETADINE® BRAND
First Aid Antibiotics
+ Moisturizer Ointment**

Actions: Topical broad-spectrum antibiotics polymyxin B sulfate and bacitracin zinc in a cholesterolized ointment* (moisturizer) base to help prevent infection. Formulated with a special blend of waxes and oils to help retain vital moisture needed to aid in healing.

Uses: First aid to help prevent infection in minor cuts, scrapes and burns.

Directions: Clean affected area. Apply small amount of this product (an amount equal to the surface area of the tip of the finger) on the area 1 to 3 times daily. May be covered with a sterile bandage.

Warnings: For External Use Only. Do not use in the eyes or apply over large areas of the body. In case of deep or puncture wounds, animal bites, or serious burns, consult a physician. Stop use and consult a physician if the condition persists or gets worse, or if a rash or other allergic reaction develops. Do not use this product if you are allergic to any of the ingredients. Do not use longer than 1 week unless directed by a physician. Keep this and all medications out of the reach of children. In case of accidental ingestion, seek professional assistance or contact a Poison Control Center immediately.

Active Ingredients: Per gram: Polymyxin B Sulfate (10,000 IU) and Bacitracin Zinc (500 IU).

How Supplied: 1/2 oz. plastic tube with applicator tip. Store at room temperature.
* Formulated with Aquaphor®—a registered trademark of Beiersdorf AG.

Copyright 1998, 2002, The Purdue Frederick Company
Shown in Product Identification Guide, page 523

**BETADINE® BRAND PLUS
First Aid Antibiotics + Pain Reliever
Ointment**
[bā 'tăh-dīn"]

Actions: Topical broad-spectrum antibiotics polymyxin B sulfate and bacitracin zinc plus topical anesthetic in a cholesterolized ointment* (moisturizer) base to help prevent infection and relieve pain.

Uses: First aid to help prevent infection and provide temporary pain relief in minor cuts, scrapes and burns.

Directions: Clean affected area. Apply small amount of this product (an amount equal to the surface area of the tip of the finger) on the area 1 to 3 times daily. May be covered with a sterile bandage. Children under 2 years of age: Consult a physician.

Warnings: For External Use Only. Do not use in the eyes or apply over large areas of the body. In case of deep or puncture wounds, animal bites, or serious burns, consult a physician. Stop use and consult a physician if the condition persists or gets worse, or if a rash or other allergic reaction develops. Do not use this product if you are allergic to any of the ingredients. Do not use longer than 1 week unless directed by a physician. Keep this and all medications out of the reach of children. In case of accidental ingestion, seek professional assistance or contact a Poison Control Center immediately.

Active Ingredients: Per gram: Polymyxin B Sulfate (10,000 IU), Bacitracin Zinc (500 IU), and Pramoxine HCl 10 mg.

How Supplied: 1/2 oz. plastic tube with an applicator tip. Store at room temperature.
*Formulated with Aquaphor® — a registered trademark of Beiersdorf AG.
Copyright 1998, 2002, The Purdue Frederick Company.
Shown in Product Identification Guide, page 523

BETADINE® OINTMENT
(povidone-iodine, 10%)
BETADINE® SOLUTION
(povidone-iodine, 10%)
BETADINE ® SKIN CLEANSER
(povidone-iodine, 7.5%)
Topical Antiseptic Bactericide/Virucide

Action: Topical microbicides active against organisms commonly encountered in minor skin wounds and burns.

Uses: Ointment—For the prevention of infection in minor burns, cuts and abrasions. Kills microorganisms promptly. **Solution**—Kills microorganisms in minor burns, cuts and scrapes. **Skin Cleanser**—Helps prevent infection in minor cuts, scrapes and burns. Use routinely for general hygiene.

Directions: Ointment—For the prevention of infection in minor burns, cuts and abrasions, apply directly to affected areas as needed. Nonocclusive: allows air to reach the wound. May be bandaged. **Solution**—For minor cuts, scrapes and burns, apply directly to affected area as needed. May be covered with gauze or adhesive bandage. **Skin Cleanser**—For handwashing, cleansing or bathing, wet skin and apply a sufficient amount to work up a rich, golden lather. Allow

lather to remain about 3 minutes and rinse off. Repeat 2–3 times a day or as directed by physician.

Warnings: For External Use Only. Do not use in the eyes. Do not use if you are sensitive to iodine or other product ingredients. Do not use longer than one week unless directed by a doctor. In case of deep or puncture wounds or serious burns, consult physician. If redness, irritation, swelling or pain persists or increases, or if infection occurs, discontinue use and consult physician. If swallowed, get medical help or contact a Poison Control Center right away. Keep out of reach of children.

How Supplied:
Ointment: 1/32 oz. and 1/8 oz. packettes and 1 oz. tubes
Solution: 1/2 oz., 4 oz., 8 oz., 16 oz. (1 pt.), 32 oz. (1 qt.), and 1 gal. plastic bottles
Skin Cleanser: 4 fl. oz. plastic bottles
Avoid storing at excessive heat.
Copyright 1991, 2002, The Purdue Frederick Company
Shown in Product Identification Guide, page 523

BETADINE® PREPSTICK® APPLICATOR
[bā' tăh-dīn'']
[povidone-iodine, 10%]
Topical Antiseptic Bactericide/Virucide
Hospital Use Only

Individually wrapped applicators are packaged dry with approximately 2.6 grams of microbicidal Betadine® Solution stored in the handle of the applicator. Antiseptic solution is released into the 1³/₈-inch-long, soft foam swab head by gently squeezing the 4-inch-long plastic handle.

Actions: Reduces bacterial load and the risk of infection.

Uses: For degerming skin and mucous membranes. Provides sufficient antiseptic solution for most kinds of site prepping—including prior to IM injections, venous punctures, and minor surgical procedures.

Directions: Tear wrapper on dotted line and discard top part of wrapper. With the tip still in the wrapper, gently squeeze plastic handle to break the seal. Release antiseptic solution into foam swab head by lightly squeezing handle. Apply to prep site with the moistened foam tip, working in a circular motion from inside to the outside. Apply as often as needed.

Warnings: For External Use Only. Do not use in the eyes. Do not use if you are sensitive to iodine or other product ingredients. Discontinue use if irritation and redness develop. **Do not heat prior to application.**

How Supplied: 150 individually packaged applicators per dispensing unit. Each applicator contains approximately 2.6 grams of solution.
Avoid storing at excessive heat.
Copyright 1999, 2002, The Purdue Frederick Company

BETADINE® PREPSTICK PLUS® applicator
[ba'tah-dīn'']
[povidone-iodine, 10%]
with alcohol for faster drying
Topical Antiseptic Bactericide/Virucide
Hospital Use Only

Povidone-iodine with alcohol is stored in the 4-inch-long plastic handle of these individually wrapped applicators which are packaged dry. Antiseptic solution is released into the soft foam swab head by gently squeezing the handle.

Actions: Reduces bacterial load and the risk of infection.

Uses: For preparation of the skin prior to surgery. Helps reduce bacteria that potentially can cause skin infection. For preparation of the skin prior to an injection.

Directions: Gently squeeze plastic handle. This allows the release of the antiseptic solution into the foam swab head. Apply to prep site with the moistened foam tip, working in a circular motion from inside to outside. Apply as often as needed.

Warnings: For External Use Only. Do not use in the eyes. Do not use if you are sensitive to iodine or other product ingredients. Discontinue use if irritation and redness develop. **Do not heat prior to application.** FLAMMABLE. KEEP AWAY FROM FIRE, FLAME OR ELECTRICAL SPARK. Avoid storing at excessive heat.

How Supplied: 150 individually packaged applicators per dispensing unit. Each applicator contains approximately 2.6 grams of solution.
Copyright 2002, The Purdue Frederick Company

GENTLAX®
[jent' lax]
brand of bisacodyl USP, 5 mg
Tablets
Laxative

Indications: For relief of occasional constipation (irregularity).

Actions: This product generally causes bowel movement in 6–12 hours.

Directions: Take as follows or as directed by doctor. Adults and children 12 years and older, take 1 to 3 tablets (usually 2) in a single daily dose. Children 6

Continued on next page

Gentlax—Cont.

to under 12, take 1 tablet in a single daily dose. Children under 6 years of age: ask a doctor.

Warnings: Do not give to children under 6 years of age unless told to do so by a doctor, or to persons who cannot swallow without chewing unless told to do so by a doctor. Do not take laxative products for longer than 1 week unless directed by a doctor. Ask a doctor before use if you have stomach pain, nausea, vomiting, or if you have noticed a sudden change in bowel movements that continues over a period of 2 weeks. Do not chew or crush these tablets, do not use within 1 hour after taking an antacid or milk. When using this product, you may have stomach discomfort, faintness and cramps. Stop use and ask a doctor if you have rectal bleeding or fail to have a bowel movement after use of a laxative; these may indicate a serious condition. If you are pregnant or breast-feeding, ask a health professional before use. **Keep out of the reach of children.** In case of overdose, get medical help or contact a Poison Control Center right away.

Other information: Sodium content is less than 0.2 mg/tablet. Store at temperatures not above 86°F (30°C). Avoid excessive humidity.

Inactive ingredients: calcium sulfate, carnauba wax, confectioner's sugar, croscarmellose sodium, D&C yellow no. 10, dibasic calcium phosphate, FD&C yellow no. 6, gelatin, kaolin, magnesium stearate, methacrylic acid copolymer, polyethylene glycol, powdered cellulose, pregelatinized starch, silicon dioxide, sucrose, talc, titanium dioxide, white wax.

How Supplied: Packages of 20 tablets and bottles of 100 tablets
Copyright 2002, The Purdue Frederick Company.
Shown in Product Identification Guide, page 523

SENOKOT® Tablets/Granules
SenokotXTRA® Tablets
(standardized senna concentrate)
SENOKOT® Syrup
SENOKOT® Children's Syrup
(extract of senna concentrate)
SENOKOT-S® Tablets
(standardized senna concentrate and docusate sodium)

Natural Vegetable Laxative

Actions: Senna provides a colon-specific action which is gentle, effective, and predictable, generally producing bowel movement in 6 to 12 hours. Senokot-S Tablets also contain a stool softener for smoother, easier evacuation if stools are hard and dry.

Uses: For the relief of occasional constipation. Senokot Products generally produce bowel movement in 6 to 12 hours.

Directions: Take according to product-package instructions or as directed by a doctor. Take preferably at bedtime. For use of Senokot Laxatives in children under 2 years of age, consult a doctor.

Warnings: Do not use a laxative product when stomach pain, nausea or vomiting are present unless directed by a doctor. If you have noticed a sudden change in bowel movements that persists over a period of 2 weeks, consult a doctor before using a laxative. Do not use laxative products for longer than 1 week unless directed by a doctor. Rectal bleeding or failure to have a bowel movement after the use of a laxative may indicate a serious condition. Discontinue use and consult your doctor. As with any drug, if you are pregnant or nursing a baby, seek the advice of a health professional before using this product. In case of accidental overdose, seek professional assistance or contact a Poison Control Center immediately. Keep out of children's reach.
Senokot-S Tablets: Do not use if you are now taking mineral oil unless directed by a doctor.

How Supplied: Senokot Tablets: Boxes of 20; bottles of 50, 100, and 1000; Unit Strip Packs in boxes of 100 individually sealed tablets. Each Senokot Tablet contains 8.6 mg sennosides.
SenokotXTRA Tablets: Boxes of 12 and 36. Each SenokotXTRA Tablet contains 17.2 mg sennosides.
Senokot-S Tablets: Packages of 10; bottles of 30, 60 and 1000; Unit Strip boxes of 100. Each Senokot-S Tablet contains 8.6 mg sennosides and 50 mg docusate sodium.
Senokot Granules: Cocoa-flavored in 2, 6, and 12 oz. plastic containers. Each teaspoon of Senokot Granules contains 15 mg sennosides.
Senokot Syrup: Chocolate-flavored, alcohol-free, in 2 and 8 fl. oz. bottles.
Senokot Children's Syrup: Chocolate-flavored, alcohol-free syrup in 2.5 fl. oz. plastic bottle packaged with measuring cup. Each teaspoon of Senokot Syrup or Senokot Children's Syrup contains 8.8 mg sennosides.
Copyright 1991, 2002, The Purdue Frederick Company.
Shown in Product Identification Guide, page 523

EDUCATIONAL MATERIAL

Samples Available:
1) Senokot-S® Tablets Samples– 1 display of 12 (4 tablets per packette)
2) Betadine® Brand First Aid Antibiotics + Moisturizer Ointment Samples– 1 display of 48 packettes
3) Betadine® Brand Plus First Aid Antibiotics + Pain Reliever– 1 display of 48 packettes
4) **Up-to-date Information:** www.senokot.com provides dosing information for the Senokot® Products family of laxatives, as well as pa-

tient education about constipation and its causes. A special section on toilet training, written by a pediatrician, describes the popular child-centered approach.

Schering-Plough HealthCare Products
**3 CONNELL DRIVE
BERKELEY HEIGHTS, NJ 07922**

Direct Product Requests to:
Schering-Plough HealthCare Products
3 Connell Drive
Berkeley Heights, NJ 07922
For Medical Emergencies Contact:
Consumer Relations Department
P.O. Box 377
Memphis, TN 38151
(901) 320-2998 (Business Hours)
(901) 320-2364 (After Hours)

CLARITIN® NON-DROWSY 24 HOUR TABLETS
Brand of Loratadine

Drug Facts:

Active Ingredient (in each tablet):   **Purpose:**
Loratadine 10 mg .... Antihistamine

Uses: temporarily relieves these symptoms due to hay fever or other upper respiratory allergies:
• runny nose • itchy, watery eyes
• sneezing • itching of the nose or throat

Warnings:
Do not use if you have ever had an allergic reaction to this product or any of its ingredients.
Ask a doctor before use if you have liver or kidney disease. Your doctor should determine if you need a different dose.
When using this product do not take more than directed. Taking more than directed may cause drowsiness.
Stop use and ask a doctor if an allergic reaction to this product occurs. Seek medical help right away.
If pregnant or breast-feeding, ask a health professional before use.
Keep out of reach of children. In case of overdose, get medical help or contact a Poison Control Center right away.

Directions:

adults and children 6 years and over	1 tablet daily; not more than 1 tablet in 24 hours
children under 6 years of age	ask a doctor
consumers with liver or kidney disease	ask a doctor

Other Information:
• safety sealed: do not use if the individual blister unit imprinted with Claritin® is open or torn

- store between 2° and 3° C (36° and 86° F)
- protect from excessive moisture

Inactive Ingredients: corn starch, lactose monohydrate, magnesium stearate

How Supplied: Boxes of 5, 10 and 20 tablets

Questions or comments?
1-800-CLARITIN (1-800-252-7484) or www.claritin.com

Shown in Product Identification Guide, page 523

CLARITIN-D NON-DROWSY 12 HOUR TABLETS

Drug Facts:

Active Ingredients (in each tablet): **Purpose:**
Loratadine 5 mg .... Antihistamine
Pseudoephedrine sulfate 120 mg .... Nasal decongestant

Uses:
- temporarily relieves these symptoms due to hay fever or other upper respiratory allergies:
  - nasal congestion • runny nose
  - sneezing • itchy, watery eyes
  - itching of the nose or throat
- reduces swelling of nasal passages
- temporarily relieves sinus congestion and pressure
- temporarily restores freer breathing through the nose

Warnings:
Do not use
- if you have ever had an allergic reaction to this product or any of its ingredients
- if you are now taking a prescription monoamine oxidase inhibitor (MAOI) (certain drugs for depression, psychiatric, or emotional conditions, or Parkinson's disease), or for 2 weeks after stopping the MAOI drug. If you do not know if your prescription drug contains an MAOI, ask a doctor or pharmacist before taking this product.

Ask a doctor before use if you have
- heart disease • thyroid disease
- high blood pressure • diabetes
- trouble urinating due to an enlarged prostate gland
- liver or kidney disease. Your doctor should determine if you need a different dose.

When using this product do not take more than directed. Taking more than directed may cause drowsiness.

Stop use and ask a doctor if
- an allergic reaction to this product occurs. Seek medical help right away.
- symptoms do not improve within 7 days or are accompanied by a fever
- nervousness, dizziness or sleeplessness occurs

If pregnant or breast-feeding, ask a health professional before use.

Keep out of reach of children. In case of overdose, get medical help or contact a Poison Control Center right away.

Directions:
- do not divide, crush, chew or dissolve the tablet

adults and children 12 years and over	1 tablet every 12 hours; not more than 2 tablets in 24 hours
children under 12 years of age	ask a doctor
consumers with liver or kidney disease	ask a doctor

Other Information:
- safety sealed: do not use if the individual blister unit imprinted with Claritin-D® 12 Hr. is open or torn
- store between 15° and 25°C (59° and 77°F)
- keep in a dry place

Inactive Ingredients: croscarmellose sodium, dibasic calcium phosphate, hypromellose, lactose monohydrate, magnesium stearate, pharmaceutical ink, povidone, titanium dioxide

How Supplied: Boxes of 10 and 20 tablets

Questions or comments?
1-800-CLARITIN (1-800-252-7484) or www.claritin.com

Shown in Product Identification Guide, page 523

CLARITIN-D NON–DROWSY 24 HOUR TABLETS

Drug Facts:

Active Ingredients (in each tablet): **Purpose:**
Loratadine 10 mg .... Antihistamine
Pseudoephedrine sulfate 240 mg .... Nasal decongestant

Uses:
- temporarily relieves these symptoms due to hay fever or other upper respiratory allergies:
  - nasal congestion • runny nose
  - sneezing • itchy, watery eyes
  - itching of the nose or throat
- reduces swelling of nasal passages
- temporarily relieves sinus congestion and pressure
- temporarily restores freer breathing through the nose

Warnings:
Do not use
- if you have ever had an allergic reaction to this product or any of its ingredients
- if you are now taking a prescription monoamine oxidase inhibitor (MAOI) (certain drugs for depression, psychiatric, or emotional conditions, or Parkinson's disease), or for 2 weeks after stopping the MAOI drug. If you do not know if your prescription drug contains an MAOI, ask a doctor or pharmacist before taking this product.

Ask a doctor before use if you have
- heart disease
- thyroid disease
- high blood pressure
- diabetes
- trouble urinating due to an enlarged prostate gland
- liver or kidney disease. Your doctor should determine if you need a different dose.

When using this product do not take more than directed. Taking more than directed may cause drowsiness.

Stop use and ask a doctor if
- an allergic reaction to this product occurs. Seek medical help right away.
- symptoms do not improve within 7 days or are accompanied by a fever
- nervousness, dizziness or sleeplessness occurs

If pregnant or breast-feeding, ask a health professional before use.

Keep out of reach of children. In case of overdose, get medical help or contact a Poison Control Center right away.

Directions:
- do not divide, crush, chew or dissolve the tablet

adults and children 12 years and over	1 tablet daily with a full glass of water; not more than 1 tablet in 24 hours
children under 12 years of age	ask a doctor
consumers with liver or kidney disease	ask a doctor

Other Information:
- safety sealed: do not use if the individual blister unit imprinted with Claritin-D® 24 hour is open or torn
- store between 20° C to 25° C (68° F to 77° F)
- protect from light and store in a dry place

Inactive Ingredients: carnauba wax, dibasic calcium phosphate, ethylcellulose, hydroxypropyl cellulose, hypromellose, magnesium stearate, pharmaceutical ink, polyethylene glycol, povidone, silicon dioxide, sugar, titanium dioxide, white wax

How Supplied: Boxes of 5 and 10 Tablets

Questions or comments?
1-800-CLARITIN (1-800-252-7484) or www.claritin.com

Shown in Product Identification Guide, page 523

CLARITIN® CHILDREN'S 24 HOUR NON-DROWSY ALLERGY SYRUP

Drug Facts:

Active Ingredient (in each 5 mL): **Purpose:**
Loratadine 5 mg .... Antihistamine

Uses: temporarily relieves these symptoms due to hay fever or other upper respiratory allergies.

Continued on next page

Information on Schering-Plough HealthCare Products appearing on these pages is effective as of November 2002.

Claritin Children's—Cont.

• runny nose • itchy, watery eyes
• sneezing • itching of the nose or throat

Warnings:
Do not use if you have ever had an allergic reaction to this product or any of its ingredients.
Ask a doctor before use if you have liver or kidney disease. Your doctor should determine if you need a different dose.
When using this product do not take more than directed. Taking more than directed may cause drowsiness.
Stop use and ask a doctor if an allergic reaction to this product occurs. Seek medical help right away.
If pregnant or breast-feeding, ask a health professional before use.
Keep out of reach of children. In case of overdose, get medical help or contact a Poison Control Center right away.

Directions:

adults and children 6 years and over	2 teaspoonfuls daily; do not take more than 2 teaspoonfuls in 24 hours
children 2 to under 6 years of age	1 teaspoonful daily; do not take more than 1 teaspoonful in 24 hours
consumers with liver or kidney disease	ask a doctor

Other Information:
• safety sealed: do not use if Schering-Plough HealthCare imprinted bottle wrap is torn or missing
• store between 2° and 25° C (36° and 77° F)

Inactive Ingredients: citric acid, edetate disodium, flavor, glycerin, propylene glycol, sodium benzoate, sugar, water

How Supplied: 4 fl oz bottle
Questions or comments?
1-800-CLARITIN (1-800-252-7484) or www.claritin.com
Shown in Product Identification Guide, page 523

CLARITIN REDITABS 24 HOUR NON-DROWSY ORALLY DISINTEGRATING TABLETS
Brand of Loratadine

Drug Facts:

Active ingredient
(in each tablet):　　　　　　**Purpose:**
Loratadine 10 mg .... Antihistamine

Uses: temporarily relieves these symptoms due to hay fever or other upper respiratory allergies:
• runny nose • itchy, watery eyes
• sneezing • itching of the nose or throat

Warnings: Do not use if you have ever had an allergic reaction to this product or any of its ingredients.

Ask a doctor before use if you have liver or kidney disease. Your doctor should determine if you need a different dose.
When using this product do not take more than directed. Taking more than directed may cause drowsiness.
Stop use and ask a doctor if an allergic reaction to this product occurs. Seek medical help right away.
If pregnant or breast-feeding, ask a health professional before use.
Keep out of reach of children. In case of overdose, get medical help or contact a Poison Control Center right away.

Directions:
• place 1 tablet on tongue; tablet disintegrates, with or without water

adults and children 6 years and over	1 tablet daily; not more than 1 tablet in 24 hours
children under 6 years of age	ask a doctor
consumers with liver or kidney disease	ask a doctor

Other Information:
• safety sealed: do not use if interior foil pouch or individual blister unit imprinte Claritin® RediTabs® inside the foil pouch is open or torn
• store between 2° and 25° C (36° and 77° F)
• keep in a dry place
• use within 6 months of opening foil pouch
• use tablet immediately after opening individual blister

Inactive Ingredients: citric acid, gelatin, mannitol, mint flavor

How Supplied: Boxes of 4 and 10 tablets
Questions or comments?
1-800-CLARITIN (1-800-252-7484) or www.claritin.com
Shown in Product Identification Guide, page 523

Clear Away®
LIQUID WART REMOVER
Clear Away®
GEL with Aloe Wart Remover

Active Ingredient:　　　　　　**Purpose:**
Salicylic acid 17% (w/w) .. Wart remover

Uses:
• for removal of common and plantar warts
• common warts can be easily recognized by the rough cauliflower-like appearance of the surface
• plantar warts can be recognized by its location only on the bottom of the foot, its tenderness, and the interruption of the footprint pattern

Warnings: For external use only
Flammable: Keep away from fire or flame.
Do not use:
• if you are a diabetic
• if you have poor blood circulation

• on irritated skin or any area that is infected or reddened
• on moles, birthmarks, warts with hair growing from them, genital warts, or warts on the face or mucous membranes

When using this product:
• if product gets in eye, flush with water for 15 minutes
• do not inhale vapors
• cap bottle/tube tightly and store at room temperature away from heat
Stop use and ask a doctor if discomfort lasts
Keep out of reach of children. If swallowed, get medical help or contact a Poison Control Center right away.

Directions:
• wash affected area
• may soak wart in warm water for 5 minutes
• dry area thoroughly
• apply one drop of liquid or a thin layer of gel at a time to sufficiently cover each wart
• let dry
• self-adhesive cover-up discs may be used to conceal wart
• repeat procedure once or twice daily as needed (until wart is removed) for up to 12 weeks

Inactive Ingredients:
(Clear Away Liquid Wart Remover): acetone, alcohol SD-32 (17% w/w), balsam oregon, ether (52% w/w), flexible collodion.
(Clear Away Gel with Aloe Wart Remover): alcohol SD-40 (58% w/w), aloe barbadensis extract, ether (16% w/w), ethyl lactate, flexible collodion, hydroxypropyl cellulose, polybutene

How Supplied:
Clear Away® Liquid Wart Remover System: Available in a 1/3 fluid ounce liquid with dropper. Cover up discs help to hide wart while it is removed.

Clear Away® Gel with Aloe Wart Remover: Available in a ½ ounce tube. Cover up discs help to hide wart while it is removed.

CLEAR AWAY®
ONE STEP WART REMOVER
CLEAR AWAY®
ONE STEP WART REMOVER FOR KIDS
CLEAR AWAY®
ONE STEP PLANTAR WART REMOVER
CLEAR AWAY® SYSTEM WART REMOVER
CLEAR AWAY® SYSTEM WART REMOVER WITH INVISIBLE STRIP
CLEAR AWAY® SYSTEM PLANTAR WART REMOVER

Active Ingredient:　　　　　　**Purpose:**
Salicylic Acid 40% .... Wart remover

Uses:
• for removal of common and plantar warts
• common warts can be easily recognized by the rough cauliflower-like appearance of the surface
• plantar warts can be recognized by its location only on the bottom of the foot,

its tenderness, and the interruption of the footprint pattern

Warnings: For external use only
Do not use:
- on children under 2 years of age unless directed by a doctor
- if you are a diabetic
- if you have poor blood circulation
- on irritated skin or any area that is infected or reddened
- on moles, birthmarks, warts with hair growing from them, genital warts, or warts on the face or mucous membranes

Stop use and ask a doctor if discomfort lasts

Keep out of reach of children. If swallowed, get medical help or contact a Poison Control Center right away.

Directions:
- parents should supervise use by children
- wash affected area
- may soak wart in warm water for 5 minutes
- dry area thoroughly
- apply medicated disc/strip/cushioning pad directly over wart
- for Clear Away System wart removers, cover-up discs/adhesive strips/cushioning pads may be used to conceal medicated disc and wart
- repeat procedure every 48 hours as needed (until wart is removed) for up to 12 weeks

Other Information: Store between 15° and 30°C (59° and 86°F)

Inactive Ingredients: Antioxidant (CAS 991-84-4), iron oxides, mineral oil, petroleum hydrocarbon resin, silicon dioxide, synthetic polyisoprene rubber, talc

How Supplied: Clear Away One Step Wart Remover and Clear Away One Step Wart Remover for Kids contain 14 all-in-one medicated strips, Clear Away One Step Plantar Wart Remover contains 16 all-in-one medicated cushioning pads, Clear Away System Wart Remover contains 18 medicated discs and 20 cover-up pads, Clear Away System Plantar Wart Remover contains 24 medicated discs and 24 cushioning pads, Clear Away System Wart Remover with Invisible Strip contains 18 medicated discs and 18 cover-up pads that protect and conceal while treatment is ongoing. Conceals as it Heals™.

Shown in Product Identification Guide, page 524

LOTRIMIN® AF ANTIFUNGAL
[lo-tre-min]
Clotrimazole
Cream 1%
Solution 1%
Lotion 1%
Jock Itch Cream 1%

Description: Lotrimin® AF Cream 1% is a white fully vanishing homogeneous cream containing 1% clotrimazole. The cream contains no sensitizing parabens and is totally grease free and nonstaining.

Lotrimin® AF Solution is a nonaqueous liquid, containing 1% clotrimazole. Also contains polyethylene glycol.
Lotrimin® AF Lotion is a light penetrating buffered emulsion containing 1% clotrimazole. Does not contain common sensitizing agents. Also is greaseless and nonstaining.

Indications: Lotrimin AF Cream, Solution and Lotion cure athlete's foot (tinea pedis), jock itch (tinea cruris) and ringworm (tinea corporis). For effective relief of the itching, cracking, burning, scaling and discomfort which can accompany these conditions.

Directions: Cleanse skin with soap and water and dry thoroughly. Apply a thin layer over affected area morning and evening or as directed by a doctor. For athlete's foot, pay special attention to the spaces between the toes. It is also helpful to wear well-fitting, ventilated shoes and to change shoes and socks at least once daily. Best results in athlete's foot and ringworm are usually obtained with 4 weeks use of this product, and in jock itch with 2 weeks use. If satisfactory results have not occurred within these times, consult a doctor or pharmacist. Children under 12 years of age should be supervised in the use of this product. This product is not effective on the scalp or nails.

Warnings: For external use only. Avoid contact with the eyes. Do not use on children under 2 years of age except under the advice and supervision of a doctor. If irritation occurs or if there is no improvement within 4 weeks (for athlete's foot or ringworm) or within 2 weeks (for jock itch), discontinue use and consult a doctor or pharmacist. Keep this and all drugs out of the reach of children. In case of accidental ingestion, seek professional assistance or contact a Poison Control Center immediately.

How Supplied: Lotrimin® AF Antifungal Cream is available in a 0.42 oz. tube (12 grams) and a 0.84 oz. tube (24 grams). Lotrimin® AF Jock Itch Cream is available in a 0.42 oz tube (12 grams). Inactive ingredients include: cetearyl alcohol, cetyl esters wax, octyldecanol, polysorbate, sorbitan monostearate and water and as a preservative, benzyl alcohol (1%).

Lotrimin® AF Antifungal Solution is available in a 0.33 fl. oz. (10 milliliters) bottle. Inactive ingredient is PEG.

Lotrimin® AF Antifungal Lotion is available in a 0.66 fl. oz. (20 milliliters) bottle. Inactive ingredients include cetearyl alcohol, cetyl esters wax, octyldodecanol, polysorbate, sodium biphosphate, sodium phosphate dibasic, sorbitan monostearate and water and as a preservative, benzyl alcohol (1%).

Storage: Keep Lotrimin® AF Cream and Solution products between 2° and 30°C (36° and 86°F), and Lotrimin® AF

Lotion product between 2° and 25°C (36° and 77°F).

Shown in Product Identification Guide, page 524

LOTRIMIN® AF ANTIFUNGAL
Miconazole Nitrate 2%
Athlete's Foot Spray Liquid
Athlete's Foot Spray Powder
Athlete's Foot Spray Deodorant Powder
Athlete's Foot Powder
Jock Itch Spray Powder

Active Ingredients: SPRAY LIQUID contains Miconazole Nitrate 2%. Also contains: Alcohol SD-40 (17% w/w), Cocamide DEA, Isobutane, Propylene Glycol, Tocopherol (vitamin E).
SPRAY POWDER (Athlete's Foot) contains Miconazole Nitrate 2%. Also contains: Alcohol SD-40 (10% w/w), Isobutane, Starch/Acrylates/Acrylamide Copolymer, Stearalkonium Hectorite, Talc.
SPRAY POWDER (Jock Itch) contains Miconazole Nitrate 2%. Also contains Alcohol SD-40 (10% w/w), Isobutane, Stearalkonium Hectorite, Talc.
SPRAY DEODORANT POWDER contains Miconazole Nitrate 2%. Also contains: Isobutane, Alcohol SD-40 (10% w/w), Talc, Starch/Acrylates/Acrylamide Copolymer, Stearalkonium Hectorite, Fragrance.
POWDER contains Miconazole Nitrate 2%. Also contains: Benzethonium Chloride, Corn Starch, Kaolin, Sodium Bicarbonate, Starch/Acrylates/Acrylamide Copolymer, Zinc Oxide.

Indications: LOTRIMIN® AF Athlete's Foot Spray Liquid, Spray Powder, Spray Deodorant Powder and Powder are proven clinically effective in the treatment of athlete's foot (tinea pedis), jock itch (tinea cruris) and ringworm (tinea corporis). For effective relief of the itching, cracking, burning, scaling and discomfort that can accompany these conditions.
LOTRIMIN AF Powder also aids in the drying of naturally moist areas.
LOTRIMIN® AF Jock Itch Spray Powder cures jock itch (tinea cruris). For effective relief of the itching, burning, scaling and discomfort associated with jock itch.

Warnings: For Athlete's Foot Spray Powder, Spray Liquid, Spray Deodorant Powder and Jock Itch Spray Powder: Do not use on children under 2 years of age unless directed by a doctor. For external use only. Avoid contact with the eyes. If irritation occurs or if there is no improvement within 4 weeks (for athlete's foot and ringworm) or 2 weeks (for

Continued on next page

Information on Schering-Plough HealthCare Products appearing on these pages is effective as of November 2002.

Lotrimin AF Spray—Cont.

jock itch), discontinue use and consult a doctor. Flammable. Do not use while smoking or near heat or flame. Avoid spraying in eyes. Contents under pressure. Do not puncture or incinerate. Do not store at temperature above 120°F. Use only as directed. Intentional misuse by deliberately concentrating and inhaling contents can be harmful or fatal. Keep this and all drugs out of the reach of children. In case of accidental ingestion, seek professional assistance or contact a Poison Control Center immediately.

Lotrimin® AF Powder: Do not use on children under 2 years of age unless directed by a doctor. For external use only. Avoid contact with the eyes. If irritation occurs, or if there is no improvement within 4 weeks (for athlete's foot or ringworm) or within 2 weeks (for jock itch), discontinue use and consult a doctor. Keep this and all drugs out of the reach of children. In case of accidental ingestion, seek professional assistance or contact a Poison Control Center immediately.

Directions: For Athlete's Foot Spray Liquid, Spray Powder, Spray Deodorant Powder and Jock Itch Spray Powder: Wash affected area and dry thoroughly. Shake can well. Spray a thin layer of product over affected area twice daily (morning and night) or as directed by a doctor. Supervise children in the use of this product. For athlete's foot, pay special attention to the spaces between the toes; wear well-fitting, ventilated shoes and change shoes and socks at least once daily. For athlete's foot and ringworm use daily for 4 weeks; for jock itch use daily for 2 weeks. If condition persists longer, consult a doctor. This product is not effective on the scalp or nails.

Powder: Wash affected area and dry thoroughly. Sprinkle a thin layer of product over affected area twice daily (morning and night) or as directed by a doctor. Supervise children in the use of this product. For athlete's foot, pay special attention to the spaces between the toes; wear well-fitting, ventilated shoes and change shoes and socks at least once daily. For athlete's foot and ringworm use daily for 4 weeks; for jock itch use daily for 2 weeks. If condition persists longer, consult a doctor. This product is not effective on the scalp or nails.

Store between 2° and 30° C (36° and 86°F).

How Supplied: LOTRIMIN® AF Athlete's Foot Spray Powder, Spray Deodorant Powder and Jock Itch Spray Powder—3.5 oz. cans. LOTRIMIN® AF Spray Liquid—4 oz. can. LOTRIMIN® AF Powder—3 oz. plastic bottle.

Shown in Product Identification Guide, page 524

LOTRIMIN® ULTRA™

[lo-tre-min]
Butenafine Hydrochloride Cream 1%
Antifungal
Athlete's Foot Cream
Jock Itch Cream

Drug Facts:

Active Ingredient: **Purpose:**
Butenafine
  hydrochloride 1% .... Antifungal

Uses:
Athlete's Foot Cream:
• cures most athlete's foot between the toes. Effectiveness on the bottom or sides of foot is unknown.
• cures most jock itch and ringworm
• relieves itching, burning, cracking, and scaling which accompany these conditions
Jock Itch Cream:
• cures most jock itch
• relieves itching, burning, cracking, and scaling which accompany this condition

Warnings:
For external use only
Do not use
• on nails or scalp
• in or near the mouth or the eyes
• for vaginal yeast infections
When using this product do not get into the eyes. If eye contact occurs, rinse thoroughly with water.
Stop use and ask a doctor if too much irritation occurs or gets worse
Keep out of reach of children. If swallowed, get medical help or contact a Poison Control Center right away.

Directions:
Athlete's Foot Cream:
• adults and children 12 years and older
  • use the tip of the cap to break the seal and open the tube
  • wash the affected skin with soap and water and dry completely before applying

Apply between and
around
the toes

1 week twice a day or
4 weeks once a day

  • **for athlete's foot between the toes:** apply to affected skin between and around the toes twice a day for 1 week (morning and night), or once a day for 4 weeks, or as directed by a doctor. Wear well-fitting, ventilated shoes. Change shoes and socks at least once daily.
  • **for jock itch and ringworm** apply once a day to affected skin for 2 weeks or as directed by a doctor
  • wash hands after each use
• children under 12 years: ask a doctor
Jock Itch Cream:
• adults and children 12 years and over
  • use the tip of the cap to break the seal and open the tube
  • wash the affected skin with soap and water and dry completely before applying
  • apply once a day to affected skin for 2 weeks or as directed by a doctor
  • wash hands after each use
• children under 12 years: ask a doctor

Other Information:
• do not use if seal on tube is broken or is not visible
• store at 5°–30°C (41°–86°F)

Inactive Ingredients: Benzyl alcohol, cetyl alcohol, diethanolamine, glycerin, glyceryl monostearate SE, polyoxyethylene (23) cetyl ether, propylene glycol dicaprylate, purified water, sodium benzoate, stearic acid, white petrolatum

How Supplied: Available in 0.42 oz (12 gram) tubes for both athlete's foot and jock itch. Also available in a 0.85 oz (24 gram) tube for athlete's foot.
Shown in Product Identification Guide, page 524

Standard Homeopathic Company

210 WEST 131st STREET
BOX 61067
LOS ANGELES, CA 90061

Direct Inquiries to:
Jay Borneman
(800) 624-9659 x20

HYLAND'S ARNISPORT™

Formula: Arnica Montana 30X HPUS, Hypericum Perefoliatium 6X HPUS, Ruta Graveolens 6X HPUS, Ledum Palustre 6X HPUS, Bellis Perennis 6X HPUS, plus Hyland's Bioplasma™ in a base of Lactose, N.F.
Hyland's Bioplasma™ contains: Calcarea Fluorica 6X HPUS, Calcarea Phosphorica 3X HPUS, Calcarea Sulphurica 3X HPUS, Ferrum Phosphoricum 3X HPUS, Kali Muriaticum 3X HPUS, Kali Phosphoricum 3X HPUS, Kali Sulphuricum 3X HPUS, Magnesia Phosphorica 3X HPUS, Natrum Muriaticum 6X HPUS, Natrum Phosphoricum 3X HPUS, Natrum Sulphuricum 3X HPUS, Silicea 6X HPUS.

Indications: Natural relief for muscle pain and soreness from overexertion.

Directions: Adults: Dissolve 3–4 tablets in mouth every 2 hours until relieved. Children 2 years or older: Dissolve 1–2 tablets in mouth every 2 hours until relieved.

Warnings: Do not use if imprinted cap band is broken or missing. If symptoms persist for more than 7 days or worsen, contact a licensed health care professional. As with any drug, if you are pregnant or nursing a baby, consult a licensed health care professional before using this or any other medication. Keep this and all medications out of the reach of children. In case of accidental overdose, contact a poison control center immediately. In case of emergency, the manufacturer may be contacted 24 hours a day, 7 days a week by calling 800/624-9659.

How Supplied: Bottles of 50 three-grain sublingual tablets (NDC 54973-0232-01). Store at room temperature.

HYLAND'S BACKACHE WITH ARNICA

Active Ingredients: BENZOICUM ACIDUM 3X HPUS, COLCHICUM AUTUMNALE 3X HPUS, SULPHUR 3X HPUS, ARNICA MONTANA 6X HPUS, RHUS TOXICODENDRON 6X HPUS.

Inactive Ingredients: Lactose, N.F.

Indications: A homeopathic medicine for the temporary relief of symptoms of low back pain due to strain or overexertion.

Directions: Adults and children over 12 years of age: Take 1–2 caplets with water every 4 hours or as needed.

Warnings: Do not use if imprinted cap band is broken or missing. If symptoms persist for more than seven days or worsen, contact a licensed health care professional. As with any drug, if you are pregnant or nursing a baby, seek the advice of a licensed health care professional before using this product. Keep this and all medications out of the reach of children. In case of accidental overdose, contact a poison control center immediately. In case of emergency, the manufacturer may be reached 24 hours a day, 7 days a week at 800/624-9659.

How Supplied: Bottles of 40 5.5 grain caplets (NDC 54973-2965-2). Store at room temperature.

HYLAND'S BUMPS 'N BRUISES™ TABLETS

Active Ingredients: Arnica Montana 6X HPUS, Hypericum Perforatum 6X HPUS, Bellis Perennis 6X HPUS, Ruta Graveolens 6X HPUS.

Inactive Ingredients: Lactose, N.F.

Indications: A homeopathic medicine for the temporary relief of symptoms of bruising and swelling from falls, trauma or overexertion. Easy to take soft tablets dissolve instantly in the mouth.

Directions: For over 1 year of age: Dissolve 3–4 tablets in a teaspoon of water or on the tongue at the time of injury. May be repeated as needed every 15 minutes until relieved.

Warnings: Do not use if imprinted cap band is broken or missing. If symptoms persist for more than 7 days or worsen, consult a licensed health care professional. As with any drug, if you are pregnant or nursing a baby, consult a health care professional before using this product. Keep this and all medications out of the reach of children. In case of accidental overdose, contact a poison control center immediately. In case of emergency,

the manufacturer may be reached 24 hours a day, 7 days a week at 800/624-9659.

How Supplied: Bottles of 125 1-grain sublingual tablets (NDC 54973-7508-1). Store at room temperature.

HYLAND'S CALMS FORTÉ™

Active Ingredients: *Passiflora* (Passion Flower) 1X triple strength HPUS, *Avena Sativa* (Oat) 1X double strength HPUS, *Humulus Lupulus* (Hops) 1X double strength HPUS, *Chamomilla* (Chamomile) 2X HPUS, *Calcarea Phosphorica* (Calcium Phosphate) 3X HPUS, *Ferrum Phosphorica* (Iron Phosphate) 3X HPUS, *Kali Phosphoricum* (Potassium Phosphate) 3X HPUS, *Natrum Phosphoricum* (Sodium Phosphate) 3X HPUS, *Magnesia Phosphoricum* (Magnesium Phosphate) 3X HPUS.

Inactive Ingredients: Lactose, N.F., Calcium Sulfate, Starch (Corn and Tapiocal), Magnesium Stearate.

Indications: Temporary symptomatic relief of simple nervous tension and sleeplessness.

Directions: Adults: As a relaxant: Swallow 1–2 tablets with water as needed, three times daily, preferably before meals. For insomnia: 1 to 3 tablets ½ to 1 hour before retiring. Repeat as needed without danger of side effects. Children: As a relaxant: Swallow 1 tablet with water as needed, three times daily, preferably before meals. For insomnia: 1 to 2 tablets ½ to 1 hour before retiring. Repeat as needed without danger of side effects.

Warning: Do not use if imprinted cap band is broken or missing. If symptoms persist for more than seven days or worsen, consult a licensed health care professional. As with any drug, if you are pregnant or nursing a baby, seek the advice of a licensed health care professional before using this product. Keep this and all medications out of the reach of children. In case of accidental overdose, contact a Poison Control Center immediately. In case of emergency, the manufacturer may be reached 24 hours a day, 7 days a week by calling 800/624-9659.

How Supplied: Bottles of 100 4-grain tablets (NDC 54973-1121-02), 50 4-grain tablets (NDC 54973-1121-01) and 32 5.5-grain caplets (NDC 54973-1121-48). Store at room temperature.

HYLAND'S COLIC TABLETS

Active Ingredients: *Disocorea* (Wild Yam) 3X HPUS, *Chamomilla* (Chamomile) 3X HPUS, *Colocynthinum* (Bitter Apple) 3X HPUS.

Inactive Ingredients: Lactose N.F.

Indications: A homeopathic combination for the temporary relief of symptoms of colic and gas pains caused by irritating food, feeding too quickly, swallowing air and similar conditions during teething, colds and other minor upset periods in children.

Directions: For children up to 2 years of age: Dissolve 2 tablets under the tongue every 15 minutes for up to 8 doses until relieved; then every 2 hours as required. If you prefer, tablets may first be dissolved in a teaspoon of water and then given to the child. Children over 2 years: Dissolve 3 tablets under the tongue as above; or as recommended by a licensed health care professional. Colic Tablets are very soft and dissolve almost instantly under the tongue. If your baby has been crying or has been very upset, your baby may fall asleep after using this product. This is because pain has been relieved and your child can rest.

Warnings: Do not use if imprinted cap band is broken or missing. If symptoms persist for more than seven days or worsen, consult a licensed health care professional. As with any drug, if you are pregnant or nursing a baby, seek the advice of a licensed health care professional before using this product. Keep this and all medications out of the reach of children. In case of accidental overdose, contact a poison control center immediately. In cases of emergency, the manufacturer may be contacted 24 hours a day, 7 days a week at 800/624-9659

How Supplied: Bottles of 125—one grain sublingual tablets (NDC 54973-7502-1). Store at room temperature.

HYLAND'S EARACHE TABLETS

Active Ingredients: Pulsatilla (Wind Flower) 30C, HPUS; Chamomilla (Chamomile) 30C, HPUS; Sulphur 30C, HPUS; Calcarea Carbonica (Carbonate of Lime) 30C, HPUS; Belladonna 30C, HPUS; (3×10^{-60} % Alkaloids) and Lycopodium (Club Moss) 30C, HPUS.

Inactive Ingredients: Lactose NF

Indications: For the relief of symptoms of fever, pain, irritability and sleeplessness associated with earaches in children after diagnosis by a physician. If symptoms persist for more than 48 hours or if there is a discharge from the ear, discontinue use and contact your health care professional.

Directions: Dissolve 4 tablets under the tongue 3 times per day for 48 hours or until symptoms subside. If you prefer, tablets may be dissolved in a teaspoon of water and then given to the child. Earache Tablets are very soft and dissolve almost instantly under the tongue.

Warnings: Do not use if imprinted blisters are broken or damaged. If symptoms persist for more than 48 hours, or if there is a discharge from the ear, discontinue

Continued on next page

Hyland's Earache—Cont.

use and consult a licensed health care professional. As with any drug, if you are pregnant or nursing a baby, seek the advice of a licensed health care professional before using this product. Keep this and all medications out of the reach of children. In case of accidental overdose, contact a poison control center immediately. In cases of emergency, the manufacturer may be contacted 24 hours a day, 7 days a week at 800/624-9659.

How Supplied: Blister pack of 40 tablets (NDC 54973-7507-1). Store at room temperature.

HYLAND'S LEG CRAMPS WITH QUININE

Active Ingredients: Cinchona Officinalis 3X, HPUS (Quinine), Viscum Album 3X, HPUS; Gnaphalium Polycephalum 3X, HPUS; Rhus Toxicodendron 6X, HPUS; Aconitum Napellus 6X, HPUS; Ledum Palustre 6X, HPUS; Magnesia Phosphorica 6X, HPUS.

Inactive Ingredients: Lactose, N.F.

Indications: Hyland's Leg Cramps is a traditional homeopathic formula for the relief of symptoms of cramps and pains in lower back and legs often made worse by damp weather. Working without contraindications or side effects, Hyland's Leg Cramps stimulates your body's natural healing response to relieve symptoms. Hyland's Leg Cramps is safe for adults and can be used in conjuction with other medications.

Directions: Adults: Dissolve 2–3 tablets under tongue every 4 hours as needed.

Warnings: Do not use if imprinted cap band is missing or broken. If symptoms persist for more than seven days or worsen, contact a licensed health care professional. As with any drug, if you are pregnant or nursing a baby, seek the advice of a licensed health care professional before using this product. Do not use if pregnant, sensitive to quinine or under 12 years of age. Keep this and all medications out of the reach of children. In case of accidental overdose, contact a poison control center immediately. In case of emergency, the manufacturer may be reached 24 hours a day, 7 days a week at 800-624-9659.

How Supplied: Bottles of 100 three-grain sublingual tablets (NDC 54973-2956-02), Bottles of 50 three-grain sublingual tablets (NDC 54973-2956-01), Bottles of 40 5.5 grain caplets (NDC 54973-2956-68). Store at room temperature.

HYLAND'S MIGRAINE HEADACHE RELIEF TABLETS

Active Ingredients:
Glononium 12X HPUS, Belladonna 6X HPUS, Gelsemium 6X HPUS, Nux Vomica 6X HPUS, Iris Versicolor 6X HPUS, Sanguinaria Canadensis 6X HPUS.

Inactive Ingredients: Lactose NF.

Indications: Temporarily relieves the symptoms of migraine pain.

Directions: Adults and Children over 12 years of age: Dissolve 1 to 2 tablets on tongue every 4 hours or as needed.

Warnings: Ask a doctor before use if pregnant or nursing. Consult a physician if symptoms persist for more than 7 days or worsen. Keep out of the reach of children. Do not use if imprinted tamper band is broken or missing. In case of accidental overdose, contact a poison control center immediately. In case of emergency, the manufacturer may be contacted 24 hours a day, 7 days a week at 800/624-9659.

How Supplied: Bottles of 60 3-grain tablets. (NDC 54973-3013-01). Store at room temperature.
Hyland's, Inc.
Los Angeles, CA 90061
800/624-9659
www.hylands.com

HYLAND'S MENOCALM™

Ingredients: AMYL NITROSUM 6X HPUS, SANGUINARIA CAN. 3X HPUS, LACHESIS MUTA 12X HPUS, CIMICIFUGA RACEMOSA 10MG RHIZOME (AS 40 MG CIMIPURE STANDARDIZED TO PROVIDE 4 MG TRITERPENE GLYCOSIDES DAILY), CALCIUM CITRATE USP 953 MG (TO PROVIDE 800MG CALCIUM PER DAY) EXCIPIENTS 5% (CELLULOSE, CROSCARMELLOSE SODIUM, VEGETABLE STEARIC ACID, SILICA, VEGETABLE MAGNESIUM STEARATE WITH A CELLULOSE COATING.)

Indications: Symptomatic relief for hot flashes, moodiness and irritability associated with menopause.

Directions: Take 2 tablets two times per day. Due to the calcium in MenoCalm™, the tablets are large. You may break the tablets along the score line without affecting the product's effectiveness. If symptoms persist for more than 14 days, discontinue use and contact your health care provider.

Warnings: Do not use if imprinted cap band is broken or missing. If symptoms persist for more than 14 days or worsen, consult a licensed health care practitioner. Do not use this product if your are pregnant or nursing. Keep this and all medications out of the reach of children. In case of accidental overdose, contact a poison control center immediately. In cases of emergency, the manufacturer may be contacted 24 hours a day, 7 days a week at 800/624-9659.

How Supplied: Bottles of 84 seven-grain tablets (NDC 54973-6056-1). Store at room temperature.

HYLAND'S NERVE TONIC

Active Ingredients: Calcarea Phosphorica (Calcium Phosphate) 3X HPUS; Ferrum Phosphorica (Iron Phosphate) 3X HPUS; Kali Phosphoricum (Potassium Phosphate) 3X HPUS; Natrum Phosphoricum (Sodium Phosphate) 3X HPUS; Magnesia Phosphoricum (Magnesium Phosphate) 3X HPUS.

Inactive Ingredients: Lactose, N.F.

Indications: Temporary symtomatic relief of simple nervous tension and stress.

Directions: Adults take 2–6 tablets before each meal and at bedtime. Children: 2 tablets. In severe cases take 3 tablets every 2 hours.

Warnings: Do not use if imprinted cap band is broken or missing. If symptoms persist for more than seven days or worsen, contact a licensed health care professional. As with any drug, if you are pregnant or nursing a baby, seek the advice of a licensed health care professional before using this product. Keep this and all medications out of the reach of children. In case of accidental overdose, contact a poison control center immediately. In cases of emergency, the manufacturer may be contacted 24 hours a day, 7 days a week at 800/624-9659.

How Supplied: Bottles of 32 caplets (NDC 54973-1129-68), Bottles of 500 tablets (NDC 54973-1129-1), Bottles of 1000 tablets (NDC 54973-1129-2)

SMILE'S PRID ®

Contains: Acidum Carbolicum 2X HPUS, Ichthammol 2X HPUS, Arnica Montana 3X HPUS, Calendula Off 3X HPUS, Echinacea Ang 3X HPUS, Sulphur 12X HPUS, Hepar Sulph 12X HPUS, Silicea 12X HPUS, Rosin, Beeswax, Petrolatum, Stearyl Alcohol, Methyl & Propyl Paraben.

Indications: Temporary topical relief of pain symptoms associated with boils, minor skin eruptions, redness and irritation. Also aids in relieving the discomfort of superficial cuts, scratches and wounds.

Directions: Wash affected parts with hot water, dry and apply PRID® twice daily on clean bandage or gauze. Do not squeeze or pressure irritated skin area. After irritation subsides, repeat application once a day for several days. Children under two years: consult a physician. CAUTION: If symptoms persist for more than seven days or worsen, or if fever occurs, contact a licensed health care professional. Do not use on broken skin. Keep out of reach of children. In case of

accidental ingestion, seek professional assistance or contact a poison control center. For external use only. Avoid contact with eyes.

How Supplied: 18GM tin (NDC 0619-4202-54). Keep in a cool dry place.

HYLAND'S TEETHING GEL

Active Ingredients: Calcarea Phosphorica (Calcium Phosphate) 12X, HPUS; Chamomilla (Chamomile) 6X, HPUS; Coffea Cruda (Coffee) 6X, HPUS; and Belladonna 6X, HPUS (Alkaloids 0.0000003%)

Inactive Ingredients: Deionized water, Vegetable Glycerin, Hydroxyethyl Cellulose, Methyl Paraben and Propyl Paraben.

Indications: A homeopathic combination for the temporary relief of symptoms of simple restlessness and wakeful irritability due to cutting teeth.

Directions: Apply to gums as necessary. If symptoms persist for more than seven days or worsen, discontinue use and contact your health care professional. Please note, if your baby has been crying or has been very upset, your baby may fall asleep after using this product because the pain has been relieved and your child can rest.

Warnings: Do not use if tube tip is broken or missing. If symptoms persist for more than seven days or if irritation persists, inflammation develops or fever or infection develop, discontinue use and consult a licensed health care professional. As with any drug, if you are pregnant or nursing a baby, seek the advice of a licensed health care professional before using this product. Keep this and all medications out of the reach of children. In case of accidental overdose, contact a poison control center immediately. In case of emergency, the manufacturer may be contacted 24 hours a day, 7 days a week at 800/624-9659.

How Supplied: Tubes of 1/3 OZ. (NDC 54973-7504-3). Store at room temperature.

HYLAND'S TEETHING TABLETS

Active Ingredients: *Calcarea Phosphorica* (Calcium Phosphate) 3X HPUS, *Chamomilla* (Chamomile) 3X HPUS, *Coffea Cruda* (Coffee) 3X HPUS, *Belladonna* 3X HPUS (Alkaloids 0.0003%).

Inactive Ingredients: Lactose N.F.

Indications: A homeopathic combination for the temporary relief of symptoms of simple restlessness and wakeful irritability due to cutting teeth.

Directions: Dissolve 2 to 3 tablets under the tongue 4 times per day. If you prefer, tablets may first be dissolved in a

teaspoon of water and then given to the child. If the child is restless or wakeful, 2 tablets every hour for 6 doses or as recommended by a licensed health care professional. Teething Tablets are very soft and dissolve almost instantly under the tongue. Please note, if your baby has been crying or has been very upset, your baby may fall asleep after using this product because the pain has been relieved and your child can rest.

Warning: Do Not use if imprinted cap band is broken or missing. If symptoms persist for more than seven days, or if irritation persist, inflammation develops or fever or infection develop, discontinue use and consult a licensed health care professional. As with any drug, if you are pregnant or nursing a baby, seek the advice of a health care professional before using this product. Keep this and all medications out of the reach of children. In case of accidental overdose, contact a poison control center immediately. In case of emergency, the manufacturer may be contacted 24 hours a day, 7 days a week at 800/624-9659.

How Supplied: Bottles of 125—one grain sublingual tablets (NDC 54973-7504-01). Store at room temperature.

Topical BioMedics, Inc.
**PO BOX 494
RHINEBECK, NEW YORK 12572**

Direct Inquiries to:
phone (845) 871-4900

TOPRICIN®
[tŏp 'rə-sĭn"]

Key Facts: Topricin® is an odorless non-irritating anti-inflammatory pain relief cream that provides excellent adjunctive support in medical treatments such as post surgical, physical and occupational therapy, chiropractic. Greaseless and contains no lanolin, menthol, capsaicin, or fragrances.

Active Ingredients: (HPUS) Arnica Montana 6X, Echinacea 6X, Aesculus 6X, Ruta Graveolens 6X, Lachesis 8X, Rhus Tox 6X Belladonna 6X, Crotalus 8X, Heloderma 8X, Naja 8X, Graphites 6X.

Inactive Ingredients: purified water, highly refined vegetable oils, glycerin, medium-chain-triglyceride.

Major Uses: Topical relief of inflammation & pain, and a healing treatment for soft tissue & trauma/sports injuries.
Benefits: relieves swelling, stiffness, numbness, tingling and burning pain associated with these soft tissue ailments: carpal tunnel syndrome, other neuropathic pain, arthritis, lower back pain, muscle spasm of the back, neck, legs, and feet, muscle soreness, crushing injury, and sprains. First aid: bruises, minor burns. Use before and after exercise

Directions: Apply generously 3–4 times a day or more often if needed making sure to cover the entire joint or area of pain. Massage in until absorbed. Reapply before bed and at the start of the day for best results.
For further information go to www.topicalbiomedics.com
Safety Information: For external use only, use only as directed, if pain persists for more than 7 days or worsens, Consult a doctor. This homeopathic medicine has no known side effects or contraindications. Complies with FDA standards as an OTC medicine. Safe to use for children, adults, pregnant women and the elderly.

How Supplied: 4 oz jars & 2 oz tube
Shown in Product Identification Guide, page 524

UAS Laboratories
**5610 ROWLAND RD #110
MINNETONKA, MN 55343**

Direct Inquiries To:
Dr. S.K. Dash: (952) 935-1707
(952) 935-1650

Medical Emergency Contact:
Dr. S.K. Dash: (952) 935-1707
Fax: (952) 935-1650

DDS®-ACIDOPHILUS
Capsule, Tablet & Powder free of dairy products, corn, soy, and preservatives

Description: DDS®-Acidophilus is the source of a special strain of Lactobacillus acidophilus free of dairy products, corn, soy and preservatives. Each capsule or tablet contains one billion viable DDS®-1 L.acidophilus at the time of manufacturing. One gram of powder contains two billion viable DDS®-1 L.acidophilus.

Indications and Usages: An aid in implanting the gut with beneficial Lactobacillus acidophilus under conditions of digestive disorders, acne, yeast infections, and following antibiotic therapy.

Administration: One to two capsules or tablets twice daily before meals. One-fourth teaspoon powder can be substituted for two capsules or tablets.

Continued on next page

DDS-Acidophilus—Cont.

How Supplied: Bottles of 100 capsules or tablets. 12 bottles per case. Powder is available in 2 oz. bottle; 12 bottles per case.

Storage: Keep refrigerated under 40°F.

EDUCATIONAL MATERIAL

DDS®-Acidophilus
Booklet describing superior-strain Acidophilus without dairy products, corn, soy, or preservatives. Two billion viable DDS®-1. L.acidopohilus per gram.

Upsher-Smith Laboratories, Inc.

**14905 23rd AVENUE N.
PLYMOUTH, MN 55447**

Direct inquiries to:
Professional Services
(763) 475-3023
Fax (763) 249-1832

AMLACTIN® 12% Moisturizing Lotion and Cream
[ăm-lăk-tĭn]
Cosmetic Lotion and Cream

Description: AMLACTIN® Moisturizing Lotion and Cream are special formulations of 12% lactic acid neutralized with ammonium hydroxide to provide a lotion or cream pH of 4.5–5.5. Lactic acid, an alpha-hydroxy acid, is a naturally occurring humectant for the skin. AMLACTIN® moisturizes and softens rough, dry skin.

How Supplied: 225g (8oz) plastic bottle: List No. 0245-0023-22
400g (14oz) plastic bottle: List No. 0245-0023-40
140g (4.9oz) tube: List No. 0245-0024-14

AMLACTIN® AP Anti-Itch Moisturizing Cream
[ăm-lăk'-tĭn]
1% Pramoxine HCl

Description: AMLACTIN® AP Anti-Itch Moisturizing Cream is a special formulation containing 12% lactic acid neutralized with ammonium hydroxide to provide a cream pH of 4.5–5.5 with pramoxine HCl. Lactic acid, an alpha-hydroxy acid, is a naturally occurring humectant which moisturizes and softens rough, dry skin. Pramoxine HCl, USP,

1% is an effective antipruritic ingredient used to relieve itching associated with dry skin.

How Supplied: 140g (4.9oz) tube: NDC No. 0245-0025-14

Wellness International Network, Ltd.

**5800 DEMOCRACY DRIVE
PLANO, TX 75024**

Direct Inquiries to:
Product Coordinator
(972) 312-1100
FAX: (972) 943-5250

BIO-COMPLEX 5000™
Gentle Foaming Cleanser

Uses: BIO-COMPLEX 5000™ Gentle Foaming Cleanser, with alpha-hydroxy acids, aloe vera and botanical infusions, is an advanced cleansing gel designed for all skin types. BIO-COMPLEX 5000 Gentle Foaming Cleanser protects the skin and works to restore elasticity while gently removing surface impurities, make-up and pollution.

Ingredients: Water (Aqua), Ammonium Lauryl Sulfate, Lauramidopropyl Betaine, Salvia Officinalis (Sage) Leaf Extract, Anthemis Nobilis Flower Extract, Glycerin, Lauramide DEA, Cetyl Betaine, Tocopherol (Vitamin E), Ascorbic Acid (Vitamin C), Citric Acid, Methylchloroisothiazolinone, Methylisothiazolinone, Aloe Barbadensis Leaf Juice, Lactic Acid, Malic Acid, Propylparaben, Methylparaben.

Directions: Splash warm water onto face. Place a small amount of gel on fingertips. Apply evenly to face and neck in circular motions, massaging skin gently but thoroughly. Rinse completely and pat dry with a soft towel.

How Supplied: 8 fluid ounce/236 ml. bottle.

BIO-COMPLEX 5000™
Revitalizing Conditioner

Uses: BIO-COMPLEX 5000™ Revitalizing Conditioner, with vitamins and anti-oxidants, helps restore moisture to dried-out, heat-styled hair. This advanced conditioner contains silkening agents which enhance the hair as well as detangle it after shampooing. Hair is left clean, soft, manageable, and protected against styling aids and environmental elements. BIO-COMPLEX 5000™ Revitalizing Conditioner is excellent for all hair types, especially damaged or over-processed hair.

Ingredients: Water, Stearyl Alcohol, Propylene Glycol, Stearamidopropyl Dimethylamine, Cyclomethicone, Polyquaternium - 11, Stearalkonium Chloride, Cetearyl Alcohol, PEG - 40 Hydrogenated Castor Oil, Citric Acid, Tocopherol (Vitamin E), Ascorbic Acid (Vitamin C), Retinyl Palmitate (Vitamin A), Ethylhexyl Methoxycinnamate Fragrance (Parfum), Ceteth - 20, Hydrolyzed Keratin, Sodium Chloride, Imidazolidinyl Urea, Methylparaben, Propylparaben.

Directions: After shampooing with BIO-COMPLEX 5000™ Revitalizing Shampoo, apply to wet hair. Massage through hair, paying special attention to the ends. Leave on 2–3 minutes. Rinse thoroughly. Towel dry and style as usual.

How Supplied: 12 fluid ounce bottle.

BIO-COMPLEX 5000™
Revitalizing Shampoo

Uses: BIO-COMPLEX 5000™ Revitalizing Shampoo, with vitamins and antioxidants, cleanses and moisturizes hair for excellent manageability. Specially formulated with the essence of awapuhi, a Hawaiian ginger plant extract known for its healing qualities, this formula contains the mildest blend of surfactants and a wealth of natural conditioning ingredients to provide body, luster and healthier-looking hair.

Ingredients: Water, Ammonium Lauryl Sulfate, Tea Lauryl Sulfate, Cocamidopropyl Betaine, Lauramide DEA, Cetyl Betaine, Glycerin, Ascorbic Acid (Vitamin C), Tocopherol (Vitamin E), Retinyl Palmitate (Vitamin A), Citric Acid, Hydrolyzed Wheat Protein, Fragrance (Parfum), Ethylhexyl Methoxycinnamate, PEG - 7 Glyceryl Cocoate, Methylchloroisothiazolinone, Methylisothiazolinone, Caramel.

Directions: Apply a small amount to wet hair and massage gently into scalp, creating a generous lather. Rinse and repeat if necessary. To further intensify this reconstructive process, follow with BIO-COMPLEX 5000™ Revitalizing Conditioner.

How Supplied: 12 fluid ounce bottle.

STEPHAN™ BIO-NUTRITIONAL
Daytime Hydrating Creme

Uses: Hypo-allergenic STEPHAN™ BIO-NUTRITIONAL Daytime Hydrating Creme hydrates the skin and preserves the moisture level of the upper layers of the epidermis. It is an excellent day cream for both men and women who wish to combat the visible signs of aging skin, the appearance of wrinkles or lines, and the inelastic look of facial features and contours. These light emulsions are absorbed rapidly, leaving an invisible

protective film which hydrates the epidermis, regulates moisture levels and leaves skin feeling supple and soft.

Ingredients: Water (Aqua), Stearic Acid, Isodecyl Neopentanoate, Isostearyl Stearoyl Stearate, DEA-Cetyl Phosphate, C12-15 Alkyl Benzoate, Tocopherol (Vitamin E), Aloe Barbadensis Leaf Juice, Squalane, Cetyl Esters, Benzophenone-3, Dimethicone, Fragrance (Parfum), Carbomer, Triethanolamine, Imidazolidinyl Urea, Methylparaben, Propylparaben, Annatto.

Directions: Apply in the morning and during the day to clean skin. May be used around the eye area, avoiding direct contact with the eyes. Suitable for all skin types. For best results, use in conjunction with the complete STEPHAN BIO-NUTRITIONAL Skin Care line.

Warnings: For external use only. Avoid contact with eyes.

How Supplied: Net Wt. 1.75 oz.

STEPHAN™ BIO-NUTRITIONAL
Eye-Firming Concentrate

Uses: Hypo-allergenic STEPHAN™ BIO-NUTRITIONAL Eye-Firming Concentrate is specially formulated to revitalize the delicate area around the eyes. This non-oily fluid pampers sensitive eyes while reducing the look of puffiness and dark circles, and smoothing and softening the appearance of fine lines in the eye area.

Ingredients: Purified water, Cornflower extract, Methylsilanol hydroxyproline aspirate, Methyl cluceth-20, Dimethicone copolyol, Peg-30, Glyceryl laurate, Horsetail extract, Panthenol, Propylene glycol, Carbomer, Disodium edta, Triethanolamine, Xanthan gum, Diazolidinyl urea, Methylparaben, Propylparaben

Directions: Apply in the morning, or any time of the day, in small quantities to the skin around the eyes with light, tapping motions, avoiding direct contact with the eyes. In the evening, apply gently to the entire eye contour area. For best results, use in conjunction with the complete STEPHAN BIO-NUTRITIONAL Skin Care line.

Warnings: For external use only. Avoid direct contact with eyes.

How Supplied: 1 fl. oz.

STEPHAN™ BIO-NUTRITIONAL
Nightime Moisture Creme

Uses: Hypo-allergenic STEPHAN™ BIO-NUTRITIONAL Nightime Moisture Creme is a heavier, richer cream for mature, dry or sun-damaged skin. This advanced formula is excellent for dehydrated skin, promoting suppleness and moisture, while improving the appearance of fine lines and wrinkles.

Ingredients: Water (Aqua), Caprylic/Capric Triglyceride, Propylene, Glycol/Dicaprylate/Dicaprate, Stearic Acid, Polysorbate 60, Cetyl Alcohol, Ethylhexyl Palmitate, Cera Alba (Beeswax), Sorbitan Stearate, Canola Oil, Persea Gratissima (Avocado) Oil, Carthamus Tinctorius (safflower) Seed Oil, Squalane, Lecithin (Liposomes), Soluble Collagen, Dimethicone, Bisabolol, Aloe Barbadensis Leaf Juice, Fragrance (Parfum), C12–15 Alkyl Benzoate, Hydroxyethylcellulose, Alcohol, Ethylhexyl Methoxycinnamate, Disodium EDTA, Sodium Borate, Benzophenone-3, Allantoin, Potassium Sorbate, Phenoxyethanol, Methylparaben, Propylparaben, Butylparaben, Ethylparaben, Yellow 10, Caramel.

Directions: In the evening, apply by lightly massaging onto a thoroughly cleansed face and neck. Avoid direct contact with eyes. For drier skin, it may be used during the day as a moisturizer, under make-up or after sun bathing. For best results, use in conjunction with the complete STEPHAN BIO-NUTRITIONAL Skin Care line.

Warning: For external use only. Avoid contact with eyes.

How Supplied: Net Wt. 1.75 oz.

STEPHAN™ BIO-NUTRITIONAL
Refreshing Moisture Gel

Uses: Hypo-allergenic STEPHAN™ BIO-NUTRITIONAL Refreshing Moisture Gel is specially formulated to refine pores and promote a clear, clean and smooth-looking complexion. It is designed to deeply cleanse and super-stimulate the skin. This gel is suitable for all skin types, especially problem areas. A quick "pick-me-up," STEPHAN BIO-NUTRITIONAL Refreshing Moisture Gel immediately restores the radiant, firm and youthful appearance of the face while acting as a cumulative, revitalizing beauty treatment.

Ingredients: Water (Aqua), Propylene Glycol, Glycerin, Hydroxyethylcellulose, Saccharum Officinarum (Sugar Cane) Extract, Citrus Unshiu Extract, Pyrus Malus (Apple) Extract, Camellia Oleifera Leaf Extract, Hydrolyzed Wheat Protein, Yeast Extract, Saccharomyces Lysate Extract, Panthenol, Aloe Barbadensis Leaf Juice, Phenethyl Alcohol, Laureth-4, Magnesium Aluminum Silicate, Tetrasodium EDTA, Benzophenone-3, Imidazolidinyl Urea, Methylchloroisothiazolinone, Methylisothiazolinone, Methylparaben, Propylparaben, Yellow 10, Red 40, Yellow 5.

Directions: Apply to clean skin at anytime. Remove after 20 minutes with warm water. Can be used around the eye area, avoiding direct contact with the eyes. Suitable for all skin types. For best results, use in conjunction with the complete STEPHAN BIO-NUTRITIONAL Skin Care line.

Warnings: For external use only. Avoid contact with eyes.

How Supplied: Net Wt. 1.75 oz.

STEPHAN™ BIO-NUTRITIONAL
Ultra Hydrating Fluid

Uses: Hypo-allergenic STEPHAN™ BIO-NUTRITIONAL Ultra Hydrating Fluid is a complete treatment formulated to soften fine lines and preserve youthful-looking, radiant skin. By utilizing ingredients focused on revitalization, STEPHAN BIO-NUTRITIONAL Ultra Hydrating Fluid possesses a progressive firming effect, helping to combat the aged look of skin due to external negative conditions.

Ingredients: Water (Aqua), Methylsilanol Hydroxyproline Aspartate, Methyl Gluceth-20, Dimethicone Copolyol, Peg-30 Glyceryl Laurate, Panthenol Saccharum Officinarum (Sugar Cane) Extract, Citrus Unshiu Extract, Pyrus Malus (Apple) Extract, Cammelia Oleifera Leaf Extract, Saccharomyces Lysate Extract, Laureth-4, Yeast Extract, Hydrolyzed Wheat Protein, Methylchloroisothiazolinone, Methylisothiazolinone, Phenethyl Alcohol, 2-Bromo-2-Nitropropane-1, 3Diol, Xanthan Gum, Disodium EDTA, Methylparaben, Propylparaben.

Directions: Gently apply all over the face, neck and eye contour area, preferably in the morning. Make-up can be applied afterwards. Use as a part of a regular daily skin care routine or as an occasional preventive treatment. For best results, use in conjunction with the complete STEPHAN BIO-NUTRITIONAL Skin Care line.

Warnings: For external use only. Avoid direct contact with eyes.

How Supplied: 1 fl. oz.

Wyeth Consumer Healthcare
Wyeth

FIVE GIRALDA FARMS
MADISON, NJ 07940

Direct Inquiries to:
Wyeth Consumer Healthcare Product Information 800-322-3129

ADVIL®
Ibuprofen Tablets, USP
Ibuprofen Caplets (Oval-Shaped Tablets)
Ibuprofen Gel Caplets (Oval-Shaped Gelatin Coated Tablets)
Ibuprofen Liqui-Gel Capsules
Fever reducer/Pain reliever

Active Ingredient: Each tablet, caplet, or liquigel capsule contains Ibuprofen 200 mg

Uses: temporarily relieves minor aches and pains due to the common cold, headache, toothache, muscular aches, backache, minor pain of arthritis, menstrual cramps; and temporarily reduces fever.

Warnings
Allergy alert: ibuprofen may cause a severe allergic reaction which may include:
- hives
- facial swelling
- asthma (wheezing)
- shock

Alcohol warning: if you consume 3 or more alcoholic drinks every day, ask your doctor whether you should take ibuprofen or other pain relievers/fever reducers. Ibuprofen may cause stomach bleeding.

Do not use if you have ever had an allergic reaction to any other pain reliever/fever reducer

Ask a doctor before use if you have
- had problems or side effects with any pain reliever/fever reducer
- stomach pain

Ask a doctor or pharmacist before use if you are
- under a doctor's care for any continuing medical condition
- taking other drugs on a regular basis
- taking any other product containing ibuprofen, or any other pain reliever/fever reducer

When using this product take with food or milk if stomach upset occurs

Stop use and ask a doctor if
- an allergic reaction occurs. Seek medical help right away.
- fever gets worse or lasts more than 3 days
- pain gets worse or lasts more than 10 days
- stomach pain occurs with the use of this product
- the painful area is red or swollen
- any new or unexpected symptoms occur

If pregnant or breast-feeding, ask a health professional before use. It is especially important not to use ibuprofen during the last 3 months of pregnancy unless definitely directed to do so by a doctor because it may cause problems in the unborn child or complications during delivery.

Keep out of reach of children. In case of overdose, get medical help or contact a Poison Control Center right away.

Dosage and Administration:
Directions—Do not take more than directed
Adults:
- take 1 tablet, caplet, gelcap or liquigel capsule every 4 to 6 hours while symptoms occur
- if pain or fever does not respond to 1 tablet, caplet, gelcap, or liquigel capsule, 2 tablets, caplets, gelcaps or liquigel capsules may be used, but do not exceed 6 tablets, caplets, gelcaps or liquigel capsules in 24 hours, unless directed by a doctor
- the smallest effective dose should be used

Children: do not give to children under 12 unless directed by a doctor

Inactive Ingredients:
Tablets and Caplets: acetylated monoglyceride, beeswax and/or carnauba wax, croscarmellose sodium, iron oxides, lecithin, methylparaben, microcrystalline cellulose, pharmaceutical glaze, povidone, propylparaben, silicon dioxide, simethicone, sodium benzoate, sodium lauryl sulfate, starch, stearic acid, sucrose, titanium dioxide.

Gel Caplets: croscarmellose sodium, FD&C red no. 40, FD&C yellow no. 6, gelatin, glycerin, hypromellose, iron oxides, medium chain triglycerides, pharmaceutical ink, propyl gallate, silicon dioxide, sodium lauryl sulfate, starch, stearic acid, titanium dioxide, triacetin

Liqui-Gels: FD&C green no. 3, gelatin, pharmaceutical ink, polyethylene glycol, potassium hydroxide, purified water, sorbitan, sorbitol.

Storage: Store at 20–25°C (68–77°F) Avoid excessive heat 40°C (above 104°F)

How Supplied:
Coated tablets in bottles of 6, 8, 24, 50, 100, 165 (non-child resistant), and 225.
Coated caplets in bottles of 24, 50, 100, 165 (non-child resistant), and 225.
Gel caplets in bottles of 24, 50, 100, 165 (non-child resistant) and 225.
Liqui-Gels in bottles of 20, 40, 80, 135 (non-child resistant) and 180.

ADVIL® ALLERGY SINUS CAPLETS
Pain Reliever/Fever Reducer
Nasal Decongestant
Antihistamine

Active Ingredients (in each caplet):
Chlorpheniramine maleate 2 mg
Ibuprofen 200 mg
Pseudoephedrine HCl 30 mg

Uses:
- temporarily relieves these symptoms associated with hay fever or other upper respiratory allergies, and the common cold:
  - runny nose • sneezing • headache • itchy, watery eyes
  - nasal congestion • minor aches and pains • itching of the nose or throat
  - sinus pressure • fever

Warnings:
Allergy alert: Ibuprofen may cause a severe allergic reaction which may include:
- hives • facial swelling • asthma (wheezing) • shock

Stomach bleeding warning: Taking more than recommended may cause stomach bleeding.

Alcohol warning: If you consume 3 or more alcoholic drinks every day, ask your doctor whether you should take ibuprofen or other pain relievers/fever reducers. Ibuprofen may cause stomach bleeding.

Do not use
- if you have ever had an allergic reaction to any other pain reliever/fever reducer
- if you are now taking a prescription monoamine oxidase inhibitor (MAOI) (certain drugs for depression, psychiatric, or emotional conditions, or Parkinson's disease), or for 2 weeks after stopping the MAOI drug. If you do not know if your prescription drug contains an MAOI, ask a doctor or pharmacist before taking this product.

Ask a doctor before use is you have
- a breathing problem such as emphysema or chronic bronchitis
- heart disease • high blood pressure • thyroid disease • diabetes • kidney disease • ulcers • bleeding problems • glaucoma
- problems or serious side effects from taking pain relievers or fever reducers
- stomach problems that last or come back, such as heartburn, upset stomach, or pain
- trouble urinating due to an enlarged prostate gland

Ask a doctor or pharmacist before use if you are
- under a doctor's care for any serious condition
- taking sedatives or tranquilizers
- over 65 years of age
- taking any other product that contains ibuprofen, or any other pain reliever/fever reducer
- taking any other product that contains pseudoephedrine, chlorpheniramine or any other nasal decongestant or antihistamine
- taking a prescription drug for anticoagulation (blood thinning), or a diuretic
- taking any other drug

When using this product
- do not use more than directed
- avoid alcoholic drinks
- be careful when driving a motor vehicle or operating machinery
- drowsiness may occur
- take with food or milk if stomach upset occurs
- alcohol, sedatives, and tranquilizers may increase drowsiness

Stop use and ask a doctor if
- an allergic reaction occurs. Seek medical help right away.
- nasal congestion lasts for more than 7 days
- fever lasts for more than 3 days
- you get nervous, dizzy, or sleepless
- symptoms continue or get worse

- stomach pain occurs with the use of this product even if mild pain persists
- any new symptoms appear

If pregnant or breast-feeding, ask a health professional before use. It is especially important not to use this product during the last 3 months of pregnancy unless definitely directed to do so by a doctor because it may cause problems in the unborn child or complications during delivery.

Keep out of reach of children. In case of overdose, get medical help or contact a Poison Control Center right away.

Directions:
- adults: take 1 caplet every 4–6 hours while symptoms persist.
- do not take more than 6 caplets in any 24-hour period, unless directed by a doctor
- children under 12 years of age: consult a doctor

Other Information:
- read all warnings and directions before use. Keep carton.
- store in a dry place 20–25°C (68–77°F)
- avoid excessive heat above 40°C (104°F)

Inactive Ingredients: carnauba wax, croscarmellose sodium, FD&C red no. 40 aluminum lake, FD&C yellow no. 6 aluminum lake, glyceryl behenate, hypromellose, iron oxide black, microcrystalline cellulose, polydextrose, polyethylene glycol, pregelatinized starch, propylene glycol, silicon dioxide, starch, titanium dioxide

How Supplied: Packages of 10 and 20 caplets

ADVIL® COLD & SINUS
Caplets, Tablets and Liqui-Gels
Pain Reliever/Fever Reducer/Nasal Decongestant

Active Ingredients (in each tablet, caplet or liqui-gel):
Ibuprofen 200 mg
Pseudoephedrine HCl 30 mg

Uses: Temporarily relieves these symptoms associated with the common cold, sinusitis or flu:
- headache • fever • nasal congestion
- minor body aches and pains

Warnings:
Allergy Alert: Ibuprofen may cause a severe allergic reaction which may include: • hives • facial swelling • asthma (wheezing) • shock

Alcohol warning: If you consume 3 or more alcoholic drinks every day, ask your doctor whether you should take ibuprofen or other pain relievers/fever reducers. Ibuprofen may cause stomach bleeding.

Do not use
- if you have ever had an allergic reaction to any other pain reliever/fever reducer
- if you are now taking a prescription monoamine oxidase inhibitor (MAOI) (certain drugs for depression, psychiatric, or emotional conditions, or Parkinson's disease), or for 2 weeks after

stopping the MAOI drug. If you do not know if your prescription drug contains an MAOI, ask a doctor or pharmacist before taking this product

Ask a doctor before use if you have
- heart disease • high blood pressure
- thyroid disease • diabetes
- trouble urinating due to an enlarged prostate gland • stomach pain
- had serious side effects from any pain reliever/fever reducer

Ask a doctor or pharmacist before use if you are
- taking any other product that contains ibuprofen or pseudoephedrine
- taking any other pain reliever/fever reducer or nasal decongestant
- under a doctor's care for any continuing medical condition
- taking other drugs on a regular basis

When using this product
- do not use more than directed
- take with food or milk if stomach upset occurs

Stop use and ask a doctor if
- an allergic reaction occurs. Seek medical help right away.
- you get nervous, dizzy, or sleepless
- nasal congestion lasts for more than 7 days
- fever lasts for more than 3 days
- symptoms continue or get worse
- new or unexpected symptoms occur
- stomach pain occurs with use of this product or if even mild symptoms persist

If pregnant or breast-feeding, ask a health professional before use. It is especially important not to use this product during the last 3 months of pregnancy unless definitely directed to do so by a doctor because it may cause problems in the unborn child or complications during delivery.

Keep out of reach of children. In case of overdose, get medical help or contact a Poison Control Center right away.

Directions:
- adults and children 12 years of age and over:
  - take 1 tablet, caplet or liqui-gel every 4 to 6 hours while symptoms persist. If symptoms do not respond to 1 tablet, caplet or liqui-gel, 2 tablets, caplets or liqui-gels may be used.
  - do not use more than 6 tablets, caplets or liqui-gels in any 24-hour period unless directed by a doctor
  - the smallest effective dose should be used
- children under 12 years of age: consult a doctor

Other Information:
- store at 20–25°C (68–77°F). Avoid excessive heat above 40°C (104°F).
- read all warnings and directions before use. Keep carton.

Inactive Ingredients (tablets and caplets): carnauba or equivalent wax, croscarmellose sodium, iron oxides, methylparaben, microcrystalline cellulose, propylparaben, silicon dioxide, sodium benzoate, sodium lauryl sulfate, starch, stearic acid, sucrose, titanium dioxide

Inactive Ingredients (liqui-gels): D&C yellow no. 10, FD&C red no. 40, fractionated coconut oil, gelatin, pharmaceutical ink, polyethylene glycol,

potassium hydroxide, purified water, sorbitan, sorbitol

How Supplied: Advil® Cold and Sinus is an oval-shaped, tan-colored caplet, a tan-colored tablet or a liqui-gel. The caplet is supplied in blister packs of 20 and 40. The tablet is available in blister packs of 20. The liqui-gel is available in blister packs of 16 and 32.

ADVIL®
FLU & BODY ACHE Caplets
Pain Reliever/Fever Reducer/Nasal Decongestant

Active Ingredients (in each caplet)
Ibuprofen 200 mg
Pseudoephedrine HCl 30 mg

Uses:
- temporarily relieves these symptoms associated with the common cold, sinusitis, or flu
  - headache
  - fever
  - nasal congestion
  - minor body aches and pains

Warnings:
Allergy alert: Ibuprofen may cause a severe allergic reaction which may include: • hives • facial swelling • asthma (wheezing) • shock

Alcohol warning: If you consume 3 or more alcoholic drinks every day, ask your doctor whether you should take ibuprofen or other pain relievers/fever reducers. Ibuprofen may cause stomach bleeding.

Do not use
- if you have ever had an allergic reaction to any other pain reliever/fever reducer
- if you are now taking a prescription monoamine oxidase inhibitor (MAOI) (certain drugs for depression, psychiatric, or emotional conditions, or Parkinson's disease), or for 2 weeks after stopping the MAOI drug. If you do not know if your prescription drug contains an MAOI, ask a doctor or pharmacist before taking this product

Ask a doctor before use if you have
- heart disease • high blood pressure
- thyroid disease • diabetes
- trouble urinating due to an enlarged prostate gland • stomach pain
- had serious side effects from any pain reliever/fever reducer

Ask a doctor or pharmacist before use if you are
- taking any other product that contains ibuprofen or pseudoephedrine
- taking any other pain reliever/fever reducer or nasal decongestant
- under a doctor's care for any continuing medical condition
- taking other drugs on a regular basis

When using this product
- do not use more than directed
- take with food or milk if stomach upset occurs

Stop use and ask a doctor if
- an allergic reaction occurs. Seek medical help right away.
- you get nervous, dizzy, or sleepless
- nasal congestion lasts for more than 7 days

Continued on next page

Advil Flu/Body Ache—Cont.

- fever lasts for more than 3 days
- symptoms continue or get worse
- new or unexpected symptoms occur
- stomach pain occurs with use of this product or if even mild symptoms persist

If pregnant or breast-feeding, ask a health professional before use. It is especially important not to use this product during the last 3 months of pregnancy unless definitely directed to do so by a doctor because it may cause problems in the unborn child or complications during delivery.

Keep out of reach of children. In case of overdose, get medical help or contact a Poison Control Center right away.

Directions:

- adults and children 12 years of age and over: Take 1 caplet every 4 to 6 hours while symptoms persist. If symptoms do not respond to 1 caplet, 2 caplets may be used.
- do not use more than 6 caplets in any 24-hour period unless directed by a doctor
- the smallest effective dose should be used
- children under 12 years of age: consult a doctor

Other Information:

- store at 20–25°C (68–77°F). Avoid excessive heat above 40°C (104°F).
- read all warnings and directions before use. Keep carton.

Inactive Ingredients: carnauba or equivalent wax, croscarmellose sodium, iron oxide, methylparaben, microcrystalline cellulose, propylparaben, silicon dioxide, sodium benzoate, sodium lauryl sulfate, starch, stearic acid, sucrose, titanium dioxide

How Supplied:
Blister packs of 20 caplets.

ADVIL®
MIGRAINE Liquigels

Use: Treats migraine

Active Ingredient:
Each brown, oval capsule contains solubilized ibuprofen, a pain reliever, equal to 200 mg ibuprofen (present as the free acid and potassium salt)

Warnings:
Allergy alert: Ibuprofen may cause a severe allergic reaction which may include:
- hives
- facial swelling
- asthma (wheezing)
- shock

Alcohol warning: If you consume 3 or more alcoholic drinks every day, ask your doctor whether you should take ibuprofen or other pain relievers/fever reducers. Ibuprofen may cause stomach bleeding.
Do not use if you have ever had an allergic reaction to any other pain reliever/fever reducer

Ask a doctor before use if you have
- never had migraines diagnosed by a health professional
- a headache that is different from your usual migraines
- the worse headache of your life
- fever and stiff neck
- headaches beginning after, or caused by head injury, exertion, coughing or bending
- experienced your first headache after the age of 50
- daily headaches
- a migraine so severe as to require bed rest
- problems or serious side effects from taking pain relievers or fever reducers
- stomach pain

Ask a doctor or pharmacist before use if you are
- under a doctor's care for any continuing medical condition
- taking other drugs on a regular basis
- taking another product containing ibuprofen, or any other pain reliever/fever reducer

Stop use and ask a doctor if
- an allergic reaction occurs. Seek medical help right away.
- migraine headache pain is not relieved or gets worse after first dose
- stomach pain occurs with the use of this product
- new or unexpected symptoms occur

If pregnant or breast-feeding, ask a health professional before use. It is especially important not to use ibuprofen during the last 3 months of pregnancy unless definitely directed to do so by a doctor because it may cause problems in the unborn child or complications during delivery.

Keep out of reach of children. In case of overdose, get medical help or contact a Poison Control Center right away.

Directions:

Adults:	• take 2 capsules with a glass of water • if symptoms persist or worsen, ask your doctor • do not take more than 2 capsules in 24 hours, unless directed by a doctor
Under 18 years of age:	• ask a doctor

Other information:

- read all directions and warnings before use. Keep carton.
- store at 20–25°C (68–77°F)
- avoid excessive heat 40°C (above 104°F)

Inactive Ingredients:
D&C yellow no. 10, FD&C green no. 3, FD&C red no. 40, gelatin, light mineral oil, pharmaceutical ink, polyethylene glycol, potassium hydroxide, purified water, sorbitan, sorbitol

How Supplied: Bottles of 20, 40, & 80 liquigels.

JUNIOR STRENGTH ADVIL
CHEWABLE TABLETS
Fever Reducer/Pain Reliever

Active Ingredient:
(in each tablet)
Ibuprofen 100 mg

Uses: temporarily:
- reduces fever
- relieves minor aches and pains due to the common cold, flu, sore throat, headaches and toothaches

Warnings:
Allergy alert: Ibuprofen may cause a severe allergic reaction which may include:
- hives • asthma (wheezing)
- facial swelling • shock

Sore throat warning: Severe or persistent sore throat or sore throat accompanied by high fever, headache, nausea, and vomiting may be serious. Consult doctor promptly. Do not use more than 2 days or administer to children under 3 years of age unless directed by doctor.
Do not use if the child has ever had an allergic reaction to any other fever reducer/pain reliever

Ask a doctor before use if the child has
- not been drinking fluids
- lost a lot of fluid due to continued vomiting or diarrhea
- stomach pain
- problems or serious side effects from taking fever reducers or pain relievers

Ask a doctor or pharmacist before use if the child is
- under a doctor's care for any serious condition
- taking any other drug
- taking any other product that contains ibuprofen, or any other pain reliever/fever reducer

When using this product give with food or milk if stomach upset occurs

Stop use and ask a doctor if
- an allergic reaction occurs. Seek medical help right away.
- fever or pain gets worse or lasts more than 3 days
- the child does not get any relief within first day (24 hours) of treatment
- stomach pain or upset gets worse or lasts
- redness or swelling is present in the painful area
- any new symptoms appear

Keep out of reach of children. In case of overdose, get medical help or contact a Poison Control Center right away.

Directions:
- do not give more than directed
- find right dose on chart below. If possible, use weight to dose; otherwise use age.
- repeat dose every 6–8 hours, if needed
- do not use more than 4 times a day

[See table at top of next page]

Dosing Chart

Weight (lb)	Age (yr)	Dose (tablets)
under 48 lb	under 6 yr	ask a doctor
48–59 lb	6–8 yr	2 tablets
60–71 lb	9–10 yr	2 ½ tablets
72–95 lb	11 yr	3 tablets

Other Information
- **Phenylketonurics:** contains phenylalanine 4.2 mg per tablet
- one dose lasts 6–8 hours
- store in a dry place at 20–25°C (68–77°F) (for blisters)
- store at 20–25°C (68–77°F) (for bottles and pouches)

Inactive Ingredients (GRAPE FLAVOR) artificial flavor, aspartame, cellulose acetate phthalate, D&C red no. 30 lake, FD&C blue no. 2 lake, gelatin, magnasweet, magnesium stearate, mannitol, microcrystalline cellulose, silicon dioxide, sodium starch glycolate

Inactive Ingredients (FRUIT FLAVOR) aspartame, cellulose acetate phthalate, D&C red no. 27 lake, FD&C red no. 40 lake, gelatin, magnasweet, magnesium stearate, mannitol, microcrystalline cellulose, natural and artificial flavors, silicon dioxide, sodium starch glycolate

How Supplied:
Chewable Tablets: bottles of 24 (fruit and grape flavors).

JUNIOR STRENGTH ADVIL SWALLOW TABLETS
Fever Reducer/Pain Reliever

Active Ingredient:
(in each tablet)
Ibuprofen 100 mg

Uses: temporarily:
- reduces fever
- relieves minor aches and pains due to the common cold, flu, sore throat, headaches and toothaches

Warnings:
Allergy alert: Ibuprofen may cause a severe allergic reaction which may include:
- hives • asthma (wheezing)
- facial swelling • shock

Sore throat warning: Severe or persistent sore throat or sore throat accompanied by high fever, headache, nausea, and vomiting may be serious. Consult doctor promptly. Do not use more than 2 days or administer to children under 3 years of age unless directed by doctor.

Do not use if the child has ever had an allergic reaction to any other fever reducer/pain reliever

Ask a doctor before use if the child has
- not been drinking fluids
- lost a lot of fluid due to continued vomiting or diarrhea
- stomach pain
- problems or serious side effects from taking fever reducers or pain relievers

Ask a doctor or pharmacist before use if the child is
- under a doctor's care for any serious condition
- taking any other drug
- taking any other product that contains ibuprofen, or any other pain reliever/fever reducer

When using this product give with food or milk if stomach upset occurs

Stop use and ask a doctor if
- an allergic reaction occurs. Seek medical help right away.
- fever or pain gets worse or lasts more than 3 days
- the child does not get any relief within first day (24 hours) of treatment
- stomach pain or upset gets worse or lasts
- redness or swelling is present in the painful area
- any new symptoms appear

Keep out of reach of children. In case of overdose, get medical help or contact a Poison Control Center right away.

Directions:
- do not give more than directed
- find right dose on chart below. If possible, use weight to dose; otherwise use age.
- repeat dose every 6–8 hours, if needed
- do not use more than 4 times a day

Dosing Chart

Weight (lb)	Age (yr)	Dose (tablets)
under 48 lb	under 6 yr	ask a doctor
48–71 lb	6–10 yr	2 tablets
72–95 lb	11 yr	3 tablets

Other Information:
- one dose lasts 6–8 hours
- store at 20–25°C (68–77°F)
- avoid excessive heat 40°C (104°F) – (for blisters and pouches only)

Inactive Ingredients: acetylated monoglycerides, carnauba wax, colloidal silicon dioxide, croscarmellose sodium, iron oxides, methylparaben, microcrystalline cellulose, povidone, pregelatinized starch, propylene glycol, propylparaben, shellac, sodium benzoate, starch, stearic acid, sucrose, titanium dioxide

How Supplied: Coated Tablets in bottles of 24.

CHILDREN'S ADVIL CHEWABLE TABLETS
Fever Reducer/Pain Reliever

Active Ingredient:
(in each tablet)
Ibuprofen 50 mg

Uses: temporarily:
- reduces fever
- relieves minor aches and pains due to the common cold, flu, sore throat, headaches and toothaches

Warnings:
Allergy alert: Ibuprofen may cause a severe allergic reaction which may include:
- hives • asthma (wheezing)
- facial swelling • shock

Sore throat warning: Severe or persistent sore throat or sore throat accompanied by high fever, headache, nausea, and vomiting may be serious. Consult doctor promptly. Do not use more than 2 days or administer to children under 3 years of age unless directed by doctor.

Do not use if the child has ever had an allergic reaction to any other fever reducer/pain reliever

Ask a doctor before use if the child has
- not been drinking fluids
- lost a lot of fluid due to continued vomiting or diarrhea
- stomach pain
- problems or serious side effects from taking fever reducers or pain relievers

Ask a doctor or pharmacist before use if the child is
- under a doctor's care for any serious condition
- taking any other drug
- taking any other product that contains ibuprofen, or any other pain reliever/fever reducer

When using this product give with food or milk if stomach upset occurs

Stop use and ask a doctor if
- an allergic reaction occurs. Seek medical help right away.
- fever or pain gets worse or lasts more than 3 days
- the child does not get any relief within first day (24 hours) of treatment
- stomach pain or upset gets worse or lasts
- redness or swelling is present in the painful area
- any new symptoms appear

Keep out of reach of children. In case of overdose, get medical help or contact a Poison Control Center right away.

Directions:
- do not give more than directed
- find right dose on chart below. If possible, use weight to dose; otherwise use age.
- repeat dose every 6–8 hours, if needed
- do not use more than 4 times a day
[See table at top of next page]

Other Information:
- **Phenylketonurics:** contains phenylalanine 2.1 mg per tablet
- one dose lasts 6–8 hours

Continued on next page

Dosing Chart

Weight (lb)	Age (yr)	Dose (tablets)
under 24 lb	under 2 yr	ask a doctor
24–35 lb	2–3 yr	2 tablets
36–47 lb	4–5 yr	3 tablets
48–59 lb	6–8 yr	4 tablets
60–71 lb	9–10 yr	5 tablets
72–95 lb	11 yr	6 tablets

[See chart below]

Dosing Chart

Weight (lb)	Age (yr)	Dose (teaspoons)
under 24	under 2 yr	ask a doctor
24–47	2–5 yr	1 teaspoon
48–95	6–11 yr	2 teaspoons

Children's Advil Chewable—Cont.

- store at 20–25°C (68–77°F) (for bottles and pouches)
- store in a dry place at 20–25°C (68–77°F) (for blisters)

Inactive Ingredients: (GRAPE FLAVOR) artificial flavor, aspartame, cellulose acetate phthalate, D&C red no. 30 lake, FD&C blue no. 2 lake, gelatin, magnasweet, magnesium stearate, mannitol, microcrystalline cellulose, silicon dioxide, sodium starch glycolate

Inactive Ingredients: (FRUIT FLAVOR) aspartame, cellulose acetate phthalate, D&C red no. 27 lake, FD&C red no. 40 lake, gelatin, magnasweet, magnesium stearate, mannitol, microcrystalline cellulose, natural and artifical flavors, silicon dioxide, sodium starch glycolate

How Supplied: Blister of 24 (fruit and grape flavors).

CHILDREN'S ADVIL COLD SUSPENSION
Pain Reliever/Fever Reducer/Nasal Decongestant

Active Ingredients:
(in each 5mL teaspoon)
Ibuprofen 100 mg
Pseudoephedrine HCl 15mg

Uses: temporarily relieves these cold, sinus and flu symptoms:
- nasal and sinus congestion • headache
- stuffy nose • sore throat
- minor aches and pains • fever

Warnings:
Allergy alert: Ibuprofen may cause a severe allergic reaction which may include: • hives • facial swelling • asthma (wheezing) • shock
Sore throat warning: Severe or persistent sore throat or sore throat accompanied by high fever, headache, nausea, and vomiting may be serious. Consult a doctor right away. Do not use more than 2 days or give to children under 3 years of age unless directed by a doctor.
Do not use:
- if the child has ever had an allergic reaction to any pain reliever, fever reducer or nasal decongestant
- in a child who is taking a prescription monoamine oxidase inhibitor (MAOI) (certain drugs for depression, psychiatric, or emotional conditions, or Parkinson's disease), or for 2 weeks after stopping the MAOI drug. If you do not know if your child's prescription drug contains an MAOI, ask a doctor or pharmacist before giving this product.
Ask a doctor before use if the child has:
- not been drinking fluids
- lost a lot of fluid due to continued vomiting or diarrhea
- problems or serious side effects from taking any pain reliever, fever reducer or nasal decongestant
- stomach pain • heart disease
- diabetes
- thyroid disease • high blood pressure
Ask a doctor or pharmacist before use if the child is
- under a doctor's care for any continuing medical condition
- taking any other drug
- taking any other product that contains ibuprofen or pseudoephedrine
- taking any other pain reliever, fever reducer or nasal decongestant
When using this product
- do not use more than directed
- give with food or milk if stomach upset occurs
Stop use and ask a doctor if
- an allergic reaction occurs. Seek medical help right away.
- the child does not get any relief within first day (24 hours) of treatment
- fever or pain or nasal congestion gets worse or lasts for more than 3 days
- stomach pain or upset gets worse or lasts
- symptoms continue or get worse
- redness or swelling is present in the painful area
- the child gets nervous, dizzy, sleepless or sleepy
- any new symptoms appear
Keep out of reach of children. In case of overdose, get medical help or contact a Poison Control Center right away.

Directions:
- do not give more than directed
- shake well before using
- find right dose on chart. If possible, use weight to dose; otherwise use age.
- if needed, repeat dose every **6 hours**
- do not use more than **4 times a day**
- replace original bottle cap to maintain child resistance
- measure only with dosing cup provided. Dosing cup to be used with Children's Advil Cold Suspension only. Do not use with other products. Dose lines account for product remaining in cup due to thickness of suspension.

Other information:
- store a room temperature 20–25°C (68–77°F)
- alcohol free

Inactive ingredients: carboxymethylcellulose sodium, citric acid, edetate disodium, FD&C blue no. 1, FD&C red no. 40, flavor, glycerin, microcrystalline cellulose, polysorbate 80, purified water, sodium benzoate, sorbitol solution, sucrose, xanthan gum

How Supplied: Bottles of 4 fl. oz. in grape flavor.

CHILDREN'S ADVIL SUSPENSION
Fever Reducer/Pain Reliever

Active Ingredient:
(in each 5 mL)
Ibuprofen 100 mg

Uses: temporarily:
- reduces fever
- relieves minor aches and pains due to the common cold, flu, sore throat, headaches and toothaches

Warnings:
Allergy alert: Ibuprofen may cause a severe allergic reaction which may include:
- hives • asthma (wheezing)
- facial swelling • shock
Sore throat warning: Severe or persistent sore throat or sore throat accompanied by high fever, headache, nausea, and vomiting may be serious. Consult doctor promptly. Do not use more than 2 days or administer to children under 3 years of age unless directed by doctor.
Do not use if the child has ever had an allergic reaction to any other fever reducer/pain reliever
Ask a doctor before use if the child has
- not been drinking fluids
- lost a lot of fluid due to continued vomiting or diarrhea
- stomach pain
- problems or serious side effects from taking fever reducers or pain relievers
Ask a doctor or pharmacist before use if the child is
- under a doctor's care for any serious condition
- taking any other drug
- taking any other product that contains ibuprofen, or any other pain reliever/fever reducer
When using this product give with food or milk if stomach upset occurs

Dosing Chart

Weight (lb)	Age (yr)	Dose (tsp)
under 24 lb	under 2 yr	ask a doctor
24–35 lb	2–3 yr	1 tsp
36–47 lb	4–5 yr	1½ tsp
48–59 lb	6–8 yr	2 tsp
60–71 lb	9–10 yr	2½ tsp
72–95 lb	11 yr	3 tsp

Dosing Chart

Weight (lb)	Age (mos)	Dose (mL)
under 6 mos		ask a doctor
12–17 lb	6–11 mos	1.25 mL
18–23 lb	12–23 mos	1.875 mL

Stop use and ask a doctor if
- an allergic reaction occurs. Seek medical help right away.
- fever or pain gets worse or lasts more than 3 days
- the child does not get any relief within first day (24 hours) of treatment
- stomach pain or upset gets worse or lasts
- redness or swelling is present in the painful area
- any new symptoms appear

Keep out of reach of children. In case of overdose, get medical help or contact a Poison Control Center right away.

Directions:
- do not give more than directed
- shake well before using
- find right dose on chart below. If possible, use weight to dose; otherwise use age.
- repeat dose every 6–8 hours, if needed
- do not use more than 4 times a day
- measure only with the blue dosing cup provided. Blue dosing cup to be used with Children's Advil Suspension only. Do not use with other products. Dose lines account for product remaining in cup due to thickness of suspension.
[See first table above]

Other Information:
- one dose lasts 6–8 hours
- store at 20–25°C (68–77°F)

Inactive Ingredients: (FRUIT FLAVOR) artifical flavors, carboxymethylcellulose sodium, citric acid, edetate disodium, FD&C red no. 40, glycerin, microcrystalline cellulose, polysorbate 80, purified water, sodium benzoate, sorbitol solution, sucrose, xanthan gum

Inactive Ingredients: (GRAPE FLAVOR) artifical flavor, carboxymethylcellulose sodium, citric acid, edetate disodium, FD&C blue no. 1, FD&C red no. 40, glycerin, microcrystalline cellulose, polysorbate 80, purified water, sodium benzoate, sorbitol solution, sucrose, xanthan gum

Inactive Ingredients: (BLUE RASPBERRY FLAVOR) carboxymethylcellulose sodium, citric acid, edetate disodium, FD&C blue no. 1, flavors, glycerin, microcrystalline cellulose, polysorbate 80, purified water, sodium benzoate, sodium citrate, sorbitol solution, sucrose, xanthan gum

How Supplied: Bottles of 2 fl. oz. and 4 fl. oz. in grape, fruit, and blue raspberry flavors.

INFANTS' ADVIL CONCENTRATED DROPS
Fever Reducer/Pain Reliever

Active Ingredient:
(in each 1.25 mL)
Ibuprofen 50 mg

Uses: temporarily:
- reduces fever
- relieves minor aches and pains due to the common cold, flu, headaches and toothaches

Warnings:
Allergy Alert: Ibuprofen may cause a severe allergic reaction which may include:
- hives • asthma (wheezing)
- facial swelling • shock
Do not use if the child has ever had an allergic reaction to any other fever reducer/pain reliever
Ask a doctor before use if the child has
- not been drinking fluids
- lost a lot of fluid due to continued vomiting or diarrhea
- stomach pain
- problems or serious side effects from taking fever reducers or pain relievers
Ask a doctor or pharmacist before use if the child is
- under a doctor's care for any serious condition
- taking any other drug
- taking any other product that contains ibuprofen, or any other pain reliever/fever reducer
When using this product give with food or milk if upset stomach occurs
Stop use and ask a doctor if
- an allergic reaction occurs. Seek medical help right away.

- fever or pain gets worse or lasts more than 3 days
- the child does not get any relief within first day (24 hours) of treatment
- stomach pain or upset gets worse or lasts
- redness or swelling is present in the painful area
- any new symptoms appear

Keep out of reach of children. In case of overdose, get medical help or contact a Poison Control Center right away.

Directions:
- do not give more than directed
- shake well before using
- find right dose on chart below. If possible, use weight to dose; otherwise use age.
- repeat dose every 6–8 hours, if needed
- do not use more than 4 times a day
- measure with the dosing device provided. Do not use with any other device.
[See second table above]

Other Information:
- one dose lasts 6–8 hours
- store at 20–25°C (68–77°F)

Inactive Ingredients: (FRUIT FLAVOR) artificial flavors, caroboxymethylcellulose sodium, citric acid, edetate disodium, FD&C red no. 40, glycerin, microcrystalline cellulose, polysorbate 80, purified water, sodium benzoate, sorbitol solution, sucrose, xanthan gum

Inactive Ingredients: (GRAPE FLAVOR) artificial flavor, caroboxymethylcellulose sodium, citric acid, edetate disodium, FD&C blue no. 1, FD&C red no. 40, glycerin, microcrystalline cellulose, polysorbate 80, purified water, sodium benzoate, sorbitol solution, sucrose, xanthan gum

How Supplied: Bottles of ½ fl. oz. in grape and fruit flavors.

ALAVERT
Loratadine orally disintegrating tablets
Antihistamine

Active Ingredient (in each tablet):
Loratadine 10 mg

Uses:
- temporarily relieves these symptoms due to hay fever or other upper respiratory allergies:
  - runny nose • sneezing • itchy, watery eyes
  - itching of the nose or throat

Warnings:
Do not use if you have ever had an allergic reaction to this product or any of its ingredients
Ask a doctor before use if you have liver or kidney disease. Your doctor should determine if you need a different dose.
When using this product do not use more than directed. Taking more than recommended may cause drowsiness.
Stop use and ask a doctor if an allergic reaction to this product occurs. Seek medical help right away.

Continued on next page

Alavert—Cont.

If pregnant or breast-feeding, ask a health professional before use.
Keep out of reach of children. In case of overdose, get medical help or contact a Poison Control Center right away.

Directions:
- tablet melts in mouth. Can be taken with or without water.

Age	Dose
adults and children 6 years and over	1 tablet daily; do not use more than 1 tablet daily
children under 6	ask a doctor
consumers who have liver or kidney disease	ask a doctor

Other Information:
- Phenylketonurics: Contains Phenylalanine 8.4 mg per tablet
- store at 20–25°C (68–77°F)
- keep in a dry place

Inactive Ingredients: artificial & natural flavor, aspartame, citric acid, colloidal silicon dioxide, corn syrup solids, crospovidone, magnesium stearate, mannitol, microcrystalline cellulose, modified food starch, sodium bicarbonate

How Supplied: Packages of 6, 12, 24 & 48 orally disintegrating tablets

---

MAXIMUM STRENGTH
ANBESOL® Gel and Liquid
Oral Anesthetic

ANBESOL JUNIOR® Gel
Oral Anesthetic

BABY ANBESOL®
Grape Flavor
Oral Anesthetic

Active Ingredients: Anbesol is an oral anesthetic which is available in a Maximum Strength gel and liquid. Anbesol Junior, available in a gel, is an oral anesthetic. Baby Anbesol, available in a grape-flavored gel, is an oral anesthetic and is alcohol-free.
Maximum Strength Anbesol Gel and Liquid contain Benzocaine 20%.
Anbesol Junior Gel contains Benzocaine 10%.
Baby Anbesol Gel contains Benzocaine 7.5%.

Uses: Maximum Strength Anbesol temporarily relieves pain associated with toothache, canker sores, minor dental procedures, sore gums, braces, and dentures. Anbesol Junior temporarily relieves pain associated with braces, sore gums, canker sores, toothaches, and minor dental procedures. Baby Anbesol Gel temporarily relieves sore gums due to teething in infants and children 4 months of age and older.

Warnings: Allergy alert: Do not use these products if you have a history of allergy to local anesthetics such as procaine, butacaine, benzocaine, or other "caine" anesthetics.
Baby Anbesol: **Do not use** to treat fever and nasal congestion. These are not symptoms of teething and may indicate the presence of infection. If these symptoms persist, consult your doctor.
Maximum Strength Anbesol, Anbesol Junior and Baby Anbesol:
When using this product
- avoid contact with the eyes
- do not exceed recommended dosage
- do not use for more than 7 days unless directed by a doctor/dentist
Stop use and ask a doctor if
- sore mouth symptoms do not improve in 7 days
- irritation, pain, or redness persists or worsens
- swelling, rash, or fever develops
Keep out of reach of children. If more than used for pain is accidentally swallowed, get medical help or contact a Poison Control Center right away.

Directions: Maximum Strength Anbesol: Gel—
- to open tube, cut tip of the tube on score mark with scissors
- adults and children 2 years of age and older: apply to the affected area up to 4 times daily or as directed by a doctor/dentist
- children under 12 years of age: adult supervision should be given in the use of this product
- children under 2 years of age: consult a doctor/dentist
- for denture irritation:
  - apply thin layer to the affected area
  - do not reinsert dental work until irritation/pain is relieved
  - rinse mouth well before reinserting
Do not refrigerate.
Tamper-Evident: Do Not Use if tube tip is cut prior to opening.
Liquid—
- adults and children 2 years of age and older:
  - wipe liquid on with cotton, or cotton swab, or fingertip
  - apply to the affected area up to 4 times daily or as directed by a doctor/dentist
- children under 12 years of age: adult supervision should be given in the use of this product
- children under 2 years of age; consult a doctor/dentist
Tamper-Evident: Safety Sealed Bottle. Do Not Use if neck seal imprinted "SEALED FOR SAFETY" on bottle is broken or missing.
Anbesol Junior Gel:
- to open tube, cut tip of the tube on score mark with scissors
- adults and children 2 years of age and older: apply to the affected area up to 4 times daily or as directed by a doctor/dentist
- children under 12 years of age: adult supervision should be given in the use of this product
- children under 2 years of age: consult a doctor/dentist

Tamper-Evident: Safety Sealed Bottle. Do Not Use if neck seal imprinted "SEALED FOR SAFETY" on bottle is broken or missing.
Grape Baby Anbesol Gel:
- to open tube, cut tip of the tube on score mark with scissors
- children 4 months of age and older: apply to the affected area not more than 4 times daily or as directed by a doctor/dentist
- infants under 4 months of age: no recommended dosage or treatment except under the advice and supervision of a doctor/dentist
Tamper-Evident: Safety Sealed Tube. Do Not Use if tube tip is cut prior to opening.

Inactive Ingredients:
Maximum Strength Gel: carbomer 934p, D&C yellow no. 10, FD&C blue no. 1, FD&C red no. 40, flavor, glycerin, methylparaben, phenylcarbinol, polyethylene glycol, propylene glycol, saccharin.
Maximum Strength Liquid: D&C yellow no. 10, FD&C blue no. 1, FD&C red no. 40, flavor, methylparaben, polyethylene glycol, propylene glycol, saccharin.
Junior Gel: artificial flavor, benzyl alcohol, carbomer 934P, D&C red no. 33, glycerin, methylparaben, polyethylene glycol, potassium acesulfame
Grape Baby Gel: benzoic acid, carbomer 934P, D&C red no. 33, edetate disodium, FD&C blue no. 1, flavor, glycerin, methylparaben, polyethylene glycol, propylparaben, saccharin, water

Storage: Store at 20–25°C (68–77°F)

How Supplied: All Gels in .25 oz (7.1 g) tubes, Maximum Strength Liquid in .31 fl oz (9 mL) bottle.

ANBESOL COLD SORE THERAPY
Fever blister/Cold sore treatment

Active Ingredients:
Allantoin 1%,
Benzocaine 20%,
Camphor 3%,
White petrolatum 64.9%

Uses:
- temporarily relieves pain associated with fever blisters and cold sores
- relieves dryness and softens fever blisters and cold sores

Warnings: For external use only
Allergy Alert: Do not use this product if you have a history of allergy to local anesthetics such as procaine, butacaine, benzocaine, or other "caine" anesthetics.
Do not use over deep or puncture wounds, infections, or lacerations. Consult a doctor.
When using this product • avoid contact with the eyes
- do not exceed recommended dosage
Stop use and ask a doctor if
- condition worsens
- symptoms persist for more than 7 days
- symptoms clear up and occur again within a few days
Keep out of reach of children. If swallowed, get medical help or contact a Poison Control Center right away.

Directions:
- to open tube, cut tip of the tube on score mark with scissors
- adults and children 2 years of age and older: apply to the affected area not more than 3 to 4 times daily
- children under 12 years of age: adult supervision should be given in the use of this product
- children under 2 years of age: consult a doctor

Taper-Evident:
Safety Sealed Tube.
Do Not Use if tube tip is cut prior to opening.

Inactive Ingredients: aloe extract, benzyl alcohol, butylparaben, glyceryl stearate, isocetyl stearate, menthol, methylparaben, propylparaben, sodium lauryl sulfate, vitamin E, white wax

Other Information
- store at 20–25°C (68–77°F)

How Supplied: 0.25 oz Tube

DIMETAPP® Cold & Allergy Elixir
Nasal Decongestant, Antihistamine

Active Ingredients:
Each 5 mL (1 teaspoonful) contains:
Brompheniramine Maleate, USP 1 mg
Pseudoephedrine Hydrochloride, USP 15 mg

Uses:
- temporarily relieves nasal congestion due to the common cold, hay fever or other upper respiratory allergies, or associated with sinusitis
- temporarily relieves these symptoms due to hay fever (allergic rhinitis):
  - runny nose
  - sneezing
  - itchy, watery eyes
  - itching of the nose or throat
- temporarily restores freer breathing through the nose

Warnings:
Do not use if you are now taking a prescription monoamine oxidase inhibitor (MAOI) (certain drugs for depression, psychiatric, or emotional conditions, or Parkinson's disease), or for 2 weeks after stopping the MAOI drug. If you do not know if your prescription drug contains an MAOI, ask a doctor or pharmacist before taking this product.

Ask a doctor before use if you have
- heart disease
- high blood pressure
- thyroid disease
- diabetes
- trouble urinating due to an enlarged prostate gland
- glaucoma
- a breathing problem such as emphysema or chronic bronchitis

Ask a doctor or pharmacist before use if you are taking sedatives or tranquilizers.

When using this product
- **do not use more than directed**
- drowsiness may occur
- avoid alcoholic beverages
- alcohol, sedatives, and tranquilizers may increase drowsiness
- be careful when driving a motor vehicle or operating machinery
- excitability may occur, especially in children

Stop use and ask a doctor if
- you get nervous, dizzy, or sleepless
- symptoms do not get better within 7 days or are accompanied by fever

If pregnant or breast-feeding, ask a health professional before use.

Keep out of reach of children. In case of overdose, get medical help or contact a Poison Control Center right away.

Directions:
- do not take more than 4 doses in any 24-hour period

age	dose
adults and children 12 years and over	4 tsp every 4 hours
children 6 to under 12 years	2 tsp every 4 hours
children under 6 years	ask a doctor

Store at Controlled Room Temperature, between 20°C and 25°C (68°F and 77°F). Product color may change over time.

Inactive ingredients: artificial flavor, citric acid, FD&C blue no. 1, FD&C red no. 40, glycerin, high fructose corn syrup, propylene glycol, saccharin sodium, sodium benzoate, sorbitol, water

How Supplied: Purple, grape-flavored liquid in bottles of 4 fl oz, 8 fl oz, and 12 fl oz. Not a USP elixir.

DIMETAPP® DM COLD & COUGH Elixir
Nasal Decongestant, Antihistamine, Cough Suppressant

Active Ingredients: Each 5 mL (1 teaspoonful) of DIMETAPP DM Elixir contains:
Brompheniramine Maleate, USP 1 mg
Pseudoephedrine Hydrochloride 15 mg
Dextromethorphan Hydrobromide, USP 5 mg

Uses:
- temporarily relieves cough due to minor throat and bronchial irritation occurring with a cold, and nasal congestion due to the common cold, hay fever or other upper respiratory allergies, or associated with sinusitis
- temporarily relieves these symptoms due to hay fever (allergic rhinitis):
  - runny nose
  - sneezing
  - itchy, watery eyes
  - itching of the nose or throat
- temporarily restores freer breathing through the nose

Warnings:
Do not use if you are now taking a prescription monoamine oxidase inhibitor (MAOI) (certain drugs for depression, psychiatric, or emotional conditions, or Parkinson's disease), or for 2 weeks after stopping the MAOI drug. If you do not know if your prescription drug contains an MAOI, ask a doctor or pharmacist before taking this product.

Ask a doctor before use if you have
- heart disease
- high blood pressure
- thyroid disease
- diabetes
- trouble urinating due to an enlarged prostate gland
- glaucoma
- cough that occurs with too much phlegm (mucus)
- a breathing problem or persistent or chronic cough that lasts or as occurs with smoking, asthma, chronic bronchitis, or emphysema

Ask a doctor or pharmacist before use if you are taking sedatives or tranquilizers.

When using this product
- **do not use more than directed**
- marked drowsiness may occur
- avoid alcoholic beverages
- alcohol, sedatives, and tranquilizers may increase drowsiness
- be careful when driving a motor vehicle or operating machinery
- excitability may occur, especially in children

Stop use and ask a doctor if
- you get nervous, dizzy, or sleepless
- symptoms do not get better within 7 days or are accompanied by fever
- cough lasts more than 7 days, comes back, or is accompanied by fever, rash, or persistent headache. These could be signs of a serious condition

If pregnant or breast-feeding, ask a health professional before use.

Keep out of reach of children. In case of overdose, get medical help or contact a Poison Control Center right away.

Directions:
- do not take more than 4 doses in any 24-hour period

Age	Dose
adults and children 12 years and over	4 tsp every 4 hours
children 6 to under 12 years	2 tsp every 4 hours
children under 6 years	ask a doctor

Store at Controlled Room Temperature, Between 20°C and 25°C (68°F and 77°F)

Inactive Ingredients: artificial flavor, citric acid, FD&C blue no. 1, FD&C red no. 40, glycerin, high fructose corn syrup, propylene glycol, saccharin sodium, sodium benzoate, sorbitol, water

How Supplied: Red, grape-flavored liquid in bottles of 4 fl oz and 8 fl oz. Not a USP Elixir. Dosage cup provided.

Continued on next page

CHILDREN'S DIMETAPP® LONG ACTING COUGH PLUS COLD SYRUP
Cough suppressant/Nasal decongestant

Active Ingredients (in each 5 mL tsp):
Dextromethorphan HBr, USP 7.5 mg
Pseudoephedrine HCl, USP 15 mg

Uses:
- temporarily relieves these symptoms occurring with a cold:
  - nasal congestion
  - cough due to minor throat and bronchial irritation

Warnings:
Do not use if you are now taking a prescription monoamine oxidase inhibitor (MAOI) (certain drugs for depression, psychiatric, or emotional conditions, or Parkinson's disease), or for 2 weeks after stopping the MAOI drug. If you do not know if your prescription drug contains an MAOI, ask a doctor or pharmacist before taking this product.
Ask a doctor before use if you have
- heart disease • high blood pressure
- thyroid disease • diabetes
- trouble urinating due to an enlarged prostate gland
- cough that occurs with too much phlegm (mucus)
- cough that lasts or is chronic such as occurs with smoking, asthma, or emphysema

When using this product do not use more than directed.
Stop use and ask a doctor if
- you get nervous, dizzy, or sleepless
- symptoms do not get better within 7 days or are accompanied by fever
- cough lasts more than 7 days, comes back, or is accompanied by fever, rash, or persistent headache. These could be signs of a serious condition.

If pregnant or breast-feeding, ask a health professional before use.
Keep out of reach of children. In case of overdose, get medical help or contact a Poison Control Center right away.

Directions:
- do not take more than 4 doses in any 24-hour period
- repeat every 6 hours

age	dose
12 years and older	4 teaspoonfuls
6 to under 12 years	2 teaspoonfuls
2 to under 6 years	1 teaspoonful
under 2 years	ask a doctor

Other Information: • store at 20–25°C (68–77°F)
• dosage cup provided
Inactive Ingredients: citric acid, FD&C red no. 40, flavor, glycerin, high fructose corn syrup, propylene glycol, purified water, saccharin sodium, sodium benzoate, sodium chloride, sodium citrate
How Supplied: Bottles of 4 fl. oz.

DIMETAPP® Infant Drops Decongestant
Nasal Decongestant

Alcohol-Free

Active Ingredients: Each 0.8 mL (1 dropperful) contains: 7.5 mg Pseudoephedrine Hydrochloride, USP.

Uses: For temporary relief of nasal congestion due to the common cold, hay fever, other upper respiratory allergies, or associated with sinusitis.

Warnings:
Do not use in a child who is taking a prescription monoamine oxidase inhibitor (MAOI) (certain drugs for depression, psychiatric, or emotional conditions, or Parkinson's disease), or for 2 weeks after stopping the MAOI drug. If you do not know if your child's prescription drug contains an MAOI, ask a doctor or pharmacist before giving this product.
Ask a doctor before use if your child has
- heart disease
- high blood pressure
- thyroid disease
- diabetes

When using this product
- **do not use more than directed**
Stop use and ask a doctor if
- your child gets nervous, dizzy, or sleepless
- symptoms do not get better within 7 days or are accompanied by fever

Keep out of reach of children. In case of overdose, get medical help or contact a Poison Control Center right away.

Directions:
- do not give more than 4 doses in any 24-hour period
- children 2 to 3 years: 1.6 mL every 4 to 6 hours or as directed by a physician
- children under 2 years: ask a doctor
- measure with dosing device provided. Do not use with any other device.
Storage: Store at Controlled Room Temperature, between 20°C and 25°C (68°F and 77°F).

Inactive Ingredients: caramel, citric acid, D&C red no. 33, FD&C blue no. 1, flavors, glycerin, high fructose corn syrup, maltol, menthol, polyethylene glycol, propylene glycol, sodium benzoate, sorbitol, sucrose, water

How Supplied: ½ oz bottle with oral dosing device.

DIMETAPP®
Infant Drops Decongestant Plus Cough
Nasal decongestant/cough suppressant
Alcohol-Free/non-staining

Active Ingredient: Each 0.8 mL (1 dropperful) contains: 7.5 mg Pseudoephedrine Hydrochloride, USP; 2.5 mg Dextromethorphan Hydrobromide, USP.

Indications: Temporarily relieves cough occurring with the common cold and temporarily relieves nasal congestion due to a cold, hay fever, or other upper respiratory allergies.

Warnings:
Do not use in a child who is taking a prescription monoamine oxidase inhibitor (MAOI) (certain drugs for depression, psychiatric, or emotional conditions, or Parkinson's disease), or for 2 weeks after stopping the MAOI drug. If you do not know if your child's prescription drug contains an MAOI, ask a doctor or pharmacist before giving this product.
Ask a doctor before use if your child has
- heart disease
- high blood pressure
- thyroid disease
- diabetes
- cough that occurs with too much phlegm (mucus)
- cough that lasts or is chronic such as occurs with asthma
When using this product
- **do not use more than directed**
Stop use and ask a doctor if
- your child gets nervous, dizzy, or sleepless
- symptoms do not get better within 7 days or are accompanied by fever
- cough lasts more than 7 days, comes back, or is accompanied by fever, rash, or persistent headache. These could be signs of a serious condition.
Keep out of reach of children. In case of overdose, get medical help or contact a Poison Control Center right away.

Directions: do not give more than 4 doses in any 24-hour period
- children 2–3 years: 1.6 mL every 4–6 hours or as directed by a physician
- children under 2 years: ask a doctor
- measure with dosing device provided. Do not use with any other device.
Storage: Store at Controlled Room Temperature, between 20°C and 25°C (68°F and 77°F).
Inactive Ingredients: citric acid, flavors, glycerin, high fructose corn syrup, maltol, menthol, polyethylene glycol, propylene glycol, sodium benzoate, sorbitol, sucrose, water.

How Supplied: Infant Drops ½ oz with oral dosing device.

FIBERCON®
Calcium Polycarbophil
Bulk-Forming Laxative

Active ingredient (in each caplet)
Calcium polycarbophil 625 mg (equivalent to 500 mg polycarbophil)

Uses:
- relieves constipation to help restore and maintain regularity
- this product generally produces bowel movement in 12 to 72 hours

Warnings:
Choking: Taking this product without adequate fluid may cause it to swell and block your throat or esophagus and may cause choking. Do not take this product if you have difficulty in swallowing. If you experience chest pain, vomiting, or difficulty in swallowing or breathing after taking this product, seek immediate medical attention.

Age	Recommended dose	Daily maximum
adults & children 12 years of age and over	2 caplets once a day	up to 4 times a day
children under 12 years	consult a physician	

age	recommended dose	daily maximum
adults and children 12 years of age and over	2 caplets	up to 4 caplets a day
children under 12 years	consult a physician	

Ask a doctor before use if you have
- abdominal pain, nausea, or vomiting
- a sudden change in bowel habits that persists over a period of 2 weeks

Ask a doctor or pharmacist before use if you are taking any other drug. Take this product 2 or more hours before or after other drugs. All laxatives may affect how other drugs work.

When using this product
- do not use for more than 7 days unless directed by a doctor
- do not take caplets more than 4 times in a 24 hour period unless directed by a doctor

Stop use and ask a doctor if rectal bleeding occurs or if you fail to have a bowel movement after use of this or any other laxative These could be signs of a serious condition.

Keep out of reach of children. In case of overdose, get medical help or contact a Poison Control Center right away.

Directions:
- take each dose of this product with at least 8 ounces (a full glass) of water or other fluid. Taking this product without enough liquid may cause choking. See choking warning
- FiberCon works naturally so continued use for one to three days is normally required to provide full benefit. Dosage may vary according to diet, exercise, previous laxative use or severity of constipation.

[See first table above]

Inactive ingredients: calcium carbonate, caramel, crospovidone, hypromellose, magnesium stearate, microcrystalline cellulose, mineral oil, povidone, silica gel and sodium lauryl sulfate

Each caplet contains: 122 mg calcium.

Storage Protect contents from moisture. Store at 20–25°C (68–77°F)

How Supplied: Film-coated scored caplets.
Package of 36 caplets, and
Bottles of 60, 90, 140 and 200 caplets.

FREELAX
Magnesium hydroxide
Saline laxative

Active Ingredient (in each caplet):
Magnesium hydroxide 1200 mg (equivalent to magnesium 500 mg)

Uses:
for relief of occasional constipation (irregularity)

this product generally produces bowel movement in ½ to 6 hours

Warnings:
Ask a doctor before us if you have
- kidney disease
- been told to follow a magnesium-restricted diet
- abdominal pain, nausea, or vomiting
- a sudden change in bowel habits that persists over a period of 2 weeks

Ask a doctor or pharmacist before use if you are taking any other drug. Take this product 2 or more hours before or after other drugs. All laxatives may affect how other drugs work.

When using this product do not use for more than 7 days unless directed by a doctor

Stop use and ask a doctor if rectal bleeding occurs or if you fail to have a bowel movement after use of this or any other laxative. These could be signs of a serious condition.

If pregnant or breast-feeding, ask a health professional before use.

Keep out of reach of children. In case of overdose, get medical help or contact a Poison Control Center right away.

Directions
Take each dose of this product with at least 8 ounces (a full glass) of water or other fluid
[See second table above]

Other Information:
each caplet contains: 500 mg magnesium
store at 20–25°C (68–77°F)

Inactive Ingredients: crospovidone, D&C yellow no. 10 aluminum lake, FD&C yellow no. 6 aluminum lake, glyceryl behenate, hydroxypropyl cellulose, hypromellose, microcrystalline cellulose, polydextrose, polyethylene glycol, silicon dioxide, titanium dioxide, triacetin

How Supplied:
packages of 30 caplets

PREPARATION H®
Hemorrhoidal Ointment and Cream
PREPARATION H®
Hemorrhoidal Suppositories
PREPARATION H®
Hemorrhoidal Cooling Gel

Active Ingredients: Preparation H is available in ointment, cream, gel, and suppository product forms. The **Oint-**

ment contains Petrolatum 71.9%, Mineral Oil 14%, Shark Liver Oil 3% and Phenylephrine HCl 0.25%.
The **Cream** contains Petrolatum 18%, Glycerin 12%, Shark Liver Oil 3% and Phenylephrine HCl 0.25%.
The **Suppositories** contain Cocoa Butter 85.5%, Shark Liver Oil 3%, and Phenylephrine HCl 0.25%.
The **Cooling Gel** contains Phenylephrine HCl 0.25% and Witch Hazel 50%.

Uses: Preparation H Ointment, Cream, and Suppositories
- help relieve the local itching and discomfort associated with hemorrhoids
- temporarily shrink hemorrhoidal tissue and relieve burning
- temporarily provide a coating for relief of anorectal discomforts
- temporarily protect the inflamed, irritated anorectal surface to help make bowel movements less painful

Cooling Gel
- helps relieve the local itching and discomfort associated with hemorrhoids
- temporarily relieves irritation and burning
- temporarily shrinks hemorrhoidal tissue
- aids in protecting irritated anorectal areas

Warnings:
For all product forms:
Ask a doctor before use if you have
- heart disease
- high blood pressure
- thyroid disease
- diabetes
- difficulty in urination due to enlargement of the prostate gland

Ask a doctor or pharmacist before use if you are presently taking a prescription drug for high blood pressure or depression.

When using this product do not exceed the recommended daily dosage unless directed by a doctor.

Stop use and ask a doctor if
- bleeding occurs
- condition worsens or does not improve within 7 days

If pregnant or breast-feeding, ask a health professional before use.

Keep out of reach of children. If swallowed, get medical help or contact a Poison Control Center right away.

Ointment: Stop use and ask a doctor if introduction of applicator into the rectum causes additional pain. For external and/or intrarectal use only.

Cream/Cooling Gel: For external use only. Do not put into the rectum by using fingers or any mechanical device or applicator.

Suppositories: For rectal use only.

Directions:
Ointment—
- adults: when practical, cleanse the affected area by patting or blotting with an appropriate cleansing wipe. Gently dry by patting or blotting with a tissue or a soft cloth before applying ointment.
- when first opening the tube, puncture foil seal with top end of cap

Continued on next page

Preparation H—Cont.

- apply to the affected area up to 4 times daily, especially at night, in the morning or after each bowel movement
- intrarectal use:
  - remove cover from applicator, attach applicator to tube, lubricate applicator well and gently insert applicator into the rectum
  - thoroughly cleanse applicator after each use and replace cover
- also apply ointment to external area
- regular use provides continual therapy for relief of symptoms
- children under 12 years of age: ask a doctor

Tamper-Evident: Do Not Use if tube seal under cap embossed with "H" is broken or missing.

Cream—

- adults: when practical, cleanse the affected area by patting or blotting with an appropriate cleansing wipe. Gently dry by patting or blotting with a tissue or a soft cloth before applying cream.
- when first opening the tube, puncture foil seal with top end of cap
- apply externally or in the lower portion of the anal canal only
- apply externally to the affected area up to 4 times daily, especially at night, in the morning or after each bowel movement
- for application in the lower anal canal: remove cover from dispensing cap. Attach dispensing cap to tube. Lubricate dispensing cap well, then gently insert dispensing cap partway into the anus.
- thoroughly cleanse dispensing cap after each use and replace cover
- children under 12 years of age: ask a doctor

Tamper-Evident: Do Not Use if tube seal under cap embossed with "H" is broken or missing.

Suppositories—

- adults: when practical, cleanse the affected area by patting or blotting with an appropriate cleansing wipe. Gently dry by patting or blotting with a tissue or a soft cloth before insertion of this product.
- detach one suppository from the strip; remove the foil wrapper before inserting into the rectum as follows:
  - hold suppository with rounded end up
  - carefully separate foil tabs by inserting tip of fingernail at end marked "peel down"
  - slowly and evenly peel apart (do not tear) foil by pulling tabs down both sides, to expose the suppository
  - remove exposed suppository from wrapper
  - insert one suppository into the rectum up to 4 times daily, especially at night, in the morning or after each bowel movement
- children under 12 years of age: ask a doctor

Tamper-Evident: Individually quality sealed for your protection. Do Not Use if foil imprinted "PREPARATION H" is torn or damaged.

Cooling Gel—

- adults: when practical, cleanse the affected area by patting or blotting with an appropriate cleansing wipe. Gently dry by patting or blotting with a tissue or a soft cloth before applying gel.

- when first opening the tube, puncture foil seal with top end of cap
- apply externally to the affected area up to 4 times daily, especially at night, in the morning or after each bowel movement
- children under 12 years of age: ask a doctor

Tamper-Evident: Do Not Use if tube seal under cap embossed with "H" is broken or missing.

Inactive Ingredients: Ointment— benzoic acid, BHA, BHT, corn oil, glycerin, lanolin, lanolin alcohol, methylparaben, paraffin, propylparaben, thyme oil, tocopherol, water, wax

Cream—BHA, carboxymethylcellulose sodium, cetyl alcohol, citric acid, edetate disodium, glyceryl oleate, glyceryl stearate, lanolin, methylparaben, propyl gallate, propylene glycol, propylparaben, simethicone, sodium benzoate, sodium lauryl sulfate, stearyl alcohol, tocopherol, water, xanthan gum.

Suppositories—methylparaben, propylparaben, starch

Cooling Gel—benzophenone-4, edetate disodium, hydroxyethylcellulose, methylparaben, propylene glycol, propylparaben, sodium citrate, water

Storage: Store at 20–25°C (68–77°F).

How Supplied: Ointment: Net Wt. 1 oz and 2 oz **Cream:** Net Wt. 0.9 oz and 1.8 oz **Suppositories:** 12's, 24's and 48's. **Cooling Gel:** Net Wt. 0.9 oz and 1.8 oz

---

PREPARATION H HYDROCORTISONE CREAM
Anti-itch cream

Active ingredient:
Hydrocortisone 1%

Uses:
- temporary relief of external anal itching
- temporary relief of itching associated with minor skin irritations and rashes
- other uses of this product should be only under the advice and supervision of a doctor

Warnings:
For external use only
Do not use for the treatment of diaper rash. Consult a doctor.
When using this product
- avoid contact with the eyes
- do not exceed the recommended daily dosage unless directed by a doctor
- do not put into the rectum by using fingers or any mechanical device or applicator

Stop use and ask a doctor if
- bleeding occurs
- condition worsens
- symptoms persist for more than 7 days or clear up and occur again within a few days. Do not begin use of any other hydrocortisone product unless you have consulted a doctor.
Keep out of reach of children. If swallowed, get medical help or contact a Poison Control Center right away.

Directions:
- adults: when practical, cleanse the affected area by patting or blotting with an appropriate cleansing wipe. Gently dry by patting or blotting with a tissue or soft cloth before application of this product.
- when first opening the tube, puncture foil seal with top end of cap
- adults and children 12 years of age and older: apply to the affected area not more than 3 to 4 times daily
- children under 12 years of age: do not use, consult a doctor

Tamper-Evident: Do Not Use if tube seal under cap embossed with "H" is broken or missing.

Inactive Ingredients: BHA, carboxymethylcellulose sodium, cetyl alcohol, citric acid, edetate disodium, glycerin, glyceryl oleate, glyceryl stearate, lanolin, methylparaben, petrolatum, propyl gallate, propylene glycol, propylparaben, simethicone, sodium benzoate, sodium lauryl sulfate, stearyl alcohol, water, xanthan gum.

Storage: Store at 20–25 °C (68–77 °F)

How Supplied: 0.9 oz. tubes

PREPARATION H® MEDICATED WIPES

Active Ingredient: Soft pads are premoistened with a solution containing Witch Hazel 50%.

Uses:
- helps relieve the local itching and discomfort associated with hemorrhoids
- temporary relief of irritation and burning
- aids in protecting irritated anorectal areas
- **for vaginal care**—cleanse the area by gently wiping, patting or blotting. Repeat as needed.
- **for use as a moist compress**—if necessary, first cleanse the area as previously described. Fold wipe to desired size and place in contact with tissue for a soothing and cooling effect. Leave in place for up to 15 minutes and repeat as needed.

Warnings:
For external use only
When using this product
- do not exceed the recommended daily dosage unless directed by a doctor
- do not put this product into the rectum by using fingers or any mechanical device or applicator

Stop use and ask a doctor if
- bleeding occurs
- condition worsens or does not improve within 7 days
If pregnant or breast-feeding, ask a health professional before use. **Keep out of reach of children.** If swallowed, get medical help or contact a Poison Control Center right away.

Directions:
- remove tab on right side of wipes pouch label and peel back to open
- grab the top wipe at the edge of the center fold and pull out of pouch
- carefully reseal label on pouch after each use to retain moistness

- adults: unfold wipe and cleanse the area by gently wiping, patting or blotting. If necessary, repeat until all matter is removed from the area.
- use up to 6 times daily or after each bowel movement and before applying topical hemorrhoidal treatments
- children under 12 years of age: consult a doctor
- store at 20–25°C (68–77°F)
- for best results, flush only one or two wipes at a time

Tamper-Evident: Pouch quality sealed for your protection. Do Not Use if tear strip imprinted "Safety Sealed" is torn or missing

Inactive ingredients: aloe barbadensis gel, capryl/capramidopropyl betaine, citric acid, diazolidinyl urea, glycerin, methylparaben, propylene glycol, propylparaben, sodium citrate, water.

How Supplied: Containers of 48 wipes. Refills of 48 wipes. 8 count travel pack.

PRIMATENE® Mist
Epinephrine Inhalation Aerosol
Bronchodilator

Active Ingredient: (in each inhalation)
Epinephrine 0.22 mg

Uses:
- temporarily relieves shortness of breath, tightness of chest, and wheezing due to bronchial asthma
- eases breathing for asthma patients by reducing spasms of bronchial muscles

Warnings:
For inhalation only
Do not use
- unless a doctor has said you have asthma
- if you are now taking a prescription monoamine oxidase inhibitor (MAOI) (certain drugs for depression, psychiatric, or emotional conditions, or Parkinson's disease), or for 2 weeks after stopping the MAOI drug If you do not know if your prescription drug contains an MAOI, ask a doctor or pharmacist before taking this product

Ask a doctor before use if you have
- heart disease • thyroid disease
- diabetes • high blood pressure
- ever been hospitalized for asthma
- trouble urinating due to an enlarged prostate gland

Ask a doctor or pharmacist before use if you are taking any prescription drug for asthma
When using this product
- overuse may cause nervousness, rapid heart beat, and heart problems
- **do not continue to use, but seek medical assistance immediately if symptoms are not relieved within 20 minutes or become worse**
- do not puncture or throw into incinerator. Contents under pressure.
- do not use or store near open flame or heat above 120°F (49°C). May cause bursting.

Contains CFC 12, 114, substances which harm public health and environment by destroying ozone in the upper atmosphere
If pregnant or breast-feeding, ask a health professional before use.

Keep out of reach of children. In case of overdose, get medical help or contact a Poison Control Center right away.

Directions:
- **do not use more often or at higher doses unless directed by a doctor**
- supervise children using this product
- adults and children 4 years and over: start with one inhalation, then wait at least 1 minute. If not relieved, use once more. Do not use again for at least 3 hours.
- children under 4 years of age: ask a doctor

Directions For Use of Mouthpiece:
The Primatene Mist mouthpiece, which is enclosed in the Primatene Mist 15 mL size (not the refill size), should be used for inhalation only with Primatene Mist.
1. Take plastic cap off mouthpiece. (For refills, use mouthpiece from previous purchase.)
2. Take plastic mouthpiece off bottle.
3. Place other end of mouthpiece on bottle.
4. Turn bottle upside down. Place thumb on bottom of mouthpiece over circular button and forefinger on top of vial. Empty the lungs as completely as possible by exhaling.
5. Place mouthpiece in mouth with lips closed around opening. Inhale deeply while squeezing mouthpiece and bottle together. Release immediately and remove unit from mouth. Complete taking the deep breath, drawing the medication into your lungs and holding breath as long as comfortable.
6. Exhale slowly keeping lips nearly closed. This helps distribute the medication in the lungs.
7. Replace plastic cap on mouthpiece.

Care of the Mouthpiece:
The Primatene Mist mouthpiece should be washed once daily with soap and hot water, and rinsed thoroughly. Then it should be dried with a clean, lint-free cloth.

Other Information:
- store at room temperature, between 20–25°C (68–77°F) • contains no sulfites

Inactive Ingredients: ascorbic acid, dehydrated alcohol (34%), dichlorodifluoromethane (CFC 12), dichlorotetrafluoroethane (CFC 114), hydrochloric acid, nitric acid, purified water

How Supplied:
$1/2$ Fl oz (15 mL) With Mouthpiece.
$1/2$ Fl oz (15 mL) Refill
$3/4$ Fl oz (22.5 mL) Refill

PRIMATENE® Tablets
Bronchodilator, Expectorant

Active Ingredients (in each tablet):
Ephedrine HCl, USP   12.5 mg
Guaifenesin   200 mg

Uses:
- temporarily relieves shortness of breath, tightness of chest, and wheezing due to bronchial asthma
- eases breathing for asthma patients by reducing spasms of bronchial muscles
- helps loosen phlegm (mucus) and thin bronchial secretions to rid bronchial

passageways of bothersome mucus, and to make coughs more productive

Warnings:
Do not use
- unless a diagnosis of asthma has been made by a doctor
- if you are now taking a prescription monoamine oxidase inhibitor (MAOI) (certain drugs for depression, psychiatric, or emotional conditions, or Parkinson's disease), or for 2 weeks after stopping the MAOI drug If you do not know if your prescription drug contains an MAOI, ask a doctor or pharmacist before taking this product

Ask a doctor before use if you have
- heart disease • high blood pressure
- thyroid disease • diabetes
- trouble urinating due to an enlarged prostate gland
- ever been hospitalized for asthma
- cough that occurs with too much phlegm (mucus)
- cough that lasts or is chronic such as occurs with smoking, asthma, chronic bronchitis, or emphysema

Ask a doctor or pharmacist before use if you are taking any prescription drug for asthma
When using this product some users may experience nervousness, tremor, sleeplessness, nausea, and loss of appetite

Stop use and ask a doctor if
- symptoms are not relieved within 1 hour or become worse
- nervousness, tremor, sleeplessness, nausea, and loss of appetite persist or become worse
- cough lasts more than 7 days, comes back, or occurs with fever, rash, or persistent headache These could be signs of a serious condition

If pregnant or breast-feeding, ask a health professional before use.
Keep out of reach of children. In case of overdose, get medical help or contact a Poison Control Center right away.

Directions:
- do not use more than dosage below unless directed by a doctor
- adults and children 12 years and over: take 2 tablets initially, then 2 tablets every 4 hours, as needed, not to exceed 12 tablets in 24 hours
- children under 12 years: ask a doctor

Other Information:
- store at 20–25°C (68–77°F)

Inactive Ingredients: crospovidone, D&C yellow no. 10 aluminum lake, FD&C yellow no. 6 aluminum lake, magnesium stearate, microcrystalline cellulose, povidone, silicon dioxide (colloidal).

How Supplied: Available in 24 and 60 tablet thermoform blister cartons.

ROBITUSSIN® Expectorant

Active Ingredient: (in each 5mL tsp)
Guaifenesin, USP 100 mg

Use: helps loosen phlegm (mucus) and thin bronchial secretions to make coughs more productive

Continued on next page

Robitussin Exp.—Cont.

Warnings:
Ask a doctor before use if you have
• cough that occurs with too much phlegm (mucus)
• cough that lasts or is chronic such as occurs with smoking, asthma, chronic bronchitis, or emphysema
Stop use and ask a doctor if cough lasts more than 7 days, comes back, or is accompanied by fever, rash, or persistent headache. These could be signs of a serious condition.
If pregnant or breast-feeding, ask a health professional before use.
Keep out of reach of children. In case of overdose, get medical help or contact a Poison Control Center right away.

Directions:
• repeat dose every 4 hrs, as needed
• do not take more than 6 doses in any 24-hour period.
• adults and children 12 yrs. and over: 2–4 tsp
• children 6 to under 12 yrs.: 1–2 tsp
• children 2 to under 6 yrs.: ½–1 tsp
• children under 2 yrs.: ask a doctor

Other Information
• store at 20–25°C (68–77°F)
• alcohol-free
• dosage cup provided

Inactive Ingredients: caramel, citric acid, FD&C red no. 40, flavors, glucose, glycerin, high fructose corn syrup, menthol, saccharin sodium, sodium benzoate, water.

How Supplied: Robitussin (wine-colored) in bottles of 4 fl oz, 8 fl oz.

ROBITUSSIN® ALLERGY & COUGH SYRUP
Nasal Decongestant, Cough Suppressant, Antihistamine

Active Ingredients: (in each 5 mL tsp)
Brompheniramine maleate, USP 2 mg
Dextromethorphan HBr, USP 10 mg
Pseudoephedrine HCl, USP 30 mg

Uses:
• temporarily relieves these symptoms due to hay fever (allergic rhinitis):
• runny nose • sneezing • itchy, watery eyes • itching of the nose or throat
• nasal congestion
• temporarily controls cough due to minor throat and bronchial irritation associated with inhaled irritants
• temporarily restores freer breathing through the nose

Warnings:
Do not use if you are now taking a prescription monoamine oxidase inhibitor (MAOI) (certain drugs for depression, psychiatric, or emotional conditions, or Parkinson's disease), or for 2 weeks after stopping the MAOI drug. If you do not know if your prescription drug contains an MAOI, ask a doctor or pharmacist before taking this product.

Ask a doctor before use if you have
• heart disease • high blood pressure
• thyroid disease • diabetes
• trouble urinating due to an enlarged prostate gland • glaucoma
• cough that occurs with too much phlegm (mucus)
• cough that lasts or is chronic such as occurs with smoking, asthma, chronic bronchitis or emphysema
Ask a doctor or pharmacist before use if you are taking sedatives or tranquilizers
When using this product
• do not use more than directed
• marked drowsiness may occur
• avoid alcoholic beverages
• alcohol, sedatives, and tranquilizers may increase drowsiness
• be careful when driving a motor vehicle or operating machinery
• excitability may occur, especially in children
Stop use and ask a doctor if
• you get nervous, dizzy, or sleepless
• symptoms do not get better within 7 days or are accompanied by fever
• cough lasts more than 7 days, comes back, or is accompanied by fever, rash, or persistent headache. These could be signs of a serious condition.
If pregnant or breast-feeding, ask a health professional before use.
Keep out of reach of children. In case of overdose, get medical help or contact a Poison Control Center right away.

Directions:
• repeat dose every 4 hrs, as needed
• do not take more than 4 doses in any 24-hour period
• adults and children 12 yrs and over: 2 tsp
• children 6 to under 12 yrs: 1 tsp
• children under 6 yrs: ask a doctor
Other Information:
• store at 20–25°C (68–77°F)
• alcohol free
• dosage cup provided

Inactive Ingredients: artificial flavor, citric acid, glycerin, propylene glycol, saccharin sodium, sodium benzoate, sorbitol, water

How Supplied: Bottles of 4 fl. oz.

ROBITUSSIN® COLD COLD & CONGESTION
Softgels, Caplets
Nasal Decongestant, Expectorant, Cough Suppressant

Active Ingredients (in each softgel, caplet)
Dextromethorphan HBr, USP 10 mg
Guaifenesin, USP 200 mg
Pseudoephedrine HCl, USP 30 mg

Uses:
• temporarily relieves nasal congestion, and cough due to minor throat and bronchial irritation occurring with the common cold
• helps loosen phlegm (mucus) and thin bronchial secretions to make coughs more productive
• temporarily relieves nasal congestion associated with hay fever or other upper respiratory allergies, or associated with sinusitis

Warnings:
Do not use if you are now taking a prescription monoamine oxidase inhibitor (MAOI) (certain drugs for depression, psychiatric, or emotional conditions, or Parkinson's disease), or for 2 weeks after stopping the MAOI drug. If you do not know if your prescription drug contains an MAOI, ask a doctor or pharmacist before taking this product.

Ask a doctor before use if you have
• heart disease • high blood pressure
• thyroid disease • diabetes
• trouble urinating due to an enlarged prostate gland
• cough that occurs with too much phlegm (mucus)
• cough that lasts or is chronic such as occurs with smoking, asthma, chronic bronchitis, or emphysema
When using this product do not use more than directed
Stop use and ask a doctor if
• you get nervous, dizzy, or sleepless
• symptoms do not get better within 7 days or are accompanied by fever
• cough lasts more than 7 days, comes back, or is accompanied by fever, rash, or persistent headache. These could be signs of a serious condition.
If pregnant or breast-feeding, ask a health professional before use.
Keep out of reach of children. In case of overdose, get medical help or contact a Poison Control Center right away.

Directions:
• repeat dose every 4 hrs, as needed
• do not exceed 4 doses in any 24-hr period
• adults and children 12 yrs and over: 2 softgels or caplets
• children 6 to under 12 yrs.: 1 softgel or caplet
• children under 6: ask a doctor
Other Information:
• store at 20–25°C (68–77°F)

Inactive Ingredients (Softgels): FD&C blue no. 1, FD&C red no. 40, gelatin, glycerin, mannitol, pharmaceutical glaze, polyethylene glycol, povidone, propylene glycol, sorbitan, sorbitol, titanium dioxide, water

Inactive Ingredients (Caplets): calcium stearate, croscarmellose sodium, FD&C red no. 40 aluminum lake, hydroxypropyl methylcellulose, maltodextrin, microcrystalline cellulose, polydextrose, polyethylene glycol, povidone, pregelatinized starch, silicon dioxide, stearic acid, titanium dioxide, triacetin

How Supplied: Softgels in packages of 12 (individually packaged). Caplets in packages of 20 (individually packaged).

ROBITUSSIN® COLD MULTI-SYMPTOM COLD & FLU
Softgels, Caplets
Pain Reliever/Fever Reducer, Cough Suppressant, Nasal Decongestant, Expectorant

Active Ingredients (in each softgel):
Acetaminophen, USP 250 mg
Dextromethorphan HBr, USP 10 mg

Guaifenesin, USP 100 mg
Pseudoephedrine HCl, USP 30 mg

Active Ingredients (in each caplet):
Acetaminophen, USP 325 mg
Dextromethorphan HBr, USP 10 mg
Guaifenesin, USP 200 mg
Pseudoephedrine HCl, USP 30 mg

Uses:
- temporarily relieves these symptoms associated with a cold, or flu:
  - headache • sore throat • fever
  - muscular aches • minor aches and pains
- temporarily relieves nasal congestion, and cough due to minor throat and bronchial irritation occurring with a cold
- helps loosen phlegm (mucus) and thin bronchial secretions to make coughs more productive

Warnings:
Alcohol warning: If you consume 3 or more alcoholic drinks every day, ask your doctor whether you should take acetaminophen or other pain relievers/fever reducers. Acetaminophen may cause liver damage.

Sore throat warning: If sore throat is severe, persists for more than two days, is accompanied or followed by fever, headache, rash, nausea, or vomiting, consult a doctor promptly

Do not use
- if you are now taking a prescription monoamine oxidase inhibitor (MAOI) (certain drugs for depression, psychiatric, or emotional conditions, or Parkinson's disease), or for 2 weeks after stopping the MAOI drug. If you do not know if your prescription drug contains an MAOI, ask a doctor or pharmacist before taking this product.
- with any other product containing acetaminophen as this may lead to an overdose. Overdose requires prompt medical attention even if you do not notice any signs or symptoms.

Ask a doctor before use if you have
- heart disease • high blood pressure
- thyroid disease • diabetes
- trouble urinating due to an enlarged prostate gland
- cough that occurs with too much phlegm (mucus)
- cough that lasts or is chronic such as occurs with smoking, asthma, chronic bronchitis, or emphysema

When using this product do not use more than directed

Stop use and ask a doctor if
- you get nervous, dizzy, or sleepless
- new symptoms occur
- you need to use for more than 7 days (adults) or 5 days (children)
- symptoms do not get better, get worse, or are accompanied by fever more than 3 days
- redness or swelling is present
- cough lasts more than 7 days, comes back, or is accompanied by fever, rash, or persistent headache. These could be signs of a serious condition.

If pregnant or breast-feeding, ask a health professional before use.

Keep out of reach of children. In case of overdose, get medical help or contact a Poison Control Center right away.

Prompt medical attention is critical for adults as well as for children, even if you do not notice any signs or symptoms.

Directions:
- repeat dose every 4 hrs, as needed
- do not use more than 4 doses in any 24-hour period
- do not exceed recommended dosage. Taking more than the recommended dose (overdose) may cause serious liver damage.
- adults and children 12 yrs and over: 2 softgels or caplets
- children 6 to under 12 yrs: 1 caplet
- children under 6 yrs: ask a doctor

Other Information
- store at 20–25°C (68–77°F)

Inactive Ingredients (Softgels): D&C yellow no. 10, FD&C red no. 40, gelatin, glycerin, iron oxides, lecithin, mannitol, pharmaceutical glaze, polyethylene glycol, povidone, propylene glycol, simethicone, sorbitan, sorbitol, water

Inactive Ingredients (Caplets): calcium stearate, croscarmellose sodium, D&C yellow no. 10 aluminum lake, FD&C yellow no. 6 aluminum lake, hydroxypropyl methylcellulose, maltodextrin, microcrystalline cellulose, polydextrose, polyethylene glycol, povidone, pregelatinized starch, silicon dioxide, stearic acid, titanium dioxide, triacetin

How Supplied: Softgels are available in blister packs of 12's.
Caplets are available in blister packs of 20's.

ROBITUSSIN® COLD SEVERE CONGESTION Softgels
Nasal Decongestant, Expectorant

Active Ingredients:
(in each softgel)
Guaifenesin, USP 200 mg
Pseudoephedrine HCl USP 30 mg

Uses:
- temporarily relieves nasal congestion associated with
  - the common cold
  - hay fever
  - upper respiratory allergies
  - sinusitis
- helps loosen phlegm (mucus) and thin bronchial secretions to make coughs more productive

Warnings:
Do not use if you are now taking a prescription monoamine oxidase inhibitor (MAOI) (certain drugs for depression, psychiatric, or emotional conditions, or Parkinson's disease), or for 2 weeks after stopping the MAOI drug. If you do not know if your prescription drug contains an MAOI, ask a doctor or pharmacist before taking this product.

Ask a doctor before use if you have
- heart disease • high blood pressure
- thyroid disease • diabetes
- trouble urinating due to an enlarged prostate gland
- cough that occurs with too much phlegm (mucus)
- cough that lasts or is chronic such as occurs with smoking, asthma, chronic bronchitis, or emphysema

When using this product do not use more than directed
Stop use and ask a doctor if
- you get nervous, dizzy, or sleepless
- symptoms do not get better within 7 days or are accompanied by fever
- cough lasts more than 7 days, comes back, or is accompanied by fever, rash, or persistent headache. These could be signs of a serious condition.

If pregnant or breast-feeding, ask a health professional before use.

Keep out of reach of children. In case of overdose, get medical help or contact a Poison Control Center right away.

Directions:
- repeat dose every 4 hrs, as needed
- do not exceed 4 doses in any 24-hr. period
- adults and children 12 yrs. and over: 2 softgels
- children 6 to under 12 yrs: 1 softgel
- children under 6 yrs: ask a doctor

Other Information: • store at 20–25°C (68°F).

Inactive Ingredients: FD&C green no. 3, gelatin, glycerin, mannitol, pharmaceutical glaze, polyethylene glycol, povidone, propylene glycol, sorbitan, sorbitol, titanium dioxide, water

How Supplied: Blister Packs of 12's.

ROBITUSSIN® COUGH DROPS
Menthol Eucalyptus, Cherry, and Honey-Lemon Flavors

Active Ingredient: (in each drop)
Menthol Eucalyptus:
Menthol, USP 10 mg
Cherry and Honey-Lemon:
Menthol, USP 5 mg

Uses:
- temporarily relieves
  - occasional minor irritation, pain, sore mouth, and sore throat
  - cough associated with a cold or inhaled irritants

Warnings:
Sore throat warning: Severe or persistent sore throat or sore throat accompanied by high fever, headache, nausea, and vomiting may be serious. Consult a doctor right away. Do not use more than 2 days or give to children under 3 years of age unless directed by a doctor

Ask a doctor before use if you have
- cough that occurs with too much phlegm (mucus)
- cough that lasts or is chronic such as occurs with smoking, asthma, or emphysema

Stop use and ask a doctor if cough lasts more than 7 days, comes back, or is accompanied by fever, rash, or persistent headache. These could be signs of a serious condition.

If pregnant or breast-feeding, ask a health professional before use.
Keep out of reach of children.

Continued on next page

Robitussin Cough Drops—Cont.

Directions:
- adults and children 4 years and over: allow 1 drop to dissolve slowly in the mouth
  - for sore throat: may be repeated every 2 hours, as needed, or as directed by a doctor
  - for cough: may be repeated every hour, as needed, or as directed by a doctor
- children under 4 years of age: ask a doctor

Other Information: store at 20–25°C (68–77°F).

Inactive Ingredients:
Menthol Eucalyptus: corn syrup, eucalyptus oil, flavor, sucrose
Cherry: corn syrup, FD&C red no. 40, flavor, methylparaben, propylparaben, sodium benzoate, sucrose
Honey-Lemon: citric acid, corn syrup, D&C yellow no. 10, FD&C yellow no. 6, honey, lemon oil, methylparaben, povidone, propylparaben, sodium benzoate, sucrose

How Supplied: All 3 flavors of Robitussin Cough Drops are available in bags of 25 drops.

ROBITUSSIN® FLU
Pain Reliever/Fever Reducer, Nasal Decongestant, Cough Suppressant, Antihistamine

Active Ingredients: (in each 5 mL tsp)
Acetaminophen, USP 160 mg
Chlorpheniramine maleate, USP 1 mg
Dextromethorphan HBr, USP 5 mg
Pseudoephedrine HCl, USP 15 mg

Uses:
- temporarily relieves these symptoms occurring with a cold or flu, hay fever, or other upper respiratory allergies:
- headache • cough • runny nose • itching of the nose or throat • nasal congestion • muscular aches • sneezing • sore throat • minor aches and pains • itchy, watery eyes • fever

Warnings:
Alcohol warning: If you consume 3 or more alcoholic drinks every day, ask your doctor whether you should take acetaminophen or other pain relievers/fever reducers. Acetaminophen may cause liver damage.
Sore throat warning: If sore throat is severe, persists for more than 2 days, is accompanied or followed by fever, headache, rash, nausea, or vomiting, consult a doctor promptly
Do not use:
- if you are now taking a prescription monoamine oxidase inhibitor (MAOI) (certain drugs for depression, psychiatric, or emotional conditions, or Parkinson's disease), or for 2 weeks after stopping the MAOI drug. If you do not know if your prescription drug contains an MAOI, ask a doctor or pharmacist before taking this product.
- with any other product containing acetaminophen as this may lead to an

overdose. Overdose requires prompt medical attention even if you do not notice any signs or symptoms.
Ask a doctor before use if you have
- heart disease • thyroid disease
- trouble urinating due to an enlarged prostate gland • diabetes
- cough that occurs with too much phlegm (mucus) • glaucoma
- a breathing problem or chronic cough that lasts or as occurs with smoking, asthma, chronic bronchitis, or emphysema • high blood pressure
Ask a doctor or pharmacist before use if you are taking sedatives or tranquilizers
When using this product
- do not use more than directed
- marked drowsiness may occur
- alcohol, sedatives, and tranquilizers may increase drowsiness
- be careful when driving a motor vehicle or operating machinery
- excitability may occur, especially in children • avoid alcoholic drinks
Stop use and ask a doctor if
- you get nervous, dizzy, or sleepless
- new symptoms occur
- symptoms do not get better within 7 days or are accompanied by fever
- symptoms do not get better, get worse, or are accompanied by fever more than 3 days • redness or swelling is present
- cough lasts more than 7 days, comes back, or is accompanied by fever, rash, or persistent headache. These could be signs of a serious condition.
If pregnant or breast-feeding, ask a health professional before use.
Keep out of reach of children. In case of overdose, get medical help or contact a Poison Control Center right away. Quick medical attention is critical for adults as well as for children, even if you do not notice any signs or symptoms.

Directions:
- repeat dose every 4 hrs, as needed
- do not take more than 4 doses in any 24-hour period
- do not exceed recommended dosage. Taking more than the recommended dose (overdose) may cause serious liver damage.
- adults and children 12 yrs and over: 4 tsp
- children 6 to under 12 yrs: 2 tsp
- children under 6 yrs: ask a doctor

Other Information:
- store at 20–25°C (68–77°F)
- alcohol free

Inactive Ingredients: citric acid, D&C red no. 33, FD&C yellow no. 6, flavor, glycerin, high fructose corn syrup, polyethylene glycol, purified water, sodium benzoate, sodium citrate, sorbitol solution, sucralose

How Supplied: Bottles of 4 fl. oz.

ROBITUSSIN®
HONEY CALMERS THROAT DROPS (BERRY)
Oral Pain Reliever

**Active Ingredient
(in each drop):**
Menthol, USP 1 mg

Use: Temporarily relieves occasional minor irritation, pain, sore mouth, and sore throat.

Warnings
Sore throat warning: Severe or persistent sore throat or sore throat accompanied by high fever, headache, nausea, and vomiting may be serious. Consult a doctor right away. Do not use more than 2 days or give to children under 3 years of age unless directed by a doctor.
If pregnant or breast-feeding, ask a health professional before use.
Keep out of reach of children.

Directions:
- adults and children 4 years and over: allow 2 drops to dissolve slowly in the mouth. May be repeated every 2 hours, as needed, or as directed by a doctor.
- children under 4 years of age: ask a doctor

Other Information: store at 20–25°C (68–77°F)

Inactive Ingredients carmine, citric acid, cochineal extract, corn syrup, glycerin, natural flavor blend, natural grade A wildflower honey, sucrose

How Supplied: Packages of 25 drops.

ROBITUSSIN®
HONEY COUGH™
Cough Suppressant

Active Ingredient: (in each 5 mL tsp) Dextromethorphan HBr, USP 10 mg

Use: temporarily relieves cough due to minor throat and bronchial irritation as may occur with a cold

Warnings:
Do not use if you are now taking a prescription monoamine oxidase inhibitor (MAOI) (certain drugs for depression, psychiatric, or emotional conditions, or Parkinson's disease), or for 2 weeks after stopping the MAOI drug. If you do not know if your prescription drug contains an MAOI, ask a doctor or pharmacist before taking this product.
Ask a doctor before use if you have
- cough that occurs with too much phlegm (mucus)
- cough that lasts or is chronic such as occurs with smoking, asthma, or emphysema
Stop use and ask a doctor if cough lasts more than 7 days, comes back, or is accompanied by fever, rash, or persistent headache. These could be signs of a serious condition
If pregnant or breast-feeding, ask a health professional before use.
Keep out of reach of children. In case of overdose, get medical help or contact a Poison Control Center right away.

Directions:
- repeat dose every 6–8 hours, as needed
- do not take more than 4 doses in any 24-hr period
- adults and children 12 yrs. and over: 3 tsp
- children 6 to under 12 yrs: 1.5 tsp
- children under 6 yrs: not recommended

Other Information: • store at 20–25°C (68°–77°F)

- alcohol-free
- dosage cup provided

Inactive Ingredients: flavors, glucose, glycerin, honey, maltol, methylparaben, propylene glycol, sodium benzoate, water

How Supplied: Bottles of 4 fl. oz. and 8 fl. oz.

ROBITUSSIN® HONEY COUGH Drops
Honey-Lemon Tea, Herbal Honey Citrus, Herbal and Herbal Almond with Natural Honey Center

Active Ingredient (in each drop)
Herbal with Natural Honey Center and *Honey-Lemon Tea:*
Menthol, USP 5 mg
Herbal Honey Citrus and Herbal Almond with Natural Honey Center:
Menthol, USP 2.5 mg

Uses
- temporarily relieves
  - occasional minor irritation, pain, sore mouth, and sore throat
  - cough associated with a cold or inhaled irritants

Warnings
Sore throat warning: Severe or persistent sore throat or sore throat accompanied by high fever, headache, nausea, and vomiting may be serious. Consult a doctor right away. Do not use more than 2 days or give to children under 3 years of age unless directed by a doctor.
Ask a doctor before use if you have
- cough that occurs with too much phlegm (mucus)
- cough that lasts or is chronic such as occurs with smoking, asthma, or emphysema
Stop use and ask a doctor if cough lasts more than 7 days, comes back, or is accompanied by fever, rash, or persistent headache. These could be signs of a serious condition.
If pregnant or breast-feeding, ask a health professional before use.
Keep out of reach of children.
Other Information store at 20–25°C (68–77°F).
Directions:
- adults and children 4 years and over:
  - for sore throat: allow 1 drop to dissolve slowly in the mouth. May be repeated every 2 hours, as needed, or as directed by a doctor.
  - for cough: *Honey-Lemon Tea and Herbal with Natural Honey Center*—allow 1 drop to dissolve slowly in mouth.
    Herbal Honey Citrus and Herbal Almond with Natural Honey Center—allow 2 drops to dissolve slowly in mouth.
    May be repeated every hour, as needed, or as directed by a doctor.
- children under 4 years: ask a doctor
Inactive Ingredients:
Herbal with Natural Honey Center: caramel, corn syrup, glycerin, high fructose corn syrup, honey, natural herbal flavor, sorbitol, sucrose
Honey Lemon Tea: caramel, citric acid, corn syrup, honey, natural flavor, sucrose, tea extract
Herbal Honey Citrus: citric acid, corn syrup, flavors, honey, sucrose
Herbal Almond with Natural Honey Center: caramel, corn syrup, glycerin, honey, natural almond flavor, natural anise flavor, natural coriander flavor, natural fennel flavor, natural honey flavor and other natural flavors, sorbitol, sucrose

How Supplied: Honey Lemon Tea and Herbal Honey Citrus in bags of 25 drops. Herbal and Herbal Almond with Natural Honey center in bags of 20 drops.

ROBITUSSIN® MULTI SYMPTOM HONEY FLU™
Non-Drowsy Cough Formula
Cough Suppressant, Nasal Decongestant, Pain Reliever/Fever Reducer

Active Ingredients: (in each 5 mL tsp)
Acetaminophen, USP 166.6 mg
Dextromethorphan HBr, USP 6.6 mg
Pseudoephedrine HCl, USP 20 mg

Uses: • temporarily relieves these symptoms associated with a cold or flu: • nasal congestion • minor aches and pains • sore throat • cough • fever • headache • muscular aches

Warnings:
Alcohol warning: If you consume 3 or more alcoholic drinks every day, ask your doctor whether you should take acetaminophen or other pain relievers/fever reducers. Acetaminophen may cause liver damage.
Sore throat warning: If sore throat is severe, persists for more than two days, is accompanied or followed by fever, headache, rash, nausea, or vomiting, consult a doctor promptly.
Do not use
- if you are now taking a prescription monoamine oxidase inhibitor (MAOI) (certain drugs for depression, psychiatric, or emotional conditions, or Parkinson's disease), or for 2 weeks after stopping the MAOI drug. If you do not know if your prescription drug contains an MAOI, ask a doctor or pharmacist before taking this product.
- with any other product containing acetaminophen as this may lead to an overdose. Overdose requires prompt medical attention even if you do not notice any signs or symptoms.
Ask a doctor before use if you have
- heart disease • high blood pressure
- thyroid disease • diabetes
- trouble urinating due to an enlarged prostate gland
- cough that occurs with too much phlegm (mucus)
- a breathing problem or chronic cough that lasts or as occurs with smoking, asthma, or emphysema

When using this product do not use more than directed
Stop use and ask a doctor if
- you get nervous, dizzy, or sleepless
- new symptoms occur
- you need to use for more than 7 days
- symptoms do not get better, get worse, or are accompanied by fever more than 3 days • redness or swelling is present
- cough lasts more than 7 days, comes back, or is accompanied by fever, rash, or persistent headache. These could be signs of a serious condition.
If pregnant or breast-feeding, ask a health professional before use.
Keep out of reach of children. In case of overdose, get medical help or contact a Poison Control Center right away. Quick medical attention is critical for adults as well as for children, even if you do not notice any signs or symptoms.

Directions: • do not take more than 4 doses in any 24-hour period
- adults and children 12 yrs and over: 3 tsp every 4 hours, as needed
- children under 12 years: not recommended
- do not use in children under 2 years of age
- do not exceed recommended dosage. Taking more than the recommended dose (overdose) may cause serious liver damage

Other Information: • store at 20–25°C (68–77°F).
- not labeled USP due to microbial content of natural honey
- dosage cup provided

Inactive Ingredients: citric acid, flavors, glucose, glycerin, high fructose corn syrup, menthol, natural grade A honey, polyethylene glycol, propylene glycol, saccharin sodium, sodium benzoate, water

How Supplied: Bottles of 4 fl. oz.

ROBITUSSIN® PM Cough & Cold
Nasal Decongestant, Cough Suppressant, Antihistamine

Active Ingredients: (in each 5 mL tsp):
Chlorpheniramine maleate, USP 1 mg
Dextromethorphan HBr, USP 7.5 mg
Pseudoephedrine HCl, USP 15 mg

Uses:
- temporarily relieves these symptoms associated with a cold:
  - cough due to minor throat and bronchial irritation
  - nasal congestion
- temporarily relieves these symptoms due to hay fever or other upper respiratory allergies: • runny nose • sneezing • itchy, watery eyes • itching of the nose or throat

Warnings:
Do not use if you are now taking a prescription monoamine oxidase inhibitor (MAOI) (certain drugs for depression, psychiatric, or emotional conditions, or Parkinson's disease), or for 2 weeks after stopping the MAOI drug. If you do not

Continued on next page

Robitussin PM—Cont.

know if your prescription drug contains an MAOI, ask a doctor or pharmacist before taking this product.

Ask a doctor before use if you have
• heart disease • high blood pressure • thyroid disease • diabetes • trouble urinating due to an enlarged prostate gland • glaucoma • cough that occurs with too much phlegm (mucus) • a breathing problem or chronic cough that lasts or as occurs with smoking, asthma, chronic bronchitis, or emphysema

Ask a doctor or pharmacist before use if you are taking sedatives or tranquilizers

When using this product
• do not use more than directed
• marked drowsiness may occur
• avoid alcoholic drinks
• alcohol, sedatives, and tranquilizers may increase drowsiness
• be careful when driving a motor vehicle or operating machinery
• excitability may occur, especially in children

Stop use and ask a doctor if
• you get nervous, dizzy, or sleepless
• symptoms do not get better within 7 days or are accompanied by fever
• cough lasts more than 7 days, comes back, or is accompanied by fever, rash, or persistent headache. These could be signs of a serious condition.

If pregnant or breast-feeding, ask a health professional before use.

Keep out of reach of children. In case of overdose, get medical help or contact a Poison Control Center right away.

Directions:
• do not take more than 4 doses in any 24-hour period
• repeat dose every 6 hours, as needed
• adults and children 12 years and over: 4 tsp
• children 6 to under 12 years: 2 tsp
• children under 6 years: ask a doctor

Other Information
• store at 20–25°C (68–77°F).
• not USP. Meets specifications when tested with a validated non-USP assay method
• dosage cup provided

Inactive Ingredients: citric acid, FD&C red no. 40, glycerin, high fructose corn syrup, natural and artificial flavors, propylene glycol, purified water, saccharin sodium, sodium benzoate, sodium chloride, sodium citrate

How Supplied:
Bottles of 4 fl. oz.

ROBITUSSIN®-PE Syrup
Nasal Decongestant, Expectorant

Active Ingredients:
(in each 5 mL tsp):

Guaifenesin, USP 100 mg
Pseudoephedrine HCl, USP 30 mg

Uses: • temporarily relieves nasal congestion due to a cold • helps loosen phlegm (mucus) and thin bronchial secretions to make coughs more productive.

Warnings:
Do not use if you are now taking a prescription monoamine oxidase inhibitor (MAOI) (certain drugs for depression, psychiatric, or emotional conditions, or Parkinson's disease), or for 2 weeks after stopping the MAOI drug. If you do not know if your prescription drug contains an MAOI, ask a doctor or pharmacist before taking this product.

Ask a doctor before use if you have
• heart disease • high blood pressure
• thyroid disease • diabetes
• trouble urinating due to an enlarged prostate gland
• cough that occurs with too much phlegm (mucus)
• cough that lasts or is chronic such as occurs with smoking, asthma, chronic bronchitis, or emphysema

When using this product do not use more than directed

Stop use and ask a doctor if
• you get nervous, dizzy, or sleepless
• symptoms do not get better within 7 days or are accompanied by fever
• cough lasts more than 7 days, comes back, or is accompanied by fever, rash, or persistent headache. These could be signs of a serious condition.

If pregnant or breast-feeding, ask a health professional before use.

Keep out of reach of children. In case of overdose, get medical help or contact a Poison Control Center right away.

Directions:
• repeat dose every 4 hrs, as needed
• do not exceed 4 doses in any 24-hr period
• adults and children 12 yrs. and over: 2 tsp
• children 6 to under 12 yrs.: 1 tsp
• children 2 to under 6 yrs.: ½ tsp
• children under 2 yrs.: ask a doctor

Other Information:
• store at 20–25°C (68–77°F)
• alcohol-free
• dosage cup provided

Inactive Ingredients:
citric acid, FD&C red no. 40, flavors, glucose, glycerin, high fructose corn syrup, maltol, menthol, propylene glycol, saccharin sodium, sodium benzoate, water

How Supplied: Robitussin-PE (orange-red) in bottles of 4 fl oz, and 8 fl oz.

ROBITUSSIN® SINUS & CONGESTION Caplets
Pain Reliever/Fever Reducer, Nasal Decongestant, Expectorant

Active Ingredients: (in each caplet)
Acetaminophen, USP 325 mg
Guaifenesin, USP 200 mg
Pseudoephedrine HCl, USP 30 mg

Uses:
• temporarily relieves these symptoms associated with a cold, or flu:
  • headache • sore throat • fever
  • muscular aches • minor aches and pains
• temporarily relieves nasal congestion occurring with a cold
• helps loosen phlegm (mucus) and thin bronchial secretions to make coughs more productive

Warnings:
Alcohol warning: If you consume 3 or more alcoholic drinks every day, ask your doctor whether you should take acetaminophen or other pain relievers/fever reducers. Acetaminophen may cause liver damage.

Sore throat warning: If sore throat is severe, persists for more than 2 days, is accompanied or followed by fever, headache, rash, nausea, or vomiting, consult a doctor promptly.

Do not use
• if you are now taking a prescription monoamine oxidase inhibitor (MAOI) (certain drugs for depression, psychiatric, or emotional conditions, or Parkinson's disease), or for 2 weeks after stopping the MAOI drug. If you do not know if your prescription drug contains an MAOI, ask a doctor or pharmacist before taking this product.
• with any other product containing acetaminophen as this may lead to an overdose. Overdose requires prompt medical attention even if you do not notice any signs or symptoms.

Ask a doctor before use if you have
• heart disease • high blood pressure
• thyroid disease • diabetes
• trouble urinating due to an enlarged prostate gland
• cough that occurs with too much phlegm (mucus)
• cough that lasts or is chronic such as occurs with smoking, asthma, chronic bronchitis, or emphysema

When using this product do not use more than directed

Stop use and ask a doctor if
• you get nervous, dizzy, or sleepless
• new symptoms occur
• you need to use for more than 7 days (adults) or 5 days (children)
• symptoms do not get better, get worse, or are accompanied by fever more than 3 days • redness or swelling is present
• cough lasts more than 7 days, comes back, or is accompanied by fever, rash, or persistent headache. These could be signs of a serious condition.

If pregnant or breast-feeding, ask a health professional before use.

Keep out of reach of children. In case of overdose, get medical help or contact a Poison Control Center right away. Prompt medical attention is critical for adults as well as for children, even if you do not notice any signs or symptoms.

Directions:
• repeat dose every 4 hrs, as needed
• do not use more than 4 doses in any 24-hour period
• do not exceed recommended dosage. Taking more than the recommended dose (overdose) may cause serious liver damage.
• adults and children 12 yrs and over: 2 caplets
• children 6 to under 12 yrs: 1 caplet
• children under 6 yrs: ask a doctor

Other Information:
• store at 20–25°C (68–77°F)

Inactive ingredients: calcium stearate, croscarmellose sodium, FD&C blue no. 2 aluminum lake, hydroxypropyl methylcellulose, lactose, microcrystalline cellulose, povidone, pregelatinized

starch, silicon dioxide, stearic acid, titanium dioxide, triacetin

How Supplied: Packages of 24

ROBITUSSIN®-DM SYRUP
ROBITUSSIN® SUGAR FREE COUGH
ROBITUSSIN® DM INFANT DROPS
Cough Suppressant, Expectorant

Active Ingredients: (in each 5 mL tsp: Robitussin DM, Robitussin Sugar Free Cough)
Dextromethorphan HBr, USP 10 mg
Guaifenesin, USP 100 mg

Active Ingredients: (in each 2.5 mL Robitussin DM Infant Drops)
Dextromethorphan HBr, USP 5 mg
Guaifenesin, USP 100 mg

Uses:
- temporarily relieves cough due to minor throat and bronchial irritation as may occur with a cold
- helps loosen phlegm (mucus) and thin bronchial secretions to make coughs more productive

Warnings:
Do not use if you or your child are now taking a prescription monoamine oxidase inhibitor (MAOI) (certain drugs for depression, psychiatric, or emotional conditions, or Parkinson's disease), or for 2 weeks after stopping the MAOI drug. If you do not know if your prescription drug contains an MAOI, ask a doctor or pharmacist before taking this product.
Ask a doctor before use if you or your child has
- cough that occurs with too much phlegm (mucus)
- cough that lasts or is chronic such as occurs with smoking, asthma, chronic bronchitis, or emphysema
Stop use and ask a doctor if cough lasts more than 7 days, comes back, or is accompanied by fever, rash, or persistent headache. These could be signs of a serious condition.
If pregnant or breast-feeding, ask a health professional before use.
Keep out of reach of children. In case of overdose, get medical help or contact a Poison Control Center right away.

Directions: (Robitussin DM, Robitussin Sugar Free Cough):
- repeat dose every 4 hrs, as needed
- do not take more than 6 doses in any 24-hour period
- adults and children 12 yrs and over: 2 tsp
- children 6 to under 12 yrs: 1 tsp
- children 2 to under 6 yrs: ½ tsp
- children under 2 yrs: ask a doctor
Directions: (Robitussin DM Infant Drops):
- repeat dose every 4 hrs, as needed
- do not use more than 6 doses in any 24-hr period
- choose by weight (if weight not known, choose by age)
- measure with the dosing device provided. Do not use with any other device
- 24–47 lbs (2 to under 6 yrs): 2.5 mL
- under 24 lbs (under 2 yrs): ask a doctor

Inactive Ingredients: (Robitussin DM): citric acid, FD&C red no. 40, flavors, glucose, glycerin, high fructose corn syrup, menthol, saccharin sodium, sodium benzoate, water
Inactive Ingredients: (Robitussin Sugar Free Cough): acesulfame potassium, citric acid, flavors, glycerin, methylparaben, polyethylene glycol, povidone, propylene glycol, saccharin sodium, sodium benzoate, water
Inactive Ingredients: (Robitussin DM Infant Drops): citric acid, FD&C red no. 40, flavors, glycerin, high fructose corn syrup, maltitol, maltol, polyethylene glycol, povidone, propylene glycol, saccharin sodium, sodium benzoate, sodium chloride, sodium citrate, water
Other Information:
- store at 20–25°C (68–77°F)
- alcohol-free
- dosage cup or oral dosing device provided

How Supplied: Robitussin DM (cherry-colored) in bottles of 4, 8 and 12, and single doses (premeasured doses 1/3 fl oz each)
Robitussin Sugar Free Cough in bottles of 4 fl oz
Robitussin DM Infant Drops (berry flavor) in 1 fl oz bottles

ROBITUSSIN®
SUGAR FREE Throat Drops
(Natural Citrus and Tropical Fruit Flavors)

Active Ingredient (in each drop):
Menthol, USP 2.5 mg

Uses:
- temporarily relieves
  - occasional minor irritation, pain, sore mouth, and sore throat
  - cough associated with a cold or inhaled irritants

Warnings:
Sore throat warning: Severe or persistent sore throat or sore throat accompanied by high fever, headache, nausea, and vomiting may be serious. Consult a doctor right away. Do not use more than 2 days or give to children under 3 years of age unless directed by a doctor.
Ask a doctor before use if you have
- cough that occurs with too much phlegm (mucus)
- cough that lasts or is chronic such as occurs with smoking, asthma, or emphysema
When using this product excessive use may have a laxative effect
Stop use and ask a doctor if cough lasts more than 7 days, comes back, or is accompanied by fever, rash, or persistent headache. These could be signs of a serious condition.
If pregnant or breast-feeding, ask a health professional before use.
Keep out of reach of children.

Directions:
- adults and children 4 years and over: allow 2 drops to dissolve slowly in the mouth

- for sore throat: may be repeated every 2 hours, as needed, up to 9 drops per day, or as directed by a doctor
- for cough: may be repeated every hour, as needed, up to 9 drops per day, as or as directed by a doctor
- children under 4 years: ask a doctor

Other Information:
- each drop contains: **phenylalanine 3.37 mg**
- store at 20–25°C (68–77°F)
- does not promote tooth decay
- product may be useful in a diabetic's diet on the advice of a doctor.
  Exchange information*:
  3 Drops = FREE Exchange
  9 Drops = 1 Fruit
*The dietary exchanges are based on Exchange Lists for Meal Planning. Copyright 1995 by the American Diabetes Association Inc. and the American Dietetic Association.

Inactive Ingredients: aspartame, canola oil, citric acid, D&C yellow no. 10 aluminum lake (natural citrus only), FD&C blue no. 1 (natural citrus only), FD&C yellow no. 5 (tropical fruit only), isomalt, maltitol, natural flavor

How Supplied: Packages of 18 drops.

ROBITUSSIN SUNNY ORANGE and RASPBERRY VITAMIN C SUPPLEMENT DROPS

Each soothing, refreshing drop provides a great tasting and convenient way to get 100% of the Daily Value of Vitamin C.
Made with 5% real orange juice.

Supplement Facts:
Serving Size: 1 drop

Amount Per Drop		% Daily Value
Calories		
Sunny Orange	15	
Sunny Raspberry	10	
Total Carbohydrate	3 g	1%†
Sugars	3 g	*
Vitamin C (as sodium ascorbate and ascorbic acid)	60 mg	100%
Sodium		
Sunny Orange	10 mg	<1%†
Sunny Raspberry	8 mg	

*Daily Value (%DV) not established.
†Percent Daily Values are based on a 2,000 calorie diet.

Other Ingredients: Corn syrup, sucrose.
Contains less than 2 % of the following (Sunny Orange): ascorbyl palmitate, beta carotene, citric acid, citrus aurantium dulcis (orange) juice (concentrate), corn oil, gelatin, menthol, methylparaben, natural flavor, phosphoric acid, potassium sorbate, propylparaben, sodium benzoate, sorbitol, tocopherols.

Continued on next page

Robitussin Sunny Orange—Cont.

(Sunny Raspberry): citric acid, citrus aurantium dulcis (orange) juice (concentrate), FD&C blue no. 1, FD&C red no. 40, menthol, methylparaben, natural and artificial raspberry flavor, potassium sorbate, povidone, propylparaben, sodium benzoate

Directions: Take a minimum of 3 to 4 drops a day, not to exceed 15 drops per day. Allow drop to dissolve fully in mouth and swallow. Not formulated for use in children.

Warnings: Keep out of reach of children.
If you are pregnant or nursing a baby, contact your physician before taking this product.
Storage: Store at 20–25°C (68–77°F)

How Supplied: 25 Drops

ROBITUSSIN® MAXIMUM STRENGTH COUGH
ROBITUSSIN® PEDIATRIC COUGH Formula
Cough Suppressant

Active Ingredients (in each 5 mL tsp Robitussin Maximum Strength Cough):
Dextromethorphan HBr, USP 15 mg
(in each 5 mL tsp Robitussin Pediatric Cough Formula):
Dextromethorphan HBr, USP 7.5 mg

Uses: temporarily relieves cough due to minor throat and bronchial irritation as may occur with a cold

Warnings:
Do not use if you are now taking a prescription monoamine oxidase inhibitor (MAOI) (certain drugs for depression, psychiatric, or emotional conditions, or Parkinson's disease), or for 2 weeks after stopping the MAOI drug. If you do not know if your prescription drug contains an MAOI, ask a doctor or pharmacist before taking this product.
Ask a doctor before use if you have
• cough that occurs with too much phlegm (mucus)
• cough that lasts or is chronic such as occurs with smoking, asthma, or emphysema
Stop use and ask a doctor if cough lasts more than 7 days, comes back, or is accompanied by fever, rash, or persistent headache. These could be signs of a serious condition.
If pregnant or breast-feeding, ask a health professional before use.
Keep out of reach of children. In case of overdose, get medical help or contact a Poison Control Center right away.

Directions:
• repeat dose every 6–8 hrs, as needed
• do not exceed 4 doses in any 24-hr period

Robitussin Maximum Strength Cough Suppressant
• adults and children 12 yrs. and over: 2 tsp
• children under 12 yrs.: ask a doctor
Robitussin Pediatric Cough Suppressant
• choose by weight (if weight is not known, choose by age)
  • under 24 lbs (2 yrs): ask a doctor
  • 24–47 lbs (2 to 6 yrs): 1 tsp
  • 48–95 lbs (6–12 yrs): 2 tsp
  • over 95 lbs (over 12 yrs): 4 tsp

Other Information:
• store at 20–25°C (68–77°F)
• dosage cup provided

Inactive Ingredients (Robitussin Maximum Strength Cough): alcohol, citric acid, FD&C red no. 40, flavors, glucose, glycerin, high fructose corn syrup, menthol, saccharin sodium, sodium benzoate, water

Inactive Ingredients (Robitussin Pediatric Cough Formula): citric acid, FD&C red no. 40, flavor, glycerin, high fructose corn syrup, saccharin sodium, sodium benzoate, sodium chloride, sodium citrate, water

How Supplied: Robitussin Maximum Strength (dark red-colored) in bottles of 4 and 8 fl oz.

How Supplied: Robitussin Pediatric (cherry-colored) in bottles of 4 fl oz.

ROBITUSSIN® MAXIMUM STRENGTH COUGH& COLD
ROBITUSSIN® PEDIATRIC COUGH & COLD Formula
Cough Suppressant, Nasal Decongestant

Active Ingredients: (in each 5 mL tsp Robitussin Maximum Strength Cough & Cold)
Dextromethorphan HBr, USP 15 mg
Pseudoephedrine HCl, USP 30 mg

Active Ingredients: (in each 5 mL tsp Robitussin Pediatric Cough & Cold Formula)
Dextromethorphan HBr, USP 7.5 mg
Pseudoephedrine HCl, USP 15 mg

Uses:
• temporarily relieves these symptoms occurring with a cold:
  • nasal congestion • cough due to minor throat and bronchial irritation

Warnings:
Do not use if you are now taking a prescription monoamine oxidase inhibitor (MAOI) (certain drugs for depression, psychiatric, or emotional conditions, or Parkinson's disease), or for 2 weeks after stopping the MAOI drug. If you do not know if your prescription drug contains an MAOI, ask a doctor or pharmacist before taking this product.
Ask a doctor before use if you have
• heart disease • high blood pressure
• thyroid disease • diabetes
• trouble urinating due to an enlarged prostate gland
• cough that occurs with too much phlegm (mucus)

• cough that lasts or is chronic such as occurs with smoking, asthma, or emphysema
When using this product do not use more than directed
Stop use and ask a doctor if
• you get nervous, dizzy, or sleepless
• symptoms do not get better within 7 days or are accompanied by fever
• cough lasts more than 7 days, comes back, or is accompanied by fever, rash, or persistent headache. These could be signs of a serious condition.
If pregnant or breast-feeding, ask a health professional before use.
Keep out of reach of children. In case of overdose, get medical help or contact a Poison Control Center right away.

Directions:
• repeat dose every 6 hrs, as needed
• do not exceed 4 doses in any 24-hr period
Robitussin Maximum Strength Cough & Cold. • adults and children 12 yrs and over: 2 tsp • children under 12 yrs: ask a doctor
Robitussin Pediatric Cough & Cold Formula • choose by weight (if weight is not known, choose by age)
• under 24 lbs (2 yrs): ask a doctor
• 24–47 lbs (2 to 6 yrs): 1 tsp
• 48–95 lbs (6 to 12 yrs): 2 tsp
• over 95 lbs (over 12 yrs): 4 tsp

Other Information: • store at 20–25°C (68–77°F)
• dosage cup provided

Inactive Ingredients (Robitussin Maximum Strength Cough & Cold): alcohol, citric acid, FD&C red no. 40, flavors, glucose, glycerin, high fructose corn syrup, menthol, saccharin sodium, sodium benzoate, water

Inactive Ingredients (Robitussin Pediatric Cough & Cold Formula): citric acid, FD&C red no. 40, flavor, glycerin, high fructose corn syrup, saccharin sodium, sodium benzoate, sodium chloride, sodium citrate, water

How Supplied:
Robitussin Maximum Strength Cough & Cold: Red syrup in bottles of 4 fl oz and 8 fl oz.
How Supplied: Robitussin Pediatric Cough & Cold Formula: (bright red) in bottles of 4 fl oz.

ROBITUSSIN®-CF Syrup
ROBITUSSIN® COUGH & COLD INFANT DROPS
Nasal Decongestant, Cough Suppressant, Expectorant

Active Ingredients: (in each 5 mL tsp Robitussin CF)
Dextromethorphan HBr, USP 5 mg
Guaifenesin, USP 100 mg
Pseudoephedrine HCl, USP 15 mg

Active Ingredients: (in each 2.5 mL Robitussin Cough & Cold Infant Drops)
Dextromethorphan HBr, USP 5 mg
Guaifenesin, USP 100 mg
Pseudoephedrine HCl, USP 15 mg

Uses:
- temporarily relieves these symptoms occurring with a cold:
  - nasal congestion
  - cough due to minor throat and bronchial irritation
- helps loosen phlegm (mucus) and thin bronchial secretions to make coughs more productive

Warnings:

Do not use if you or your child are taking a prescription monoamine oxidase inhibitor (MAOI) (certain drugs for depression, psychiatric, or emotional conditions, or Parkinson's disease), or for 2 weeks after stopping the MAOI drug. If you do not know if your child's prescription drug contains an MAOI, ask a doctor or pharmacist before giving this product.

Ask a doctor before use if you or your child has
- heart disease • high blood pressure
- thyroid disease • diabetes
- trouble urinating due to an enlarged prostate gland
- cough that occurs with too much phlegm (mucus)

- cough that lasts or is chronic such as occurs with asthma

When using this product do not use more than directed

Stop use and ask a doctor if
- you or your child gets nervous, dizzy, or sleepless
- symptoms do not get better within 7 days or are accompanied by fever
- cough lasts more than 7 days, comes back, or is accompanied by fever, rash, or persistent headache. These could be signs of a serious condition.

If pregnant or breast-feeding, ask a health professional before use.

Keep out of reach of children. In case of overdose, get medical help or contact a Poison Control Center right away.

Directions:
- repeat dose every 4 hrs, as needed
- do not use more than 4 doses in any 24-hr period
- adults and children 12 yrs and over: 2 tsp
- children 6 to under 12 yrs: 1 tsp
- children 2 to under 6 yrs: ½ tsp or 2.5 mL

- children under 2 yrs: ask a doctor

Other Information:
- store at 20–25°C (68–77°F)
- alcohol-free
- dosage cup or oral dosing device provided

Inactive Ingredients: (Robitussin CF) citric acid, FD&C red no. 40, flavors, glycerin, propylene glycol, saccharin sodium, sodium benzoate, sorbitol, water

Inactive Ingredients: (Robitussin Cough & Cold Infant Drops) citric acid, FD&C red no. 40, flavors, glycerin, high fructose corn syrup, maltitol, maltol, polyethylene glycol, povidone, propylene glycol, saccharin sodium, sodium benzoate, sodium citrate, water

How Supplied: Robitussin CF (red-colored) in bottles of 4, 8, and 12 fl oz. Robitussin Cough & Cold Infant Drops in 1 fl oz bottles

DIETARY SUPPLEMENT INFORMATION

This section presents information on natural remedies and nutritional supplements marketed under the Dietary Supplement Health and Education Act of 1994. It is made possible through the courtesy of the manufacturers whose products appear on the following pages. The information concerning each product has been prepared, edited, and approved by the manufacturer's professional staff.

Products found in this section include vitamins, minerals, herbs and other botanicals, amino acids, other substances intended to supplement the diet, and concentrates, metabolites, constituents, extracts, and combinations of these ingredients. The descriptions of these products are designed to provide all information necessary for informed use, including, when applicable, active ingredients, inactive ingredients, actions, warnings, cautions, interactions, symptoms and treatment of oral overdosage, dosage and directions for use, and how supplied. Descriptions in this section must be in full compliance with the Dietary Supplement Health and Education Act, which permits claims regarding a product's effect on the structure or functioning of the body, but forbids claims regarding a product's ability to treat, diagnose, cure, or prevent any specific disease. Descriptions of products marketed under the act do not receive formal evaluation or approval from the Food and Drug Administration.

In compiling this section, the publisher has emphasized the necessity of describing products comprehensively. The descriptions seen here include all information made available by the manufacturer. The publisher does not warrant or guarantee any product described here, and does not perform any independent analysis of the information provided. Inclusion of a product in this book does not represent an endorsement, and the publisher does not necessarily advocate the use of any product listed.

A & Z Pharmaceutical Inc.

180 OSER AVENUE, SUITE 300 HAUPPAUGE, NY 11788

Direct Inquiries to:
Customer Service
(631) 952-3800
Fax: (631) 952-3900

D-CAL™
Calcium Supplement with Vitamin D Chewable Caplets

Ingredients: Calcium Carbonate, Vitamin D, Sorbitol, Flavor, D&C Red #27 Lake, Magnesium Stearate. No sugar, No salt, No lactose, No preservative.

Supplement Facts

Serving Size One Caplet

Each Caplet Contains		% Daily Value
Calcium (as calcium carbonate)	300 mg	30%
Vitamin D	100 IU	25%

Recommended Intake: Take two caplets daily for adult and one caplet for child, or as directed by your physician.

Warnings: KEEP OUT OF REACH OF CHILDREN. Do not accept if safely seal under cap is broken or missing.

Actions: D-Cal™ provides a concentrated form of calcium to help build healthy bones. It contains Vitamin D to help the body absorb calcium. D-Cal™ can also help prevent osteoporosis. It is helpful to pregnant and nursing women, children's growth, and calcium deficiency at all ages.

How Supplied: Bottles of 30 and 60 caplets
Shown in Product Identification Guide, page 503

AkPharma Inc.
**P.O. BOX 111
PLEASANTVILLE, NJ
08232-0111**

Direct Inquiries To:
Elizabeth Klein: (609) 645-5100
FAX: (609) 645-0767

Medical Emergency Contact:
Alan E. Kligerman: (609) 645-5100

PRELIEF®

PRODUCT OVERVIEW
Key Facts: Prelief is AkPharma's brand name for calcium glycerophos-phate. It is used to take acid out of acidic foods and beverages for more comfortable consumption. Prelief tablets are swallowed with the first bite or drink of acidic food or beverage. Prelief granulate is added to each serving of acidic food or beverage. It is classified as a dietary supplement.

Major Uses: Takes acid out of acidic foods such as tomato sauce, citrus, fruit drinks, coffee, wine, beer and colas. Acid foods are now established as problematic for persons with interstitial cystitis, overactive bladder and are suspect in some situations of intestinal irritation. Those with interstitial cystitis or overactive bladder, whose symptoms may be exacerbated by acidic foods, may particularly benefit.

Safety Information: Prelief is made from an FDA Generally Recognized as Safe (GRAS)[1] dietary supplement ingredient and is also listed as a food ingredient in the US Government Food Chemicals Codex (FCC)[2]

PRODUCT INFORMATION
Prelief®

Description: Prelief Tablets: Each tablet contains 333 mg of calcium glycerophosphate. The tablets also contain 0.025% magnesium stearate as a processing aid. Two tablets should be swallowed with the average serving of food or beverage. (See chart)

Prelief Granulate: Each packet contains 333 mg of calcium glycerophosphate. Add 2 packets of granulate to each average serving of acidic food or beverage. The granulate dissolves rapidly in acidic food or non-alcoholic beverages. Tablets are recommended for taking with alcoholic beverages. An additional 1–2 tablets or packets may be needed on foods that may be particularly high in acid. (See chart)

One tablet or packet of granulate supplies 6% (65 mg) of the US Recommended Daily Intake (RDI) for calcium and 5% (50 mg) of the RDI for phosphorus. No sodium; no aluminum; no sugar.

[1]reference 21 CFR §184.1201
[2]reference Food Chemicals Codex, 3rd Edition, pp 51–52

Reasons for Use: Prelief is for use with acidic foods and beverages. It is a dietary intervention used to take acid out of these foods for persons who identify acid discomfort with the ingestion of acidic foods and beverages.

Action: Prelief neutralizes the acid found in a large number of foods which many people find cause them discomfort. **See Table.**

Usage: 2 tablets or 2 granulate packets per average serving of acidic food, beverage or snack.

How Supplied: Prelief is supplied in both tablet form (30, 60, 120 and 300 tablet bottle sizes and 24 tablets in 12–2 tablet packets), and granulate form (36 packets and 150 serving granulate shaker).

Kosher: Prelief is Kosher and Pareve.
Use Limitations: None, except as may apply below.

Adverse Reactions: None known
Toxicity: None known
Interactions with Drugs: Calcium may interfere with efficacy of some medications. Check with drug publications.

Precautions: None, except for people who have been advised by their physician not to take calcium, phosphorus or glycerin/glycerol.
Prelief is classified as a dietary supplement, not a drug.
For more information and samples, please write or call toll-free 1-800-994-4711.

Typical Food Acid Removal by Prelief			
Product	1 Packet or 1 Tablet	2 Packets or 2 Tablets	3 Packets or 3 Tablets
Pepsi Cola® – 8 oz.	98%	99.8%	–
Mott's® 100% Apple Juice – 4 oz.	49.8%	74.9%	90%
Tropicana® Orange Juice – 4 oz.	20.6%	36.9%	60%
Coors Light® Beer – 12 oz.	80.1%	95%	96.8%
Monty's Hill® Chardonnay – 4 oz.	37%	60.1%	80%
Ireland® Coffee – 6 oz.	93.7%	96.8%	98%
Tetley® Iced Tea – 8 oz.	99%	99.5%	–
Seven Seas® Red Wine & Vinegar Salad Dressing – 31 gm	90%	95%	98%
Old El Paso® Thick'n Chunky Salsa Medium – 2 Tbsp.	80.1%	95%	97.5%
Heinz® Tomato Ketchup – 1 Tbsp.	68.4%	87.4%	92.1%
Kraft® Original Barbeque Sauce 2 Tbsp.	60.2%	80%	90%
Ragu® Old World Style Traditional Sauce – 125 gm	20.6%	36.9%	60.2%
Dannon® Strawberry Lowfat Yogurt (fully mixed) – 116 gm	49.9%	68.4%	80.1%
Grapefruit Sections – 150 gm	36.9%	50%	68.3%
Sauerkraut – 2 Tbsp.	60.3%	80%	92.1%
Red Cabbage – 130 gm	49.7%	68.3%	74.8%

[See table at bottom of previous page]
Shown in Product Identification Guide, page 503

American Longevity
**2400 BOSWELL ROAD
CHULA VISTA, CA 91914**

Direct Inquiries to:
Customer Service
800-982-3189
Fax:
619-934-3205
www.americanlongevity.net

Plant Derived Minerals

Description: Minerals which are so important to our health are not so readily available. Minerals never occured in a uniform blanket on the crust of the Earth. Therefore, unless you supplement with minerals, you can't guarantee that you will get all you need through the 4 food groups. Our Plant Derived Mineral products are liquid concentrates containing a natural assortment of up to 77 minerals from prehistoric plants in their unaltered colloidal form. A mineral deficiency can lead to disease or even death. Plant Derived Minerals can help you in your fight against deficiencies. Now, it even comes in a great tasting cherry flavor.

Supplement Facts:
Calories <5
Majestic Earth Plant   600mg *
  Derived Minerals
*daily value not established

Directions:
1) Store in cool environment after opening
2) Suggested as a dietary supplement. For adults, mix 1 or 2 ounces in a small glass of fruit or vegetable juice of your choice. Drink during or after meals, 1 to 3 times a day or as desired. For children reduce amount by two-thirds

Other Ingredients: Calcium, Chlorine, Magnesium, Phosphorus, Potassium, Sodium, Sulfur, Antimony, Arsenic, Aluminum Hydroxide, Barium, Beryllium, Bismuth, Boron, Bromine, Cadmium, Carbon, Cerium Cesium, Chromium, Cobalt, Copper, Dysprosium, Erbium, Europium, Fluorine, Gadolinium, Gallium, Germanium, Gold, Hafnium, Holmium Hydrogen, Indium, Iodine, Iridium, Iron, Lanthanum, Lead, Lithium, Lutetium, Manganese, Mercury, Molybdenum, Neodymium, Nickel, Niobium, Nitrogen, Osmium, Oxygen, Palladium, Platinum, Praseodymium, Rhenium, Rhodium, Rubidium, Ruthenium, Samarium, Scandium, Selenium, Silicon, Silver, Strontium, Tantalum, Tellurium, Terbium, Thallium, Thorium, Thulium, Tin, Titanium, Tungsten, Vanadium, Ytterbium, Zinc, Zirconium.

MAJESTIC EARTH
(Ultimate Osteo-FX)

Description: *Majestic Earth Ultimate Osteo-FX was formulated to support healthy bones and joints. With todays fast paced life styles it is becoming increasingly difficult to get enough nutrients in our diets. For many people Majestic Earth Osteo-FX fills the gap! American Longevity is proud to include Majestic Earth Ultimate Osteo-FX in our popular line of Majestic Earth products. Note Majestic Earth Ultimate Osteo-FX goes great with an Ultimate Natures Whey Chocolate or Vanilla shake also. Each quart of Majestic Earth Ultimate Osteo-FX contains Majestic Earth plant derived minerals. These minerals come from a unique source in Southern Utah. They are leached from humic shale with purified water only. The balance of Majestic Earth Ultimate Osteo-FX contains vitamins, major minerals and other beneficial nutrients.

Supplement Facts:

Calories	0
Calories from Fat	0
Total Fat	0
Saturated Fat	0g
Cholesterol	0g
Total Carbohydrates	0g
Dietary Fiber	0g
Sugars	0g
Sodium	0g
Protein	0g
Vitamin D3	100 IU
25% of Daily Value	
Calcium (as tricalcium phosphate, calcium citrate)	1200mg
120% of Daily Value	
Magnesium (as citrate)	200mg
50% of Daily Value	
Zinc (as gluconate)	5mg
33% of Daily Value	
Boron (as chelated amino acid complex)	1mg T
MSM (methyl sulffonyl methane)	250mg T
Glucosamine sulphate KCl	100mg T

*Percent Daily values are based on a 2,000 calorie diet.
T Daily value not established

Directions:
1) Shake well before using.
2) Store in cool environment after opening.
3) Suggested as a food for special dietary use.
4) As with any nutritional supplement program, seek the advice of your health care professional.

Other Ingredients: Water, Majestic Earth Plant Derived Minerals complex, citric acid, potassium benzoate, sodium benzoate, vanillain, natural flavors, sucralose.

Amerifit Nutrition, Inc.
**166 HIGHLAND PARK DRIVE
BLOOMFIELD, CT 06002**

Direct Inquiries to:
Consumer Affairs
(800) 722-3476
FAX: (860) 243-9400
www.amerifit.com

ESTROVEN®
Dietary supplement for perimenopause, menopause and postmenopause

Uses: Estroven contains natural ingredients to help reduce physical and psychological effects of hormonal imbalance. Clinical studies of the specific ingredients in Estroven when used by women experiencing climateric symptoms have shown significant reduction in vasomotor symptoms including night sweats and hot flashes; reduction of menopause-related irritability; support for a restful sleep; and protective effects on bones and the cardiovascular system.

Directions: Take one caplet or gelcap daily before bedtime with food.

Precautions: Do not take if pregnant, lactating or trying to conceive. Keep out of reach of children.

Ingredients: Each caplet or gelcap contains: Vitamin E 30IU; Thiamin 2mg; Riboflavin 2mg; Niacin 20mg; Vitamin B-6 10mg; Folate 400mcg; Vitamin B-12 6mcg; Calcium 150mg; Selenium 70mcg; Boron 1.5mg; Purified isoflavones (from GMO-free soybeans and other plants) 55mg; Estroven Calming Herbal Blend (proprietary blend of Date seed extract [*Zizyphus spinosa*] and Magnolia bark extract) 150mg; Black cohosh root standardized extract 40mg.

Other Ingredients: pueraria lobata root extract, cellulose, croscarmellose sodium, silica, vegetable magnesium stearate, titanium dioxide (natural mineral source), vanilla and caramel color. Estroven contains no artificial dyes, colors, preservatives, flavors, yeast, wheat, gluten or lactose.

How Supplied: Box of 30 Caplets Box of 40 Easy-to-Swallow Gelcaps
Shown in Product Identification Guide, page 503

VITABALL® VITAMIN GUMBALLS
Multi-vitamin supplement

Uses: Vitaball is a fun and great tasting way to take vitamins. Each bubble gum gumball delivers 100% of the Daily Value of 11 essential vitamins. Offered in a variety of flavors.

Continued on next page

Vitaball—Cont.

Directions: For adults and children over five years of age, chew one gumball daily for 5–10 minutes to ensure release of vitamins. Best taken near mealtime. Adults should supervise children's use.

Serving Size 1 Gumball

Total Calories 15
Total Fat 0g
Total Carbohydrates 4g
    Sugars 4g

	Amount Per Serving	% Daily Value
Vitamin A	5000IU	100
Vitamin C	60mg	100
Vitamin D	400IU	100
Vitamin E	30IU	100
Thiamin	1.5mg	100
Riboflavin	1.7mg	100
Niacin	20mg	100
Vitamin B-6	2mg	100
Folic Acid	400mcg	100
Vitamin B-12	6mcg	100
Biotin	45mcg	15
Pantothenic Acid	10mg	100

*Percent Daily Values (DV) for adults and children 4 years of age and over, based on a 2000 caloric diet.
Not a significant source of dietary fiber, calcium or iron.

Other Ingredients: sugar, gum base, corn syrup, additional ingredient**, tapioca dextrin, artificial flavors, sucralose, confectioners glaze, carnauba wax, corn starch, artificial colors†, BHT (to maintain freshness).

**Cherry additional ingredient: citric acid
†Cherry—FD&C Red 40; Bubble gum—FD&C Red 40, Red 3; Grape—FD&C Blue 1, Red 3; Watermelon—FD&C Blue 1, Yellow 5
Vitaball contains no yeast, wheat, gluten, nuts or dairy products.

Precautions: Keep out of reach of children. Store at room temperature. Secure lid tightly.
Shown in Product Identification Guide, page 503

Awareness Corporation/ dba AwarenessLife
25 SOUTH ARIZONA PLACE, SUITE 500
CHANDLER, ARIZONA 85225

Direct Inquiries to:
1-800-69AWARE
www.awarecorp.com
www.awarenesslife.com

AWARENESS CLEAR™

Description: May help with Candida, mold, and general microbial conditions.*

Ingredients: Proprietary blend of Green Hull Black Walnut, Cloves, Pumpkin Seed, Gentian Root, Hyssop, Black Seed, Cramp Bark, Peppermint Leaf, Thyme Leaf, Fennel, Grapefruit Seed.

Directions: Take 2 capsules each morning on an empty stomach, 1–2 hours before eating with 1 glass of water, for a minimum of 90 days.

Warnings: Do not use if Pregnant or Breastfeeding. Stop taking product if you experience allergic reaction. Keep out of reach of children.

How Supplied: 90 Capsules (Vegetarian) per Bottle

*These statements have not been evaluated by the Food and Drug Administration. These products are not intended to diagnose, treat, cure, or prevent any disease.
Shown in Product Identification Guide, page 503

AWARENESS FEMALE BALANCE™

Description: May help with symptoms of Menopause and PMS.* 75 year old Mediterranean product.

Ingredients: Black Cohosh Root, Cramp Bark, Squaw Vine, King Solomon Seed, Valerian Root, Dandelion Root, Chaste Tree Berry, Rosemary Leaves Caraway Seeds (Black Seed), Queen of the Meadow, Epimedium Leaf, Chuanxiong Rhizome, Schizandra Berry, Peppermint leaves, Red Raspberry leaves.

Directions: Symptoms of Menopause: take 1 or 2 capsules morning and evening with 1 glass of water. Symptoms of PMS: take approx. 7 days before and during menstruation.

Warnings: Do not use this product if you are pregnant or breastfeeding. Consult your doctor prior to using this product if you are taking any medication. Keep out of reach of children.

How Supplied: 60 Capsules per Bottle, Clinically Tested, & 100% Vegetarian

*These statements have not been evaluated by the Food and Drug Administration. These products are not intended to diagnose, treat, cure, or prevent any disease.
Shown in Product Identification Guide, page 503

DAILY COMPLETE®

Description: Whole-food liquid supplement. 100% vegetarian ingredients delivers 211 vitamins, minerals, antioxidants, enzymes, fruits and vegetables, amino acids and herbs, in one ounce liquid a day* (great orange taste).

Ingredients: Proprietary blend of 24 essential vitamins & major minerals, 70 organic ionic plant minerals, botanical antioxidants with phenalgin(tm), enzyme active fruits, enzyme active vegetables, essential fatty acids with lipotropic factors, amino acids protein complex, 23 natural herbal ingredients, 22 homeopathic micronutrients, aloe vera, 100% vegetarian.

Directions: Take 1 ounce (30 ml) per day, during or immediately after a meal.

Warnings: Do not use if pregnant breast-feeding. Keep out of reach of children.

How Supplied: 30 ounces per Bottle, Clinically tested

*These statements have not been evaluated by the Food and Drug Administration. These products are not intended to diagnose, treat, cure, or prevent any disease.
Shown in Product Identification Guide, page 503

EXPERIENCE®

Description: Known to help with digestion, regularity, energy, and weight. 100 year old Mediterranean product. 100% Natural/Vegetarian.

Ingredients: Proprietary blend of Psyllium Seed Husk, Rhubarb Root, Fennel Seed, Cornsilk, King Solomon's Seed, and Kelp.

Directions: Take 1 to 3 Capsules before bedtime with a full glass of water. Or take 20 minutes after each meal.

Warnings: Do not use if pregnant or breast-feeding or if you have colitis. Keep out of reach of children.

How Supplied: 90 Capsules per Bottle, Clinically Tested

*These statements have not been evaluated by the Food and Drug Administration These products are not intended diagnose, treat, cure, or prevent any disease.
Shown in Product Identification Guide, page 503

PURE GARDEN CREAM®

Description: 100% natural, may help to improve dry problem skin, fine lines, and age spots.*

Ingredients: Proprietary blend of chamomile oil, calendula oil, bee's wax, rhubarb root oil, aloe vera leaf, almond oil, flax seed oil, cold press virgin olive oil, sesame seed oil, vitamin C and vitamin E.

Directions: Application for both body and face

Warning: External use only

How Supplied: 2 ounce jar, Clinically tested

*These statements have not been evaluated by the Food and Drug Administration These products are not intended diagnose, treat, cure, or prevent any disease.

Shown in Product Identification Guide, page 503

Bayer HealthCare LLC
Consumer Care
Division
36 COLUMBIA ROAD
P.O. BOX 1910
MORRISTOWN, NJ 07962-1910

Direct Inquiries to:
Consumer Relations
(800) 331-4536
www.bayercare.com

For Medical Emergency Contact:
Bayer HealthCare LLC
Consumer Care Division
(800) 331-4536

FERGON®
Ferrous Gluconate
Iron Supplement
High Potency

Fergon Tablets are for use as a dietary iron supplement.

Directions: Adults: One tablet daily, with food.

Serving Size: One tablet

	Amount Per Serving	% Daily Value
Iron	27 mg	150%

Ingredients: Ferrous Gluconate Sucrose, Corn Starch, Hydroxypropyl Methylcellulose, Talc, Maltodextrin, Magnesium Stearate, Silicon Dioxide, Titanium Dioxide, Polyethylene Glycol, FD&C Yellow #5 Aluminum Lake (tartrazine), FD&C Blue #1 Aluminum Lake, Polysorbate 80, Carnauba Wax.

AVOID EXCESSIVE HEAT
USP: Fergon meets the USP standards for strength, quality, and purity.

> **Warning:** Accidental overdose of iron-containing products is a leading cause of fatal poisoning in children under 6. Keep this product out of reach of children. In case of accidental overdose, call a doctor or Poison Control Center immediately.

If pregnant or breast feeding, ask a health professional before use.

How Supplied: Bottle of 100 Easy to Swallow Tablets
Questions? Comments?
Please call 1-800-331-4536.
Visit our website at
www.bayercare.com
Bayer Corporation
Consumer Care Division
Morristown, NJ 07960 USA
Shown in Product Identification Guide, page 504

FLINTSTONES® COMPLETE
Children's Chewable Multivitamin/Multimineral Supplement

Directions: 2 & 3 years of age —**Chew** one-half tablet daily. Adults and children 4 years of age and older—**Chew** one tablet daily.

Serving Size: $^1/_2$ tablet (2 & 3 years of age); 1 tablet (4 years of age and older)

Amount Per Tablet	% Daily Value for Children 2 & 3 Years of Age ($^1/_2$ Tablet)	% Daily Value for Adults and Children 4 Years of Age and older (1 Tablet)
Vitamin A 5000 IU	100%	100%
Vitamin C 60 mg	75%	100%
Vitamin D 400 IU	50%	100%
Vitamin E 30 IU	150%	100%
Thiamin (B_1) 1.5 mg	107%	100%
Riboflavin (B_2) 1.7 mg	106%	100%
Niacin 20 mg	111%	100%
Vitamin B_6 2 mg	143%	100%
Folic Acid 400 mcg	100%	100%
Vitamin B_{12} 6 mcg	100%	100%
Biotin 40 mcg	13%	13%
Pantothenic Acid 10 mg	100%	100%
Calcium (elemental) 100 mg	6%	10%
Iron 18 mg	90%	100%
Phosphorus 100 mg	6%	10%
Iodine 150 mcg	107%	100%
Magnesium 20 mg	5%	5%
Zinc 15 mg	94%	100%
Copper 2 mg	100%	100%

Ingredients:
Dicalcium Phosphate, Sorbitol, Magnesium Phosphate, Sodium Ascorbate, Gelatin, Ferrous Fumarate, Natural and Artificial Flavors (including fruit acids), Starch, Stearic Acid, Vitamin E Acetate, Carrageenan, Magnesium Stearate, Niacinamide, Zinc Oxide, Hydrogenated Vegetable Oil, Calcium Pantothenate, FD&C Red #40 Lake, FD&C Yellow #6 Lake, Xylitol, Aspartame* (a sweetener), FD&C Blue #2 Lake, Cupric Oxide, Pyridoxine Hydrochloride, Vitamin A Acetate, Riboflavin, Thiamine Mononitrate, Monoammonium Glycyrrhizinate, Beta Carotene, Folic Acid, Potassium Iodide, Vitamin D, Biotin, Magnesium Oxide, Vitamin B_{12}.* **PHENYLKETONURICS: CONTAINS PHENYLALANINE.**

> **Warning:** Accidental overdose of iron-containing products is a leading cause of fatal poisoning in children under 6. Keep this product out of reach of children. In case of accidental overdose, call a doctor or Poison Control Center immediately.

KEEP OUT OF REACH OF CHILDREN.

How Supplied: Bottles of 60s.
THE FLINTSTONES and all related characters and elements are trademarks of Hanna-Barbera © 2000.
Questions or comments?
Please call 1-800-800-4793
Visit our website at www.bayercare.com
Bayer Corporation
Consumer Care Division
P.O. Box 1910
Morristown, NJ 07962-1910 USA
Shown in Product Identification Guide, page 504

MY FIRST FLINTSTONES®
Children's Multivitamin Supplement

#1 Pediatricians' Choice
For children's chewable vitamins
- Specially formulated for children 2 and 3 years of age.
- Provides 10 essential vitamins, including A, D, and C, important for your child's healthy growth and development.
- Small, easy to chew tablets
- **GREAT TASTING** flavors
- **FUN CHARACTER SHAPES**
THE NUTRIENTS NEEDED TO GROW-UP STRONG AND HEALTHY.
B VITAMINS

Continued on next page

My First Flintstones—Cont.

Aid in the release of energy from food.*
VITAMIN C
Helps support the immune system.*
VITAMIN D
Helps absorption of Calcium for strong bones and teeth.*

---

*These statements have not been evaluated by the FDA. This product is not intended to diagnose, treat, cure, or prevent any disease.

Directions: Children 2–3 years of age – **Chew** one tablet daily. Tablet should be fully chewed or crushed for children who cannot chew.

Serving Size: One tablet

	Amount Per Tablet	% Daily Value for Children 2 & 3 Years of Age
Vitamin A	2500 IU	100%
Vitamin C	60 mg	150%
Vitamin D	400 IU	100%
Vitamin E	15 IU	150%
Thiamin (B$_1$)	1.05 mg	150%
Riboflavin (B$_2$)	1.2 mg	150%
Niacin	13.5 mg	150%
Vitamin B$_6$	1.05 mg	150%
Folic Acid	300 mcg	150%
Vitamin B$_{12}$	4.5 mcg	150%

Ingredients: Sucrose (a natural sweetener), Sodium Ascorbate, Stearic Acid, Invert Sugar, Artificial Flavors (including fruit acids), Gelatin, Vitamin E Acetate, Niacinamide, FD&C Red #40 Lake, FD&C Yellow #6 Lake, FD&C Blue #2 Lake, Pyridoxine Hydrochloride, Riboflavin, Thiamine Mononitrate, Vitamin A Acetate, Folic Acid, Beta Carotene, Vitamin D, Vitamin B$_{12}$.

USP: My First Flintstones formula meets the USP standards for strength, quality, and purity for Oil- and Water-soluble Vitamins Tablets. Complies with USP Method 2: Vitamins A, D, E, B12, Thiamin, Riboflavin, Niacin, and B6.

Keep out of reach of children.

How Supplied: Flintstones in bottles of 60 Chewable Tablets.

THE FLINTSTONES and all related characters and elements are trademarks of and © Hanna-Barbera.

(s01)

Questions or comments?
Please call 1-800-800-4793.
Visit our website at
www.bayercare.com
Bayer Corporation Consumer Care Division
P.O. Box 1910
Morristown, NJ 07962-1910
Shown in Product Identification Guide, page 504

ONE-A-DAY® ACTIVE DIETARY SUPPLEMENT
Energy enhancing multivitamin tailored for active lifestyles—Feel your best

Complete with 32 ingredients formulated to help you keep up with your active lifestyle.
- More Ginseng than any leading multivitamin.
- More cell protective antioxidants Vitamin C and E plus Beta Carotene and Selenium.*
- More essential B vitamins for energy metabolism plus Chromium to help your body regulate fuel stores for energy.*

*These statements have not been evaluated by the Food and Drug Administration. This product is not intended to diagnose, treat, cure, or prevent any disease.

Directions: Adults: One tablet daily, with food.

Serving Size: One tablet

	Amount Per Serving	% Daily Value
Vitamin A	5000 IU	100%
Vitamin C	120 mg	200%
Vitamin D	400 IU	100%
Vitamin E	60 IU	200%
Vitamin K	25 mcg	31%
Thiamin (B$_1$)	4.5 mg	300%
Riboflavin (B$_2$)	5.1 mg	300%
Niacin	40 mg	200%
Vitamin B$_6$	6 mg	300%
Folic Acid	400 mcg	100%
Vitamin B$_{12}$	18 mcg	300%
Biotin	40 mcg	13%
Pantothenic Acid	10 mg	100%
Calcium (elemental)	110 mg	11%
Iron	9 mg	50%
Phosphorus	48 mg	4%
Iodine	150 mcg	100%
Magnesium	40 mg	10%
Zinc	15 mg	100%
Selenium	45 mcg	64%
Copper	2 mg	100%
Manganese	2 mg	100%
Chromium	100 mcg	83%
Molybdenum	25 mcg	33%
Chloride	180 mg	5%
Potassium	200 mg	5%
Nickel	5 mcg	*
Tin	10 mcg	*
Silicon	6 mg	*
Vanadium	10 mcg	*
Boron	150 mcg	*
American Ginseng Standardized Extract (*Panax quinquefolius*) (root)	55 mg	*

*Daily Value not established

Ingredients: Potassium Chloride, Dicalcium Phosphate, Ascorbic Acid, Calcium Carbonate, Cellulose, Gelatin, Magnesium Oxide, dl-alpha Tocopheryl Acetate, American Ginseng Extract, Niacinamide, Ferrous Fumarate, Croscarmellose Sodium, Silicon Dioxide, Zinc Oxide, Stearic Acid, Hydroxypropyl Methylcellulose, Dextrin, d-Calcium Pantothenate, Pyridoxine Hydrochloride, Magnesium Stearate, Acacia, Manganese Sulfate, Riboflavin, Titanium Dioxide, Thiamine Mononitrate, Polyethylene Glycol, FD&C Yellow #6 Lake, Starch, FD&C Red #40 Lake, Mannitol, Cupric Oxide, Resin, Dextrose, Lecithin, Beta Carotene, Vitamin A Acetate, Sodium Borate, Potassium Borate, Chromium Chloride, FD&C Blue #2 Lake, Folic Acid, Potassium Iodide, Sodium Selenate, Sodium Molybdate, Sodium Metavanadate, d-Biotin, Sodium Metasilicate, Phytonadione, Nickelous Sulfate, Cyanocobalamin, Stannous Chloride, Ergocalcerifol.

USP: One-A-Day Active formula meets the USP standards of strength, quality, and purity for Oil- and Water-Soluble Vitamins with Minerals Tablets.

> **WARNING:** Accidental overdose of iron-containing products is a leading cause of fatal poisoning in children under 6. Keep this product out of reach of children. In case of accidental overdose, call a doctor or Poison Control Center immediately.

If pregnant or breast-feeding, ask a health professional before use.

How Supplied: Bottle of 50 Tablets. Questions? Comments? Please call 1-800-800-4793. Visit out website at www.oneaday.com
Distributed by:
Bayer Corporation Consumer Care Division
P.O. Box 1910
Morristown, NJ 07962-1910
Shown in Product Identification Guide, page 504

ONE-A-DAY® ENERGY FORMULA
Dietary Supplement

Directions: Adults (18 years and older): Take one tablet daily, with food.

Serving Size: One Tablet

	AMOUNT PER SERVING	% DAILY VALUE
Thiamin (B$_1$)	2.25 mg	150%
Niacin	20 mg	100%
Vitamin B$_6$	3 mg	150%
Folic Acid	200 mcg	50%
Pantothenic Acid	10 mg	100%
Chromium (as Picolinate)	100 mcg	83%
American Ginseng Standardized Extract (*Panax quinquefolius*) (root)	200 mg	*

*Daily Value not established.

Ingredients: Calcium Carbonate, American Ginseng Extract, Cellulose, Maltodextrin, Hydroxypropyl Methylcellulose, Nicotinic Acid, Croscarmellose So-

dium, d-Calcium Pantothenate, Crospovidone, Stearic Acid, Silicon Dioxide, Titanium Dioxide, Pyridoxine Hydrochloride, Magnesium Stearate, Starch, Thiamine Mononitrate, Hydroxypropyl Cellulose, Acacia, Polyethylene Glycol, FD&C Yellow #6 Lake, Chromium Picolinate, FD&C Blue #1 Lake, Folic Acid, Polysorbate 80.

Warnings: Seek the advice of a health professional before use if you are taking medication for high blood pressure or anticoagulation (blood-thinning) or if you have diabetes. **Do not use if pregnant or breast-feeding.** If using for more than 6 months, consult your doctor. Before any surgery, ask your doctor about continued use of this product. Keep out of reach of children.

How Supplied: Bottles of 30.
Questions or comments?
Please call 1-800-800-4793
Visit our website at www.oneaday.com
Distributed by:
Bayer Corporation
Consumer Care Division
P.O. Box 1910
Morristown, NJ 07962-1910 USA

ONE-A-DAY® KIDS
BUGS BUNNY AND FRIENDS COMPLETE
SUGAR FREE
CHILDREN'S MULTIVITAMIN/ MULTIMINERAL SUPPLEMENT

Complete with 19 essential vitamins and minerals, including Vitamin C, Iron, and Calcium for your child's healthy growth and development.

Directions: 2 & 3 years of age—**Chew** one-half tablet daily. Adults and children 4 years of age and older—**Chew** one tablet daily.
Serving Size: ½ tablet – (2 & 3 years of age); 1 tablet – (4 years of age and older) [See first table above]

Ingredients: Dicalcium Phosphate, Sorbitol, Magnesium Phosphate, Sodium Ascorbate, Gelatin, Ferrous Fumarate, Natural and Artificial Flavors (including fruit acids), Starch, Stearic Acid, FD&C Red #40 Lake, Vitamin E Acetate, Carrageenan, Niacinamide, Magnesium Stearate, Hydrogenated Vegetable Oil, Zinc Oxide, FD&C Yellow #6 Lake, FD&C Blue #2 Lake, Calcium Pantothenate, Aspartame** (a sweetener), Cupric Oxide, Pyridoxine Hydrochloride, Vitamin A Acetate, Riboflavin, Thiamine Mononitrate, Beta Carotene, Folic Acid, Potassium Iodide, Vitamin D, Biotin, Magnesium Oxide, Vitamin B₁₂.
** PHENYLKETONURICS: CONTAINS PHENYLALANINE
KEEP OUT OF REACH OF CHILDREN

| WARNING: Accidental overdose of iron-containing products is a leading cause of fatal poisoning in children under 6. Keep this product out of reach of children. In case of acciden- |

Amount Per Tablet	% Daily Value for Children 2 & 3 Years of Age (½ Tablet)	% Daily Value for Adults and Children 4 Years of Age and Older (1 Tablet)
Vitamin A 5000 IU	100%	100%
Vitamin C 60 mg	75%	100%
Vitamin D 400 IU	50%	100%
Vitamin E 30 IU	150%	100%
Thiamin (B₁) 1.5 mg	107%	100%
Riboflavin (B₂) 1.7 mg	106%	100%
Niacin 20 mg	111%	100%
Vitamin B₆ 2 mg	143%	100%
Folic Acid 400 mcg	100%	100%
Vitamin B₁₂ 6 mcg	100%	100%
Biotin 40 mcg	13%	13%
Pantothenic Acid 10 mg	100%	100%
Calcium (elemental) 100 mg	6%	10%
Iron 18 mg	90%	100%
Phosphorus 100 mg	6%	10%
Iodine 150 mcg	107%	100%
Magnesium 20 mg	5%	5%
Zinc 15 mg	94%	100%
Copper 2 mg	100%	100%

Amount Per Tablet	% Daily Value for Children 2 & 3 Years of Age (½ Tablet)	% Daily Value for Adults and Children 4 Years of Age and older (1 Tablet)
Vitamin A 5000 IU	100%	100%
Vitamin C 60 mg	75%	100%
Vitamin D 400 IU	50%	100%
Vitamin E 30 IU	150%	100%
Thiamin (B₁) 1.5 mg	107%	100%
Riboflavin (B₂) 1.7 mg	106%	100%
Niacin 20 mg	111%	100%
Vitamin B₆ 2 mg	143%	100%
Folic Acid 400 mcg	100%	100%
Vitamin B₁₂ 6 mcg	100%	100%
Biotin 40 mcg	13%	13%
Pantothenic Acid 10 mg	100%	100%
Calcium (elemental) 100 mg	6%	10%
Iron 18 mg	90%	100%
Phosphorus 100 mg	6%	10%
Iodine 150 mcg	107%	100%
Magnesium 20 mg	5%	5%
Zinc 15 mg	94%	100%
Copper 2 mg	100%	100%

tal overdose, call a doctor or Poison Control Center immediately.

USP: Bugs Bunny Complete formula meets the USP standards for strength, quality, and purity for Oil- and Water-soluble Vitamins and Minerals Tablets.

How Supplied: Contains 60 chewable tablets
Cartoon Network and logo are trademarks of Cartoon Network ©2001
LOONEY TUNES, characters, names and all related indicia are trademarks of Warner Bros. ©2001.
Questions or comments?
Please call 1-800-800-4793
Visit our website at www.oneaday.com
Bayer Corporation
Consumer Care Division
P.O. Box 1910
Morristown, NJ 07962-1910 USA

ONE-A-DAY® KIDS
SCOOBY-DOO!™ COMPLETE
CHILDREN'S MULTIVITAMIN/ MULTIMINERAL SUPPLEMENT

Provides 19 essential vitamins and minerals, including Vitamin C, Iron, and Calcium for your child's healthy growth and development.

Directions: 2 & 3 years of age—**Chew** one-half tablet daily. Adults and children 4 years of age and older—**Chew** one tablet daily.
Serving Size: ½ tablet (2 & 3 years of age); 1 tablet (4 years of age and older) [See second table above]

Ingredients: Dicalcium Phosphate, Sorbitol, Magnesium Phosphate, Sodium Ascorbate, Gelatin, Ferrous Fumarate, Natural and Artificial Flavors (including fruit acids), Starch, Stearic Acid, Vitamin E Acetate, Carrageenan, Magnesium

Continued on next page

One-A-Day Kids Scooby—Cont.

Stearate, Niacinamide, Zinc Oxide, Hydrogenated Vegetable Oil, Calcium Pantothenate, FD&C Red #40 Lake, FD&C Yellow #6 Lake, Xylitol, Aspartame* (a sweetener), FD&C Blue #2 Lake, Cupric Oxide, Pyridoxine Hydrochloride, Vitamin A Acetate, Riboflavin, Thiamine Mononitrate, Monoammonium Glycyrrhizinate, Beta Carotene, Folic Acid, Potassium Iodide, Vitamin D, Biotin, Magnesium Oxide, Vitamin B_{12}.

***PHENYLKETONURICS: CONTAINS PHENYLALANINE**

> **WARNING:** Accidental overdose of iron-containing products is a leading cause of fatal poisoning in children under 6. Keep this product out of reach of children. In case of accidental overdose, call a doctor or Poison Control Center immediately.

Scooby-Doo Complete formula meets the USP standards for strength, quality, and purity for Oil- and Water-soluble Vitamins and Minerals Tablets.
KEEP OUT OF REACH OF CHILDREN

How Supplied: ONE-A-DAY® KIDS SCOOBY-DOO COMPLETE contains 50 chewable tablets.
SCOOBY-DOO, characters, names and all related indicia are trademarks of Hanna-Barbera © 2001.
CARTOON NETWORK and logo are trademarks of Cartoon Network © 2001
Questions or comments?
Please call 1-800-800-4793.
Visit our website at www.oneaday.com
Bayer Corporation
Consumer Care Division
P.O. Box 1910
Morristown, NJ 07962-1910 USA
Shown in Product Identification Guide, page 504

ONE-A-DAY® KIDS SCOOBY-DOO™ PLUS CALCIUM
CHILDREN'S MULTIVITAMIN SUPPLEMENT

Provides 10 essential vitamins plus calcium for your child's healthy growth and development. Contains as much calcium as one 5 oz glass of milk.

Directions: Adults and children 2 years of age and older—**Chew** one tablet daily.

Serving Size: One tablet

Amount Per Tablet	% Daily Value for Children 2 & 3 Years of Age	% Daily Value for Adults and Children 4 Years of Age and older
Vitamin A 2500 IU	100%	50%
Vitamin C 60 mg	150%	100%

Vitamin D 400 IU	100%	100%
Vitamin E 15 IU	150%	50%
Thiamin (B_1) 1.05 mg	150%	70%
Riboflavin (B_2) 1.2 mg	150%	70%
Niacin 13.5 mg	150%	67%
Vitamin B_6 1.05 mg	150%	52%
Folic Acid 300 mcg	150%	75%
Vitamin B_{12} 4.5 mcg	150%	75%
Calcium (elemental) 200 mg	25%	20%

Ingredients: Calcium Carbonate, Sorbitol, Starch, Sodium Ascorbate, Natural and Artificial Flavors (including fruit acids), Stearic Acid, Gelatin, Magnesium Stearate, Vitamin E Acetate, Niacinamide, FD&C Red #40 Lake, FD&C Yellow #6 Lake, Aspartame* (a sweetener), FD&C Blue #2 Lake, Pyridoxine Hydrochloride, Riboflavin, Thiamine Mononitrate, Vitamin A Acetate, Monoammonium Glycyrrhizinate, Folic Acid, Beta Carotene, Vitamin D, Vitamin B_{12}.
***PHENYLKETONURICS: CONTAINS PHENYLALANINE**
KEEP OUT OF REACH OF CHILDREN
USP: Scooby-Doo Plus Calcium formula meets the USP standards for strength, quality, and purity for Oil- and Water-soluble Vitamins and Minerals Tablets.

How Supplied: Contains 50 Chewable Tablets.
SCOOBY-DOO, characters, names and all related indicia are trademarks of Hanna-Barbera ©2001.
CARTOON NETWORK and logo are trademarks of Cartoon Network ©2001
Questions or comments?
Please call 1-800-800-4793.
Visit our website at www.oneaday.com
Made in U.S.A.
Bayer Corporation
Consumer Care Division
P.O. Box 1910
Morristown, NJ 07962-1910 USA
Shown in Product Identification Guide, page 504

ONE-A-DAY® MEMORY & CONCENTRATION
Dietary Supplement

Directions: Adults (18 years and older): Take one to two tablets daily, with food.

Serving Size: 1 Tablet

	Amount Per Serving	% Daily Value
Vitamin B_6	1 mg	50%
Vitamin B_{12}	3 mcg	50%
Choline	30 mg	*
Ginkgo Biloba Extract (*Ginkgo biloba*) (leaf) (Standardized to 24% Ginkgo Flavone Glycosides and 6% Terpene Lactones)	60 mg	*

*Daily Value not established.

Ingredients: Calcium Carbonate, Cellulose, Choline Bitartrate, Ginkgo Biloba Leaf Extract, Maltodextrin, Hydroxypropyl Methylcellulose, Polyethylene Glycol, Silicon Dioxide, Croscarmellose Sodium, Magnesium Stearate, Acacia, Titanium Dioxide, Crospovidone, FD&C Yellow #5 (Tartrazine) Lake, Starch, Hydroxypropyl Cellulose, Pyridoxine Hydrochloride, Resin, FD&C Yellow #6 Lake, Polysorbate 80, Cyanocobalamin.

Warnings: Do not take this product, without first consulting a health professional, if you are taking medication for anticoagulation (thinning the blood). **If pregnant or breast-feeding, ask a health professional before use.** Before any surgery ask your doctor about continued use of this product. Keep out of reach of children.

How Supplied: Bottles of 30.
Questions or comments?
Please call 1-800-800-4793
Visit our website at www.oneaday.com
Distributed by:
Bayer Corporation
Consumer Care Division
P.O. Box 1910
Morristown, NJ 07962-1910 USA

ONE-A-DAY® MEN'S HEALTH FORMULA
MULTIVITAMIN/MULTIMINERAL SUPPLEMENT

Directions: Adults: One tablet daily, with food.

Serving Size: One Tablet

	AMOUNT PER SERVING		% DAILY VALUE
Vitamin A (14% as beta carotene)	3500	IU	70%
Vitamin C	90	mg	150%
Vitamin D	400	IU	100%
Vitamin E	45	IU	150%
Vitamin K	20	mcg	25%
Thiamin (B_1)	1.2	mg	80%
Riboflavin (B_2)	1.7	mg	100%
Niacin	16	mg	80%
Vitamin B_6	3	mg	150%
Folic Acid	400	mcg	100%
Vitamin B_{12}	18	mcg	300%
Biotin	30	mcg	10%
Pantothenic Acid	5	mg	50%
Calcium (elemental)	210	mg	21%
Magnesium	120	mg	30%
Zinc	15	mg	100%
Selenium	105	mcg	150%
Copper	2	mg	100%
Manganese	2	mg	100%
Chromium	120	mcg	100%

Potassium	100 mg	3%
Lycopene	600 mcg	*

*Daily value not established

Ingredients: Calcium Carbonate, Magnesium Oxide, Potassium Chloride, Cellulose, Ascorbic Acid, dl-Alpha Tocopheryl Acetate, Gelatin, Croscarmellose Sodium, Acacia, Dicalcium Phosphate, Zinc Oxide, Niacinamide, Stearic Acid, Silicon Dioxide, Dextrin, Magnesium Stearate, Starch, d-Calcium Pantothenate, Manganese Sulfate, Calcium Silicate, Pyridoxine Hydrochloride, Sucrose, Mannitol, Hypromellose, Cupric Oxide, Resin, Riboflavin, Thiamine Mononitrate, Vitamin A Acetate, Dextrose, Lecithin, Chromium Chloride, Lycopene, Sodium Carboxymethylcellulose, Folic Acid, Ascorbyl Palmitate, Beta Carotene, Sodium Selenate, Sodium Ascorbate, Sodium Citrate, dl-Alpha Tocopherol, Biotin, Phytonadione, Cyanocobalamin, Ergocalciferol.

KEEP OUT OF REACH OF CHILDREN

How Supplied: Bottles of 60's & 100's.

USP: One-A-Day Men's Health formula meets the USP standards of strength, quality, and purity for Oil- and Water-Soluble Vitamins with Minerals Tablets.

Questions or comments?
Please call 1-800-800-4793.
Visit our website at www.oneaday.com
Distributed by:
Bayer Corporation
Consumer Care Division
P.O. Box 1910
Morristown, NJ 07962-1910 USA
Shown in Product Identification Guide, page 504

ONE-A-DAY® PROSTATE HEALTH
Dietary Supplement

Directions: Adults (18 years and older): Take two softgels daily, with food.

Serving Size:	Two softgels	
	AMOUNT PER SERVING	% DAILY VALUE
Vitamin E	9 IU	30%
Zinc	15 mg	100%
Selenium	35 mcg	50%
Saw Palmetto Standardized Extract (*Serenoa repens*) (fruit)	320 mg	*
Lycopene (*Lycoperiscon esculentum*) (fruit)	3 mg	*

*Daily Value not established.

Ingredients: Saw Palmetto Berry Extract, Gelatin, Glycerin, Zinc Gluconate Chelate, Soybean Oil, Yellow Beeswax, Tomato Oleoresin, Dicalcium Phosphate, Lecithin, dl-Alpha Tocopheryl, Titanium Dioxide, FD&C Yellow #5 (tartrazine), FD&C Red #40, Sodium Selenate, FD&C Blue #1, FD&C Yellow #6

Warnings: If you are experiencing urinary problems, or are being treated for prostate problems, consult your doctor. Keep out of reach of children.

How Supplied: Bottles of 30.
Questions or comments?
Please call 1-800-800-4793.
Visit our website at www.oneaday.com
Distributed by:
Bayer Corporation
Consumer Care Division
P.O. Box 1910
Morristown, NJ 07962-1910 USA

ONE-A-DAY® TODAY
Specially designed for ACTIVE WOMEN 50 and over
Dietary Supplement

Directions: Adults: One tablet daily, with food.
[See table below]

Ingredients: Calcium Carbonate, Magnesium Oxide, Potassium Chloride, Cellulose, Ascorbic Acid, dl-alpha Tocopheryl Acetate, Acacia, Croscarmellose Sodium, Zinc Oxide, Dicalcium Phosphate, Stearic Acid, Dextrin, Titanium Dioxide, Niacinamide, Silicon Dioxide, Hypromellose, Gelatin, Soy Extract, Magnesium Stearate, Calcium Silicate, d-Calcium Pantothenate, Manganese Sulfate, Polyethylene Glycol, Corn Starch, Pyridoxine Hydrochloride, Mannitol, Cupric Oxide, Resin, Lecithin, Riboflavin, Thiamine Mononitrate, Vitamin A Acetate, Chromium Chloride, Folic Acid, Dextrose, Beta Carotene, FD&C Red #40 Lake, FD&C Blue #2 Lake, Sodium Selenate, Biotin, Phytonadione, Cyanocobalamin, Ergocalciferol.

If pregnant or breast-feeding, ask a health professional before use.
USP: One-A-Day Today Formula meets the USP standards of strength, quality, and purity for Oil- and Water-Soluble Vitamins with Minerals Tablets.
KEEP OUT OF REACH OF CHILDREN

How Supplied: Bottles of 55 Tablets.
Questions or comments?
Please call 1-800-800-4793.
Visit our website at www.oneaday.com
Made in the U.S.A.
Distributed by:
Bayer Corporation
Consumer Care Division
P.O. Box 1910
Morristown, NJ 07962-1910 USA
Shown in Product Identification Guide, page 504

Continued on next page

Serving Size: One tablet

	Amount Per Serving	% Daily Value	% of NAS Recommended Value for Women Over 50**
Vitamin A (17% as beta carotene)	3000 IU	60%	129%
Vitamin C	75 mg	125%	100%
Vitamin D	400 IU	100%	100%†
Vitamin E	33 IU	110%	100%
Vitamin K	20 mcg	25%	22%
Thiamin (B₁)	1.1 mg	73%	100%
Riboflavin (B₂)	1.7 mg	100%	154%
Niacin	14 mg	70%	100%
Vitamin B₆	3 mg	150%	200%
Folic Acid	400 mcg	100%	100%
Vitamin B₁₂	18 mcg	300%	750%
Biotin	30 mcg	10%	100%
Pantothenic Acid	5 mg	50%	100%
Calcium (elemental)	240 mg	24%	20%
Magnesium	120 mg	30%	38%
Zinc	15 mg	100%	187%
Selenium	70 mcg	100%	127%
Copper	2 mg	100%	222%
Manganese	2 mg	100%	111%
Chromium	120 mcg	100%	600%
Potassium	100 mg	3%	N/A
Soy Extract (*Glycine max.* bean) (Standardized to 40% Isoflavones)	10 mg	*	N/A

*Daily Value not established
**Percentages based upon Dietary Reference Intakes (DRIs) for women over 50, National Academy of Sciences (NAS), Institute of Medicine, 2001
†DRI for women over 70 is 600 IU

ONE-A-DAY® WOMEN'S
Multivitamin/Multimineral Supplement

Directions: Adults: One tablet daily with food.
Serving Size: One tablet

	AMOUNT PER SERVING		% DAILY VALUE
Vitamin A (20% as beta carotene)	2500	IU	50%
Vitamin C	60	mg	100%
Vitamin D	400	IU	100%
Vitamin E	30	IU	100%
Thiamine (B$_1$)	1.5	mg	100%
Riboflavin (B$_2$)	1.7	mg	100%
Niacin	10	mg	50%
Vitamin B$_6$	2	mg	100%
Folic Acid	400	mcg	100%
Vitamin B$_{12}$	6	mcg	100%
Pantothenic Acid	5	mg	50%
Calcium (elemental)	450	mg	45%
Iron	18	mg	100%
Magnesium	50	mg	12%
Zinc	15	mg	100%

Ingredients: Calcium Carbonate, Cellulose, Magnesium Oxide, Ascorbic Acid, Acacia, Ferrous Fumarate, dl-alpha Tocopheryl Acetate, Croscarmellose Sodium, Zinc Oxide, Magnesium Stearate, Titanium Dioxide, Dextrin, Hypromellose, Niacinamide, Gelatin, Starch, d-Calcium Pantothenate, Calcium Silicate, Polyethylene Glycol, Silicon Dioxide, Dextrose, Pyridoxine Hydrochloride, Lecithin, Riboflavin, Thiamine Mononitrate, Vitamin A Acetate, Resin, Folic Acid, Beta Carotene, FD&C Yellow #5 (tartrazine) Lake, FD&C Yellow #6 Lake, FD&C Blue #2 Lake, Cyanocobalamin.

USP: One-A-Day Women's formula meets the USP standards of strength, quality, and purity for Oil- and Water-Soluble Vitamins with Minerals Tablets.

Warning: Accidental overdose of iron-containing products is a leading cause of fatal poisoning in children under 6. Keep this product out of reach of children. In case of accidental overdose, call a doctor or Poison Control Center immediately.

KEEP OUT OF REACH OF CHILDREN

How Supplied: Bottles of 60 and 100. Questions or comments?
Please call 1-800-800-4793.
Visit our website at www.oneaday.com
Distributed by:
Bayer Corporation
Consumer Care Division
P.O. Box 1910
Morristown, NJ 07962-1910 USA
Shown in Product Identification Guide, page 504

Beach Pharmaceuticals
Division of Beach Products, Inc.
5220 SOUTH MANHATTAN AVE. TAMPA, FL 33611

Direct Inquiries to:
Richard Stephen Jenkins, Exec. V.P.:
(813) 839-6565

BEELITH Tablets
MAGNESIUM SUPPLEMENT with PYRIDOXINE HCL

Description: Each tablet contains magnesium oxide 600 mg and pyridoxine hydrochloride (Vitamin B$_6$) 25 mg equivalent to Vitamin B$_6$ 20 mg.

Supplement Facts
Serving Size: 1 Tablet

	Amount Per Tablet	% Daily Value
Magnesium	362 mg	90%
Vitamin B$_6$	20 mg	1000%

Inactive Ingredients: D&C Yellow No. 10, FD&C Yellow No. 6 (Sunset Yellow), hydroxypropylmethylcellulose, magnesium stearate, microcrystalline cellulose, polyethylene glycol, sodium starch glycolate, titanium dioxide, and water.

Indications: As a dietary supplement for patients with magnesium and/or Vitamin B$_6$ deficiencies resulting from malnutrition, alcoholism, magnesium depleting drugs, chemotherapy, and inadequate nutritional intake or absorption. Also, increases urinary magnesium levels.

Dosage: One tablet daily or as directed by a physician.

Warnings: Do not take this product if you are presently taking a prescription drug without consulting your physician or other health professional. If you have kidney disease, take only under the supervision of a physician. Excessive dosage may cause laxation. If pregnant or breast-feeding, ask a health professional before use. **KEEP OUT OF THE REACH OF CHILDREN.**

How Supplied: Golden yellow, film-coated tablet with the letters **BP** and the number **132** imprinted on each tablet. Packaged in bottles of 100 (NDC 0486-1132-01) tablets.

Earthspring, LLC
7620 E McKELLIPS RD., SUITE 4 PMB 86 SCOTTSDALE, ARIZONA USA 85257

Direct Inquiries to:
www.pharmabetic.com
888-841-7363

PHARMABETIC™

Description: A 100% natural dietary supplement formulated to help nourish the body.*

Ingredients: proprietary blend Sage Leaves, Horsetail, Mullein, Coriander Seed, Black Seed, Corn Silk, Neem Leaves, Gymnema Sylvestre, Bitter Melon, Fenugreek, Guava Leaves, Bilberry, Mulberry Leaves, Olive Leaves

Directions: Only take this product with water. Take 1 or 2 capsules First thing in the morning or 1 to 2 capsules before bedtime. Contact your healthcare practitioner for further advice.

Warnings: Do not use if pregnant or breast-feeding. Keep out of reach of children. Consult your doctor prior to using this product if you are taking any prescription medication.

How Supplied: 30 Capsules (Vegetarian) per Bottle

*These statements have not been evaluated by the Food and Drug Administration. This product is not intended to diagnose, treat, cure, or prevent any disease.

Fleming & Company
1600 FENPARK DR. FENTON, MO 63026

Direct Inquiries to:
Tom Fleming
636 343-8200
FAX (636) 343-9865
e-mail: info@flemingcompany.com

MAGONATE® Tablets
MAGONATE® Liquid
MAGONATE NATAL Liquid
Magnesium Gluconate (Dihydrate), USP
(Dietary Supplement)

Description: Each 2 tablets contain magnesium 54 mgs (from 1000 mg magnesium gluconate dihydrate) calcium 175 mg and phosphorous 182 mg (from 752 mgs dibasic calcium phosphate dihydrate). Each 5 mL of MAGONATE®

liquid contains magnesium (elemental) 54 mgs. (Each 5 ml contains the same amount of magnesium as contained in 1000 mgs of magnesium gluconate dihydrate). Each ml of MAGONATE NATAL Liquid (magnesium gluconate) contains 3.52 mg (0.29 mEq) of magnesium as the gluconate in a sugarless and flavor free isotonic base.

Suggested Uses: Magonate® Tablets and Liquid are indicated to maintain magnesium levels when the dietary intake of magnesium is inadequate or when excretion and loss are excessive. Magonate® is recommended during and for three weeks after a course in chemotherapy, then monitored regularly. MAGONATE NATAL Liquid is indicated for newborns with magnesium deficiency and for the restoration of magnesium in infants.

Precautions: Excessive dosage may cause loose stools.

Contraindications: Patients with kidney disease should not take magnesium supplements without the supervision of a physician.

Dosages And Administration: Two Magonate® tablets or 1 teaspoon Magonate® Liquid three times a day (mid-morning, mid-afternoon and bedtime) on an empty stomach with a glass of water. MAGONATE Natal Liquid usual dose is 1 ml per kg of body weight daily, divided into two doses or 10 drops per kg twice a day.

How Supplied: Magonate® Tablets are orange scored, and supplied in bottles of 100 (NDC 256-0172-01), and 1000 (NDC 256-0172-02) tablets. Magonate® Liquid is supplied in pints, (NDC 256-0184-01). MAGONATE NATAL Liquid is supplied 90 mL bottles.
Rev. 7/00

NICOTINEX Elixir
Niacin Dietary Supplement

Composition: Contains niacin 50 mg./tsp. in a sherry wine base (amber color).

Action and Uses: Produces peripheral flushing. To increase micro-circulation of inner-ear in Meniere's, tinnitus and labyrinthine syndromes. For 'cold hands & feet', and as a vehicle for additives.

Administration and Dosage: One or two teaspoonsful on fasting stomach, or as directed by physician.

Side Effects: Patients should be warned of dermal flush. Ulcer and gout patients may be affected by 10% alcoholic content.

Contraindications: Severe hypotension and hemorrhage.

How Supplied: Plastic pints.

4Life Research
**9850 SOUTH 300 WEST
SANDY, UT 84070**

Direct Inquiries to:
Ph: (801) 562-3600
Fax: (801) 562-3699
Email: productsupport@4-life.com
Website: www.4-life.com

TRANSFER FACTOR CARDIO

*Description: Transfer Factor Cardio combines Targeted Transfer Factor™ derived from egg yolks, (U.S. patent 6,468,534) with scientifically validated nutrients that are designed to address (via immune system response) the pathogens that cause cardiovascular tissue damage and inflammation. Transfer Factor Cardio supports healthy cardiac function with Targeted Transfer Factors—immune system identification codes for specific cardio viruses and bacteria and suppressor cells that help the immune system control inflammation. Additional cardiovascular support ingredients protect the heart against cholesterol, homocysteine, oxidative damage, and unhealthy blood pressure levels include vitamins A, C, E, B6, B12 and phytochemicals from herbs such as garlic, red rice yeast, hawthorn, ginkgo biloba and butchers broom.

Summary of Research: Research indicates that elevated homocysteine levels and infections that cause inflammation are some of the most common causes of cardiovascular (atherosclerotic-arteria plaque collection) risk factors. Other risk factors for cardiovascular disease (CVD) include: unhealthy cholesterol levels, hardening of the arteries, blood vessel constriction, toxin and oxidative damage and inefficient pumping of the heart. Transfer Factor Cardio contains key ingredients to support the body's efforts to block oxidative damage, improve toxin clearance, maintain cholesterol balance, activate the immune response against inflammation, relax the blood vessels and support the pumping efficiency of the heart. Transfer Factor Cardio is formulated to support and strengthen these specific cardiovascular processes.

Directions for Use: Take 4–8 capsules daily with 8 oz of fluid.

How Supplied: Transfer Factor Cardio is supplied in encapsulated form.

---

*Transfer Factor is not intended to diagnose, treat, cure or prevent any disease. These statements have not been evaluated by the Food and Drug Administration.
Shown in Product Identification Guide, page 524

TRANSFER FACTOR PLUS

*Description: Transfer factors are small peptides of approximately 44 amino acids that "transfer" or have the ability to express cell-mediated immunity from immune donors to non-immune recipients. 4Life™ Transfer Factor™ is derived from colostrum extracts containing antigens. The extraction of Transfer Factor from colostrum is protected by US patent 4,816,563.

Transfer Factor Plus combines Transfer Factor with a proprietary formulation of innate and adaptive immune system enhancers such as Inositol Hexaphosphate, Cordyceps, Beta Glucans, Maitake and Shiitake Mushrooms. These ingredients work together to trigger and enhance the various immune protective mechanisms of the body. Clinical studies show that Transfer Factor Plus can increase Natural Killer cell activity up to 248% above baseline.

Summary of Research: In 1949 transfer factors were discovered by Dr. HS Lawrence. Since that time hundreds of studies have been completed involving transfer factors effect on various diseases. Transfer factors have been shown to be immune modulators effective in providing immune system support for people with cancer, immune disorders and infections. Recent studies completed:
Rak, AV et al. Effectiveness of Transfer Factor (TF) in the Treatment of Osteomyelitis Patients. *International Symposium in* Moscow 2002, Nov 5–7, 62–63.
Granitov, VM et al. Usage of Transfer Factor Plus in Treatment of HIV – Infected Patients. *Russian Journal of HIV, AIDS and Related Problems* 2002, 1, 79–80.
Karbysheva, NV et al. Enhanced Transfer Factor in the Complex Treatment of Patients with Opisthorchiasis. *International Symposium in* Moscow 2002, May, 104–105.
Luikova, SG et al. Transfer Factor in Dermatovenerology. *Syberian Journal of Dermatology and Venerology* 2002, 3, 34–35.

Directions for Use: Transfer Factor Plus – Take two (2) capsules daily with 8 oz. of fluid.

How Supplied: Transfer Factor is supplied encapsulated, chewable, oral spray, and cream.
Shown in Product Identification Guide, page 524

IF YOU SUSPECT AN INTERACTION. . .
The 1,800-page
PDR Companion Guide™ can help.
Use the order form
in the front of this book.

**GlaxoSmithKline
Consumer Healthcare,
L.P.**

P.O. BOX 1467
PITTSBURGH, PA 15230

Direct Inquiries to:
Consumer Affairs
1-800-245-1040

For Medical Emergencies Contact:
Consumer Affairs
1-800-245-1040

ALLUNA™ SLEEP
Herbal Supplement Tablet

Use: **Alluna Sleep** is an herbal supplement that can relieve occasional sleeplessness.* It works by helping you relax, so you can drift off to sleep naturally.*
Alluna Sleep has been clinically tested and shown to be effective in actually promoting your body's own natural sleep pattern – safely and gently.* This is a natural process. Depending upon your particular circumstances, benefits are typically seen within a few nights with more consistent results within two weeks.
Alluna Sleep is not habit forming and is safe to take over time. You can expect to wake up refreshed, with no groggy side effects, because you experience a natural, healthy sleep through the night.*

Supplement Facts:
Serving Size: 2 Tablets

	Amount Per 2 Tablets	% Daily Value
Calories	5	
Valerian Root Extract	500 mg	†
Hops Extract	120 mg	†

†Daily Value Not Established

Other Ingredients: microcrystalline cellulose, soy polysaccharide, hydrogenated castor oil, hypromellose. Contains less than 2% of titanium dioxide, propylene glycol, magnesium stearate, silica, polyethylene glycol (400, 6,000 and 20,000), blue 2 lake, artificial flavoring.

Directions: Take **two** (2) tablets one hour before bedtime with a glass of water.

Warning: As with all dietary supplements, contact your doctor before use if you are pregnant or lactating. Keep this and all dietary supplements out of the reach of children. Driving or operating machinery while using this product is not recommended. Chronic insomniacs should consult their doctor before using this product.

Please Note: The herbs in this product have a distinct natural aroma.
Store in a cool, dry place. Avoid temperatures above 86°F.

How Supplied: Packets of 28 and 56 Tablets

BEANO®
[bēan ō]
Food Enzyme Dietary Supplement

PRODUCT INFORMATION

Description:
Beano drops: each 5 drop dosage follows Food Chemical Codex (FCC) standards for activity and contains 150 GalU (galactosidase units) of alpha-D-galactosidase derived from *Aspergillus niger* mold. The enzyme is in a liquid carrier of water and xylitol. Add about 5 drops on the first bite of problem food serving, but remember a normal meal has 2-3 servings of the problem foods.
Beano tablets: each tablet follows Food Chemical Codex (FCC) standards for activity and contains 150 GalU (galactosidase units) of alpha-D-galactosidase derived from *Aspergillus niger* mold. The enzyme is in a carrier of cellulose gel, mannitol, invertase, potato starch, magnesium stearate, gelatin (fish), colloidal silica. 3 tablets swallowed, chewed, or crumbled onto food should be enough for a normal meal of 3 servings of problem foods (1 tablet per ½ cup serving). Beano® will hydrolyze complex sugars, raffinose, stachyose and verbascose, into the simple sugars - glucose, galactose and fructose, and the easily digestible disaccharide, sucrose. (Sucrose hydrolysis happens simultaneously with normal digestion.) In some cases, more enzyme than 5 drops or 3 tablets will be required, and this is a function of the quantity of food eaten, the levels of alpha-linked sugars in the food, and the gas-producing propensity of the person.

Use: Helps prevent flatulence and/or bloat from a variety of grains, cereals, nuts, seeds, and vegetables containing the sugars raffinose, stachyose and/or verbascose. This includes all or most legumes and all or most cruciferous vegetables. Examples of such foods are oats, wheat, beans of all kinds, chickpeas, peas, lentils, peanuts, soy-content foods, broccoli, brussel sprouts, cabbage, carrots, corn, leeks, onions, parsnips, squash. Note: Most vegetables and beans also contain fiber, which is gas productive in some people, but usually far less so than the alpha-linked sugars. Beano® has no effect on fiber.

Usage: About 5 drops per food serving or 3 tablets per meal (1 tablet per ½ cup serving) of 3 servings of problem foods; higher levels depending on symptoms.

Precautions: If you are pregnant or nursing, ask your doctor before product use. Beano is made from a safe, food-grade mold. However, if a rare sensitivity occurs, discontinue use. Galactosemics should not use without physician's advice, since one of the breakdown sugars is galactose.

How Supplied: Beano® is supplied in both a liquid form (30 and 75 serving sizes, at 5 drops per serving), and a tablet form (30, 60, and 100 tablet sizes as well as 24 tablets in packets of 3). These statements have not been evaluated by the Food and Drug Administration. This product is not intended to diagnose, treat, cure or prevent any disease.
For more information and free samples, please write or call toll-free 1-800-257-8650 or visit www.beano.net.

FEOSOL® Caplets
Hematinic
Iron Supplement

Description: FEOSOL Caplets contain pure iron micro particles called carbonyl iron. Replacing FEOSOL Capsules, this advanced formula is specially designed to be well absorbed, gentle on the stomach and offers enhanced safety in the event of an accidental overdose. Each FEOSOL carbonyl iron caplet delivers 45 mg of pure elemental iron, the same amount of elemental iron contained in the 225 mg ferrous sulfate capsule. At equivalent doses, carbonyl iron and ferrous sulfate were shown to be equally efficacious in correcting hemoglobin, hematocrit and serum iron levels in iron-deficient patients[1].

Safety: According to the American Association of Poison Control Centers, iron containing supplements are the leading cause of pediatric poisoning deaths for children under six in the United States[2]. Widely used as a food additive, carbonyl iron must be gastrically solubilized before it can be absorbed, giving it lower toxicity and enhancing its safety versus any of the ferrous salts[3]. As a result, carbonyl iron presents less chance of harm from accidental overdose. In addition, at equivalent doses, carbonyl iron side effects are no greater than those experienced with ferrous sulfate[4].

Warnings: Do not exceed recommended dosage. The treatment of any anemic condition should be under the advice and supervision of a physician. Since oral iron products interfere with absorption of oral tetracycline antibiotics, these products should not be taken within two hours of each other. Occasional gastrointestinal discomfort (such as nausea) may be minimized by taking with meals. Iron containing medication may occasionally cause constipation or diarrhea. If you are pregnant or nursing a baby, seek the advice of a health professional before using this product.
WARNING: Accidental overdose of iron-containing products is a leading cause of fatal poisoning in children under 6. Keep this product out of reach of children. In case of accidental overdose, call a doctor or poison control center immediately.

SUPPLEMENT FACTS

Serving Size: 1 Caplet

Amount per Caplet	% Daily Value
Iron 45 mg	250%

Ingredients: Lactose, Sorbitol, Carbonyl Iron, Hypromellose. Contains 1% or less of the following ingredients: Carnauba Wax, Crospovidone, FD&C Blue #2 Al Lake, FD&C Red #40 Al Lake, FD&C Yellow #6 Al Lake, Magnesium Stearate, Polydextrose, Polyethylene Glycol, Polyethylene Glycol 8000 (Powder), Stearic Acid, Titanium Dioxide, Triacetin.

Directions: Adults—one caplet daily or as directed by a physician. Children under 12 years: Consult a physician.

Tamper-Evident Feature: Each caplet is encased in a plastic cell with a foil back; do not use if cell or foil is broken.

References: [1]Devasthali SD, Gordeuk VR, Brittenham GM, et al, "Bioavailability of Carbonyl Iron: A randomized, double-blind study." Eur J Haematology, 1991; 46:272–278.
[2]FDA Consumer; March 1996:7
[3]Heubers, JA, Brittenham GM, Csiba E and Finch CA. "Absorption of carbonyl iron." J Lab Clin Med 1986; 108:473–78.
[4]Devasthali SD, Gordeuk VR, Brittenham GM, et al, "Bioavailability of a Carbonyl Iron: A randomized, double-blind study." Eur J Haematology, 1991; 46:272–278.
Store at room temperature, avoid excessive heat (greater than 100°F) or humidity.

How Supplied: Boxes of 30 and 60 caplets in blisters. Also available in single unit packages of 100 caplets intended for institutional use

Also available: Feosol Tablets.

Comments or Questions? Call Toll-Free 1-800-245-1040 Weekdays.

GlaxoSmithKline Consumer Healthcare, L.P.

Pittsburgh, PA 15230   Made in USA
Shown in Product Identification Guide, page 506

FEOSOL® TABLETS
Hematinic
Iron Supplement

Description: Feosol tablets provide the body with ferrous sulfate—an iron supplement for iron deficiency and iron deficiency anemia when the need for such therapy has been determined by a physician.

SUPPLEMENT FACTS

Serving Size: 1 Tablet

Amount per Tablet	% Daily Value
Iron 65 mg	360%

Supplement Facts
Serving Size 1 Tablet

Amount Per Serving	% Daily Value for Pregnant or Lactating Women	% Daily Value for Adults and Children 4 or more years of age
Calories 5		
Calcium 500 mg	38%	50%

Amount Per Tablet	% Daily Value for Pregnant or Lactating Women	% Daily Value for Adults and Children 4 or More Years of Age
Vitamin D 125 IU	31%	31%
Calcium 250 mg	19%	25%

Ingredients: Dried ferrous sulfate 200 mg (65 mg of elemental iron) equivalent to 325 mg of ferrous sulfate per tablet. Lactose, Sorbitol, Crospovidone, Magnesium Stearate, Carnauba Wax. Contains 2% or less of the following ingredients: FD&C Blue #1, FD&C Yellow #6, Hypromellose, Polydextrose, Polyethylene Glycol, Titanium Dioxide, Triacetin.

Directions: Adults and children 12 years and over—One tablet daily or as directed by a physician. Children under 12 years—Consult a physician.

Tamper-Evident Feature: Each tablet is encased in a plastic cell with a foil back; do not use if cell or foil is broken.

Warnings: Do not exceed recommended dosage. The treatment of any anemic condition should be under the advice and supervision of a physician. Since oral iron products interfere with absorption of oral tetracycline antibiotics, these products should not be taken within two hours of each other. Occasional gastrointestinal discomfort (such as nausea) may be minimized by taking with meals. Iron containing medication may occassionally cause constipation or diarrhea.

If you are pregnant or nursing a baby, seek the advice of a health professional before using this product.

WARNING: Accidental overdose of iron-containing products is a leading cause of fatal poisoning in children under 6. Keep this product out of reach of children. In case of accidental overdose, call a doctor, or poison control center immediately.

Store at room temperature (59–86°F).

Not USP for dissolution.

How Supplied: Cartons of 100 tablets in child-resistant blisters.

Previously packaged in bottles.

Also available: Feosol caplets.

Comments or Questions?
Call toll-free 1-800-245-1040 weekdays.

GlaxoSmithKline Consumer Healthcare, L.P.

Pittsburgh, PA 15230   Made in USA
Shown in Product Identification Guide, page 506

OS-CAL® CHEWABLE
Calcium Supplement

Description: Calcium supplement to help reduce the risk of osteoporosis. Osteoporosis affects middle-aged and older persons, especially Caucasian and Asian women, and those whose families tend to have fragile bones in later years. A lifetime of regular exercise and eating a healthful diet that includes enough calcium, especially during teen and early adult years, builds and maintains good bone health and may reduce the risk of osteoporosis in later life.

Adequate calcium intake is important, but daily intakes above 2000 mg are not likely to provide any additional benefit. [See first table above]

Ingredients: Calcium carbonate, dextrose monohydrate, maltodextrin, microcrystalline cellulose, magnesium stearate, artificial flavors, sodium chloride. Each tablet provides 500 mg of elemental calcium

Directions: One tablet two to three times a day with meals, or as recommended by your physician.

How Supplied: Bottle of 60 tablets
Store at room temperature.
Keep out of reach of children.
Shown in Product Identification Guide, page 508

OS-CAL® 250 + D
Calcium with Vitamin D Supplement

Description: Calcium supplement to help reduce the risk of osteoporosis (see below*). Also contains Vitamin D.

Supplement Facts
Serving Size 1 Tablet
[See second table above]

Ingredients: Oyster shell powder, corn syrup solids, talc, corn starch, hypromellose. Contains less than 1% of calcium stearate, polysorbate 80, titanium dioxide, polyethylene glycol, Vitamin D, propylparaben and methylparaben (preservative), simethicone, yellow 5 lake, blue 1 lake, carnauba wax, edetate sodium.

Continued on next page

Os-Cal 250+D—Cont.

Directions: One tablet three times a day with meals, or as recommended by your physician.

How Supplied: Bottle of 100 and 240 tablets

Store at room temperature.

Keep out of reach of children.

*Osteoporosis affects middle-aged and older persons, especially Caucasian andAsian women, and those whose families tend to have fragile bones in later years.

A lifetime of regular exercise and eating a healthful diet that includes enough calcium, especially during teen and early adult years, builds and maintains good bone health and may reduce the risk of osteoporosis in later life.

Adequate calcium intake is important, but daily intakes above 2000 mg are not likely to provide any additional benefit.

Shown in Product Identification Guide, page 508

OS-CAL® 500
Calcium Supplement

Description: Calcium supplement to help reduce the risk of osteoporosis.

Osteoporosis affects middle-aged and older persons, especially Caucasian and Asian women, and those whose families tend to have fragile bones in later years.

A lifetime of regular exercise and eating a healthful diet that includes enough calcium, especially during teen and early adult years, builds and maintains good bone health and may reduce the risk of osteoporosis in later life.

Adequate calcium intake is important, but daily intakes above 2000 mg are not likely to provide any additional benefit.

Supplement Facts
Serving Size 1 Tablet
[See table above]

Ingredients: Oyster shell powder, corn syrup solids, talc, corn starch. Contains less than 1% of sodium starch glycolate, calcium stearate, polysorbate 80, hypromellose, polydextrose, titanium dioxide, propylparaben and methylparaben (preservative), triacetin, yellow 5 lake, blue 1 lake, polyethylene glycol, carnauba wax.

Directions: One tablet two to three times a day with meals, or as recommended by your physician.

How Supplied: Bottles of 75 and 160 tablets

Store at room temperature.

Keep out of reach of children.

Shown in Product Identification Guide, page 508

Amount Per Tablet	% Daily Value for Pregnant or Lactating Women	% Daily Value for Adults and children 4 or more years of age
Calcium 500 mg	38%	50%

OS-CAL® 500 + D
Calcium with Vitamin D Supplement

Description: Calcium supplement to help reduce the risk of osteoporosis (see below*). Also contains Vitamin D.

[See table at bottom of next page]

Ingredients: Oyster shell powder, corn syrup solids, talc, corn starch. Contains less than 1% of sodium starch glycolate, calcium stearate, polysorbate 80, hypromellose, polydextrose, titanium dioxide, Vitamin D, propylparaben and methylparaben (preservative), triacetin, yellow 5 lake, blue 1 lake, polyethylene glycol, carnauba wax.

Directions: One tablet two to three times a day with meals, or as recommended by your physician.

How Supplied: Bottle of 75 and 160 tablets

Store at room temperature.

Keep out of reach of children.

*Osteoporosis affects middle-aged and older persons, especially Caucasian and Asian women, and those whose families tend to have fragile bones in later years.

A lifetime of regular exercise and eating a healthful diet that includes enough calcium, especially during teen and early adult years, builds and maintains good bone health and may reduce the risk of osteoporosis in later life.

Adequate calcium intake is important, but daily intakes above 2000 mg are not likely to provide any additional benefit.

Shown in Product Identification Guide, page 508

REMIFEMIN Menopause
Drug Free
Herbal Supplement

A safe, natural, effective way to help ease the physical and emotional symptoms of menopause*

Remifemin Menopause **is a unique, natural formula. For over 40 years in Europe, it has helped reduce the unpleasant physical and emotional symptoms associated with menopause, such as hot flashes, night sweats and mood swings. Clinically shown to be safe and effective. Not a drug.**

Remifemin Menopause **helps you approach menopause with confidence – naturally.***

Supplement Facts
Serving Size 1 tablet

Ingredients:	Amount Per Tablet:	% Daily Value:
Black Cohosh Extract (Root and Rhizome) Equivalent to	20 mg	†

†Daily Value Not Established.

Other Ingredients: Lactose, Cellulose, Potato Starch, Magnesium Stearate, and Natural Peppermint Flavor. Standardized to be equivalent to 20 mg Black Cohosh (*Cimicifuga racemosa*) root and rhizome.
Contains no salt, yeast, wheat, gluten, corn, soy, coloring, or preservatives.

Directions: Take one tablet in the morning and one tablet in the evening, with water. You can expect to notice improvements within a few weeks with full benefits after using Remifemin twice a day for 4 to 12 weeks. This product is intended for use by women who are experiencing menopausal symptoms. Does not contain estrogen. Remifemin is not meant to replace any drug therapy.

Warnings: This product should not be used by women who are pregnant or considering becoming pregnant or are nursing. As with any dietary supplement, always keep out of reach of children. For a few consumers, gastric discomfort may occur but should not be persistent. If gastric discomfort persists, discontinue use and see your health care practitioner. As part of an overall good health care program, we encourage you to see your health care practitioner on a regular basis.

Making Sense Out of Menopause with Remifemin Menopause
Today, women are leading very dynamic and diverse lifestyles. Despite this diversity, there is one constant. They are all experiencing physiological changes. They will all experience menopause. The time when you have menopausal symptoms is a multiphasic period. Technically, the change or transitional process of menopause is known as the *"Climacteric"*. There are different phases of the climacteric that a woman experiences:

1. Perimenopause is the transitional phase when hormone levels begin to drop. This phase lasts typically 3 to 5 years but can last up to 10 years. This gradual decline in estrogen levels causes the troublesome effects of menopause.

2. Menopause is the permanent cessation of menstruation. The average age at menopause is 51, but there is considerable variation in this timing among women. Menopause is medically defined as one year without menstruation.

3. Postmenopause is the phase following menopause. During this phase, your body gets used to the loss of estrogen and eventually the symptoms such as hot flashes go away.

Some Commonly Asked Questions Regarding Remifemin Menopause

1. What is Remifemin Menopause? Remifemin Menopause is a uniquely formulated natural herbal supplement derived from the black cohosh plant. It is formulated to work with your body to promote physical and emotional balance during menopause. Over 40 years of clinical research has shown Remifemin Menopause helps reduce hot flashes, night sweats, related occasional sleeplessness, irritability and mood swings. In a recent clinical study, on average, women experienced the following overall improvements:

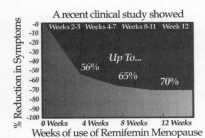

A recent clinical study showed

% Reduction in Symptoms

Weeks 2-3 Weeks 4-7 Weeks 8-11 Week 12

Up To...

56%   65%   70%

Weeks of use of Remifemin Menopause

2. What makes Remifemin Menopause so special? Remifemin Menopause contains an **exclusive** extract of black cohosh. Unlike many other black cohash products, it is developed with specific modern analytical techniques which produce a standardized extract of the black cohosh root and rhizome. In addition, Remifemin is estrogen free and does not influence hormone levels, unlike estrogens and phytoestrogens such as soy.

3. With so many products out there claiming to be "natural," how can I be sure that this product is safe and effective? Remifemin Menopause's formulation is supported by over 40 years of clinical research, and millions of women in Europe have safely used it. Remifemin Menopause is drug free and estrogen free. And it is brought to you from a world-renowned health care company.

4. How does Remifemin Menopause work? Remifemin Menopause contains a proprietary standardized extract taken from the rootstock of the black cohosh plant. Studies have shown that the compounds found within this standardized herbal extract seem to interact with certain hormone receptors – without influencing hormone levels.*

5. How long does it take for Remifemin Menopause to work? Remifemin Menopause is a natural herbal supplement, not a drug. It will take time for your body's cycles to respond to its gentle onset. Personally, you may notice improvements within a few weeks. But for some women, it may take 4 to 12 weeks to benefit fully from Remifemin Menopause. Since the effects of Remifemin Menopause increase after extended twice daily use, we recommend that you take Remifemin Menopause for at least 12 weeks. If you do not find any difference in your well being after 12 weeks, please consult your physician to discuss other options.

6. Can I take it over a long period of time, since the menopausal period lasts for years? Every woman's menopause symptoms are different. Depending on your particular circumstances, you should expect that over time your body will be adjusted to its lower level of estrogen and you may find that you no longer need to take Remifemin. You should listen to your body. We recommend that you take Remifemin Menopause twice daily for up to 6 months continuously. If, after discontinuing use your symptoms return, you may start taking Remifemin Menopause again. Keep in mind that Remifemin Menopause is a natural herbal supplement that supports a natural change that may take you years to go through. As part of an overall good healthcare program, we encourage you to see your health care practitioner on a regular basis.

7. Are there any known side effects? When used properly following the package directions, Remifemin Menopause has few side effects, if any. In clinical research, there was a small percentage of gastric discomfort complaints. If you have been taking Remifemin Menopause and find that this or any other condition develops and persists, please discontinue use and see your physician.

8. Is there a certain time of the day when I should take this product? Do I need to take it with food? You can take Remifemin Menopause with or without food any time of the day. We recommend that you take one tablet in the morning with your breakfast and one tablet in the evening with water.

9. Can I take my herbal tea, vitamins, or other dietary supplements with Remifemin Menopause? Typically, dietary supplements can be taken with other dietary supplements. Always follow package directions. If you should notice any undesirable effects, discontinue taking them together.

Expiration and Storage Information

The expiration date of this package is printed on the side panel flap of the outer carton as well as on the blister packs. Do not use this product after this date.

Store this product in a cool, dry place. Keep out of the reach of children. Avoid storing at temperatures above 86°F.

*These statements have not been evaluated by the Food and Drug Administration. This product is not intended to diagnose, treat, cure, or prevent any disease.

Questions or Comments? Call toll-free 1-800-965-8804 weekdays, or visit www.remifemin.com anytime.

Remifemin ® is a trademark of Schaper & Brümmer GmbH & Co. KG, licensed to GlaxoSmithKline.

Kyowa Engineering-Sundory

6-964 NAKAMOZU-CHO, SAKAI-CITY, OSAKA, JAPAN

Direct Inquiries to:
Consumer Relations
Tel: 81-722-57-8568
Osaka
Fax: 81-722-57-8655
URL: http://www.sundory.co.jp

SEN-SEI-RO LIQUID GOLD™
Kyowa's *Agaricus blazei Murill*
Mushroom Extract
100 ml liquid
Dietary Supplement

Description: Sen-Sei-Ro Liquid Gold™, a dietary supplement containing an exclusive all-natural, standardized extract of the Kyowa's cultured *Agaricus blazei Murill* mushroom is primarily used to reduce symptoms of fatigue, to promote vitality, overall well-being, and to support immune functions.[†] Normal immune function can decline with age, and are necessary for maintenance of vitality, energy, good health, and quality of life. A few major biomarkers for decreased immune functions are decreased natural killer cell (NK) activity, and the number of lymphocytes and macrophage cells. These cells, primarily attack diseased cells and thereby, maintain body homeostasis, promote health and quality of life. For the past half a century in Brazil and other countries, *Agaricus blazei Murill* mushroom has been used to restore vitality, and energy, and to serve as a potent tonic conducive to general health and aging concerns.[†]

Clinical Trials: The effectiveness of ABMK22 in Sen-Sei-Ro Gold™ for health benefits were tested in several controlled pre- and clinical trials in animals and in humans.[†] Recent studies in Japan led researchers to report that in humans, ABMK22 in Sen-Sei-Ro Gold™ enhanced NK cell activity, promoted maturation and activation of dendritic cells indicated

Supplement Facts
Serving Size 1 Tablet

Amount Per Tablet	% Daily Value for Pregnant or Lactating Women	% Daily Value for Adults and Children 4 or more years of age
Vitamin D 200 IU	50%	50%
Calcium 500 mg	38%	50%

Continued on next page

Sen-Sei-Ro Liquid—Cont.

by increased cell kill, elevated expression of CD80 and CD83 expressions (Biotherapy 15(4): 503–507, 2001), increased the number of macrophage (Anticancer Research 17(1A): 274–284, 1997; Japanese Association of Cancer Research, no. 2268, 1999) and tumor necrosis factor α (TNF-α)(Japanese Association of Cancer Research, no. 1406, 1999; Japanese J. Veterinary Clin. Medicine 17(2):31–42, 1998).[†] Further clinical studies with Sen-Sei-Ro Gold™ among 100 cancer patients undergoing chemotherapy in Korea have shown that NK cell activity were significantly enhanced, while NK cell activity in the placebo group was markedly diminished.[†] Earlier and recent both pre-and clinical studies in Japan, and Korea, led researchers to report that Kyowa's *Agaricus blazei Murill* mushroom extract can be part of an effective treatment for supporting the immune systems of cancer patients by stimulating host defense system (Biotherapy 15(4): 503–507, 2001; Carbohydrate Res. 186(2): 267–273, 1989; Japanese J. Pharmacology 662: 265–271, 1994; Agricultural and Biological Chemistry 54: 2889–2905, 1990).[†]

Ingredients: Each 100ml heat-treated high pressure pack of all natural Kyowa's *Agaricus blazei Murill* water extract is scientifically standardized to contain 300mg% carbohydrate, 700mg% protein, 0mg% fat,; 1.4mg% sodium, 0% food quality cellulose, and 4 Kcal energy. Molecular weights of polysaccharopeptides ranges between 600∼8,000. Water: 99.2g%,; includes a variety of amino acids and vitamins (arginine 12mg%, lysine 6mg%, histidine 2mg%, phenylalanine 4mg%, tyrosine 4mg%, leucine 5mg%, isoleucine 3mg%, methionine 1mg%, valine 5mg%, alanine 13mg%, glycine 7mg%, proline 13mg%, glutamic acid 53mg%, serine 6mg%, threonine 5mg%, and asparagine 10mg%).

Recommended Use: As a dietary supplement, take 1∼3 packs per day. Pour the liquid content into a cup or drink directly from the pack. Do not heat the pack either in a microwave oven or heating range or leave the pack open since the product does not contain any preservatives. If warming is necessary, place the pack in warm to mildly hot water for desired length of time. Once the pack is open, drink immediately.

Adverse Reactions: No subjects have reported any side effects since the dietary supplement was placed for consumers in Japan, and Korea for the past 9, and 4 years, respectively. The use of this dietary supplement is generally safe based on two-year chronic toxicity studies of the product carried out by the Good Laboratory Practice (GLP) and American Association of Accreditation of Laboratory Animal Certification (AAALAC) certified Toxicology Research Center. No toxicity of general, CNS, reproductive

and developmental, cardiovascular, immunology, and the two-year bioassay for carcinogenicity was negative. Recent clinical studies with 100 cancer patients undergoing chemotherapy in Korea have shown no known side effects or contraindications.[†]

Warnings: Sen-Sei-Ro Liquid Gold™ has not been evaluated in pregnant and breast feeding mothers or children and should consult a physician prior to use. Also consult a physician prior to use if taking a prescription medication. **Keep this product out of the reach of children. Do not use if you are pregnant, can become pregnant or breast feeding.**

How Supplied: Sen-Sei-Ro Liquid Gold™ 100ml water extract is high pressure heat sealed. A box contains 30, 100ml packs, and can be purchased directly from company representatives, health food stores, and independent pharmacies. Storage condition keep at room temperature and avoid any direct heat or sun light.

[†]These statements have not been evaluated by the Food and Drug Administration. These products are not intended to diagnose, treat, cure or prevent any disease.

Shown in Product Identification Guide, page 509

SEN-SEI-RO POWDER GOLD™
KYOWA'S *Agaricus blazei Murill* Mushroom
1800mg standard granulated powder
Dietary Supplement

Description: Sen-Sei-Ro Powder Gold™ slim pack, a dietary supplement containing an exclusively all natural and prepared from Kyowa's *Agaricus blazei Murill* mushroom is primarily used to reduce symptoms of fatigue, to promote vitality, overall well-being, and to support immune functions.[†] Normal immune function can decline with age, and are necessary for maintenance of vitality, energy, good health, and quality of life. A few major biomarkers for decreased immune functions are decreased natural killer cell (NK) activity, and the number of lymphocytes and macrophage cells. These cells, primarily attack diseased cells and thereby, maintain body homeostasis, promote health and quality of life. For the past half a century in Brazil and other countries, *Agaricus blazei Murill* mushroom has been used to restore vitality, and energy, and to serve as a potent tonic conducive to general health and aging concerns.[†]

Clinical Trials: The effectiveness of Sen-Sei-Ro Powder Gold™ for health benefits were tested in several controlled pre- and clinical trials in animals and in humans.[†] Recent studies in Japan, and Korea led researcher to report that in humans, Sen-Sei-Ro Powder Gold™ en-

hanced NK cell activity, increased the number of macrophage cells (Anticancer Research 17 (1A): 274–284, 1997; Japanese Association of Cancer Research, no. 2268, 1999) and tumor necrosis factor α (TNF-α)(Japanese Association of Cancer Research, no. 1406, 1999).[†] Antitumor effects of Sen-Sei-Ro against various murine and dog tumors were thought to be mediated by stimulation of NK cell activity, increased number of macrophage cells, and increased activity of tumor necrosis factor α (TNF-α)(Japanese J. Veterinary Clin. Medicine 17(2):31–42, 1998).[†] Recent clinical studies in Japan, and Korea, led researchers to report that *Agaricus blazei Murill* mushroom extract can be part of an effective treatment for supporting the immune systems of cancer patients by stimulating host defense system (Biotherapy 15(4): 503–507, 2001; Carbohydrate Res. 186(2): 267–273, 1989; Japanese J. Pharmacology 662: 265–271, 1994; Agricultural and Biological Chemistry 54: 2889–2905, 1990).[†]

Ingredients: Each 1800mg granulated powder in a slim pack contains 488 mg protein, 820 mg carbohydrate, 47 mg fat, 0.19 mg Sodium; 284 mg food grade cellulose; 5.7 kcal energy.

Water: 68mg, includes 0.1 mg Fe, 0.24 mg Ca, 37 mg K, 0.01mg thiamine, 0.04mg ergosterol, 0.59mg niacin.

Recommended Use: As a dietary supplement, take 1∼3 packs per day. Pour the content into a cup containing warm water or other desirable beverage and mix and drink. Do not heat the pack either in a microwave oven or heating range or leave the pack open since the product does not contain any preservatives. Once the pack is open, drink immediately.

Adverse Reactions: No subjects have reported any side effects since the dietary supplement was placed for consumers in Japan and Korea for the past 9, and 4 years, respectively. The use of this dietary supplement is generally safe based on two-year chronic toxicity studies of the product by the Good Laboratory Practice (GLP) and American Association of Accreditation of Laboratory Animal Certification (AAALAC) certified Toxicology Research Center. Toxicity evaluation of general, CNS, reproductive and developmental, cardiovascular, immunology, and the two-year bioassay for carcinogenicity was negative.[†]

Warnings: Sen-Sei-Ro Powder Gold™ has not been evaluated in pregnant and breast feeding mothers or children and should consult a physician prior to use. Also consult a physician prior to use if taking a prescription medications. **Keep this product out of the reach of children. Do not use if you are pregnant, can become pregnant or breast feeding.** Quality of the dietary supplement is guaranteed for 2 years

from the manufactured date, but for more information, please write or call 81-72-257-8568 or 81-3-3512-5032.

How Supplied: Sen-Sei-Ro Powder Gold™ is high pressure heat sealed. A box contains 30 slim packs of each with 1800mg per pack, and can be purchased directly from company representatives, health food stores, and independent pharmacies. Storage condition keep at room temperature and avoid any direct heat or sun light.

†These statements have not been evaluated by the Food and Drug Administration. These products are not intended to diagnose, treat, cure or prevent any disease.
Shown in Product Identification Guide, page 509

Legacy for Life, LLC
P.O. BOX 410376
MELBOURNE, FL 32941-0376

Direct Inquiries to:
(800) 557-8477
(321) 951-8815
www.legacyforlife.net

IMMUNE[26®]
IMMUNE SUPPORT

Description: These immune[26®] products contain hyperimmune egg powder, pure egg product derived from hens hyperimmunized with over 26 inactivated enteric pathogens of human origin.

Clinical Background: Upon oral administration, immune[26®] specific immunoglobulins and immunomodulatory factors are passively transferred. immune[26®] and Immune Support modulate autoimmune responses, plus support and balance cardiovascular function, healthy cholesterol levels, a vital circulatory system, a fully functional digestive tract, flexible and healthy joints and energy levels.

How Supplied: immune[26®] is available as immune[26®], hyperimmune egg in powder and capsule form, and as immune[26®] Immune Support, hyperimmune egg enriched with minerals and 100% of the daily value of more than 13 essential vitamins.

Precautions: Those with known allergies to eggs should consult with a health practitioner before consuming this product.
Note: immune[26®] is not intended to diagnose, treat, cure, or prevent any disease. These statements have not been evaluated by the Food and Drug Administration.

Maitake Products, Inc.
PO BOX 1534
PARAMUS, NJ 07653

Direct Inquiries to:
800-747-7418
www.maitake.com

GRIFRON®-PRO
Maitake Mushroom
D-Fraction® Extract

Description: Maitake D-fraction® is a standardized extract based on active β-glucan/protein compound of Maitake mushroom. Water soluble β-1,3 and 1,6 glucans derived from Maitake are confirmed to have activity to enhance cellular immune function. Maitake D-fraction® is designed and developed to be optimal for oral administration. Recent studies indicate that it enhances apoptosis inducing activity on aggressive prostate cancer cell line. This product has been given an Investigational New Drug (IND) status from the FDA for Phase II pilot study against advanced breast and prostate cancer patients. Because of its established safety, Phase I toxicity study was exempted by the FDA. This product does not contain sugar, yeast, mold, artificial colors, dairy foods, preservatives, and chemical pesticides or fertilizers.

Supplement Fact:
Serving size: 6 drops

Serving per container: 135
Amount per 6 drops: % Daily Value:
Maitake Mushroom
  Standardized Extract: 22mg*
  (D-fraction 30%)

*Daily Value not established

Every 6 drops contains a minimum of pure and active 6.6mg of Beta-glucan in a standardized extract from organically ground Maitake fruit body in a vegetable glycerin base.

Other Ingredients:
Vegetable Glycerine
Water

Directions for use: As a dietary supplement, take 6 drops three times a day for health maintenance or as directed by your practitioner. Therapeutic total daily amount would be one drop per kilo of body weight.

How Supplied: Bottles of 30ml and 60ml.
This product is safety sealed for your protection. Do not use if seal is missing or broken.
Keep out of reach of children. Consult a physician before using if pregnant or nursing. Store in a cool, dry place.

Mannatech, Inc.
600 S. ROYAL LANE
SUITE 200
COPPELL, TX 75019

For Medical Professional Inquiries Contact:
Kia Gary, RN LNCC
(972) 471-8189
Kgary@mannatech.com

Direct Inquiries to:
Customer Service
(972) 471-8111

Product Information:
www.mannatech.com

Ingredient Information:
www.glycoscience.com

AMBROTOSE®
A Glyconutritional Dietary Supplement

Supplement Facts:
Ambrotose® powder:
Serving Size 0.44 g (approx. ¼ teaspoon)
Powder canister: 100g or 50g
Amount
  Per   % Daily
Serving   Value
0.44g   *

* Daily Values not established.

Ambrotose® capsules:
Serving Size: two capsules
Capsules per container: 60
Amount
  Per   % Daily
Serving   Value
2 capsules   *

* Daily Values not established.

Ambrotose® with Lecithin capsules:
Ambrotose® with Lecithin
Supplement Facts:
Serving Size: two capsules
Capsules per container: 60
Amount
  Per   % Daily
Serving   Value
1–2 capsules   *

* Daily Values not established.

Ingredients:
Ambrotose® Powder
(patent pending)
Arabinogalactan (Larix decidua) (gum), Rice starch, Aloe vera extract, (inner leaf gel)- Manapol® powder, Ghatti (Anogeissus latifolia)(gum), Glucosamine HCl, Tragacanth (Astragalus Gummifer) (gum).
Ambrotose® capsules
(patent pending)
Arabinogalactan (Larix decidua) (gum), Rice starch, Aloe vera extract, (inner leaf

Continued on next page

Ambrotose—Cont.

gel)- Manapol® powder, Ghatti (Anogeis-sus latifolia) (gum), Tragacanth (Astragalus gummifer) (gum).

Ambrotose® with Lecithin capsules
(patent pending)
Arabinogalactan (Larix decidua) (gum), Rice starch, Aloe vera extract, (inner leaf gel) - Manapol® powder, Ghatti (Anogeissus latifolia) (gum), Tragacanth (Astragalus gummifer) (gum).
Other ingredients: Calcium, lecithin powder
For additional information on ingredients, visit www.glycoscience.com

Use: Ambrotose complex is a proprietary formula designed to help provide saccharides used in glycoconjugate synthesis to promote cellular communication and immune support.** Consumers who are healthy may notice improved concentration, more energy, better sleep, improved athletic performance, and a greater sense of well-being.

Directions: The recommended intake of Ambrotose powder is ¼ teaspoon two times a day; the recommended intake of Ambrotose capsules or Ambrotose with Lecithin is two capsules three times a day. If desired, you may begin by taking less than the recommended intake. If well tolerated, you may gradually increase to the recommended intake. As a blend of plant saccharides, Ambrotose complex is safe in amounts well in excess of the label recommendations. Children between the ages of 12 and 48 months with growth/nutritional problems (failure to thrive) have been given 1 tablespoon a day of Ambrotose powder for 3 months with no adverse effects. Individuals have reported taking as much as 10 tablespoons of Ambrotose powder (approx. 50 grams) each day for several months with no adverse effects. The amount needed by each individual may vary with time, age, genetic makeup, metabolic rate, and activities, stress level, current dietary intake, and health challenges of the moment. A health care professional experienced with use of Ambrotose complex may be helpful.

Warning: Anyone who is taking medication may wish to advise his/her physician. One teaspoon of Ambrotose powder (equivalent to 12 Ambrotose capsules) contains the amount of glucose equivalent to 1/25 teaspoon of sucrose (table sugar)
KEEP BOTTLE TIGHTLY CLOSED. STORE IN A COOL, DRY PLACE.

How Supplied: Bottle of 3.50 oz (100g) powder. Bottle of 1.75 oz (50g) powder. Bottle of 60 (150mg) capsules.

** This statement has not been evaluated by the Food and Drug Administration. This product is not intended to diagnose, treat, cure or prevent any disease.

Mannatech Inc.
600 S. Royal Lane, Suite 200
Coppell, Texas 75019
www.mannatech.com
Shown in Product Identification Guide, page 509

PHYTALOE® with Ambrotose® Complex
A Dietary Supplement of Dried Fruits and Vegetables

Supplement Facts:

Serving size: 1 capsule or ¼ teaspoon
Capsules per container: 60 capsules
Powder canister: 3.5 oz. (100g)

	Amount Per Serving	% Daily Value
PhytAloe	490mg	*
Ambrotose complex	50mg	*

Broccoli, Brussels sprout, cabbage, carrot, cauliflower, garlic, kale, onion, tomato, turnip, papaya, pineapple. Ambrotose complex, naturally occurring plant polysaccharides including freeze-dried Aloe vera (inner leaf gel extract) – Manapol® powder.

---
*Percent Daily Values not established.

Other Ingredients: Magnesium stearate. This product contains no sugar, starch, preservatives, synthetic colorants or chemical stabilizers.

Use: PhytAloe is a blend of dehydrated fruits and vegetables in combination with Ambrotose complex for immune system support.** PhytAloe contains no synthetic additives and is supplied as powder and as capsules.

Directions: The recommended intake of PhytAloe powder is ¼ teaspoon twice a day; the recommended intake of PhytAloe capsules is one capsule twice a day.

Warnings: If any one of the fruits or vegetables in PhytAloe has caused stomach upset or any other adverse reaction in the past, start below the recommended amount and gradually increase to the recommended intake as tolerated.
KEEP BOTTLE TIGHTLY CLOSED. STORE IN A COOL, DRY PLACE.

How Supplied: Bottle of 60 capsules. Bottle of 3.5 oz (100g) powder.

** This statement has not been evaluated by the Food and Drug Administration. This product is not intended to diagnose, treat, cure or prevent any disease.

Shown in Product Identification Guide, page 509

PLUS with Ambrotose® Complex
Dietary Supplement Caplets

Supplement Facts:
Serving Size - 1 Caplet

	Amount Per Serving	% Daily Value
Iron	1mg	5
Wild Yam (root)	200mg	*
Standardized for Phytosterols	25mg	
L-Glutamic acid	200mg	*
L-Glycine	200mg	*
L-Lysine	200mg	*
L-Arginine	100mg	*
Beta Sitosterol	25mg	*
Ambrotose® Complex (patent pending)	2.5mg	*

Naturally occurring plant polysaccharides including freeze-dried Aloe vera inner gel extract-Manapol® powder.

Other Ingredients: Microcrystalline cellulose, silicon dioxide, croscarmellose sodium, magnesium stearate, titanium dioxide coating.

---
*Daily value not established.

For additional information on ingredients, visit www.glycoscience.com

Use: PLUS caplets provide nutrients to help support the endocrine system's production and balance of hormones.** A well-functioning endocrine system works in harmony with the body's immune system, helps support the efficient metabolism of fat, and supports natural recovery from physical or emotional stress.** The functional components of PLUS caplets are wild yam extract, amino acids, and beta sitosterol. PLUS caplets contain no hormones.

Directions: The recommended intake of PLUS caplets is two caplets per day.

Warning: After an extensive review of the literature, no documented evidence was found linking the ingredients in PLUS caplets with any form of human cancer or with any problems associated with pregnancy. However, as with all supplements, you should consult your health care professional if you are pregnant.

KEEP BOTTLE TIGHTLY CLOSED. STORE IN A COOL, DRY PLACE.

How Supplied: Bottle of 90 caplets.

** This statement has not been evaluated by the Food and Drug Administration. This product is not intended to diagnose, treat, cure or prevent any disease.

Shown in Product Identification Guide, page 509

Matol Botanical International Ltd.

**290 LABROSSE AVENUE
POINTE-CLAIRE, QUEBEC,
CANADA, H9R 6R6**

Direct Inquiries to:
Ph: (800) 363-1890
website: www.matol.com

BIOMUNE OSF™ PLUS
**Dietary supplement for immune
system support**

Description: Biomune OSF™ Plus is
an immune system support product for
all ages. Biomune OSF™ Plus is a combination of a special extract of antigen infused colostrum and whey with the herb
Astragalus. The exclusive colostrum/
whey extract (Ai/E$^{10™}$) is prepared using
a patented and proprietary process
unique to the nutritional industry.
Astragalus is a traditional Chinese herb
that is known for its immune enhancing
properties. Clinical studies show that
Biomune OSF™ Plus is effective in con-
sistently and dramatically increasing
Natural Killer cell activity. Medical research has shown that low NK cell activity is present in most illness. A double
blind study with antigen infused dialyzable bovine colostrum/whey shows its effectiveness as an immune system modulator.

Summary of clinical studies:
**The Use of Dialyzable Bovine Colos-
trum/Whey Extract in Conjunction
with a Holistic Treatment Model for
Natural Killer Cell Stimulation in
Chronic Illness by Jesse A. Stoff,
MD**
This clinical study consists of 107 pa-
tients with an average treatment time of
13.2 months. The average initial
Natural Killer (NK) cell activity was 18
Lytic Units (LU) and the average final
NK cell activity was 246 LU. All patients
in the study greatly improved, went into
remission or recovered.
Conclusions: The Study Group demonstrated that increased NK activity paral-
leled restored resistance to illness and
recovery from illness.
**An Examination of Immune Response
Modulation in Humans by Antigen Infused Dialyzable Bovine Colostrum/
Whey Extract Utilizing a Double Blind
Study by Jesse A. Stoff, MD.**
This study provides double blind evidence that the cytokines, peptide neuro-
hormones and other informational molecules in Antigen Infused Dialyzable Bovine Colostrum/Whey Extract modulate
and normalize immune function. Further, Antigen Infused Dialyzable Bovine
Colostrum/Whey Extract demonstrates
its effectiveness as a Biological Immune
Response Modulator for increasing the
protective functions of the immune system.

Both studies are available from Matol
Botanical International Ltd. upon re-
quest.

Use: Dietary Supplement

Directions for Use: Take one capsule
daily for maintenance and one or two
capsules every 2–3 hours when additional immune support is needed. The
product can be taken daily for maintenance or as above for extended periods of
time. There is no known toxicity.

How Supplied: One bottle contains
30 capsules.

*Shown in Product Identification
Guide, page 509*

Mayor Pharmaceutical Laboratories

**2401 S. 24TH ST.
PHOENIX, AZ 85034**

Direct Inquiries to:
Medical Director
(602) 244-8899

www.vitamist.com

B-PRODUCT DAILY DIETARY SUPPLEMENTS

B-Young:
High potency calcium and mineral dietary supplement drink mix.

Description: B-Young contains high
levels of calcium, potassium, phosphorous, magnesium and zinc, together with
vitamin D3, a vitamin essential for calcium absorption. B-Young is a water soluble powder, making it an ideal calcium
supplement for people of all ages. Calcium deficiency has been linked to many
diseases, including osteoporosis. Approximately 25 million American women currently have some degree of osteoporosis
and the disease will affect more than one-
third of post-menopausal women. In addition, more than 5 million American
men suffer from osteoporosis. Calcium
supplements may help to reduce the risk
of osteoporosis and other diseases associated with calcium deficiency.

B-Slim:
Appetite suppressant and weight loss
formula.

Description: B-Slim is a unique product combining herbal extracts with vitamins and minerals. Obesity has reached
epidemic proportions in the United
States. B-Slim contains ingredients that
have been shown in scientific studies to
help control appetite as well as improve
the levels of cholesterol and other vital
factors in your blood.

B-Fit:
Electrolyte replacement and exercise formula.

Description: During exercise the body
loses essential electrolytes that are necessary for normal physiological processes. If these electrolytes are not
replaced the body can suffer serious consequences. B-Fit can help replace these
lost electrolytes quickly and effectively.
B-Fit is ideal for adding to water to be
consumed during periods of exertion.

Directions: Add the contents of each
packet to 8–16 oz water. Stir until dissolved, and drink. Each B-Product can
also be added to your choice of fruit juice
or iced tea. Use 3–4 times per day.

How Supplied: All three B-Products
are available in boxes of 24 individual
serving packets.

VITAMIST® Intra-Oral Spray
[vĭt '-ə-mĭst]
Nutraceuticals/Dietary Supplements

Description: VitaMist® products are
patented, intra-oral sprays for the delivery of vitamins, minerals, and other nutritional supplements, directly into the
oral cavity. A 55 microliter spray delivers
high concentrations of nutrients directly
onto the mouth's sensitive tissue. The
buccal mucosa transfers the nutrients
into the bloodstream. (U.S. Patent
4,525,341—Foreign patents issued and
pending.)

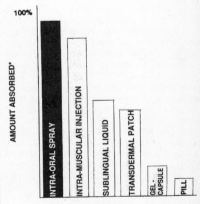

METHOD OF DELIVERY
*Representative of the product class.

Benefits:
- Spray supplementation provides an
  absorption rate approximately nine
  times greater than that of pills.
- Once the formula is sprayed into the
  mouth, the nutrients reach the bloodstream within minutes.
- No fillers or binders are added; the
  body receives only pure ingredients.
- An alternative method of supplementation for those that cannot take pills,
  or simply do not enjoy swallowing
  pills.
- Convenient administration; no water
  needed.

Continued on next page

Vitamist—Cont.

Product Overview: Multiple: vitamins and minerals in three separate formulations: adult, children's, and prenatal.

C+Zinc: with vitamin E and the amino acids L-lysine and glycine.

B12: contains 1000% of the US RDI of vitamin B12.

Stress: herbal formula with B vitamins.

St. John's Wort: St. John's wort extract with vitamin B12, ginkgo biloba, kava kava and folic acid.

E+Selenium: contains vitamin E and selenomethionine.

Anti-Oxidant: with vitamins A, C, E, niacin, folate, and beta-carotene.

VitaSight®: with vitamins A, C and E, beta-carotene, zinc, selenium, bilberry, lutein, and ginkgo biloba.

Colloidal Minerals: more than 70 trace and essential minerals from natural sources.

Smoke-Less™: herbal combination with additional nutrients designed to reduce cravings.

PMS and LadyMate: supplementation for the nutritional needs of pre-menstrual syndrome.

Folacin: vitamins B6 and B12 added to folate (folic acid).

Slender-Mist®: dietary snack supplements containing a combination of B vitamins, hydroxy-citric acid, L-carnitine and chromium. Four different flavors.

Blue-Green Sea Spray: spirulina extract, additional omega 3 fatty acids from flaxseed oil, and vitamin E.

Re-Leaf: a blend of more than 10 herbs that are recommended for minor discomfort, anxiety, and stress.

Osteo-CalMag: herbal supplement with additional vitamin D, calcium and magnesium.

Pine Bark and Grape Seed: powerful proanthocyanidins (anti-oxidants) from natural sources, with additional B vitamins.

1-Before, 2-During, 3-After: three performance sprays designed for the needs of physical activity.

CardioCare: with vitamins C and E, the amino acids L-lysine and L-proline, coenzyme Q10 and additional herbal extracts.

Melatonin: a natural hormone that is effective in re-establishing sleep patterns.

DHEA: dehydroepiandrosterone in both men's and women's formulations.

Revitalizer®: high levels of B vitamins, as well as vitamins A and E, the amino acids L-cysteine and glycine, and selenium.

GinkgoMist™: with ginkgo biloba, vitamin B12, acetyl-L-carnitine, choline, inositol, phosphatidylserine and niacin.

ArthriFlex™: with chondroitin sulfate, glucosamine sulfate, vitamins C and D, calcium, manganese, boron and dong quai.

VitaMotion-S™: dimenhydrinate with ginger and vitamin B6.

Echinacea + G: combination of echinacea, goldenseal and garlic extracts, together with honey and lemon.

Ex. O: powerful blend of cayenne and peppermint with additional herbs recommended for allergy control.

How Supplied: VitaMist dietary supplements are supplied in sealed containers fitted with a natural pump. Each container provides a 30-day supply.

Recommended Dosage: Two sprays, four times per day, for a total dosage of eight sprays per day.

McNeil Consumer & Specialty Pharmaceuticals
**Division of McNeil-PPC, Inc.
FORT WASHINGTON, PA 19034**

Direct Inquiries to:
Consumer Relationship Center
Fort Washington, PA 19034
(215) 273-7000

LACTAID® Original Strength Caplets
(lactase enzyme)

LACTAID® Extra Strength Caplets
(lactase enzyme)

LACTAID® Ultra Caplets and Chewable Tablets
(lactase enzyme)

Description: Each serving size (3 caplets) of *LACTAID® Original Strength* contains 9000 FCC (Food Chemical Codex) units of lactase enzyme (derived from *Aspergillus oryzae*).
Each serving size (2 caplets) of *LACTAID® Extra Strength* contains 9000 FCC units of lactase enzyme (derived from *Aspergillus oryzae*).
Each serving size (1 caplet) of *LACTAID® Ultra Caplet* contains 9000 FCC units of lactase enzyme (derived from *Aspergillus oryzae*).
Each serving size (1 tablet) of *LACTAID® Ultra Chewable Tablet* contains 9000 FCC units of lactase enzyme (derived from *Aspergillus oryzae*).
LACTAID® is the original lactase dietary supplement that makes milk and dairy foods more digestible for individuals with lactose intolerance. *LACTAID®* lactase enzyme hydrolyzes lactose into two digestible simple sugars: glucose and galactose. *LACTAID® Caplets/Chewable Tablets* are taken orally for *in vivo* hydrolysis of lactose.

Actions: *LACTAID® Caplets/Chewable Tablets* work by providing the enzyme that hydrolyzes the milk sugar lactose (disaccharide) into the two monosaccharides, glucose and galactose.

Uses: LACTAID contains a natural enzyme that helps your body break down lactose, the complex sugar found in dairy foods. If not properly digested, lactose can cause flatulence, bloating, cramps or diarrhea.*

---
*This statement has not been evaluated by the Food and Drug Administration. This product is not intended to diagnose, treat, cure, or prevent any disease.

Directions: Original Strength: Swallow or chew 3 caplets with the first bite of dairy food. For best results, you may have to adjust the number of caplets up or down. **Extra Strength:** Swallow or chew 2 caplets with first bite of dairy food. For best results, you may have to adjust the number of caplets up or down. **Ultra Caplets:** Swallow 1 caplet with the first bite of dairy food. If you suffer from severe digestive discomfort, you may have to take more than one caplet, but no more than two at a time. **Ultra Chewables:** Chew and swallow 1 chewable tablet with your first bite of dairy food. If you suffer from severe digestive discomfort, you may have to take more than one tablet but no more than two at a time. Don't be discouraged if at first LACTAID does not work to your satisfaction. Because the degree of enzyme deficiency naturally varies from person to person and the amount of lactose varies from food to food, you may have to adjust the number of caplets/chewable tablets up or down to find your own level of comfort. Since LACTAID Caplets/Chewable Tablets work only on the food as you eat it, use them every time you consume dairy foods.

Warnings: *Consult your doctor if* your symptoms continue after using the product or if your symptoms are unusual or seem unrelated to eating dairy. Keep out of reach of children. **Do not use if carton is open or if printed plastic neckwrap is broken or if single serve packet is open.**
LACTAID® Ultra Chewable Tablets:
Phenylketonurics: Contains Phenylalanine

Ingredients: *LACTAID® Original Strength Caplets:* Lactase Enzyme (9000 FCC Lactase units/3 caplets), Mannitol, Cellulose, Dextrose, Sodium Citrate, Magnesium Stearate.
LACTAID® Extra Strength Caplets: Lactase Enzyme (9000 FCC Lactase units/2 caplets), Mannitol, Cellulose, Dextrose, Sodium Citrate, Magnesium Stearate.
LACTAID® Ultra Caplets: Lactase Enzyme (9000 FCC Lactase units/Caplet), Cellulose, Dextrose, Sodium Citrate, Magnesium Stearate, Colloidal Silicon Dioxide.
LACTAID® Ultra Chewable Tablets: Lactase Enzyme (9000 FCC Lactase units/tablet), Mannitol, Cellulose, Sodium Citrate, Dextrose, Magnesium Stearate, Flavor, Citric Acid, Acesulfame K, Aspartame.

How Supplied: *LACTAID® Original Strength Caplets* are available in bottles

of 120 count. Store at or below room temperature (below 77°F) but do not refrigerate. Keep away from heat. *LACTAID® Extra Strength Caplets* are available in bottles of 50 count. Store at or below room temperature (below 77°F) but do not refrigerate. Keep away from heat. *LACTAID® Ultra Caplets* are available in single serve packets in 12, 32, 60 and 90 count packages. Store at or below 86°F. Keep away from heat. *LACTAID® Ultra Chewable Tablets* are available in single serve packets of 12, 32 and 60 counts. Store at or below room temperature (below 77°F), but do not refrigerate. Keep away from heat and moisture. *LACTAID® Caplets* and *LACTAID® Ultra Chewable Tablets* are certified kosher from the Orthodox Union.
Also available: 70% lactose-reduced Lactaid Milk and 100% lactose-reduced Lactaid Milk.

Shown in Product Identification Guide, page 510

MDR Fitness Corp.
MEDICAL DOCTORS' RESEARCH
14101 NW 4th STREET
SUNRISE, FL 33325

Direct Inquiries to:
1-800-637-8227 ext 5111 or 5445
www.mdri.com

MDR FITNESS TABS FOR MEN OTC
MDR FITNESS TABS FOR WOMEN

DESCRIPTION
The original AM/PM Fitness Tabs® from Medical Doctors' Research are patented because of their ability to increase blood levels of nutrients that can increase immune defenses and reduce the risk of coronary heart disease within weeks of taking the formula. MDR Fitness Tabs. The A.M. and P.M. dosage allows more absorption of the water soluble vitamins (B-complex and C) which are not readily stored by the body. The AM tablet provides more micronutrients required for energy producing reactions when physical activity is greater. The MDR formulas are free of dyes, yeast, preservatives, fillers, soy, wheat gluten, lactose and other sugars.

INDICATIONS AND USAGE
MDR Fitness Tabs are designed for the maintenance of good health and nutrition for men and women, 11 years of age or older, whenever a multi-vitamin, mineral supplement is indicated to help provide nutrients missing from the diet or to replace nutrient loss from oral contraceptives, antacids, excessive alcohol, smoking, physical or emotional stress, exercise, weight loss diets, or illness. Daily use of MDR Fitness Tabs may also play a protective role for good health by

assuring adequate intake of essential nutrients, including antioxidant nutrients shown in recent research to enhance the body's natural defenses.
Directions: After the first meal of the day, take one "AM" Fitness Tab (and one Stress Defense Performance Tab, if needed.) After lunch or dinner, take one "PM" Fitness Tab. Swallow Fitness Tab with a full glass of water.
PRECAUTIONS
Not recommended for persons with severe kidney disease or those undergoing renal dialysis, unless under a physician's supervision. Diabetics may need to adjust insulin dosage and should be monitored. Not recommended for those suffering from pernicious anemia, or Parkinson patients on levodopa therapy, due to the presence of vitamin B-6 which may decrease levodopa's efficacy. Pregnant and lactating women may need additional supplementation.
Note: MDR also provides a Stress Defense supplement to be taken with MDR Fitness Tabs when higher dosages are indicated. MDR has formulated Vital Factors for persons over 40 years of age to supply secretagogues that help enhance the body's natural release of Human Growth Hormone, and to supply other vital factors which decline with age. A majority of users report increased vitality, energy, better sleep, reduced depression, improved flexibility and greater mental function after using Vital Factors.
Also available: Nite-Cal Calcium, Vitamin B-12 Sublingual, Chondro-Pro Arthritis Formula, CardioTone Cardiovascular Nutritional Support, and Longevity Antioxidants.
For Samples, Product or Order Information Call
1-800-MDR-TABS ext. 5111 or 5445 or fax (954) 845-9505
att: L. Giordano
www.mdri.com
(MDR) Medical Doctors' Research
14101 NW 4th Street
SUNRISE, FL 33325

Memory Secret
1221 BRICKELL AVENUE
SUITE 1000,
MIAMI FL 33131 USA

For direct inquiries contact:
phone 1-412-318-4308
fax 1-305-675-2279
e-mail memorysecret@ari.es

INTELECTOL™ MEMORY ENHANCER
VINPOCETINE TABLETS MEMORY SECRET

Description: Intelectol® is a powerful memory enhancer. Scientific studies

have shown that its ingredient vinpocetine helps the body to maintain healthy circulation in the brain by decreasing cerebral vascular resistance, improving cerebral blood flow and cerebral oxygen and glucose utilization, and that vinpocetine increases the concentration of some neurotransmitters involved in the process of memory formation. Intelectol™ can be taken for enhancing the following cognitive functions: memory, attention, orientation, perception, information fixation, judgment. Clinical studies have also shown that vinpocetine helps to maintain healthy microcirculation in the inner ear and eyes.
Active ingredients: Vinpocetine 5mg (No U.S. RDA established)
Inactive ingredients: Lactose, Hydropropylcellulose, Magnesium Stearate, Talc.

Recommended Use: 1 to 2 tablets × 3 times daily with meals.

Warning: Keep out of reach of children. Do not take if you are pregnant or lactating. If you have hemophilia or are on blood thinning medication, please consult your physician before taking this product.
Interactions: Not known.

How Supplied: packs of 50 tablets.
Availability: Available at Web Site www.memorysecret.net, phone number 1 412 318 4308.

References/Function Claim:
Visit Web Site http://www.memory-secret.net
Shown in Product Identification Guide, page 509

Mission Pharmacal Company
10999 IH 10 WEST
SUITE 1000
SAN ANTONIO, TX 78230-1355

Direct Inquiries to:
PO Box 786099
San Antonio, TX 78278-6099
TOLL FREE: (800) 292-7364
(210) 696-8400
FAX: (210) 696-6010
For Medical Information Contact:
In Emergencies:
Mary Ann Walter
(830) 249-9822
FAX: (830) 249-1376

CITRACAL®Ⓤ
[*sit'ra-cal*]
Ultradense® calcium citrate dietary supplement

Ingredients: Calcium (as Ultradense® calcium citrate) 200 mg, polyethylene

Continued on next page

Citracal—Cont.

glycol, croscarmellose sodium, hydroxy-propyl methylcellulose, color added, magnesium silicate, magnesium stearate.

Sensitive Patients: CITRACAL® contains no wheat, barley, yeast or rye; is sugar, dairy and gluten free and contains no artificial colors.
One Tablet Provides:
200 mg. calcium (elemental, equaling 20% of the U.S. recommended daily allowance for adults and children 4 or more years of age).

Directions: Take 1 to 2 tablets two times daily or as recommended by a physician, pharmacist or health professional. Store at room temperature.

How Supplied: Supplied as white, rectangular (nearly oval) shaped, coated tablets in bottles of 100 UPC 0178-0800-01, and bottles of 200 UPC 0178-0800-20. ⓤ=Kosher Parvae approved by Orthodox Union.

CITRACAL® 250 MG + D
[sit 'ra-cal]
Ultradense® calcium citrate-Vitamin D dietary supplement

Ingredients: Each tablet contains: calcium (as Ultradense® calcium citrate) 250 mg., polyethylene glycol, citric acid, microcrystalline cellulose, hydroxypropyl methylcellulose, croscarmellose sodium, color added, magnesium silicate, magnesium stearate vitamin D_3 (62.5 IU).

How Supplied: Available in bottles of 150 tablets, UPC 0178-0837-15.

CITRACAL® Caplets + D
[sit ' ra-cal]
Ultradense® calcium citrate-Vitamin D dietary supplement

Ingredients: CITRACAL® Caplets + D are supplied in an ultra-dense caplet formulation, each containing calcium (as Ultradense® calcium citrate) 315 mg., polyethylene glycol, croscarmellose sodium, hydroxypropyl methylcellulose, color added, magnesium silicate, magnesium stearate, vitamin D_3 (200 IU).

How Supplied: Available in bottles of 60
UPC 0178-0815-60, and bottles of 120 UPC 0178-0815-12.
Store at room temperature.

CITRACAL® LIQUITAB® ⓤ
[sit ' ra-cal]
Effervescent calcium citrate dietary supplement

Ingredients: Each effervescent tablet contains: calcium (as calcium citrate)

500 mg., adipic acid, citric acid, sodium saccharin, artificial orange flavor, cellulose gum, aspartame.
Phenylketonurics: Contains phenylalanine.

How Supplied: Available in bottles of 30 effervescent tablets. UPC 0178-0811-30.
ⓤ=Kosher Parvae approved by Orthodox Union.

CITRACAL® PLUS
[sit 'ra-cal]
Ultradense® calcium citrate-Vitamin D-multimineral dietary supplement

Ingredients: calcium (as Ultradense® calcium citrate) 250 mg., polyethylene glycol, magnesium oxide, povidone, croscarmellose sodium, hydroxypropyl methylcellulose, color added, pyridoxine hydrochloride, zinc oxide, sodium borate, manganese gluconate, copper gluconate, magnesium stearate, magnesium silicate, maltodextrin, vitamin D_3 (125 IU).

How Supplied: Available in bottles of 150 tablets, UPC 0178-0825-15.

Novartis Consumer Health, Inc.
**200 KIMBALL DRIVE
PARSIPPANY, NJ 07054-0622**

Direct Product Inquiries to:
Consumer & Professional Affairs
(800) 452-0051
Fax: (800) 635-2801
Or write to above address.

BENEFIBER® Fiber Supplement

Benefiber® is a 100% natural fiber, that can be mixed with almost anything. It's taste free, grit-free, and will never thicken. So it won't alter the taste or texture of foods or non-carbonated beverages. It can be used in coffee, pudding, soup, or whatever is desired. From the makers of ex•lax®.

**Supplement Facts:
Serving Size: 1 tbsp (4g)
(makes 4 fl oz prepared)**

Amount Per Serving	%DV
Calories 20	
Total Carbohydrate 4g	1%*
Dietary Fiber 3g	12%*
Soluble Fiber 3g	†
Sodium 20mg	1%

*Percent Daily Values (DV) are based on a 2,000 calorie diet.
†Daily Value not established.

Ingredients: Partially Hydrolyzed Guar Gum (A 100% natural fiber).

Guar Gum is derived from the seed of the cluster bean.
ⓤ 100% Natural Fiber–Sugar Free

Directions for use: Stir 1 tablespoon (tbsp) of Benefiber into at least 4 oz. of any beverage or soft food (hot or cold). Use 8 oz. if using 2 tbsp. Stir until dissolved.††

Age	Dosage
12 yrs. to adult	1–2 tbsp up to 3 times daily*
7 to 11 yrs.	1/2–1 tbsp up to 3 times daily**
Under 6 yrs.	Ask your doctor

tbsp=tablespoon
* Not to exceed 5 tbsp per day.
**Not to exceed 2.5 tbsp per day.
††Not recommended for carbonated beverages.

Store at controlled room temperature 20–25°C (68–77°F). Protect from moisture.
Use within 6 months of opening.
Keep out of reach of children.
If you are pregnant or nursing a baby, ask a health professional before use.
Tamper Evident Feature: Do not use if printed bottle inner seal is broken or missing or if sealed packet is broken or torn.

How Supplied:
• 24 serving cannister = 3.4 oz/96 g
• 42 serving cannister = 6 oz/168 g
• 80 serving cannister = 11.3 oz/320 g
• Box of 14 ct. individual packets = 2 oz/56 g
Packaged by weight, not volume. Contents may settle during shipping and handling.
Benefiber® guarantees your satisfaction or your money back.
Questions? Call **1-800-452-0051** 24 hours a day, 7 days a week or visit us at **www.benefiber.com** for recipe ideas and additional information.
Novartis Consumer Health, Inc.
Parsippany, NJ 07054-0622 ©2003
Shown in Product Identification Guide, page 513

SLOW FE®
Slow Release Iron Tablets

**Drug Facts:
Active Ingredient
(in each tablet):** **Purpose:**
160 mg dried ferrous sulfate, USP (equivalent to 50 mg elemental iron) .... Iron deficiency

Uses: For use in the prevention of iron deficiency when the need for such therapy has been determined by a doctor.

Warnings:
- The treatment of any anemic condition should be under the advice and supervision of a doctor.
- As oral iron products interfere with absorption of oral tetracycline antibiotics, these products should not be taken within two hours of each other.
- **If pregnant or breast-feeding,** ask a health professional before use.

Warning: Accidental overdose of iron-containing products is a leading cause of fatal poisoning in children under 6. Keep this product out of reach of children. In case of accidental overdose, call a doctor or poison control center immediately.

Directions:
- Tablets must be swallowed whole.
- ADULTS: One or two tablets daily or as recommended by a doctor. A maximum of four tablets daily may be taken.
- CHILDREN UNDER 12: consult a doctor

Other Information:
- store at controlled room temperature 20–25°C (68–77°F)
- protect from moisture

Inactive Ingredients: cetostearyl alcohol, FD&C blue #2 aluminum lake, hydroxypropyl methylcellulose, lactose, magnesium stearate, polysorbate 80, talc, titanium dioxide, yellow iron oxide **Questions?** call **1-800-452-0051** 24 hours a day, 7 days a week.

How Supplied: Child-resistant blister packages of 30 ct., 60 ct. and 90 ct. NDC 0067-0125-47.

Child Resistant
Blister packaged for your protection.
Do not use if individual seals are broken.
Tablets non-USP (disintegration, content uniformity)
Tablets made in Great Britain
Distributed by:
Novartis Consumer Health, Inc.
Parsippany, NJ 07054-0622 © 2003

SLOW FE® WITH FOLIC ACID
(Slow Release Iron, Folic Acid)
Dietary Supplement

Description: Slow Fe + Folic Acid delivers 47.5 mg elemental iron as ferrous sulfate plus 350 mcg folic acid using the unique wax matrix delivery system described above (for SLOW FE® Slow Release Iron Tablets).
Provides women of childbearing potential with folic acid to help reduce the risk of neural tube birth defects. These birth defects are rare, but serious, and occur within 28 days of conception, often before a woman knows she's pregnant.

Formula: Each tablet contains: 47.5 mg elemental iron as ferrous sulfate and 350 mcg folic acid.
Other Ingredients: lactose, hydroxypropyl methylcellulose, talc, magnesium stearate, cetostearyl alcohol, polysorbate 80, titanium dioxide, yellow iron oxide.

Dosage: ADULTS—One or two tablets once a day or as recommended by a physician. A maximum of two tablets daily may be taken. CHILDREN UNDER 12—Consult a physician. Tablets must be swallowed whole.

Warning: The treatment of any anemic condition should be under the advice and supervision of a physician. As oral iron products interfere with absorption of oral tetracycline antibiotics, these products should not be taken within two hours of each other. Intake of folic acid from all sources should be limited to 1000 mcg per day to prevent the masking of Vitamin B_{12} deficiencies. Should you become pregnant while using this product, consult a physician as soon as possible about good prenatal care and the continued use of this product. If you are already pregnant or nursing a baby, seek the advice of a health care professional before using this product.

Warning: Accidental overdose of iron-containing products is a leading cause of fatal poisoning in children under 6. Keep this product out of reach of children. In case of accidental overdose, call a doctor or poison control center immediately.

How Supplied: Blister packages of 20 supplied in Child-Resistant packaging. Store at controlled room temperature 20–25°C (68°–77°F). Protect from moisture.
Tablets made in Great Britain
Novartis Consumer Health, Inc.
Parsippany, NJ 07054-0622 © 2003
Shown in Product Identification Guide, page 515

OBIKEN
JAPAN APPLIED
MICROBIOLOGY
RESEARCH
INSTITUTE LTD.

242 ido isawa-cho,
higashiyatsushiro-
gun yamanashi 406-0045 JAPAN

For Direct Inquiries contact:
TEL: 81-55-262-9861
FAX: 81-55-262-9862
E-MAIL: info@oubiken.co.jp or salo@oubiken.co.jp

ABPC (Agaricus Blazei Practical Compound)

ABPC is a processed food enzyme treated Agaricus mushroom mycelia and used as dietary supplemental products.

*Product Description: Agaricus Blazei H-1 strain, which our company originally isolated from natural Agaricus Blazei Murrill mushrooms, is used for ABPC (Enzyme treated Agaricus mushroom mycelium processed food).
ABPC is prepared from cultured mycelia of Agaricus mushroom in a large culture tank that our company originally designed.
The manufacturing method of culturing in a tank facilitates manufacturing stability content, quality and yield. The content of β-glucan contained in the natural Agaricus Blazei mushroom is 8.0%, but the content of β-glucan contained in the mycelia cultured in the tank is more than 30.0%.
It is a product, which succeeded in heightening dramatically the absorption of β-glucan, which is hard to be absorbed, cutting into absorbable molecular weights by enzyme treating polysaccharides including β-glucan contained in cell walls of Agaricus mycelia.
Agaricus Blazei Murrill Mushroom has been used habitually as mushroom to maintain the health in Brazil and other countries since olden days.
ABPC is a processed food most suitable for maintenance of the health, preventing onset of hypodynamia of body parts and suppressing the immune system, which are caused by irregular life habits and aging, and bringing out the homeostasis.
Our company has a U.S. patent concerning the mycelium culturing method.

---

*This statement has not been evaluated by the Food And Drug Administration. This products are not intended to diagnose, treat, cure OR prevent any disease.

Clinical Trials: The first publication regarding the clinical trials of ABPC (Agaricus Blazei Practical Compound) reported the treatment reports at the 35th Conference of Japan Society Clinical Oncology in 1997 where Dr. Yukie Niwa (Tosa Shimizu Hospital), Dr. Jiro Itami (Shibata Hospital) presented the cases of high survival rates of breast cancers, stomach cancers and spleen cancers among 1,260 cases of cancer patients.
The clinical cases are being worked on at hospitals including Kanazawa Medical University, Yamanashi Medical University Hospital, Juntendo University School of Medicine, Akiyama Neurosurgery Hospital and Sano Surgical Hospital.

Ingredients: The composition of contents of ABPC per pack (5 grains: 1.25 g) is as follows:

Continued on next page

Information on Novartis Consumer Health, Inc., products appearing on these pages is effective as of November 2002.

ABPC—Cont.

Glucide: 0.64 g, Protein: 0.18 g, Dietary fiber: 0.07 g, Lipid: 0.05 g, Sodium: 1.5 mg, Energy: 3.7 Kcal

Adverse Reactions: 6 years have passed since the release of ABPC in Japan. No adverse reaction have been reported with causal relation with its administration.
As a result of the acute toxicity tests of mouse administration (Attachment: December 4, 1997, Tested by the Japan Food Analysis Center, June 14, 2002, Tested by Japan Applied Microbiology Research Institute Ltd., June 26, 2002, Tested by the Japan Food Analysis Center), there is no problem at all and the safety is proved.

Recommended Intake: Take 10 grains (2 packs) per day lukewarm water. Intake by chewing is also recommendable.
Regardless of before meal or after meal, the supplement can be taken.
Can be taken before bed.

Warnings: ABPC is a safe food for adults as well as children.
But, evaluation has not been made for infants. Avoid feeding ABPC to the infant. There is no danger of adverse reaction in taking a large amount. Do not exceed 5 times of the daily dosage.

How Supplied: A box contains 60 packs (75 g). A pack contains 5 grains (1.25 g: 0.25 g/grain). It can be supplied in tablet.
Store under room temperature and avoid any direct heat or sun light.
Shown in Product Identification Guide, page 516

Pharmics, Inc.
PO BOX 27554
SALT LAKE CITY, UT 84127

Direct Inquiries to:
Customer Service: 800-456-4138
FAX: 801-966-4177
customerservice@pharmics.com
www.pharmics.com
For Medical Emergency Contact:
801-966-4138

FERRETTS
Ferrous Fumarate

Ferretts tablets are for use as a dietary iron supplement.

Each tablet contains:

Iron (from 325 mg ferrous fumarate) 106 mg

Other ingredients: Microcrystalline cellulose, sodium starch glycolate, magnesium stearate, Opadry II clear, Opadry II Red 40L15175.

Suggested use: One tablet daily or as directed by physician.

> **Warning:** Accidental overdose of iron containing products is a leading cause of fatal poisoning in children under 6. Keep this product out of the reach of children. In case of accidental overdose, call a doctor or poison control center immediately.

Caution: As with any drug, if you are pregnant or nursing a baby, seek the advise of a health care professional before using this product.

How Supplied: Ferretts are supplied in tamper evident, child resistant unit dose packages of 60 tablets (NDC 00813-0012-06). Do **not** use if blister or seal is broken. Ferretts are a scored red film coated caplet shape tablet. Embossed "P-Fe"
Store in cool dry place protected from light.
Manufactured for:
Pharmics, Inc.
Salt Lake City, UT 84119
www.pharmics.com
(800) 456-4138
Rev. 11/01

The Procter & Gamble Company
P. O. BOX 599
CINCINNATI, OH 45201

Direct Inquiries to:
Consumer Relations
(800) 832–3064
For Medical Emergencies:
Call Collect: (513) 636-5107

METAMUCIL®
DIETARY FIBER SUPPLEMENT
[*met uh-mū sil*]
(psyllium husk)
Also see Metamucil Fiber Laxative in Nonprescription Drugs section

Description: Metamucil contains psyllium husk (from the plant *Plantago ovata*), a concentrated source of soluble fiber which can be used to increase one's dietary fiber intake. When used as part of a diet low in saturated fat and cholesterol, 7g per day of soluble fiber from psyllium husk (the amount in 3 doses of Metamucil) may reduce the risk of heart disease by lowering cholesterol. Each dose of Metamucil powder and Metamucil Fiber Wafers contains approximately 3.4 grams of psyllium husk (or 2.4 grams of soluble fiber). A listing of ingredients and nutrition information is available in the listing of Metamucil Fiber Laxative in the Nonprescription Drug section. Metamucil Smooth Texture Sugar-Free Regular Flavor and

Metamucil capsules contains no sugar and no artificial sweeteners. Metamucil Smooth Texture Sugar-Free Orange Flavor contains aspartame (phenylalanine content of 25 mg per dose). Metamucil powdered products are gluten-free.

Uses: Metamucil Dietary Fiber Supplement can be used as a concentrated source of soluble fiber to increase the dietary intake of fiber. Diets low in saturated fat and cholesterol that include 7 grams of soluble fiber per day from psyllium husk, as in Metamucil, may reduce the risk of heart disease by lowering cholesterol. One adult dose of Metamucil has 2.4 grams of this soluble fiber. Consult a doctor if you are considering use of this product as part of a cholesterol-lowering program.

Warnings: Read entire Drug Facts section in listing for Metamucil Fiber Laxative in the Nonprescription Drug section.

Directions: Adults 12 yrs. & older: 1 dose in 8 oz of liquid *3 times daily*. Capsules: 2–6 capsules for increasing daily fiber intake; 6 capsules for cholesterol lowering use. Up to three times daily. Under 12 yrs.: Consult a doctor. See mixing directions in Drug Facts in listing for Metamucil Fiber Laxative in the Nonprescription Drug section.
NOTICE: Mix this product with at least 8 oz (a full glass) of liquid. Taking without enough liquid may cause choking. Do not take if you have difficulty swallowing.
For listing of ingredients and nutritional information for Metamucil Dietary Fiber Supplement, and for laxative indications and directions for use, see Metamucil Fiber Laxative in the Nonprescription Drug section.
Notice to Health Care Professionals: To minimize the potential for allergic reaction, health care professionals who frequently dispense powdered psyllium products should avoid inhaling airborne dust while dispensing these products. Handling and Dispensing: To minimize generating airborne dust, spoon product from the canister into a glass according to label directions.

How Supplied: Powder: canisters and cartons of single-dose packets. Capsules: 100 and 160 count bottles. For complete ingredients and sizes for each version, see Metamucil Table 1, page 752, Nonprescription Drug section.
Questions? 1-800-983-4237
Shown in Product Identification Guide, page 522

**IF YOU SUSPECT
AN INTERACTION. . .**
The 1,800-page
PDR Companion Guide™ can help.
Use the order form
in the front of this book.

Rexall Inc.
6111 BROKEN SOUND PKWY
BOCA RATON, FL 33487

Direct inquiries to:
1-888-VITAHELP (848-2435)
www.osteobiflex.com

OSTEO BI-FLEX®
• Triple Strength
• Plus Calcium

Helps rebuild cartilage and lubricate joints*

Description: Osteo Bi-Flex is a nutritional supplement containing glucosamine HCl and chondroitin sulfate that helps rebuild cartilage and lubricate joints.

Osteo Bi-Flex Triple Strength provides the full clinically studied dosage of glucosamine HCl (1500mg) and chondroitin sulfate (1200mg) in just two easy-to-swallow Smoothcap™ caplets (one serving).

Osteo Bi-Flex Plus Calcium provides the full clinically studied dosage of glucosamine HCl (1500mg) and chondroitin sulfate (1200mg) plus 500mg of calcium in three easy-to-swallow Smoothcap™ caplets (one serving).

Both glucosamine and chondroitin occur naturally in the body and play an important role in the production, repair and maintenance of healthy cartilage and connective tissue.

Osteo Bi-Flex Triple Strength
Supplement Facts:
Serving Size 2 Caplets

Amount Per Serving	% Daily Value
Calories 10	
Total Carbohydrate 2g	1%[†]
Dietary Fiber <1g	3%[†]
Vitamin C (as ascorbic acid) 60mg	100%
Manganese (as manganese sulfate) 2mg	100%
Sodium 105mg	4%
Glucosamine HCL 1500mg	‡
Chondroitin Sulfate 1200mg	‡
Boron (as sodium tetraborate) 3mg	‡

[†]Percent Daily Values are based on a 2,000 calorie diet.
‡Daily Value not established.

Other Ingredients: Microcrystalline cellulose, sodium carboxymethylcellulose, crospovidone, Red 40 Lake, Yellow 5 Lake, maltodexterin, magnesium state, dextrose, Yellow 6 Lake, soy lecithin, sodium citrate, Blue 1 Lake.

Caution: If you are allergic to shellfish, please consult your health care professional before taking this product.

Directions: FOR ADULT USE TAKE 2 CAPLETS PER DAY WITH FOOD. NOTE: THE SAME BENEFIT WILL RESULT BY TAKING BOTH CAPLETS TOGETHER OR SPREAD THROUGHOUT THE DAY.

How Supplied: Bottle (with flip-top cap) of 40, 80 or 120 easy-to-swallow Smoothcap™ caplets

Osteo Bi-Flex Plus Calcium
Supplement Facts:
Serving Size 3 Caplets

Amount Per Serving	% Daily Value
Calories 10	
Total Carbohydrate 2g	1%[†]
Dietary Fiber <1g	3%[†]
Vitamin C (as ascorbic acid) 60mg	100%
Vitamin D (as cholecalciferol) 400IU	100%
Calcium (as calcium carbonate) 500mg	50%
Sodium 105mg	4%
Glucosamine HCL 1500mg	‡
Chondroitin Sulfate 1200mg	‡

[†]Percent Daily Values are based on a 2,000 calorie diet.
‡Daily Value not established.

Other Ingredients: Microcrystalline cellulose, sodium carboxymethylcellulose, crospovidone, titanium oxide (color), maltodexterin, magnesium state, Yellow 5 Lake, dextrose, soy lecithin, sodium citrate, Red 40 Lake, Blue 1 Lake, Yellow 6 Lake.

Caution: If you are allergic to shellfish, please consult your health care professional before taking this product.

Directions: FOR ADULT USE TAKE 3 CAPLETS PER DAY WITH FOOD. NOTE: THE SAME BENEFIT WILL RESULT BY TAKING BOTH CAPLETS TOGETHER OR SPREAD THROUGHOUT THE DAY.

How Supplied: Bottle (with flip-top cap) of 90 easy-to-swallow Smoothcap™ caplets

Rexall Inc.
6111 Broken Sound Parkway NW
Boca Raton, FL 33487

Direct Inquiries to:
1-888-VITAHELP (848-2435)
www.osteobiflex.com

Produced under USP Good Manufacturing Practices.

*These statements have not been evaluated by the Food and Drug Administration. This product is not intended to diagnose, treat, cure or prevent any disease.

Shown in Product Identification Guide, page 523

Rotta Pharmaceuticals Inc.
1340 CAMPUS PARKWAY
NEPTUNE, NJ 07753

Direct Inquiries to:
phone (732) 751-9020
fax (732) 751-9021
info@rottapharmaceuticals.com
www.originalglucosamine.com
www.donausa.com

DONA™ Crystalline Glucosamine Sulfate Powder for Oral Solution—Maximum Strength.
DONA™ Crystalline Glucosamine Sulfate Caplets—Maximum Strength.

Helps improve joint flexibility, rebuild cartilage, and maintain joint health.[†]
Description: Dona is Crystalline Glucosamine Sulfate, a key building block for cartilage. Dona works by lubricating and rebuilding cartilage and preventing it from breaking down, keeping joints flexible and free of pain. Dona was developed by Rotta Pharmaceuticals, Inc. of Italy and is sold as a prescription medicine in over 60 countries. The recommended dose is 1500mg. Each packet or two caplets of Dona is one full daily dose.
Crystalline Glucosamine Sulfate is the derivative of the naturally occurring amino-sugar Glucosamine and is a chemically well-defined and pure substance. Glucosamine has been thoroughly studied and shown effective in promoting cartilage metabolism, protecting joint structure and supporting joint mobility. Only Dona contains the Crystalline Glucosamine Sulfate studied in more than 150 pre-clinical and clinical studies including the two landmark 3-year studies published in The Lancet and the Archive of Internal Medicine.
Dona™ Crystalline Glucosamine Sulfate Caplets
Supplement Facts:
Serving size: 2 Caplets
Servings per container: 30

	Amount Per Caplet	% DV
Calories	0	
Sodium	75 mg	3%
Glucosamine Sulfate	750 mg	*

Percent daily value (DV) based on a 2,000 calorie diet.
* Daily value not established

Other Ingredients: Microcrystalline cellulose, Polyvinyl Pyrrolidone K25, Polyethylenglycol 400, Talc, Magnesium

Continued on next page

DONA—Cont.

Stearate, Eudragit RL, Triacetin, Micronized Titanium Dioxide, Polyethylenglycol 4000

*In stabilized form.

Directions for Use: Take two caplets daily with water or juice.

Dosage: Two Caplets Daily.

DONA™ Sulfate Powder for Oral Solution

Supplement Facts:

Serving size: 1 packet

Servings per container: 30

	Amount Per Packet	% DV
Calories	10	
Sodium	150 mg	6%
Glucosamine Sulfate	1500 mg	*

Percent daily value (DV) based on a 2,000 calorie diet.
* Daily value not established.

Other Ingredients: Aspartame, Citric Acid, Sorbitol

Phenylketonurics: Contains phenylalanine.

Directions for Use: Dissolve the contents of one packet in water or juice before taking.

Dosage: One Packet Daily.

Due to its mechanism of action it may take 1–2 weeks or possibly longer, to notice any effects. Optimal effects on joint mobility have been observed after 12 weeks of daily administration.

Store in a cool, dry place.

Keep out of the reach of children.

As with any nutritional product, please consult your physician before taking. If you are pregnant or breast feeding ask your Doctor before taking.

Use only as directed.

How Supplied: Available as a 30 day supply in boxes of 60 caplets of 750 mg each or 30 packets of 1500 mg each.

†These Statements Have Not Been Evaluated By The Food & Drug Administration. This Product Is Not Intended To Diagnose, Treat, Cure, or Prevent Any Disease.

Manufactured by: Rottapharm Ltd., Ireland

Exclusively distributed in USA and Canada by:

Rotta Pharmaceuticals, Inc.

1340 Campus Parkway

Neptune, NJ 07753

1-800-214-9600

Product of Ireland

Sunpower Nutraceutical Inc.

8850 RESEARCH DRIVE
IRVINE, CA 92618

Direct Inquiries to:
Ph: (949) 553-8899

PRODUCT LISTING

Descriptions: Sunpower Nutraceutical System combined vitamins, minerals, special formulated herbs, Pycnogenol® and proprietary Traditional Chinese Medicines (TCM) from S.P. Pharmaceutical Inc. (S.P.) which manufactured at GMP facility and under FDA Act and U.S. Pharmacopeia quality, purity and potency standards.

Time-released, Double-layered tablets are made by advanced manufacturing techniques which allows nutrients to be released slowly for better absorption during digestion.

Sunpower Product Overview:

Sun Liver™: contains vitamins, minerals, Pycnogenol® and S.P. Pro-Liver Formula to help to fight free radical damage, and provide nutrients essential for healthy liver function.

Sun Cardio™: contains CoQ10, OPC, Ginkgo Biloba, Red Wine Extract and S.P. Pro-Cardio Formula to help maintain normal cardiovascular system.

Power Circulation™: contains Ginkgo Biloba, Barley Grass, Lecithin and S.P. Pro-Circulation Formula to help maintain a healthy blood circulatory system.

Sun Joint™: contains Glucosamine, Chondroitin, Wild Yam, Bee Propolis and S.P. Pro-Connection Formula to provide essential nutrients for bone, joint, ligament and cartilage function.

Power Lasting™: contains Yohimbe, Damiana, Saw Palmetto, Pumpkin Seed, Sarsaparilla Root, and S.P. Pro-Long Formula to help maintain normal kidney and sexual function and enhance endurance.

Sun Beauty™ 1: Formulated for women ages 14–28 contains Alfalfa, St. John's Wort, Cranberry, Royal Jelly, and S.P. Beauty I Formula to help establish healthy hormonal rhythms and basic immunity.

Sun Beauty™ 2: Formulated for women ages 29–42 contains Alfalfa, Selenium, Green Tea, Uva Ursi Leaves, Cranberry, and S.P. Beauty II Formula to support and balance a woman's vitality and healthy immunity during the menstrual cycle.

Sun Beauty™ 3: Formulated for women ages over 43 contains chromium, Burdock Root, Fo-Ti, Black Cohoshe, Red Clover, Chaste Tree Berries, and S.P. Beauty III Formula to support general

well-being during menopause and post-menopause.

Sun Dechole™: contains Monascus Purpureus. Green Tea Extract, Crataegus Pinnatifida and Odorless Yeast Powder.

Power Refresh™: contains Cordyceps Sinensis, American Ginseng, Grape Seeds Extract, Bee Pollen and Licorice.

5 Seng Tea™: contains Ginseng, American Ginseng, Dang-Shen Root, Red-Rooted Sage and Figwort Root.

Shown in Product Identification Guide, page 524

Tahitian Noni International

333 WEST RIVER PARK DRIVE
PROVO, UT 84604 USA

Direct Inquiries to:
Ph: (801) 234-1000
Website: www.tahitiannoni.com

TAHITIAN NONI® LIQUID DIETARY SUPPLEMENT

Description: TAHITIAN NONI® Juice has a heritage, a pedigree that distinguishes it from every other product on the market. This pedigree extends back 2,000 years to the people who used the noni fruit for its benefits. The countless benefits of this unique fruit can only be enjoyed if the fruit is revealed in its most pure form. Our proprietary formulation captures this precisely. It's no wonder that TAHITIAN NONI Juice touches the lives of millions worldwide. You'll find 2,000 years of goodness in every bottle of TAHITIAN NONI Juice! Always look for the TAHITIAN NONI Juice Footprint: Your only assurance of quality, purity, and authenticity.

Supplement Facts
Serving Size: 1 fluid ounce (30 ml)
Servings Per Container 33

Amount Per Serving	% Daily Value*
Calories 13	
Total Carbohydrate 3g	1%
Sugars 2g	†

*Percent Daily Values are based on a 2,000 calorie diet.
†Daily Value not established.

Ingredients: Reconstituted *Morinda citrifolia* fruit juice from pure juice puree from French Polynesia, natural grape juice concentrate, natural blueberry juice concentrate, and natural flavors. Not made from dried or powdered *Morinda citrifolia*.

How Supplied: 1 FL. OZ./30 mL daily. Preferably before meals

Shake well before using and refrigerate after opening

Do not use if seal around cap is broken

Packaged by Tahitian Noni International, a subsidiary of Morinda, Inc. Provo, UT 84604. USA.

101825-1 0206014-US © 2003 Tahitian Noni International

References:
Wang MY et al., Morinda citrifolia (Noni): A Literature Review and Recent Advances in Noni Research. Acta Pharmacol Sin. 2002 Dec; 23 (12): 1127–41.
Morinda citrifolia L. (NOAE) of TAHITIAN NONI® Juice has been used in folk remedies by Polynesians for over 2000 years, and is reported to have a broad range of therapeutic effects.* Including antibacterial, antiviral, antifungal, antitumor, antihelmin, analgesic, hypotensive, anti-inflammatory, and immune enhancing effects.* Includes data on allergenicity and toxicity, which shows no observed adverse effects (NOAE) for TAHITIAN NONI® Juice.
Hirazumi A, Furusawa E. An Immunomodulatory Polysaccharide-rich Substance from the Fruit Juice of Morinda citrifolia (noni) with Antitumour Activity. Phytother Res. 1999 Aug; 13(5): 380–7.
The fruit juice of *Morinda citrifolia* L. (Noni) contains a polysaccharide-rich substance (noni-ppt) with antitumor activity in the Lewis lung carcinoma (LLC) peritoneal cancinomatosis model. The therapeutic administration of noni-ppt significantly enhanced the duration of survival of inbred syngeneic LLC tumor bearing mice, which seems to suggest that noni-ppt may suppress tumor growth through activation of the host immune system and stimulate the release of certain interleukins and nitric oxide (NO).
Gerson, S. Green, L. Preliminary Evaluation of the Antimicrobial Activity of Extracts of Morinda citrifolia L. 2002 General Meeting of American Society for Microbiology.
Morinda citrifolia was shown to have antimicrobial and antifungal properties against *A. niger, C. albicans, E. coli, S. aureus* and *T. mentagrophytes.*
Opinion of the Scientific Committee on Foods on Tahitian Noni® Juice, European Commission. SCF/CS/NF/DOS/18 ADD 2 Final. 11, December 2002.
Sub-chronic and acute oral toxicity studies of TAHITIAN NONI® Juice measured clinical signs, food consumption, weight gain, hematology, clinical chemistry, selective organ weights, and tissue samples of 55 organs (for histology). The No-Observable-Adverse-Effect-Level (NOAEL) was 80 g/kg which is more than 8% of the animals' body weight.
B. A. Mueller, et al. Am J. Kidney Dis. 2000 Feb; 35(2): 330–2.
They reported that "The potassium concentration in noni juice samples was determined and found to be 56.3 mEq/L, similar to that in orange juice and to-

mato juice... [and]...may be surreptitious source of potassium in patients with renal disease." Tahitian Noni® Juice is not a significant source of potassium. B.A. Mueller in USA Today, March 28, 2000 clarified his previous conclusion, stating that his analysis was made on a different noni product and not on Tahitian Noni® Juice and the amount of potassium in the brand of noni juice he analyzed in his study was "only 65 milligrams of potassium per 1 ounce serving, as much as you'd get in 2 inches of a banana."

---

*This statement has not been evaluated by the Food and Drug Administration. This product is not intended to diagnose, treat, cure or prevent any disease.

Shown in Product Identification Guide, page 524

Wellness International Network, Ltd.
5800 DEMOCRACY DRIVE PLANO, TX 75024

Direct Inquiries to:
Product Coordinator
(972) 312-1100
FAX: (972) 943-5250

BIOLEAN®
Herbal & Amino Acid Dietary Supplement

Uses: BIOLEAN® is a unique combination of Chinese herbal extracts and pharmaceutical-grade amino acids specifically designed to help raise overall health, participate in individual life extension programs, and enhance athletic performance. It has been shown to be extremely effective in promoting the healthy loss of excess body fat while helping to maintain lean body mass and potent energy levels. BIOLEAN, when used as a daily nutritional supplement, has also been shown to stimulate immune function in individuals with blunted sympathetic nervous systems, especially overweight and obese persons. It acts as a positive stimulator to immune functions involved in protection from environmental and dietary carcinogens.
Components in BIOLEAN are known to cause fat loss through thermogenic activity and altered fuel metabolism resulting from sympathomimetic response to stimulation of beta receptors in adipose and muscle cells. The positive immune response, though not completely understood, is at least partially attributable to beta stimulation in adipocytes and the adaptogenic and tonifying activity of certain herbal extracts. This has been demonstrated in their long history

of use in traditional Chinese herbal medicine as well as current scientific research which points to, among other possibilities, the extremely potent antioxidant properties found in some of the component plants, most notably in Green Tea and Schizandrae extracts. BIOLEAN may increase athletic performance and endurance through three pathways: 1) increased oxygen uptake in the lungs as a result of expanding bronchial passages; 2) enhanced mental acuity and response resulting from sympathetic nervous system stimulus; and 3) increasing the employment of fatty acids as fuel in muscle mitochondria while simultaneously sparing muscle glycogen and nitrogen.
The herbal extracts in BIOLEAN are produced in a unique and exclusive process which is proprietary to this product. Instead of creating extracts based on a set quantity of one particular active within many which may be present in any particular plant, BIOLEAN components are concentrated to maintain the natural and complete spectrum of biologically active factors, in the same ratio presented by the unprocessed plant.

Directions: AM Serving – Adults take one white tablet and two green tablets with low calorie food. PM Serving – Adults may take one green tablet with low calorie food. If using BIOLEAN dietary supplement for the first time, limit daily intake to one white tablet and one green tablet on days one and two, and one white tablet and two green tablets on day three. Needs vary with each individual. This product has a maximum of 25mg concentrated ephedrine group alkaloids per serving in the form of herbal extracts.

Warnings: Not for use by children under the age of 18. If you are pregnant or nursing, if you have heart disease, thyroid disease, diabetes, high blood pressure, depression or other psychiatric condition, glaucoma, difficulty urinating, prostate enlargement, or seizure disorder, if you are using a monoamine oxidase inhibitor (MAOI) or any other prescription drug or over-the-counter drug containing ephedrine, pseudoephedrine or phenylpropanolamine (ingredients found in certain allergy, asthma, cough/cold and weight control products), consult a health professional before using this product. Exceeding recommended serving may cause serious adverse effects. Taking this product with other stimulants such as caffeine may cause serious side effects. Discontinue use and call a health professional immediately if you experience rapid heartbeat, dizziness, severe headache, shortness of breath, or other similar symptoms. Phenylketonurics: Contains phenylalanine. The maximum recommended daily dosage of ephedrine for a healthy, human adult is 100 mg, for not more than 12 weeks.

Continued on next page

Biolean—Cont.

Ingredients: Calcium (as calcium carbonate, dicalcium phosphate anhydrous), Ephedra Alkaloids (as ma haung), Caffeine (as green tea leaf), Schizandrae berry, Rehmannia root, Hawthorne berry, Jujube seed, Alisma root, Angelicae dahuricae root, Epemidium, Poria Cocos, Rhizoma rhei, Angelicae sinensis root, Codonopsis root, Euconium bark, Notoginseng root, L-phenylalanine, L-tyrosine, L-carnitine 85%, Cellulose, Stearic acid, Starch, Sodium lauryl sulfate, Hydroxypropyl cellulose, Magnesium stearate, Crosscarmelose sodium and Silicon dioxide.

How Supplied: One box contains 28 packets (28 daily servings), with one white tablet and three green tablets per packet.

BIOLEAN Accelerator™
Herbal & Amino Acid Formulation

Uses: BIOLEAN Accelerator™ is a unique combination of Chinese herbal extracts and pharmaceutical grade amino acids specifically designed to complement both BIOLEAN® and BIOLEAN Free® by extending and accelerating their actions. BIOLEAN and BIOLEAN Free are, in the traditional view of Chinese herbal medicine, strong Yang blends. This means that they are energy or heat-producing at their core. The addition of the amino acids and certain of the herbal components lends a very definite restorative or Yin element, as well. BIOLEAN Accelerator is a strong Yin herbal formula, intended to augment the lesser replenishing Yin elements of the other two herbal and amino acid supplements. Though the physiological actions of many herbs are complex and not totally understood, the formula in BIOLEAN Accelerator extends the adaptogenic, thermogenic, restorative and detoxifying results experienced with BIOLEAN and BIOLEAN Free, with an emphasis on the restorative and adaptogenic effects. The herbal formula is a combination of tonifiers traditionally used in China for the lungs, liver and kidneys.

Directions: For maximum effectiveness, use in conjunction with original BIOLEAN or BIOLEAN Free. (Do not consume BIOLEAN and BIOLEAN Free on the same day.) Take one tablet in the morning with original BIOLEAN or BIOLEAN Free. BIOLEAN Accelerator™ may also be taken in the afternoon with or without additional BIOLEAN or BIOLEAN Free if desired. Maximum absorption will be attained if taken with low-calorie food.

Warnings: Phenylketonurics: Contains Phenylalanine. Not for use by children. Consult your physician before using this product if you are taking appetite suppressing drugs or antidepressants, or if you are pregnant or lactating. If symptoms of allergy develop, discontinue use.

Ingredients: Each tablet contains 250 mg herbal mix (Microcrystalline Cellulose, Black Sesame Seed, Raw Chinese Foxglove Root, Chinese Wolfberry Fruit, Achyranthes Root, Cornelian Cherry Fruit, Chinese Yam, Eclipta Herb, Rose Hips, Privet Fruit, Mulberry Fruit-Spike, Polygonati Rhizome, Cooked Chinese Foxglove Root, Poria Cocos, Cuscuta Seed, Foxnut Seed, Alisma Rhizome, Moutan Bark, Phellodendron Bark, Anemarrhena Rhizome, Schisandra Berry, Royal Jelly), L-Tyrosine, L-Phenylalanine, Calcium Carbonate, Calcium Phosphate Dibasic, Partially Hydrogenated Vegetable Oil, Hydroxypropyl Cellulose, Croscarmellose Sodium, Magnesium Stearate, Silicon Dioxide and Sodium Lauryl Sulfate.

How Supplied: One bottle contains 56 tablets.

BIOLEAN Free®
Herbal & Amino Acid Dietary Supplement

Uses: BIOLEAN Free® is a strategic blend of herbs, spices, vitamins, minerals and amino acids specifically formulated to enhance fat utilization and energy production through various metabolic pathways. It has been shown to reduce body fat through its thermogenic effects and to enhance both physical and mental performance.

Thermogenesis refers to the body's ability to convert substrates such as proteins, fats and carbohydrates into heat energy. This is carried out most efficiently in the Brown Adipose Tissue of our body which uses fatty acids as its preferred fuel. Other fat cells, namely White Adipose Tissue, are concerned primarily with the storage of fat rather than its conversion to energy. The thermogenic pathway is complex and relies upon a series of reactions to occur. BIOLEAN Free utilizes many compounds which act at various locations in this pathway to ensure the maximum efficiency of the thermogenic process. Quebracho is one of these very special compounds. This South American plant contains quebrachine, aspidiospermine and other alkaloids that possess the ability to block alpha-2 adrenergic receptors in the body. This produces an enhanced sympathetic nervous system effect which, in turn, increases lipolysis (fat breakdown) within fat cells. The fatty acids released by this process can then be transported into the mitochondria to be used as a fuel. Ginger, cinnamon, horseradish, turmeric, cayenne and mustard are spices that stimulate thermogenesis in different ways. Some stimulate lipid mobilization in adipose tissue; others raise the resting metabolic rate; and some increase cAMP levels by inducing more beta receptors on fat cells and by increasing the concentration of adenylate cyclase. cAMP increases the breakdown of triglycerides to free fatty acids which are later used as fuel by the mitochondria in the cell. Methylxanthines (such as those found in green tea and yerba maté) also increase cAMP levels, but do this by inhibiting the enzyme, phosphodiesterase. These compounds have been noted to increase mental alertness, improve vitality, satisfy the appetite and increase energy. In addition to its methylxanthine content, green tea has recently been shown to possess strong antioxidant properties. Yerba maté is a plant that has been shown to produce the positive effects above without causing the insomnia seen with other methylxanthine-containing plants (such as coffee and kola nut). BIOLEAN Free also contains vitamin B-3 (niacin), vitamin B-6 (pyridoxine), chromium and vanadium, which aid in the proper metabolism of fats, proteins and carbohydrates. L-tyrosine also aids in metabolism and promotes satiety through hypothalamic release of CCK. Methionine is a precursor of L-carnitine which aids in the transport of fatty acids into the mitochondria for thermogenesis. Other herbs have been utilized in BIOLEAN Free. Ginseng and ho shou wu possess adaptogenic properties. Adaptogens help the body adapt to physiological and environmental stresses. Ginseng accomplishes this through its stabilizing effect on the hypothalamic-pituitary-adrenal-sympathetic nervous system. It can mediate an increased adrenal response to stress.

Ho shou wu has a stabilizing effect on the endocrine system and has restorative properties. It is also an antioxidant with a high flavonoid content. *Centella asiatica* contains asiaticoside and has been shown to increase activity levels and ease the body's ability to overcome fatigue when taken with ginseng and cayenne. Individually, *centella* has been shown to increase memory and mental acuity in studies abroad. Uva ursi contains the glycoside arbutin and promotes urinary health and body strength through its purifying effects. Ginkgo biloba is a tree whose leaves have been used for centuries as an herbal medicine. It contains flavonoids and is therefore a strong antioxidant. It reduces the tendency of platelets to stick together by inhibiting Platelet Activating Factor. It has been shown to increase blood flow to the heart, brain and other organs.

Directions: Adults (18 years and older) may take 4 tablets in the mid to late morning with a low-calorie food. Needs may vary with each individual. Some persons may require less than 4 caplets, or may prefer taking 3 tablets mid morning and 1 additional tablet mid afternoon to achieve optimum results. Do not exceed recommended daily amounts. It is recommended that you drink at least eight glasses of water daily.

Warnings: Not for use by children, pregnant women or lactating women. Consult your physician before using this product if you are taking appetite suppressing drugs or cardiovascular medication. Consult your physician if you have hypertension, heart disease, arrhythmias, prostatic hypertrophy, glaucoma, liver disease, renal disease or diabetes. Do not use if you have hyperthyroidism, psychosis, Parkinson's Disease, or are taking Monoamine oxidase inhibitors. BIOLEAN Free should not be taken on the same day as original BIOLEAN®. It is recommended that you minimize your caffeine intake while consuming this product. If allergic symptoms develop, discontinue use. Store in a cool, dry place. Keep out of reach of children.

Ingredients: Niacin (as niacinamide), Vitamin B6 (as pyridoxine HCl), Chromium (as chromium Chelavite® chloride), Potassium (as potassium citrate), Green tea leaf extract (10% methylxanthines), Yerba mate leaf extract (10% methylxanthines), Korean ginseng root extract (4% ginsenosides), Uva ursi leaf (20% arbutin), Guarana seed (22% methylxanthines), Quebracho bark extract (10% quebrachine), Gotu kola leaf (Centella asiatica), Ceylon cinnamon bark, Chinese horseradish root, Jamaican ginger root, Turmeric rhizome, Nigerian cayenne pepper (fruit), English mustard seed, Ho shou wu root, Ginkgo biloba leaf (24% ginkgoflavoneslycosides and 6% bilobalides), L-Tyrosine, L-Methionine, Vanadium (as BMOV), Dicalcium phosphate, Cellulose, Cellulose gum, Vegetable stearic acid, Silica, Vegetable magnesium stearate and Vegetable resin glaze.

How Supplied: One box contains 28 packets, four tablets per packet.

BIOLEAN LipoTrim™
All-Natural Dietary Supplement

Uses: LipoTrim™ is a highly active, synergistic combination of garcinia cambogia extract and chromium polynicotinate specifically created for use with the other products in the BIOLEAN® System. The method of action is by inhibition of lipogenesis and regulation of blood glucose levels. Serum glucose derived from dietary carbohydrates and not immediately converted to energy or glycogen tends to be converted into fat stores and cholesterol. In individuals with excess body fat stores or slow basal metabolism, this tendency is thought to be higher. The garcinia cambogia extract present in LipoTrim is verified by HPLC analysis to be no less than 50%(-) hydroxycitrate (HCA). HCA inhibits ATP-citrate lyase which retards Acetyl CoA synthesis, severely restricting conversion of excess glucose into fatty acids and cholesterol. Animal studies have shown a post-meal fatty acid synthesis reduction of 40–80% for an 8–12 hour period. When glucose to fat/cholesterol conversion is re-

tarded, glycogen conversion continues, increasing liver stores and causing satiety signals to be sent to the brain resulting in appetite suppression. In situations of intense physical exercise, increased glycogen stores have been shown to result in enhanced endurance and recovery.

Directions: As a dietary supplement, take one capsule three times daily, 30 minutes before each meal. LipoTrim should be used in conjunction with a healthy diet and exercise plan.

Warnings: Do not consume if you are pregnant or lactating. Not for use by young children. Consult your physician before using this product if your diet consists of less than 1,000 calories per day.

Ingredients: Garcinia Cambogia (as CitriMax™* supplying naturally occuring hydroxycitrate), Chromium Polynicotinate (as Chromemate®* supplying elemental chromium) Magnesium Stearate and silicone dioxide.

How Supplied: One bottle contains 84 easy-to-swallow capsules.

---

*CitriMax™ is a trademark of InterHealth.
ChromeMate® is a registered trademark of InterHealth.

FOOD FOR THOUGHT™
Choline-Enriched Nutritional Drink

Uses: By utilizing scientifically established "smart nutrients," Food For Thought™ is a great-tasting citrus beverage ideal for work, school or anytime peak mental performance is desired.
Choline, a member of the B-complex family, is determined to be one of the few substances that possesses the ability to penetrate the blood-brain barrier—a protectant of the brain from the onslaught of chemicals taken into the body each day—and go directly into the brain cells to produce acetylcholine.
The most abundant neurotransmitter in the body, acetylcholine is the primary neurotransmitter between neurons and muscles. It is vital because of its role in motor behavior (muscular movement) and memory. Acetylcholine helps control muscle tone, learning, and primitive drives and emotions, while also controlling the release of the pituitary hormone vasopressin—which is involved in learning and in the regulation of urine output. Studies show that low levels of acetylcholine can contribute to lack of concentration and forgetfulness, and may interfere with sleep patterns.
Food For Thought further enhances its effectiveness through the utilization of essential vitamins—required for promoting the synthesis of brain neurotransmitters—with a unique blend of minerals. The brain uses vitamins B3 (niacin) and B6 (pyridoxine), to convert the amino acid L-tryptophan into the mood-

and sleep-regulating neurotransmitter serotonin, while vitamins B1 (thiamin), B5 (pantothenic acid), B6 (pyridoxine), and C and the minerals zinc and calcium are required for the production of acetylcholine.

Directions: Add 3/4 cup of chilled water or fruit juice to one packet of mix. Stir briskly. Consume 1–2 times per day. Keep in a cool, dry place. For maximum results, combine this product with one serving of Winrgy™.

Warnings: Not for use by children, pregnant or lactating women. Persons taking medications should seek medical advice before taking this product. Persons with ulcers or a history of ulcers should consult their physician before using a choline supplement. Do not consume more than four servings per day. Avoid the use of antacids containing aluminum with this product.

Ingredients: Carbohydrates, Sugars, Vitamin C (as ascorbic acid), Vitamin E (as alpha tocopherol acetate), Thiamin (as thiamin mononitrate), Riboflavin, Niacin (as niacinamide), Vitamin B6 (as pyridoxine hydrochloride), Vitamin B12 (as cyanocobalamin), Pantothenic Acid (as calcium pantothenate), Calcium (as calcium pantothenate), Zinc (as zinc gluconate), Copper (as copper gluconate), Chromium (as chromium aspartate), Choline (as choline bitartrate), Glycine, Lysine (as L-lysine hydrochloride), Fructose, Natural Flavors, Silicon Dioxide and Magnesium Gluconate.

How Supplied: One box contains 28 packets of drink mix. Serving size equals one packet.

DHEA Plus™
Pharmaceutical-Grade Formulation

Uses: By utilizing the latest and most advanced breakthrough applications in age management, DHEA Plus™ uniquely combines dihydroxyepiandrosterone (DHEA), Bioperine® and ginkgo biloba leaf to safely and effectively aid the body.
These age management factors are mainly attributed to the properties of DHEA, a natural substance obtained from the barbasco root, also known as Mexican Wild Yam, which is synthesized in a pharmaceutical laboratory to be utilized for specific health applications. Once supplemental DHEA is orally consumed, it is quickly absorbed into the bloodstream through the intestines and binds to a sulfate compound which creates DHEA-S. DHEA-S is the ultimate substance for which the body uses to manufacture hormones. Natural DHEA levels, abundant in the bloodstream and present at an even higher level in the tissues of the brain, are known to decline with age in both sexes. Scientific re-

Continued on next page

DHEA Plus—Cont.

search proves that adequate levels of DHEA in the body can actually slow the aging process.

Bioperine, a pure piperine extract, enhances the body's natural thermogenic activity and is another important ingredient in DHEA Plus. Thermogenesis is the metabolic process that generates energy at the cellular level. While thermogenesis plays an integral role in our body's ability to properly utilize daily foods and nutrients in the body, it also sets in motion the mechanisms that lead to digestion and subsequent gastrointestinal absorption.

Known for possessing antioxidant activity, or flavonoid effects, ginkgo biloba proves to decrease platelet aggregation and increase vasodilation which appears to extend blood flow to the peripheral arteries and the brain. Some improvement in cognitive abilities has been noted as well as inhibition of lipid peroxidation, thereby stabilizing the cell wall against free-radical attack.

Directions: Adults take one capsule daily with food.

Warnings: This product should only be consumed by adults and is not intended for use by children. Do not consume if you are pregnant or lactating. Consult your physician before using this product if you are taking prescription medications. Persons with a history of prostate cancer should seek medical advice before using this product.

Ingredients: Dihydroxyepiandrosterone (DHEA), Ginkgo Biloba leaf, Bioperine*, Calcium Phosphate Dibasic, Partially Hydrogenated Vegetable Oil, Talc, Magnesium Stearate, Silicon Dioxide and Croscarmellose Sodium.

How Supplied: One bottle contains 60 enteric-coated tablets.

---

*Bioperine is a registered trademark of Sabinsa Corporation.

MASS APPEAL™
Amino Acid & Mineral Workout Supplement

Uses: Utilizing natural compounds which mimic the beneficial effects of anabolic steroids, Mass Appeal™ is specifically formulated to enhance athletic performance without the harmful side effects of steroids.

Among Mass Appeal's scientifically researched and proven ingredients is creatine, a naturally occurring substance which functions as a storage molecule for high-energy phosphate – the ultimate source of muscular energy known as adenosine triphosphate, or ATP. More than 95 percent of the body's total amount of creatine is contained within the muscles, with type II muscle fibers (fibers that generate large amounts of

force) possessing greater initial levels and higher rates of utilization. Unlike other artificial aids used to enhance performance, creatine monohydrate saturates the muscle cells and causes a muscle "cell volumizing" effect by beneficially forcing water molecules inside the muscle cell. This promotes an increase in muscle growth by helping muscles form new proteins faster while slowing down the destructive breakdown of muscle cells during exercise. Studies show that creatine loading not only improves performance during short-duration, high intensity and intermittent exercises, but it accelerates energy recovery and reduces muscle fatigue by reducing lactic acid build-up as well.

Found in high concentrations within muscle cells and proteins throughout the body, the branched chain amino acids (BCAAs) L-leucine, L-valine and L-isoleucine are also incorporated into Mass Appeal's scientifically engineered formulation. BCAAs increase protein synthesis and can be oxidized inside muscle cells as ATP, a protein-sparing effect which indirectly increases anabolism by reducing the muscle's need to burn its own proteins during bodybuilding or strenuous exercise. When dietary intake of these amino acids is inadequate, muscle protein is broken down into its individual amino acid constituents and utilized in other essential metabolic reactions within the body. Through supplementation, the catabolic breakdown of muscle can be minimized and the muscle tissue preserved.

Alpha-ketoglutaric acid and the amino acid L-glutamine also protect against muscle catabolism by assisting muscle protein synthesis and preserving the body's natural stores of glutamine in the muscle.

Another major contributor to the Mass Appeal™ formulation is the amino acid inosine. By increasing hemoglobin's affinity for binding oxygen within red blood cells, inosine supplementation enables red blood cells to carry more oxygen as they travel from the lungs to the muscles.

Vanadyl sulfate, known for its vasodilator effects, has been shown to markedly increase the blood flow to muscle cells. Researchers also believe that this mineral not only contributes to increased efficiency in the metabolic pathways controlled by the body's insulin, but also triggers certain glucose transporters much in the same way insulin does. This results in increased glucose transport into the muscle tissue, increased glycogen storage, and decreases the breakdown of muscle protein as an energy source.

Directions: Adults (18 years and older) may take a loading dose of 3 packets in the morning and 2 packets in the late afternoon for one week. This dose may be repeated every three months. Following one week of the loading dose,

begin the maintenance dose of 1 packet daily two hours after exercise. Needs may vary with each individual.

For individuals desiring enhanced effects, increase the loading dose to 3 to 4 packets, three times per day (morning, afternoon and evening). Following one week of this enhanced loading dose, begin the enhanced maintenance dose of 2 packets in the morning and 2 packets in the late afternoon. It is recommended that one maintain a low-fat, high-protein diet; drink at least eight glasses of water per day; and engage in 30 to 60 minutes of aerobic and anaerobic exercise three to four times per week. For optimal effects, take in conjunction with Phyto-Vite®, Pro-Xtreme™ and Sure2Endure™.

Warning: Not for use by children, pregnant women or lactating women. Consult your physician before using this product if you have any medical conditions. Do not take if you have kidney disease, muscle disease or are on a protein-restricted diet. Discontinue immediately if allergic symptoms develop. Keep out of the reach of children. Store in a cool, dry place.

Ingredients: Creatine Monohydrate, Inosine (phosphate-bonded), L-leucine, L-valine, L-isoleucine, Alpha-Ketoglutaric acid, KIC (calcium keto-isocaproate), L-glutamine, Vanadyl Sulfate, Dicalcium phosphate, Microcrystalline Cellulose, Stearic Acid, Croscarmellose Sodium, Silica, Magnesium Stearate and film coating (hydroxypropyl methylcellulose, hydroxypropyl cellulose, polyethylene glycol, titanium dioxide and propylene glycol).

How Supplied: One box contains 28 packets, four tablets per packet.

PRO-XTREME™
Dietary Supplement

Uses: The need for protein in the human diet has been increasingly studied, especially in the last decade. As a result of this research, several factors regarding the optimal daily requirements and sources of protein have become very clear. Even the current government published RDIs, which are based solely on minimal needs for survival, have increased to .6–.8 grams per kilogram of body weight per day.

Current clinical findings however indicate that an RDI necessary to maintain optimum health for even a sedentary adult are closer to double that. Circumstances including illness, fat-loss diets, regular exercise, accelerated adolescent growth, or chronic mental or emotional stress indicate requirements 2–3 times that. Competitive or strength athletes, post surgical patients or any situation causing wasting disease such as chemotherapy, HIV, burn trauma or radiation therapy can increase the metabolic need for protein by a factor of up to 6 times the official government RDIs.

Furthermore, these figures represent protein which has been absorbed and made available to the tissues of the body and *not* merely that which has been consumed. This is a distinction current clinical research has recognized as *critical* to proper understanding of the need for protein in the human diet.

Before protein can be absorbed and utilized it must first be digested. Following digestion the free amino acids and di and tripeptides that result from protein breakdown are absorbed at the surface of the small intestine. The process of digestion and absorption requires several steps and is most efficient in the upper portion or proximal section of the jejunum (small intestine). In order for absorption of dietary protein to occur, it must first be reduced from larger oligo and polypeptides to di and tripeptides, the smallest protein fragments consisting of only two or three peptide-bonded amino acids, and free amino acids. Di and tripeptides have been clearly shown to be preferential over free forms. This process must occur fast enough and at a rate high enough to take advantage of the proximal transporters, those that specialize in di and tripeptides and which are in abundance only in this short section of upper intestinal bowel. Once protein has passed this lumenal area, relatively no further protein breakdown or absorption occurs. The balance moves on relatively unchanged into the colon, where it is definitely a negative health factor causing minimal gas and gastrointestinal distress, and when experienced chronically, can lead to colon disease and malignancy. It is now generally believed to be the number one factor responsible for the world's highest rate of colon cancer experienced in the U.S. Pro-Xtreme™ is specifically engineered based on a new profile for protein in optimum human metabolism arising from these new clinical findings. With an exceptionally high di and tripeptide content of 40 percent, Pro-Xtreme™ not only promotes increased nitrogen retention—thereby minimizing the negative effects of increased protein intake or reduced caloric intake—but it works in harmony with natural gastrointestinal activity to produce maximum absorption as well.

Because of the fat content and the density of the bolus, meals containing tissue-source protein are released from the stomach and travel through the intestines at a rate which is naturally slower and more conducive to efficient digestion and absorption. The problems begin when too much tissue protein is consumed or the process of digestion and absorption is incomplete. It is estimated that at best only 30–35% of the protein consumed in an average protein-containing meal is absorbed allowing the balance of now detrimental undigested protein to pass into the colon.

In the case of liquid protein supplements, the problem is one not only of excessive amounts of protein being consumed but also the speed at which the bolus travels throughout the jejunum. Liquid meals, especially those with insufficient soluble fiber, have decreased transit time, leaving less time for digestion and absorption. Consequently, even in individuals with normal gastrointestinal function, liquid forms of whole proteins generally result in equally incomplete and oftentimes less absorption than their tissue food counterparts.

Pro-Xtreme™ utilizes sequentially hydrolyzed whey protein isolates of the highest quality to insure complete and rapid absorption of the highest levels of essential and branched-chain amino acids (BCAAs) in the preferred smallest peptide bonded form. These features, coupled with its industry-leading lowest average molecular weight, soluble-fiber content and delicious vanilla-cappuccino flavor, offer a primary source of protein that may be used any time a protein supplement is desired.

The combination and sequencing of amino acids in whey protein also results in increased tissue storage of glutathione, a stable tripeptide whose antioxidant activity is known to improve immune function. And, although whey protein naturally contains 5 to 7 percent of glutamine, the formula for Pro-Xtreme™ incorporates additional gram amounts of L-glutamine to its list of highly evolved ingredients as well. This extra step is designed to promote anticatabolic effects in skeletal muscle while focusing on gastrointestinal and immune function improvement. Glutamine and the critical BCAA leucine are deemed indispensable for the healthy functioning of other tissues and metabolic processes. By maintaining a rich supply of BCAAs, Pro-Xtreme™ proves protein sparing within muscle and offers the highest biological value possible.

Pro-Xtreme™ is formulated specifically for use with the other products in the BI-OLEAN® System.

Directions: Add 1 packet (36 grams) Pro-Xtreme™ to 1 cup (8 ounces) cold water and stir. There is no need for blending or shaking. Pro-Xtreme™ may also be mixed with lowfat or nonfat milk, milk substitutes or blended with ice for a delicious and nourishing dessert.

Warning: Accidental overdose of iron-containing products is a leading cause of fatal poisoning in children under 6. Keep this product out of reach of children. In case of accidental overdose, call a doctor or poison control center immediately.

Ingredients: Carbohydrates, Dietary fiber, Sugars, Protein, Calcium, Iron, Magnesium, Chloride, Sodium, Potassium, Glutamic acid (as Whey Protein Hydrolysate & L-glutamine), The following ingredients as Whey Protein Hydrolysate (Leucine, Aspartic Acid, Lysine, Threonine, Isoleucine, Proline, Valine, Alanine, Serine, Cysteine, Phenylalanine, Tyrosine, Arginine, Methionine, Glycine, Histidine, Tryptophan), Malto-

dextrin, Natural and Artificial Flavorings, Fructose, Cocoa, Salt and Sucralose.

How Supplied: One box contains 14 packets. Serving size equals one packet.

SATIETE®
Herbal and Amino Acid Supplement

Uses: With its synergistic blend of herbs and amino acids, Satiete® addresses many of today's health concerns by ensuring maximum nutritional support.

One such ingredient is 5-HTP (5-Hydroxytryptophan). 5-HTP is an amino acid derivative and the immediate precursor to serotonin, a neurotransmitter involved in regulating mood, sleep, appetite, energy level and sensitivity to pain. Like drugs known as selective serotonin reuptake inhibitors (SSRI's), 5-HTP enhances the activity of serotonin, a hormone produced by the brain that is involved in mood, sleep, and appetite. Low levels of serotonin are associated with depression, anxiety, and sleep disorders. SSRI's prevent the brain cells from using up serotonin too quickly, thereby causing a deficiency. 5-HTP increases the cell's production of serotonin, which boosts serotonin levels.

L-5-HTP is a standardized extract of Griffonia simplicifolia (containing greater than 95% anhydrous 5-HTP).

The diverse physiological functions of serotonin in the body include actions as a neurotransmitter, a regulator of smooth muscle function in the cardiovascular and gastrointestinal system, and a regulator of platelet function. Serotonin is involved in numerous central nervous system actions such as regulating mood, sleep and appetite. In the gastrointestinal system, serotonin stimulates gastric motility. Serotonin also stimulates platelet aggregation.

As a precursor to serotonin, 5-HTP helps to normalize serotonin activity in the body. Considerable research has been conducted regarding the activity of 5-HTP. Some of the clinical studies are summarized below:

Mood—Dysregulation of serotonin metabolism in the central nervous system has been shown to affect mood. 5-HTP helps to normalize serotonin levels and, thereby, positively affect mood. In a double-blind study using objective assessments of mood, researchers in Zurich reported significant improvements in mood with 5-HTP. Likewise, in a double-blind, multi-center study in Germany, researchers reported significant improvements in both objective and self-assessment indices of mood.

Sleep—Many studies have shown that depletion of serotonin results in insomnia, which is reversed by administration of 5-HTP. Likewise, Soulairac and Lam-

Continued on next page

Satiete—Cont.

binet reported that 100 mg of 5-HTP resulted in significant improvement for people who complained of trouble sleeping. Futhermore, serotonin is metabolized to the hormone melatonin, which is known to help regulate the sleep cycle; by increasing serotonin levels with 5-HTP, melatonin levels are also increased.

Appetite—Food intake is thought to suppress appetite through the production of serotonin from the amino acid tryptophan. Because it is an intermediary in the conversion process of tryptophan to serotonin, 5-HTP may reduce appetite in a similar manner as food intake, but without the calories. In a recent double-blind placebo-controlled study, subjects taking 5-HTP lost significant weight compared to control subjects. A reduction in carbohydrate intake and early satiety were seen in the 5-HTP group.

Another key ingredient in the Satiete formulation is Gymnema sylvestre, whose active ingredient "gymnemic acid" affects the taste buds in the oral cavity as the acid prevents the taste buds from being activated by any sugar molecules in the food; and the absorptive surface of the intestines where the acid prevents the intestine from absorbing sugar molecules. Practically speaking, this creates a reduced appetite for sweet tasting food, as well as reducing the metabolic effect of sugar by reducing its digestion in the intestines thus reducing the blood sugar level. In experimental and clinical trials, Gymnema sylvestre has been successful in treating both insulin-dependent and non-insulin dependent diabetics without reducing the blood sugar level to below the normal blood sugar levels, an effect seen with the use of insulin oral hypoglycemic sulphony lurea compounds.

Studies show that vanadyl sulfate is very effective in normalizing blood sugar levels and controlling conditions such as insulin resistance, or Type II diabetes.

Magnesium, malic acid and St. John's Wort are also combined in Satiete's proven formulation. Magnesium is a key mineral cofactor for many anaerobic as well as aerobic reactions that generate energy, and has an oxygen-sparing effect. It is essential for the cell's mitochondria "powerhouses" to function normally, being involved in both the production and utilization of ATP.

Malic Acid has an oxygen-sparing effect and there are a number of indications that malic acid is a very critical molecule in controlling mitochondrial function. Malate is a source of energy from the Krebs cycle and is the only metabolite of the cycle which falls in concentration during exhaustive physical activity. Depletion of malate has also been linked to physical exhaustion. By giving malic acid and magnesium as dietary supplements, flexibility to use aerobic and anaerobic energy sources can be enhanced

and energy production can be boosted. Lab studies show that many patients with fibromyalgia (or with chronic fatigue) have low magnesium levels. Magnesium supplementation enhances the treatment of both conditions. Its benefits appear to result, at least in part, from its positive impact on serotonin function.

Combining 5-HTP with St. John's Wort Extract (0.3% hypericin context), malic acid, and magnesium, is part of an overall fibromyalgia treatment plan providing excellent results, due in large measure to its improvement of sleep quality and mood.

Directions: Start by taking one hypoallergenic tablet three times per day 30 to 60 minutes before meals. If needed after two weeks of use, increase the dosage to two tablets three times per day. Do not exceed nine tablets daily without medical supervision.

Warning: If you are taking MAO inhibitor drugs, tricyclic antidepressants, SSRI antidepressants (Prozac, Paxil, Zoloft) or prescription diet drugs, do not take this product without medical supervision. If you suffer from liver or kidney diseases, serious gastrointestinal disorders or carcinoid syndrome, do not take this product without medical supervision. If gastrointestinal upset develops and persists, reduce dosage, take only with large meals or discontinue use.

Ingredients: Three enteric-coated Satieté tablets contain: Griffonia Seed Extract (Supplying 95% min. naturally occurring L-5htp), Gymnema Sylvestre, Vanadyl Sulfate, Vitamin B-2, Niacinamide, Magnesium (Oxide), Vitamin B-1, Vitamin B-6, Malic Acid, St. John's Wort Extract, Ginkgo Biloba Extract, Vitamin B-12, Folic Acid, Microcrystalline Cellulose, Stearic Acid, Croscarmelose Sodium, Magnesium Stearate, Silicon Dioxide, Ethylcellulose and Hydroxypropylcellulose.

How Supplied: One bottle contains 84 tablets.

STEPHAN Clarity™
Nutritional Supplement

Uses: STEPHAN Clarity™, designed for use by both men and women, contains selected tissue proteins in the form of nutrients important to memory and concentration.

This is achieved by utilizing such ingredients as lecithin and glutamic acid. Lecithin is a popular supplement widely embraced for memory health, while glutamic acid is an amino acid which influences the body by serving as brain fuel, and has been scientifically proven to increase the firing of neurons in the nervous system. It also metabolizes sugars and fats, as well as detoxifies.

Ginkgo biloba, a third primary ingredient in STEPHAN Clarity™, is a special additive which increases the flow of

blood to the brain and is noted for improving concentration and learning ability. A study published in the *Journal of the American Medical Association* demonstrated ginkgo biloba's effects on individuals with Alzheimer's disease and multi-infarct dementia. It was reported to stabilize and – in 20% of the cases – improve the subjects' functioning for periods of six months to a year.

Together with the support of carefully selected vitamins, minerals, amino acids, and herbs, STEPHAN Clarity™ is a natural and effective way to better one's health.

Directions: As a dietary supplement, take one capsule daily.

Warnings: Contains 9.2 mg phenylalanine per serving.

Ingredients: Proprietary blend (Lecithin, Bee Pollen, L-Glutamic Acid, Ribonucleic Acid Yeast, L-Aspartic Acid, L-Arginine HCl, L-Leucine, L-Lysine HCl, L-Phenylalanine, L-Serine, L-Proline, L-Valine, L-Isoleucine, L-Alanine, L-Glycine, L-Threonine, L-Tyrosine, L-Histidine, L-Cysteine HCl, L-Methionine, Adenosine Triphosphate, Ginkgo Biloba 50:1 Extract), Hydroxypropylmethylcellulose, Dl-Alpha Tocopheryl Acetate, Ascorbic Acid, Niacinamide, Stearic Acid, Ethylcellulose, Vitamin A Acetate, D-Calcium Pantothenate, Thiamine HCl, Silicon Dioxide, Dicalcium Phosphate, Pyridoxine HCl, Riboflavin, Folic Acid, Cholecalciferol, Biotin, Cyancobalamin.

How Supplied: One bottle contains 60 easy-to-swallow capsules.

STEPHAN™ Elasticity®
Nutritional Supplement

Uses: A nutritional food supplement for men and women, STEPHAN™ Elasticity® contains a scientifically balanced mixture of specific tissue proteins established as important for skin tone and texture.

Utilizing such scientifically respected ingredients as vitamin A and selenium, STEPHAN Elasticity is also supported by various other vitamins, minerals and amino acids dedicated to epidermal appearance.

Due to its antioxidant properties, vitamin A has been dubbed the "skin vitamin." It is commonly used as a means of preventing premature aging of the skin. In addition, synthetic derivatives of vitamin A are often used to treat acne and psoriasis.

Selenium is also considered beneficial to the skin. It was recently reported that low blood selenium in the context of low blood vitamin A increases the risk for certain types of skin cancer.

Directions: As a dietary supplement, take one capsule daily.

Warnings: Accidental overdose of iron-containing products is a leading cause of

fatal poisoning in children under 6. Keep this product out of the reach of children. In case of accidental overdose, call a doctor or poison control center immediately.

Ingredients: Proprietary Blend (Shavegrass Herb, L-Glutamic Acid, Bladderwrack Extract, Ribonucleic Acid Yeast, L-Aspartic Acid, L-Arginine HCl, L-Leucine, L-Lysine HCl, L-Phenylalanine, L-Serine, L-Proline, L-Valine, L-Isoleucine, L-Alanine, L-Glycine, L-Threonine, L-Tyrosine, L-Histidine, L-Cysteine HCl, L-Methionine, Adenosine Triphosphate), Hydroxypropylmethylcellulose, DL-Alpha Tocopheryl Acetate, Ascorbic Acid, Ethylcellulose, Stearic Acid, Silicon Dioxide, Calcium Amino Acid Chelate, Manganese Amino Acid Chelate, Iron Amino Acid Chelate, Magnesium Amino Acid Chelate, Zinc Amino Acid Chelate, Vitamin A Acetate, Selenium Amino Acid Chelate, Chromium Amino Acid Chelate.

How Supplied:　One bottle contains 60 easy-to-swallow capsules.

STEPHAN Elixir®
Nutritional Supplement

Uses:　Formulated with an exclusive blend of specific proteins, STEPHAN Elixir® is ideal for both men and women. These tissue proteins are supported by vitamins, minerals, amino acids and herbs recognized as important for general health and well-being.

Among the scientifically researched and proven ingredients utilized in STEPHAN Elixir are vitamin E and cysteine. Vitamin E protects against the ravages of aging in several ways. It is essential for the normal functioning of the body and is especially important for normal neurological functions in humans. It also serves as a potent antioxidant and has been dubbed the body's "first line of defense" against free-radical attack by helping to guard against free radicals. Cysteine has also been found to inactivate free radicals and thus protect and preserve the cells. This sulfur-containing amino acid is a precursor of glutathione, a tripeptide that is claimed to safeguard the body against various toxins and pollutants.

Directions:　As a dietary supplement, take one (1) capsule daily.

Warning:　Accidental overdose of iron-containing products is a leading cause of fatal poisoning in children under 6. Keep this product out of the reach of children. In case of accidental overdose, call a doctor or poison control center immediately. CAUTION PHENYLKETONURICS: Contains 6.9 mg phenylalanine per serving.

Ingredients:　Proprietary Blend (Isolated Soy Protein, Bee Pollen, Citric Acid, Malic Acid, Ribonucleic Acid Yeast, Ginkgo Biloba Leaf Extract, Adenosine Triphosphate), Hydroxypropylmethylcel-

lulose, Zinc Amino Acid Chelate, Iron Amino Acid Chelate, Dl-alpha tocopheryl Acetate, Starch, Ascorbic Acid, Calcium Carbonate, Niacinamide, D-calcium Pantothenate, Vitamin A Acetate, Silicon Dioxide, Thiamine HCl, dicalcium Phosphate, Pyridoxine HCl, Riboflavin, Folic Acid, Selenium Amino Acid Chelate, Cholecalciferol, Biotin, Cyano-cobalamin.

How Supplied:　One bottle contains 60 easy-to-swallow capsules.

STEPHAN Essential®
Nutritional Supplement

Uses:　STEPHAN Essential® is a nutritional food supplement which contains specific tissue proteins supported by vitamins, minerals, herbs and amino acids that are proactive to cardiovascular and circulatory management. L-carnitine, vitamin E and linoleic acid are only some of these very important components.

Scientifically researched and a major contributor to the effects of STEPHAN Essential, L-carnitine is necessary for the transport of long-chain fatty acids into the mitochondria, the metabolic furnaces of the cells. These fatty acids prove a major source for the production of energy in the heart and skeletal muscles, structures that are particularly vulnerable to L-carnitine deficiency.

While vitamin E has proven beneficial in serving to boost the immune system and protect against cardiovascular disease, it has also been established as an important therapy for disorders related to neurologic symptoms. Omega 3–Oil, another important addition to STEPHAN Essential, can lower serum cholesterol levels and decrease platelet stickiness, proving beneficial in the prevention of coronary heart disease.

STEPHAN Essential may be consumed by both men and women.

Directions:　As a dietary supplement, take one (1) capsule daily.

Warning:　Contains 6.9 mg phenylalanine per serving.

Ingredients:　Proprietary Blend (Isolated Soy Protein, L-carnitine Bitartrate, Bee Pollen, Marine Lipid Concentrate, Ribonucleic Acid Yeast, Adenosine Triphosphate), Hydroxypropylmethylcellulose, Magnesium Amino Acid Chelate, Magnesium Silicate, D-alpha Tocopheryl Succinate (Vitamin E), Selenium Amino Acid Chelate, Silicon Dioxide.

How Supplied:　One bottle contains 60 easy-to-swallow capsules.

STEPHAN Feminine®
Nutritional Supplement

Uses:　Specifically designed for women, STEPHAN Feminine® contains selected tissue proteins supported by vitamins, minerals and amino acids regarded as

important to the ever-changing female body. This is achieved through such scientifically researched ingredients as magnesium and boron.

STEPHAN Feminine utilizes magnesium as an important ingredient responsible for regulating the flow of calcium between cells. Studies reveal that women with high-calcium diets report fewer PMS symptoms including less irritability and depression, as well as fewer headaches, backaches and cramps. Magnesium allows for maximum benefits from calcium intake.

Researchers also report many promising results on the effects of dietary boron. Conclusions show that supplementary boron markedly reduces the excretion of both calcium and magnesium while increasing production of an active form of estrogen and testosterone.

Directions:　As a dietary supplement, take one (1) capsule daily.

Warning:　Contains 9.2 mg phenylalanine per serving.

Ingredients:　Proprietary blend (isolated soy protein, magnesium oxide, boron aspartate, ribonucelic acid yeast, adenosine triphosphate), hydroxypropylmethylcellulose, dl-alpha tocopheryl acetate, magnesium silicate, silicon dioxide, selenium amino acid chelate.

How Supplied:　One bottle contains 60 easy-to-swallow capsules.

STEPHAN™ Flexibility®
Nutritional Supplement

Uses:　A nutritional supplement for both men and women, STEPHAN™ Flexibility® is rich with exclusive proteins which are supported by vitamins, minerals and amino acids recognized as beneficial to the health of joint and soft tissues.

Glycine, an amino acid, is one very significant ingredient utilized in STEPHAN Flexibility. In a pilot study investigating the possibility of glycine's effect on spastic control, a 25% improvement was noted on subjects with chronic multiple sclerosis. Furthermore, all patients benefited to some degree, and no toxicity or other adverse side effects were noted.

Another important amino acid in STEPHAN Flexibility is L-histidine. Reports suggest that supplementary L-histidine may actually boost the activity of suppressor T cells. Because rheumatoid arthritis is one of the many autoimmune diseases in which T-cell activity is subnormal, these conclusions lend further support that normal levels of L-histidine are beneficial to joint health.

Vitamin E can also be found in STEPHAN Flexibility because of its ability to relieve muscular cramps. According to one popular study, supplemental

Continued on next page

Stephan Flexibility—Cont.

vitamin E caused remarkable relief from nocturnal leg and foot cramps in 82% of the 125 patients tested.

Directions: As a dietary supplement, take one capsule daily.

Warnings: Contains 9.2 mg phenylalanine per serving.

Ingredients: Proprietary Blend (Boron Gluconate, L-Glutamic Acid, Ribonucleic Acid Yeast, L-Aspartic Acid, L-Arginine HCl, L-Leucine, L-Lysine HCl, Bee Pollen, L-Phenylalanine, L-Serine, L-Proline, L-Valine, L-Isoleucine, L-Alanine, L-Glycine, L-Threonine, L-Tyrosine, L-Histidine, L-Cysteine HCl, L-Methionine, Adenosine Triphosphate), Hydroxypropylmethylcellulose, Zinc Amino Acid Chelate, Calcium Amino Acid Chelate, Stearic Acid, Ascorbic Acid, Whey, D-Alpha Tocopheryl Succinate, Magnesium Stearate, Niacinamide, Silicon Dioxide, Cellulose, Vitamin A Palmitate, D-Calcium Pantothenate, Thiamine HCl, Dicalcium Phosphate, Pyridoxine HCl, Riboflavin, Folic Acid, Selenomethionine, Cholecalciferol, Biotin, Cyanocobalamin.

How Supplied: One bottle contains 60 easy-to-swallow capsules.

STEPHAN Lovpil™
Nutritional Supplement

Uses: STEPHAN Lovpil™ is a nutritional food supplement for men and women of all ages that is formulated with vitamins, minerals, herbs, amino acids and selected proteins recognized as important for general health and sexual vitality.

Damiana, typically thought of as an aphrodisiac by those who are familiar with its effects, is an important ingredient utilized in STEPHAN Lovpil. A major herbal remedy in Mexican medical folklore, damiana is proven for its stimulating properties of male virility and libido. A number of scientific studies have shown a direct relationship between low sperm count and diets deficient in arginine.

Scientific studies on Vitamin C have uncovered that ascorbic acid may actually protect human sperm from oxidative DNA damage.

Directions: As a dietary supplement, take one (1) capsule daily.

Ingredients: Proprietary blend (damiana leaf, isolated soy protein, ribonucleic acid yeast, adenosine triphosphate), calcium carbonate, hydroxypropylmethylcellulose, ascorbic acid (Vitamin C), stearic acid, zinc amino acid chelate, magnesium stearate, manganese amino acid chelate, silicon dioxide, vitamin A acetate, dicalcium phosphate, cholecalciferol, folic acid, selenomethionine, cyanocobalamin.

How Supplied: One bottle contains 60 easy-to-swallow capsules.

STEPHAN Masculine®
Nutritional Supplement

Uses: A nutritional food supplement formulated for the adult male, STEPHAN Masculine® contains a special blend of nutrients with vitamins, minerals, herbs and amino acids. Scientifically researched ingredients have been carefully selected to help ensure STEPHAN Masculine's effectiveness. Zinc is one such ingredient. Proven to be closely interrelated with the male sex hormone, testosterone, zinc deficiency often results in regression of the male sex glands, decreased sexual interest, mental lethargy, emotional problems and even poor appetite. It has been found that in males with only a mild zinc deficiency, zinc supplementation was accompanied by increased sperm count and plasma testosterone.

Directions: As a dietary supplement, take one capsule daily.

Ingredients: Proprietary Blend (L-Histidine, Bee Pollen, Parsley Leaf, Ribonucleic Acid, Adenosine Triphosphate), Calcium Carbonate, Zinc Amino Acid Chelate, Hydroxypropylmethylcellulose, Magnesium Amino Acid Chelate, Stearic Acid, Magnesium Stearate.

How Supplied: One bottle contains 60 easy-to-swallow capsules.

PHYTO-VITE®
Advanced Antioxidant, Vitamin and Mineral Supplement

Uses: Phyto-Vite® is a state-of-the-art nutritional supplement providing chelated minerals, vitamins and a diverse group of antioxidants. It was formulated to meet the nutritional needs of our society where studies estimate only 9% consume foods in the quantities necessary to protect against the oxidative damage caused by free radicals.

The antioxidant coverage provided by Phyto-Vite is both comprehensive and diverse. First, it includes optimal amounts of vitamins A, C, and E as well as the pro-vitamins alpha and beta carotene. Vitamin A, in addition to its antioxidant capabilities, is also felt to improve immune function, protein synthesis, RNA synthesis and steroid hormone synthesis. In this product, vitamin A is derived from two sources: retinyl palmitate and lemongrass. Additional vitamin A activity is provided by the alpha and beta carotene found in *Dunaliella salina*. These carotenoids are strong antioxidants in their own right; however, they can also be converted to vitamin A. This occurs only when the body is deficient in this vitamin. Consequently, vitamin A toxicity cannot be caused by alpha or beta carotene. Vitamin C has long been associated with wound healing, collagen formation, and maintaining the structural integrity of capillaries, cartilage, dentine and bone. Phyto-Vite utilizes esterified vitamin C which has been shown to provide a quicker uptake and a decreased rate of excretion when compared with conventional vitamin C. This allows for higher, more sustained levels of this vitamin in the body. Phyto-Vite also contains 400 I.U. of vitamin E, from natural sources. The antioxidant effects of vitamin E have been shown to stabilize cell membranes, increase HDL cholesterol, and decrease platelet aggregation.

Many flavonoids are incorporated into Phyto-Vite. These substances possess antioxidant activity themselves and also potentiate the effects of vitamins C and E. This later effect is produced by decreasing the degradation of vitamin C and E into inactive metabolites. Ginkgo biloba has flavonoid activity as well as other significant effects. Among these are a decrease in platelet aggregation and an increase in vasodilation which appears to increase blood flow to the peripheral arteries and the brain. Some improvement in cognitive abilities has been noted. It also helps to inhibit lipid peroxidation, thereby stabilizing the cell wall against free radical attack.

A phytonutrient blend has been incorporated into Phyto-Vite to further enhance its antioxidant effects. Phytonutrient is a term given to the thousands of chemical compounds found in fruits and vegetables. Some of these compounds have shown great promise in aiding the cardiovascular system. Currently, much research is ongoing to isolate and identify more of these compounds, but it has already been clearly established that phytonutrients work best when the entire plant source is used rather than just the isolated compound. The phytonutrients found in Phyto-Vite are obtained from alfalfa (lutein), broccoli (indoles), cabbage (isothiocyanates), cayenne (capsanthin and capsorubin), green onion (thioallyl compounds), parsley (chlorophyll), spirulina (gamma linolenic acid), tomato (lycopene), soy isoflavones (genistein, lecithin and daidzein), aged garlic concentrate, and Pure-Gar-A-8000™ (allicin).

The antioxidant minerals copper, zinc, manganese and selenium have also been incorporated into Phyto-Vite. These minerals have been chelated via a patented process in which the mineral is wrapped within an amino acid. Once inside the body, the minerals can then be utilized in the millions of metabolic reactions that take place in the body. With this process, overall mineral absorption can approach 95% instead of the 5 to 10% absorption seen with other mineral supplements.

Phyto-Vite also provides two antioxidant enzymes (catalase and peroxidase). These help to reduce the body's free radical burden by neutralizing free radicals in the pharynx or stomach.

There are three other features that make Phyto-Vite unique among supplements. First, a small amount of canola oil was included to aid in the proper absorption of fat soluble vitamins, even on an empty stomach. Canola oil also provides essential fatty acids. Second, the product is formed into prolonged-release tablets which allow flexibility in dosing frequency. It can be taken all at once or staggered throughout the day. Dissolution testing has been performed to insure that the product will dissolve properly. Lastly, Phyto-Vite tablets are covered with a Betacoat™. This is a beta carotene coating that is designed to provide antioxidant coverage to the tablet itself. This helps to protect the integrity and activity of the product.

Directions: As a dietary supplement take six tablets per day with eight ounces of liquid. Tablets may be taken all at once or staggered throughout the day.

Warnings: If pregnant or lactating, consult physician before using. Accidental overdose of iron-containing products is a leading cause of fatal poisoning in children under 6. Keep this product out of reach of children. In case of accidental overdose, call a doctor or poison control center immediately. This hypoallergenic formula is free of dairy, yeast, wheat, sugar, starch, animal products, dyes, preservatives, artificial flavors and pesticide residues.

Ingredients: Vitamin A, Vitamin C, Vitamin D, Vitamin E, Vitamin K, Thiamin, Riboflavin, Niacin, Vitamin B6, Folate, Vitamin B12, Biotin, Pantothenic Acid, Calcium, Iron, Phosphorus, Iodine, Magnesium, Zinc, Selenium, Copper, Manganese, Chromium, Potassium, Phytonutrient Blend (alfalfa leaf, aged garlic bulb concentrate, Pur-Gar® A-10,000 [garlic bulb], soy protein isolate, broccoli floret, cabbage leaf, cayenne pepper fruit, green onion bulb, parsley leaf, tomato, spirulina), canola oil concentrate, citrus bioflavonoid complex, rutin, quercetin dehydrate, choline, Inositol, PABA, ginkgo biloba leaf standardized extract, bilberry fruit standardized extract, catalase enzymes, grape seed proanthocyanidins, red grape skin extract, boron, dicalcium phosphate, magnesium oxide, calcium carbonate, calcium ascorbate, microcrystalline cellulose, d-alpha-tocopheryl succinate, croscarmellose sodium, stearic acid, potassium citrate, choline bitartrate, beta-carotene, niacinamide, silica, d-calcium pantothenate, magnesium stearate, copper Chelazome® glycinate, zinc Chelazome® glycinate, calcium citrate, calcium lactate, magnesium amino acid chelate, inositol, L-selenomethionine, kelp, manganese Chelazome® glycinate, biotin, pyridoxine HCl, Ferrochel® iron bisglycinate, boron chelate, riboflavin, magnesium citrate, thiamin mononitrate, retinyl palmitate, chromium Chelavite® glycinate, phylloquinone, cyanocobalamin, vanillin, cholecalciferol, folic acid.

How Supplied: One bottle contains 180 Betacoat™ tablets.

STEPHAN Protector®
Nutritional Supplement

Uses: STEPHAN Protector® is a nutritional food supplement that combines specific proteins, vitamins, minerals and amino acids recognized as important for the health of areas associated with the human immune system.
Among these specially selected and scientifically researched ingredients are astragalus and kelp. Known for its strengthening effects of both the immune and digestive systems, astragalus can be combined with other herbs to increase phagocytosis, interferon production and the number of macrophages. It, in combination, enhances T-cell transformation and functions as an adaptogen to relieve stress-induced immune system suppression.
Research clearly indicates that kelp supplies dozens of important nutrients for improved cardiovascular health and function.

Directions: As a dietary supplement, take one (1) capsule daily.

Warning: Contains 9.2 mg phenylalanine per serving.

Ingredients: Proprietary blend (isolated soy protein, astragalus root, bee pollen, kelp, ribonucleic acid yeast, adenosine triphosphate), hydroxypropylmethylcellulose, cellulose, stearic acid, magnesium stearate, silicon dioxide.

How Supplied: One bottle contains 60 easy-to-swallow capsules.

STEPHAN Relief®
Nutritional Supplement

Uses: Designed for both men and women, STEPHAN Relief® has been formulated with a special combination of nutrients, vitamins, minerals, amino acids and herbs which are recognized as important to the digestive and excretory systems.
Parsley, a member of the carrot family, can be used as a carminative and an aid to digestion. While the root has a mild diuretic property, parsley has also been reported, in large doses, to affect blood pressure.
Psyllium is a gel-forming fiber used in many bulk laxatives to promote bowel regularity. In recent years, because of its affects on healthy cholesterol levels, psyllium has gained wide-spread popularity and can be found in some ready-to-eat cereals.

Directions: As a dietary supplement, take one (1) capsule daily.

Ingredients: Proprietary blend (Psyllium Seed Powder, L-isoleucine, L-leucine, L-valine, Bee Pollen, Bladderwrack

Herb 5:1 Extract, Parsley Leaf 4:1 extract, Ribonucleic Acid Yeast, Adenosine Triphosphate), Hydroxypropylmethylcellulose, Ethylcellulose, Magnesium Silicate, D-calcium Pantothenate, Silicon Dioxide.

How Supplied: One bottle contains 60 easy-to-swallow capsules.

SLEEP-TITE™
Herbal Sleep Aid

Uses: Sleep-Tite™ is a non-addicting herbal sleep aid formulated to promote a deeper, more restorative sleep without the use of pharmaceutically synthesized hormones. With the body's overall health, and proper functioning, dependent upon efficient sleep patterns in order to achieve cellular, organ, tissue and emotional repair, this powerful tool's primary function is to rejuvenate and restore by assisting the body in initiating and maintaining sleep.
Sleep-Tite is a blend of 10 highly effective, all-natural herbs. California poppy, passion flower, valerian, kava kava and skullcap have been used for centuries as a remedy for insomnia because of their calming effects and ability to relieve muscle tension. Hops and celery seed produce a generalized calming effect and are especially helpful for indigestion, gastrointestinal and smooth muscle relaxation. Chamomile also has a relaxing effect on the body and the gastrointestinal tract, but with the added benefit of producing anti-inflammatory effects on joints. Feverfew has been used as a treatment for fever, migraines and arthritic complaints dating back to ancient Greece. A study published in *Lancet* demonstrated that feverfew inhibited the body's production of prostaglandin and serotonin. These biochemicals can cause inflammation, fever and the vasoactive response that triggers migraine headaches.
By utilizing this unique blend of herbs to aid in the effective initiation and maintenance of sleep patterns, Sleep-Tite can be consumed by adults, thereby promoting physical and emotional well-being in a safe, active manner.

Directions: Adults (18 years and older) may take two Sleep-Tite caplets approximately 30 to 60 minutes prior to bedtime. Needs may vary with each individual. Some persons may require less than two caplets to achieve optimum results. Do not exceed recommended nightly amounts.

Warnings: Not for use by children, pregnant women or lactating women. Consult your physician before using this product if you have any medical condition or are taking antidepressant, sedative or hypnotic medications. Do not take this product if using Monoamine Oxidase Inhibitors (MAOI). This product may

Continued on next page

Sleep-Tite—Cont.

cause drowsiness and should not be taken with alcohol or while operating a vehicle or other machinery. If allergic symptoms develop, discontinue use. Store in a cool, dry place. Keep out of reach of children.

Ingredients: European Valerian Root 4:1 extract, Celery Seed 4:1 extract, Hops Strobile 4:1 extract, Passion Flower 4:1 extract (whole plant), California Poppy 5:1 extract (aerial parts), Chamomile Flower 5:1 extract, Chinese Fu Ling 5:1 extract (Poria Cocos), Kava Kava Root 5:1 extract, Feverfew 5:1 extract (aerial parts), Skullcap (aerial parts), Dicalcium Phosphate, Microcrystalline Cellulose, Croscarmellose Sodium, Stearic Acid, Silica, Magnesium Stearate and Sugar Coat (calcium sulfate, sucrose, kaolin, talc, gelatin, shellac, titanium dioxide, anise oil, beeswax and carnauba wax).

How Supplied: One box contains 28 packets. Two caplets per packet.

STEPHAN Tranquility™ Nutritional Supplement

Uses: Designed for both men and women, STEPHAN Tranquility™ is a nutritional food supplement which contains a blend of vitamins, minerals and amino acids recognized as important to areas involved in stress management. Myo-Inositol is among these specially researched ingredients. It has long been claimed to lower blood concentrations of triglycerides and cholesterol, as well as to generally protect against cardiovascular disease. In addition, Myo-Inositol intake can influence the phosphatidylinositol levels in the membranes of brain cells. Compounds derived from this process could conceivably have some beneficial effect on insomnia and anxiety. Valerian root contains valepotriates which are said to be the source of its sedative effects. Studies reveal that valeranon, an essential oil component of this herb, produces a pronounced smooth-muscle effect on the intestine.

Directions: As a dietary supplement, take one (1) capsule daily.

Warning: Contains 9.2 mg phenylalanine per serving.

Ingredients: Proprietary blend (isolated soy protein, choline bitartrate, inositol, lecithin, ribonucelic acid yeast, valerian root extract, adenosine triphosphate), hydroxypropylmethylcellulose, dl-alpha tocopheryl acetate, calcium aspartate, silicon dioxide, ascorbic acid, stearic acid, niacinamide, magnesium amino acid chelate, vitamin A palmitate, hydroxypropylcellulose, d-calcium pantothenate, thiamine HCl, dicalcium phosphate, pyridoxine HCl, riboflavin, folic acid, cholecalciferol, biotin, cyanocobalamin.

How Supplied: One bottle contains 60 easy-to-swallow capsules.

SURE2ENDURE™
Herbal, Vitamin & Mineral Workout Supplement

Uses: Attaining peak physical and athletic performance can be an elusive and time-consuming endeavor. It requires a conditioning process whereby the body's endurance, stamina and ability to recover are enhanced. Sure2Endure™ is formulated to aid in this process through an innovative blend of herbs, vitamins and minerals.
Among these specially selected ingredients is ciwujia (*Radix Acanthopanax senticosus*). Used in traditional Chinese medicine for almost 1,700 years to treat fatigue and boost the immune system, ciwujia has been shown to improve overall performance in aerobic exercise, endurance activities and weight lifting without any stimulant effects. According to a recent study, ciwujia increases fat metabolism during exercise by shifting toward the use of fat as an energy source instead of carbohydrates. In addition, the caffeine-free herb improves endurance by reducing lactic acid build-up in the muscles. This process delays the muscle fatigue which often leads to muscle pain and cramps.
Sure2Endure™ also provides antioxidant coverage and enzyme cofactors. Vitamins C and E address the otherwise high levels of free radicals generated from the oxidation of fuel substrates during exercise, while vitamins B1 (thiamin), B2 (riboflavin), B6 (pyridoxine), and B12 (cyanocobalamin) aid in proper carbohydrate metabolism and serve as cofactors in numerous biochemical reactions in the body. Ciwujia has been credited with antioxidant properties as well. Since tissue stress and damage are often the result of strenuous exercise, it is important to maintain proper integrity and recovery of connective tissue. Glucosamine, one of the basic constituents making up joint cartilage, is another special additive to Sure2Endure™. This substance enhances the synthesis of cartilage cells and protects against destructive enzymes. It stabilizes cell membranes and intercellular collagen thereby protecting cartilage during rest, exercise and recovery.
The anti-inflammatory activities of bromelain and boswellia further prove beneficial to the health of joint and soft tissues.

Directions: Adults (18 years and older) take 3 tablets one hour prior to exercise. Needs may vary with each individual. For optimum performance, use in conjunction with BIOLEAN® or BIOLEAN Free® one hour before exercise. Phyto-Vite® may be taken with this product to maximize the antioxidant effect necessary with exercise. Pro-Xtreme™ and Mass Appeal™ may also be consumed for maximum effectiveness.

Warning: Not for use by children, pregnant women or lactating women. Consult your physician before using this product if you have any medical conditions. Discontinue immediately if allergic symptoms develop. Keep out of the reach of children. Store in a cool, dry place.

Ingredients: Vitamin C (as ascorbic acid), Vitamin E (as d-alpha tocopheryl succinate), Thiamin (as thiamin mononitrate), Riboflavin, Vitamin B6 (as pyridoxine hydrochloride), Vitamin B12 (as cyanocobalamin), Chromium (as patented Chelavite® chromium dinicotinate glycinate), Ciwujia root standardized extract (0.8% eleutherosides) (Acanthopanax senticosus), Magnesium L-aspartate, Potassium L-aspartate, Boswellia Serrata standardized extract (40% boswellic acids (as gum resins), Bromelain (600 GDU/g), Glucosamine hydrochloride, Dicalcium Phosphate, Microcrystalline Cellulose, Croscarmellose Sodium, Stearic Acid, Silica, Magnesium Stearate and Sugar Coat (calcium sulfate, sucrose, kaolin, talc, gelatin, shellac, titanium dioxide, wintergreen oil, FD&C yellow #5, FD&C blue #1, beeswax and carnauba wax).

How Supplied: One box contains 28 packets, three tablets per packet.

WINRGY™
Nutritional Drink with Vitamin C

Uses: Through nutrients in the diet, nerves are able to send signals throughout the body called neurotransmitters. One such neurotransmitter, noradrenaline, provides individuals with the necessary alertness and energy required in day-to-day activity. A unique blend of vitamins and minerals important to the creation of noradrenaline has been incorporated into Winrgy™, making it a delicious, nutritional alternative to coffee and cola.
Studies reveal that vitamin B2 (riboflavin) helps the body release energy from protein, carbohydrates and fat, while vitamin B12 (cobalamin) is given to combat fatigue and alleviate neurological problems, including weakness and memory loss. Another important component of Winrgy, vitamin B3 (niacin), works with both thiamin and riboflavin in the metabolism of carbohydrates and is essential for providing energy for cell tissue growth. Niacin has also proven to dilate blood vessels and thereby increase the blood flow to various organs of the body, sometimes resulting in a blush of the skin and a healthy sense of warmth. Unlike caffeine, Winrgy offers the raw materials necessary to continue the production of noradrenaline and is ideal for anytime performance is required.

Directions: Add 3/4 cup of chilled water or fruit juice to one packet of mix. Stir briskly. Consume 1–2 times per day. Keep in a cool, dry place. For maximum results, combine this product with one serving size of Food For Thought.™

Warnings: Phenylketonurics: Contains Phenylalanine. Not for use by children, pregnant or lactating women. Persons taking medications should seek medical advice before taking this product. Do not consume more than four servings per day. Avoid the use of antacids containing aluminum with this product.

Ingredients: Vitamin C (as ascorbic acid), Vitamin E (as alpha tocopherol acetate), Thiamin (as thiamin mononitrate), Riboflavin, Niacin (as niacinamide), Vitamin B6 (as pyridoxine hydrochloride), Folate (as folic acid), Vitamin B12 (as cyanocobalamin), Pantothenic Acid (as calcium pantothenate), Zinc (as zinc gluconate), Copper (as copper gluconate), Manganese (as manganese aspartate), Chromium (as chromium aspartate), Potassium (as potassium aspartate), Phenylalanine (as L-phenyl-alanine), Taurine, Glycine, Caffeine, Fructose, Natural Flavor, Citric Acid and Silicon Dioxide.

How Supplied: One box contains 28 packets. Serving size equals one packet.

Wyeth Consumer Healthcare
Wyeth

FIVE GIRALDA FARMS
MADISON, NJ 07940

Direct Inquiries to:
Wyeth Consumer Healthcare Product Information 800-322-3129

CALTRATE® 600 + D
CALTRATE® 600 + SOY

Description: CALCIUM SUPPLEMENT WITH VITAMIN D, NATURE'S MOST CONCENTRATED FORM OF CALCIUM® NO SALT, NO LACTOSE; TABLET SHAPE SPECIALLY DESIGNED FOR EASIER SWALLOWING CALTRATE 600 + SOY CONTAINS SOY ISOFLAVONES

SUPPLEMENT FACTS:
Serving Size 1 Tablet

AMOUNT PER SERVING			% DAILY VALUE
CALTRATE® 600 + D	Vitamin D 200 IU		50%
	Calcium 600 mg		60%
CALTRATE® 600 + SOY	Vitamin D 200 IU		50%
	Calcium 600 mg		60%
	Soy Isoflavones 25 mg		*

*Daily Value Not Established

CALTRATE® 600 + D: Calcium Carbonate, Cholecalciferol (Vit. D), Starch. **Contains less than 2% of the following:** Croscarmellose Sodium, dl-Alpha Tocopherol, FD&C Yellow No. 6 Aluminum Lake, Gelatin, Hydroxypropyl Methylcellulose, Magnesium Stearate, Partially Hydrogenated Soybean Oil, Sucrose, Titanium Dioxide. **May contain less than 2% of the following:** Glycerin, Polydextrose.

CALTRATE® 600 + SOY: Calcium Carbonate, Maltodextrin, Soy Isoflavones Extract, Cellulose, Mineral Oil, Soy Polysaccharides, Hydroxypropyl Methylcellulose, Gelatin, Sucrose, Corn Starch, Polyethylene Glycol, Canola Oil, Carnauba Wax, Crospovidone, Magnesium Stearate, Stearic Acid, Cholecalciferol (Vit. D), dl-Alpha Tocopherol (Vit. E).

Warnings:
Caltrate® 600 + D
As with any supplement, if you are pregnant or nursing a baby, contact your healthcare professional.
Caltrate® 600 + Soy
Use only as directed. Do not exceed recommended dosage. As with any supplement, if you are taking a prescription medication, or if you are pregnant or nursing a baby, contact your physician before using this product.
Keep out of reach of children.

Suggested Use: Take one tablet twice daily with food or as directed by your physician. Not formulated for use in children.
Bottle sealed with printed foil under cap. Do not use if foil is torn.

How Supplied:
Caltrate 600 + D, Bottles of 60, 120 tablets
Caltrate 600 + SOY, Bottle of 60 tablets
Storage: Store at Room temperature. Keep bottle tightly closed.

CALTRATE® 600 PLUS™ Tablets
Calcium Carbonate

Calcium Supplement With Vitamin D & Minerals
No Salt, No Lactose

SUPPLEMENT FACTS
Serving Size: 1 Tablet

AMOUNT PER SERVING:		% Daily Value
Vitamin D	200 IU	50%
Calcium	600 mg	60%
Magnesium	40 mg	10%
Zinc	7.5 mg	50%
Copper	1 mg	50%
Manganese	1.8 mg	90%
Boron	250 mcg	*

* Daily Value not established.
† Percent daily value based on a 2000 calorie diet.

Ingredients: Calcium Carbonate, Maltodextrin, Magnesium Oxide, Cellulose, Hydroxypropyl Methylcellulose, Mineral Oil, Zinc Oxide, Soy Polysaccharides, Titanium Dioxide, Manganese Sulfate, Polysorbate 80, Sodium Borate, Cupric Oxide, Polyethylene Glycol, Gelatin, Sucrose, FD&C Yellow No. 6 Aluminum Lake, Corn Starch, Canola Oil, Carnauba Wax, FD&C Red No. 40 Aluminum Lake, FD&C Blue No. 1 Aluminum Lake, Crospovidone, Magnesium Stearate, Stearic Acid, Cholecalciferol (Vit D), dl-Alpha Tocopherol (Vit. E).

Suggested Use: Take one tablet twice daily with food or as directed by your physician. Not formulated for use in children.

Warnings: As with any supplement, if you are pregnant or nursing a baby, contact your healthcare professional.

Keep out of reach of children.

How Supplied: Bottles of 60 & 120 tablets.

Storage: Bottle sealed with printed foil under cap. Do not use if foil is torn. Store at room temperature. Keep bottle tightly closed.

© 1999

CALTRATE COLON HEALTH
Calcium Supplement with Vitamin D

Supplement Facts
Serving Size 1 Tablet

Amount Per Serving	% Daily Value
Vitamin D 200 IU	50%
Calcium 600 mg	60%

Ingredients: Calcium Carbonate, Maltodextrin. **Contains less than 2% of the following:** Carnauba Wax, Cholecalciferol (Vit. D), Crospovidone, dl-Alpha Tocopherol, FD&C Yellow No. 6 Aluminum Lake, Gelatin, Hydroxypropyl Methylcellulose, Magnesium Stearate, Mineral Oil, Partially Hydrogenated Soybean Oil, Polyethylene Glycol, Polysorbate 80, Powdered Cellulose, Starch, Stearic Acid, Sucrose, Titanium Dioxide

Suggested Use: Take one tablet twice daily with food or as directed by your physician. Replaces your daily calcium supplement.

Not formulated for use in children.

As with any supplement, if you are pregnant or nursing a baby, contact your healthcare professional

Store at room temperature. Keep bottle tightly closed.

Keep out of reach of children.

Bottle sealed with printed foil under cap. Do not use if foil is torn.

How Supplied: Bottles of 60 tablets

Continued on next page

CENTRUM®
High Potency
Multivitamin-Multimineral
Supplement, Advanced Formula
From A to Zinc®

Supplement Facts:
Serving Size 1 Tablet

Each Tablet Contains	% DV
Vitamin A 3500 IU	70%
(29% as Beta Carotene)	
Vitamin C 60 mg	100%
Vitamin D 400 IU	100%
Vitamin E 30 IU	100%
Vitamin K 25 mcg	31%
Thiamin 1.5 mg	100%
Riboflavin 1.7 mg	100%
Niacin 20 mg	100%
Vitamin B$_6$ 2 mg	100%
Folic Acid 400 mcg	100%
Vitamin B$_{12}$ 6 mcg	100%
Biotin 30 mcg	10%
Pantothenic Acid 10 mg	100%
Calcium 162 mg	16%
Iron 18 mg	100%
Phosphorus 109 mg	11%
Iodine 150 mcg	100%
Magnesium 100 mg	25%
Zinc 15 mg	100%
Selenium 20 mcg	29%
Copper 2 mg	100%
Manganese 2 mg	100%
Chromium 120 mcg	100%
Molybdenum 75 mcg	100%
Chloride 72 mg	2%
Potassium 80 mg	2%
Boron 150 mcg	*
Nickel 5 mcg	*
Silicon 2 mg	*
Tin 10 mcg	*
Vanadium 10 mcg	*
Lutein 250 mcg	*
Lycopene 300 mcg	*

*Daily Value (%DV) not established.

Ingredients: Dibasic Calcium Phosphate, Magnesium Oxide, Potassium Chloride, Microcrystalline Cellulose, Ascorbic Acid (Vit. C), Ferrous Fumarate, Calcium Carbonate, Gelatin, dl-Alpha Tocopheryl Acetate (Vit. E). **Contains less than 2% of the following:** Acacia Senegal Gum, Ascorbyl Palmitate, Beta Carotene, Biotin, Boron, Butylated Hydroxytoluene, Calcium Pantothenate, Chromic Chloride, Citric Acid, Colloidal Silicon Dioxide, Crospovidone, Cupric Acid, Cyanocobalamin (Vit. B$_{12}$), Ergocalciferol (Vit. D), FD&C Yellow No. 6 Aluminum Lake, Folic Acid, Hypromellose, Lutein, Lycopene, Magnesium Stearate, Manganese Sulfate, Niacinamide, Nickelous Sulfate, Phytonadione (Vit. K), Polysorbate 80, Potassium Iodide, Potassium Sorbate, Pregelatinized Starch, Purified Water, Pyridoxine Hydrochloride (Vit. B$_6$), Riboflavin (Vit. B$_2$), Silicon Dioxide, Sodium Ascorbate, Sodium Benzoate, Sodium Citrate, Sodium Metavanadate, Sodium Molybdate, Sodium Selenate, Sodium Silicoaluminate, Sorbic Acid, Stannous Chloride, Starch, Sucrose, Thiamine Mononitrate (Vit. B$_1$), Titanium Dioxide, Tocopherol, Tribasic Calcium Phosphate, Triethyl Citrate, Vitamin A Acetate (Vit. A), Zinc Oxide. **May also contain:** Calcium Stearate, Glucose, Lactose Monohydrate.

Suggested Use:
One tablet daily with food. Not formulated for use in children.

Warnings: Accidental overdose of iron-containing products is a leading cause of fatal poisoning in children under 6. Keep this product out of reach of children. In case of accidental overdose, call a doctor or poison control center immediately. As with any supplement, if you are pregnant or nursing a baby, contact your healthcare professional.
IMPORTANT INFORMATION: Long-term intake of high levels of vitamin A (excluding that sourced from beta-carotene) may increase the risk of osteoporosis in postmenopausal women. Do not take this product if taking other vitamin A supplements.

How Supplied: Light peach, engraved CENTRUM C1.
Bottles of 15, 50, 130, 180, 250 tablets
Storage: Store at room temperature. Keep bottle tightly closed.
Bottle sealed with printed foil under cap. Do not use if foil is torn.

CENTRUM KIDS COMPLETE
Rugrats®
Chewable Multivitamin Supplement
(Orange, Cherry, Fruit Punch)

Supplement Facts:
[See table below]

Ingredients: Sucrose, Dibasic Calcium Phosphate, Mannitol, Calcium Carbonate, Stearic Acid, Magnesium Oxide, Ascorbic Acid (Vit. C), Pregelatinized Starch, Microcrystalline Cellulose, dl-Alpha Tocopheryl Acetate (Vit. E). **Contains less than 2% of the following:** Acacia, Aspartame**, Beta Carotene, Biotin, Butylated Hydroxytoluene (BHT), Calcium Pantothenate, Carbonyl Iron, Carrageenan, Chromic Chloride, Citric Acid, Cupric Oxide, Cyanocobalamin (Vit. B$_{12}$), Dextrose, Ergocalciferol (Vit. D), FD&C Blue 2 Aluminum Lake, FD&C Red 40 Aluminum Lake, FD&C Yellow 6 Aluminum Lake, Folic Acid, Gelatin, Glucose, Guar Gum, Lactose, Magnesium Stearate, Malic Acid, Manganese Sulfate, Mono and Diglycerides, Natural and Artificial Flavors, Niacinamide, Phytonadione (Vit. K), Potassium Iodide, Potassium Sorbate, Purified Water, Pyridoxine Hydrochloride (Vit. B$_6$), Riboflavin (Vit. B$_2$), Silicon Dioxide, Sodium Ascorbate, Sodium Benzoate, Sodium Citrate, Sodium Molybdate, Sodium Silicoaluminate, Sorbic Acid, Starch, Thiamine Mononitrate (Vit. B$_1$), Tocopherol, Tribasic Calcium Phosphate, Vanillin, Vitamin A Acetate (Vit. A), Zinc Oxide. **May also contain:** Fructose, Maltodextrin.

Suggested Use: Children 2 and 3 years of age, chew approximately ½ tablet daily with food. Adults and children 4 years of age and older, chew 1 tablet daily with food. Not formulated for use in children less than 2 years of age.

Serving Size:	½ Tablet	1 Tablet
Amount Per Serving:	% DV for Children 2 and 3 Years (1/2 Tablet)	% DV for Adults and Children 4 Years and Older (1 Tablet)
Total Carbohydrate <1g	*	<1%+
Vitamin A 3500 IU	70%	70%
(29% as Beta Carotene)		
Vitamin C 60 mg	75%	100%
Vitamin D 400 IU	50%	100%
Vitamin E 30 IU	150%	100%
Vitamin K 10 mcg	*	13%
Thiamin 1.5 mg	107%	100%
Riboflavin 1.7 mg	106%	100%
Niacin 20 mg	111%	100%
Vitamin B$_6$ 2 mg	143%	100%
Folic Acid 400 mcg	100%	100%
Vitamin B$_{12}$ 6 mcg	100%	100%
Biotin 45 mcg	15%	15%
Pantothenic Acid 10 mg	100%	100%
Calcium 108 mg	7%	11%
Iron 18 mg	90%	100%
Phosphorus 50 mg	3%	5%
Iodine 150 mcg	107%	100%
Magnesium 40 mg	10%	10%
Zinc 15 mg	94%	100%
Copper 2 mg	100%	100%
Manganese 1 mg	*	50%
Chromium 20 mcg	*	17%
Molybdenum 20 mcg	*	27%

*Daily Value (%DV) not established.
+Percent Daily Values based on a 2,000 calorie diet.

Warnings: Accidental overdose of iron-containing products is a leading cause of fatal poisoning in children under 6. Keep this product out of reach of children. In case of accidental overdose, call a doctor or poison control center immediately. **CONTAINS ASPARTAME.**
** PHENYLKETONURICS: CONTAINS PHENYLALANINE.

Storage: Store at room temperature. Keep bottle tightly closed. Bottle sealed with printed foil under cap. Do not use if foil is torn.

How Supplied: Assorted Flavors— Uncoated Tablet—Bottle of 60 tablets **Also available as: Centrum® Kids™ + Extra C** (250 mg); and as: **Centrum® Kids™ + Extra Calcium** (200 mg). Marketed by: Wyeth Consumer Healthcare, Madison, NJ 07940

CENTRUM® PERFORMANCE COMPLETE MULTIVITAMIN-MULTIMINERAL SUPPLEMENT Tablets

Supplement Facts
Serving Size 1 Tablet

Each Tablet Contains	%DV
Vitamin A 3500 IU (29% as Beta Carotene)	70%
Vitamin C 120 mg	200%
Vitamin D 400 IU	100%
Vitamin E 60 IU	200%
Vitamin K 25 mcg	31%
Thiamin 4.5 mg	300%
Riboflavin 5.1 mg	300%
Niacin 40 mg	200%
Vitamin B_6 6 mg	300%
Folic Acid 400 mcg	100%
Vitamin B_{12} 18 mcg	300%
Biotin 40 mcg	13%
Pantothenic Acid 10 mg	100%
Calcium 100 mg	10%
Iron 18 mg	100%
Phosphorus 48 mg	5%
Iodine 150 mcg	100%
Magnesium 40 mg	10%
Zinc 15 mg	100%
Selenium 70 mcg	100%
Copper 2 mg	100%
Manganese 4 mg	200%
Chromium 120 mcg	100%
Molybdenum 75 mcg	100%
Chloride 72 mg	2%
Potassium 80 mg	2%
Ginseng Root (*Panax ginseng*) 50 mg Standardized Extract	*
Ginkgo Biloba Leaf (*Ginkgo biloba*) 60 mg Standardized Extract	*
Boron 60 mcg	*
Nickel 5 mcg	*
Silicon 4 mg	*
Tin 10 mcg	*
Vanadium 10 mcg	*

*Daily Value (%DV) not established.

Ingredients: Dibasic Calcium Phosphate, Potassium Chloride, Ascorbic Acid (Vit. C), Microcrystalline Cellulose, Calcium Carbonate, dl-Alpha Tocopheryl Acetate (Vit. E), Magnesium Oxide, Ginkgo Biloba Leaf (*Ginkgo biloba*) Standardized Extract, Gelatin, Ginseng Root (*Panax ginseng*) Standardized Extract, Ferrous Fumarate, Niacinamide, Crospovidone, Starch. **Contains less than 2% of the following:** Acacia Senegal Gum, Beta Carotene, Biotin, Butylated Hydroxytoluene, Calcium Pantothenate, Chromic Chloride, Citric Acid, Cupric Oxide, Cyanocobalamin (Vit. B_{12}), Ergocalciferol (Vit. D), FD&C Red No. 40 Aluminum Lake, FD&C Yellow No. 6 Aluminum Lake, Folic Acid, Glucose, Hypromellose, Lactose Monohydrate, Magnesium Borate, Magnesium Stearate, Manganese Sulfate, Nickelous Sulfate, Phytonadione (Vit.K), Polyethylene Glycol, Polysorbate 80, Potassium Iodide, Potassium Sorbate, Purified Water, Pyridoxine Hydrochloride (Vit. B_6), Riboflavin (Vit. B_2), Silicon Dioxide, Sodium Ascorbate, Sodium Benzoate, Sodium Borate, Sodium Citrate, Sodium Metavanadate, Sodium Molybdate, Sodium Selenate, Sodium Silicoaluminate, Sorbic Acid, Stannous Chloride, Sucrose, Thiamin Mononitrate (Vit. B_1), Titanium Dioxide, Tocopherol, Tribasic Calcium Phosphate, Vitamin A Acetate (Vit. A), Zinc Oxide. **May also contain:** Maltodextrin.

Suggested Use: Adults—One tablet daily with food. Not formulated for use in children.

Warning: Accidental overdose of iron-containing products is a leading cause of fatal poisoning in children under 6. Keep this product out of reach of children. In case of accidental overdose, call a doctor or poison control center immediately.

Precaution: As with any supplement, if you are taking a prescription medication, or if you are pregnant or nursing a baby, contact your physician before using this product.

Important Information: Long-term intake of high levels of vitamin A (excluding that sourced from beta-carotene) may increase the risk of osteoporosis in postmenopausal women. Do not take this product if taking other vitamin A supplements.
Store at room temperature. Keep bottle tightly closed. Bottle sealed with printed foil under cap. Do not use if foil is torn.

How Supplied: Bottles of 45, 75 and 120 Tablets.

CENTRUM® SILVER®
Multivitamin/Multimineral Dietary Supplement for Adults 50+ From A to Zinc®

Supplement Facts
Serving Size 1 Tablet

Each Tablet Contains	% DV
Vitamin A 3500 IU (29% as Beta Carotene)	70%
Vitamin C 60 mg	100%
Vitamin D 400 IU	100%
Vitamin E 45 IU	150%
Vitamin K 10 mcg	13%
Thiamin 1.5 mg	100%
Riboflavin 1.7 mg	100%
Niacin 20 mg	100%
Vitamin B_6 3 mg	150%
Folic Acid 400 mcg	100%
Vitamin B_{12} 25 mcg	417%
Biotin 30 mcg	10%
Pantothenic Acid 10 mg	100%
Calcium 200 mg	20%
Phosphorus 48 mg	5%
Iodine 150 mcg	100%
Magnesium 100 mg	25%
Zinc 15 mg	100%
Selenium 20 mcg	29%
Copper 2 mg	100%
Manganese 2 mg	100%
Chromium 150 mcg	125%
Molybdenum 75 mcg	100%
Chloride 72 mg	2%
Potassium 80 mg	2%
Boron 150 mcg	*
Nickel 5 mcg	*
Silicon 2 mg	*
Vanadium 10 mcg	*
Lutein 250 mcg	*
Lycopene 300 mcg	*

*Daily Value (%DV) not established.

Ingredients: Calcium Carbonate, Dibasic Calcium Phosphate, Magnesium Oxide, Potassium Chloride, Microcrystalline Cellulose, Ascorbic Acid (Vit. C), dl-Alpha Tocopheryl Acetate (Vit. E), Gelatin, Pregelatinized Starch, Crospovidone. **Contains less than 2% of the following:** Acacia Senegal Gum, Ascorbyl Palmitate, Beta Carotene, Biotin, Boron, Butylated Hydroxytoluene, Calcium Pantothenate, Chromic Chloride, Citric Acid, Colloidal Silicon Dioxide, Cupric Oxide, Cyanocobalamin (Vit. B_{12}), Ergo-

Continued on next page

Centrum Silver—Cont.

calciferol (Vit. D), FD&C Blue No. 2 Aluminum Lake, FD&C Red No. 40 Aluminum Lake, FD&C Yellow No. 6 Aluminum Lake, Folic Acid, Hypromellose, Lutein, Lycopene, Magnesium Stearate, Manganese Sulfate, Niacinamide, Nickelous Sulfate, Phytonadione (Vit. K), Polysorbate 80, Potassium Iodide, Potassium Sorbate, Purified Water, Pyridoxine Hydrochloride (Vit. B$_6$), Riboflavin (Vit. B$_2$), Silicon Dioxide, Sodium Ascorbate, Sodium Benzoate, Sodium Citrate, Sodium Metavanadate, Sodium Molybdate, Sodium Selenate, Sodium Silicoaluminate, Sorbic Acid, Starch, Sucrose, Thiamine Mononitrate (Vit. B$_1$), Titanium Dioxide, Tocopherol, Tribasic Calcium Phosphate, Triethyl Citrate, Vitamin A Acetate (Vit. A), Zinc Oxide. **May also contain:** Calcium Stearate, Glucose, Lactose Monohydrate.

Recommended Intake:

Adults, 1 tablet daily with food. Not formulated for use in children.

Warnings: Keep out of the reach of children. As with any supplement, if you are pregnant or nursing a baby, contact your healthcare professional.

Important Information: Long-term intake of high levels of vitamin A (excluding that sourced from beta-carotene) may increase the risk of osteoporosis in postmenopausal women. Do not take this product if taking other vitamin A supplements.

How Supplied: Bottles of 60, 100, 150, and 220 tablets

Storage: Store at Room Temperature. Keep bottle tightly closed. Bottle is sealed with printed foil under cap. Do not use if foil is torn.

YOUNGEVITY, INC.
The Anti-Aging Company

**3100 EAST PLANO PARKWAY
PLANO, TX 75074**

Direct Inquiries to:

Website: www.youngevity.com
eMail: asd@youngevity.com
Corporate Fax: 972-404-3067
Corporate Tel: 972-239-6864 ext. 108

Our Anti-Aging, Life-Changing Products Are Manufactured to Pharmaceutical Standards

The Anti-Aging Daily Premium Pak: contains 60 Packets. Each Packet contains: 3 Capsules of Daily Premium Multiple, 1 Capsule of Super Anti-Oxidant Complex, 1 Capsule of Super Cell Protector, 1 Soft Gel Capsule of EFA Complex with CoQ10, 1 Capsule of Concentrated Fruits & Vegetables and 1 Capsule of Bone Building Formula. The strongest, most complete, multi-vitamin, multi-mineral and herbal supplement on the market. Youngevity's Best Product to provide for a high energy level, boost Immunity System and slow down the aging process.

Every Capsule Contains Our Patented Anti-Aging Chelated Miracle Minerals:

Proprietary Blend: Potassium, Calcium, Magnesium, Zinc, Chromium, Selenium, Iron, Copper, Molybdenum, Vanadium, Iodine, Cobalt and Manganese.

ANTI-AGING DAILY PREMIUM PAK
The Ultimate Anti-Aging Program

Each Packet Contains:

**DAILY PREMIUM MULTIPLE
3 Capsules in Packet**

28 Anti-Aging Proprietary Complex Anti-Oxidants, Synergistic Vitamins, Synergistic Herbs & Digestive Enzymes

**SUPER ANTI-OXIDANT COMPLEX
1 Capsule in Packet**

**SUPER ANTI-OXIDANT CELL PRTCTR
1 Capsule in Packet**
Grape Seed Extract
1 Super Anti-Oxidant Cell Protector
11 Anti-Oxidant Actives

**ESSENTIAL FATTY ACIDS COMPLEX WITH CoQ10
1 Soft Gel Capsule in Packet**
Flaxseed, Evening Primrose, Borage, Marine Lipids, Omega-3, 6 and 9 Fatty Acids, CoQ10

**FRUITS & VEGETABLES
1 Capsule in Packet
Live Food Enzymes**
7 Anti-Aging Green Foods
8 Anti-Aging Fruits & Bio-Factors
6 Anti-Aging Live Plant Enzymes

**BONE BUILDING FORMULA
1 Capsule in Packet**
Building and Maintaining Bone Mass
4 Bone Building Structural Minerals:
3 Anti-Aging Activators
[See table below and at top of next page]

Supplement Facts:
Serving Size: 1 Packet (7 Capsules & 1 Softgel)
Servings Per Container: 60

Amount Per Serving			% Daily Value*
Vitamin A (as beta carotene, retinyl palmitate)	11250	I.U.	225%
Vitamin C (as calcium ascorbate)	575	mg	958%
Vitamin D (as cholecalciferol)	400	I.U.	100%
Vitamin E (as d-alpha tocopheryl succinate)	130	I.U.	433%
Vitamin K (as phytonadione)	3	mcg	4%
Vitamin B1 (as thiamine mononitrate)	9	mg	600%
Vitamin B2 (as riboflavin)	9	mg	529%
Vitamin B3 (as niacinamide)	15	mg	75%
Vitamin B6 (as pyridoxine hydrochloride)	9	mg	450%
Vitamin B9 (as folic acid)	300	mcg	75%
Vitamin B12 (as cyanocobalamin)	6	mcg	100%
Vitamin H (as biotin)	375	mcg	125%
Vitamin B5 (as d-calcium pantothenate)	9	mg	90%
Calcium (as ascorbate, carbonate, amino acid chelate, propionate)	202	mg	20%
Iron (as amino acid chelate)	7.5	mg	42%
Iodine (as potassium iodide)	75	mcg	50%
Magnesium (as magnesium oxide, amino acid chelate)	80	mg	20%
Zinc (as amino acid chelate)	7.5	mg	50%
Selenium (as amino acid chelate)	35	mcg	50%
Copper (as amino acid chelate)	0.75	mg	38%
Manganese (as amino acid chelate)	1	mg	50%
Chromium (as amino acid chelate)	60	mcg	50%
Molybdenum (as amino acid chelate)	37.5	mcg	50%
Patented Chelated Anti-Aging Miracle Minerals™ The Vilcabamba Mineral Essence® Proprietary Blend—Potassium,† Calcium, Magnesium, Zinc, Chromium, Selenium, Iron, Copper, Molybdenum, Vanadium,† Iodine, Cobalt,† Manganese	500	mg	**
Organic Flaxseed Oil	205	mg	**
Omega-3 (from evening primrose oil, borage oil, organic flaxseed oil, marine lipid oil)	154	mg	**
Omega-6 (from evening primrose oil, borage oil, organic flaxseed oil, marine lipid oil)	128	mg	**
Evening Primrose Oil	100	mg	**
Borage Oil	100	mg	**
Marine Lipid Oil	95	mg	**
Grape Seed Extract (standardized to provide 75.05mg proanthocyanidins) (Vitis vinifera) (seed)	79	mg	**

(Table continued on next page)

Supplement Facts: *(cont.)*
Serving Size: 1 Packet (7 Capsules & 1 Softgel)
Servings Per Container: 60

Amount Per Serving			% Daily Value*
Omega-9 (from evening primrose oil, borage oil, organic flaxseed oil, marine lipid oil)	59	mg	**
Rose Hips *(Rosa Canina)*(fruit)	43.33	mg	**
Broccoli *(Brassica oleracea v. botrytis)* (florets)	35	mg	**
Garlic *(Allium sativum)*(clove)	35	mg	**
Barley Grass *(Hordeum vulgare)* (young grass)	35	mg	**
Beet Juice Powder *(Beta vulgaris)* (root)	35	mg	**
Carrot Powder *(Daucus carota)*(fresh carrots)	35	mg	**
Papaya *(Carrica papaya)*(leaf)	35	mg	**
Pineapple Extract *(Ananas comosus)* (fruit)	35	mg	**
Wheat Grass *(Triticum aestivum)* (organic)	35	mg	**
Quercetin	34	mg	**
Alpha Lipoic Acid	29	mg	**
Apple Pectin *(Malus sylvestris)*	26	mg	**
Hesperidin Complex	25	mg	**
Rutin *(Sophora japonica)*	25	mg	**
Milk Thistle Extract (standardized to provide 19.2mg silymarin) *(Silyburn marianum)* (fruit)	24	mg	**
Lactobacillus Acidophilus	20	mg	**
Parsley *(Petroselinum crispum)* (aerial parts)	20	mg	**
Horsetail *(Equisetum majus)*(aerial parts)	20	mg	**
Plant Enzyme Blend	19	mg	**
Hawthorn *(Crataegus oxycantha)* (berry & leaf)	15	mg	**
Turmeric Extract *(Curcuma longa)* (rhizome)	15	mg	**
Ginkgo Biloba Extract (standardized to provide 3.6mg flavonglycosides and 0.9mg terpenes) *(Ginkgo biloba)*(leaf)	15	mg	**
Carnitine (as acetyl L-carnitine)	10	mg	**
Flavones (from citrus bioflavoniod complex) (Citrus species) (peel)	9	mg	**
Choline Bitartrate	3	mg	**
Soy Isoflavones *(Glycine max)*(seed)	1.6	mg	**
Lycopene (from tomato extract) *(Lycopersicum esculentum)* (fruit)	1.375	mg	**
Lutein (crystalline lutein) (from marigold flowers)	0.375	mg	**
Boron (as amino acid chelate)	0.2	mg	**
Vanadium (as vanadyl sulfate)	1	mcg	**

* Percent Daily Values are based on a 2,000 calorie diet
** Daily Value Not Established
†Contains less than 2% of the Daily Value of these Nutrients

Other Ingredients: Gelatin, glycerin, water, yellow beeswax, rice flour, micro- crystalline cellulose, magnesium stearate (vegetable source), silicon dioxide.

Directions: Take 1–3 Paks Daily, one after each meal

How Supplied: 30 or 60 Paks Per Box

PREMIUM HAWAIIAN NONI JUICE

WITH PATENTED ANTI-AGING CHELATED MIRACLE MINERALS:

Proprietary Blend: Potassium, Calcium, Magnesium, Zinc, Chromium, Selenium, Iron, Copper, Molybdenum, Vanadium, Iodine, Cobalt and Manganese

THE WELLNESS DRINK FOR THE WHOLE FAMILY

Noni is a fruit that is grown in Hawaii. For 2000 years it has been used for its "Miraculous Benefits" and is considered sacred by Hawaiians.

Suggested Serving Size: 1 oz.–2 oz.

Ingredients: Premium Grade Hawaiian Noni in Purified Water, Natural Pineapple Flavor, Glycerin, Citric Acid, Xanthan Gum, Potassium Sorbate & Sodium Benzoate (To preserve freshness), and The Vilcabamba Mineral Essence® (Potassium, Calcium, Magnesium, Zinc, Chromium, Selenium, Iron, Copper, Molybdenum, Vanadium, Iodine, Cobalt and Manganese).

Directions: Drink 1 oz.–2 ozs. several times a day, preferably on an empty stomach

How Supplied: 32 oz. Bottle

DRUG INFORMATION CENTERS

Drug information centers are strategically located throughout the nation to provide additional information on overdosage, adverse reactions, drug interactions, and any other medication problem. Use the following directory to find the center nearest you. Listings are alphabetical by state and city.

ALABAMA

BIRMINGHAM

Drug Information Service
University of Alabama
UAB Hospital Pharmacy
Drug Information-JT1720
619 S. 19th St.
Birmingham, AL 35249-6860
Mon.-Fri. 8 AM-5 PM
    205-934-2162
Fax: 205-934-3501
www.health.uab.edu/
pharmacy

Global Drug
Information Service
Samford University
McWhorter School
of Pharmacy
800 Lakeshore Dr.
Birmingham, AL 35229-7027
Mon.-Fri. 8 AM-4:30 PM
    205-726-2659
Fax: 205-726-4012
www.samford.edu

HUNTSVILLE

Huntsville Hospital Drug
Information Center
101 Sivley Rd.
Huntsville, AL 35801
Mon.-Fri. 8 AM-5 PM
    256-517-8288
Fax: 256-517-6558

ARIZONA

TUCSON

Arizona Poison and Drug
Information Center
Arizona Health
Sciences Center
University Medical Center
1501 N. Campbell Ave.
Room 1156
Tucson, AZ 85724
7 days/week, 24 hours
    520-626-6016
    800-362-0101 (AZ)
Fax: 520-626-2720
www.pharmacy.arizona.edu

ARKANSAS

LITTLE ROCK

Arkansas Poison and Drug
Information Center
4301 West Markham St.
Slot 522-2
Little Rock, AR 72205
Mon.-Fri. 8:30 AM-5 PM
    501-686-5072
    (for healthcare
    professionals only)
    800-228-1233
    (AR only - for health-
    care professionals
    only)
Fax: 501-686-7357

CALIFORNIA

LOS ANGELES

Los Angeles Regional
Drug Information Center
LAC & USC Medical Center
1200 N. State St.
Trailer 25
Los Angeles, CA 90033
Mon.-Fri. 8 AM-4:30 PM
    323-226-7741
Fax: 323-226-4194

MARTINEZ

Drug Information Service
VA Northern California
Health Care System
Pharmacy Service 119
150 Muir Rd.
Martinez, CA 94553
Mon.-Fri. 8 PM-4:30 PM
    925-372-2000 x2167
Fax: 925-372-2169
cherie.dillon@med.va.gov

Drug Information Service
University of California
San Diego Medical Center
200 West Arbor Dr.
MC 8925
San Diego, CA 92103-8925
Mon.-Fri. 9 AM-5 PM
    900-288-8273
Fax: 858-715-6361

SAN FRANCISCO

Drug Information Analysis
Service, University of
California, San Francisco
521 Parnassus Ave.
Room C152
San Francisco, CA
94143-0622
Mon.-Fri. 8:30 AM-4:30 PM
    415-502-9540
    (for healthcare
    professionals only)
Fax: 415-502-0792
E-mail: DIAS@itsa.ucsf.edu

STANFORD

Drug Information Center
University of California
Stanford Hospital and
Clinics
300 Pasteur Dr.
Room H-0301
Stanford, CA 94305
Mon.-Fri. 8 AM-4 PM
    650-723-6422
Fax: 650-725-5028

COLORADO

DENVER

Rocky Mountain Poison
and Drug Consultation
Center
1001 Yosemite St.
Denver, CO 80230
7 days/week, 24 hours
    303-893-3784
    (For Denver County
    residents only)
Fax: 303-739-1119
www.rmpdc.org

Drug Information Center
University of Colorado
Health Science Center
School of Pharmacy
4200 E. 9th Ave., Box C239
Denver, CO 80262
Mon.-Fri. 8:30 AM-4:30 PM
    303-315-8489
Fax: 303-315-3353

CONNECTICUT

FARMINGTON

Drug Information Service
University of Connecticut
Health Center
263 Farmington Ave.
Farmington, CT 06030
Mon.-Fri. 7:30 AM-4 PM
    860-679-2783
Fax: 860-679-1231
E-mail: badore@uchc.edu

HARTFORD

Drug Information Center
Hartford Hospital
P.O. Box 5037
80 Seymour St.
Hartford, CT 06102
Mon.-Fri. 8:30 AM-5 PM
    860-545-2221
    860-545-2961
    (After 5 PM)
Fax: 860-545-4371
www.harthosp.org

NEW HAVEN

Drug Information Center
Yale-New Haven Hospital
20 York St.
New Haven, CT 06504
Mon.-Fri. 8:30 AM-5 PM
    203-688-2248
Fax: 203-688-3691
www.ynhh.com

DISTRICT OF COLUMBIA

Drug Information Service
Howard University Hospital
Room BB06
2041 Georgia Ave. NW
Washington, DC 20060
Mon.-Fri. 8 AM-4 PM
    202-865-1325
    202-865-7413
Fax: 202-865-7410

FLORIDA

FT. LAUDERDALE

Nova Southeastern University College of Pharmacy Drug Information Center
3200 S. University Dr.
Ft. Lauderdale, FL 33328
Mon.-Fri. 9 AM-5 PM
    954-262-3103
Fax: 954-262-3170
www.pharmacy.nova.edu

GAINESVILLE

Drug Information & Pharmacy Resource Center SHANDS Hospital at University of Florida
P.O. Box 100316
Gainesville, FL 32610-0316
Mon.-Fri. 9 AM-5 PM
    352-265-0408
    (for healthcare professionals only)
Fax: 352-338-9860
www.cop.ufl.edu/vdis

JACKSONVILLE

Drug Information Service SHANDS Jacksonville
655 W. 8th St.
Jacksonville, FL 32209
Mon.-Fri. 8:30 AM-5 PM
    904-244-4185
    (for healthcare professionals only)
    904-244-4700
    (for consumers,
    Mon.-Fri. 9 AM-4 PM)
Fax: 904-244-4272

ORLANDO

Orlando Regional Drug Information Service Orlando Regional Healthcare System
1414 Kuhl Ave., MP 192
Orlando, FL 32806
Mon.-Fri. 8 AM-4 PM
    321-841-8717
Fax: 407-649-1827
E-mail: druginfo@orhs.org

TALLAHASSEE

Drug Information Education Center Florida Agricultural and Mechanical University College of Pharmacy
Tallahassee, FL 32307
Mon.-Fri. 9 AM-5 PM
    850-488-5239
    850-599-3064
    800-451-3181
Fax: 850-412-7020
www.pharmacy.samu.edu

WEST PALM BEACH

Drug Information Center Nova Southeastern University - West Palm Beach
3970 RCA Blvd., Suite 7006A
Palm Beach Gardens, FL 33410
Mon.-Fri. 9 AM-5 PM
    561-622-0658
    (for healthcare professionals only)
Fax: 561-627-0972

GEORGIA

ATLANTA

Emory University Hospital Dept. of Pharmaceutical Services-Drug Information
1364 Clifton Rd. NE
Atlanta, GA 30322
Mon.-Fri. 8:30 AM-5 PM
    404-712-7150
    (for healthcare professionals only)
Fax: 404-712-7577

Drug Information Service Northside Hospital
1000 Johnson Ferry Rd. NE
Atlanta, GA 30342
Mon.-Fri. 9 AM-4 PM
    404-851-8676
    (GA only)
Fax: 404-851-8610

AUGUSTA

Drug Information Center Medical College of Georgia Hospital and Clinic
BI2101
1120 15th St.
Augusta, GA 30912
Mon.-Fri. 8:30 AM-5 PM
    706-721-2887
Fax: 706-721-3827

COLUMBUS

Columbus Regional Drug Information Center
710 Center St.
Columbus, GA 31902
Mon.-Fri. 8 AM-5 PM
    706-571-1934
    (for healthcare professionals only)
Fax: 706-571-1625

IDAHO

POCATELLO

Drug Information Center Idaho State University School of Pharmacy
Campus Box 8092
Pocatello, ID 83209
Mon.-Thur. 8:30 AM-5 PM
Fri. 8:30 AM-2:30 PM
    208-282-4689
    800-334-7139
    (ID only)
Fax: 208-282-3003
http://rx.isu.edu/services_contacts/idis/

ILLINOIS

CHICAGO

Drug Information Center Northwestern Memorial Hospital
251 E. Huron
Feinberg LC-700B
Chicago, IL 60611
Mon.-Fri. 8 AM-5 PM
    312-926-7573
Fax: 312-926-7956

Drug Information Services University of Chicago Hospitals
5841 S. Maryland Ave.
MC 0010
Chicago, IL 60637-1470
Mon.-Fri. 8 AM-5 PM
    773-702-1388
Fax: 773-702-6631

Drug Information Center University of Illinois at Chicago
833 S. Wood St.
MC 886
Chicago, IL 60612
Mon.-Fri. 8 AM-4 PM
    312-996-3681
Fax: 312-996-0448
www.uic.edu/pharmacy/services/di/index.html

HARVEY

Drug Information Center Ingalls Memorial Hospital
1 Ingalls Dr.
Harvey, IL 60426
Mon.-Fri. 8 AM-4:30 PM
    708-915-4430
Fax: 708-915-3108

HINES

Drug Information Service Hines Veterans Administration Hospital
Pharmacy Services
MC119
P.O. Box 5000
Hines, IL 60141-5000
Mon.-Fri. 8 AM-4:30 PM
    708-202-8387,
    ext. 23780
Fax: 708-202-2675

PARK RIDGE

Drug Information Center Lutheran General Hospital
1775 Dempster St.
Park Ridge, IL 60068
Mon.-Fri. 7:30 AM-4 PM
    847-723-8128
    (for healthcare professionals only)
Fax: 847-723-2326

INDIANA

INDIANAPOLIS

Drug Information Center St. Vincent Hospital and Health Services
2001 W. 86th St.
Indianapolis, IN 46260
Mon.-Fri. 8 AM-4 PM
    317-338-3200
    (for healthcare professionals only)
Fax: 317-338-3041

Drug Information Service Clarian Health Partners
Pharmacy Department I-65 at 21st
Room CG04
Indianapolis, IN 46202
Mon.-Fri. 8 AM-4:30 PM
    317-962-1750
Fax: 317-962-1756

MUNCIE

Drug Information Center Ball Memorial Hospital
2401 University Ave.
Muncie, IN 47303
7 days/week, 24 hours
    765-747-3035
Fax: 765-751-2522
E-mail:
kwolfe@chs.cami3.com

IOWA

DES MOINES

**Regional Drug
Information Center
Mercy Medical Center-
Des Moines**
1111 Sixth Ave.
Des Moines, IA 50314
Mon.-Fri. 8 AM-4:30 PM
    515-247-3286
    (7 days/week,
    24 hours)
Fax: 515-247-3966

IOWA CITY

**Drug Information Center
University of Iowa
Hospitals and Clinics**
200 Hawkins Dr.
Iowa City, IA 52242
Mon.-Fri. 8 AM-4:30 PM
    319-356-2600
    **(for healthcare
    professionals only)**
Fax: 319-384-8840

KANSAS

KANSAS CITY

**Drug Information Center
University of Kansas
Medical Center**
3901 Rainbow Blvd.
Kansas City, KS 66160
Mon.-Fri. 8:30 AM-4:30 PM
    913-588-2328
    **(for healthcare
    professionals only)**
Fax: 913-588-2350
E-mail: druginfo@kumc.edu

KENTUCKY

LEXINGTON

**Drug Information Center
Chandler Medical Center
College of Pharmacy
University of Kentucky**
800 Rose St., C-117
Lexington, KY 40536-0293
Mon.-Fri. 8 AM-5 PM
    859-323-5320
Fax: 859-323-2049
E-mail: cgwhit1@uky.edu

LOUISIANA

MONROE

**Louisiana Drug and Poison
Information Center
University of Louisiana at
Monroe College of
Pharmacy**
Monroe, LA 71209-6430
Mon.-Fri. 8 AM-4:30 PM
    318-342-1710
Fax: 318-342-1744
E-mail: wross@ulm.edu

NEW ORLEANS

**Xavier University Drug
Information Center
Tulane University
Hospital and Clinic**
Box HC12
1415 Tulane Ave.
New Orleans, LA 70112
Mon.-Fri. 9 AM-5 PM
    504-588-5670
Fax: 504-588-5862
E-mail:
mharris6@tulane.edu

MARYLAND

ANDREWS AFB

Drug Information Services
89 MDTS/SGQP
1050 W. Perimeter Rd.
Suite D1-119
Andrews AFB, MD
20762-6660
Mon.-Fri. 7:30 AM-5 PM
    240-857-4565
Fax: 240-857-8892

ANNAPOLIS

**The Anne Arundel
Medical Center
Dept. of Pharmacy**
64 Franklin St.
Annapolis, MD 21401
7 days/week, 24 hours
    443-481-4155
    443-481-1000
    (switchboard)
Fax: 443-481-4844
www.aahs.org

BALTIMORE

**Drug Information Service
Johns Hopkins Hospital**
600 N. Wolfe St.,
Halsted 503
Baltimore, MD 21287-6180
Mon.-Fri. 8:30 AM-5 PM
    410-955-6348
Fax: 410-955-8283

**Drug Information Service
University of Maryland
School of Pharmacy**
Pharmacy Hall Room 760
20 North Pine St.
Baltimore, MD 21201
Mon.-Fri. 8:30 AM-5 PM
    410-706-7568
    (consumers only)
    410-706-0898
    **(for healthcare
    professionals only)**
Fax: 410-706-0754
www.pharmacy.umaryland.
edu/umdi

BETHESDA

**Drug Information Service
National Institutes of
Health**
Building 10, Room 1S-259
10 Center Dr. (MSC1196)
Bethesda, MD 20892-1196
Mon.-Fri. 8:30 AM-5 PM
    301-496-2407
Fax: 301-496-0210
www.cc.nih.gov/phar

EASTON

**Drug Information
Pharmacy Dept.
Memorial Hospital**
219 S. Washington St.
Easton, MD 21601
7 days/week, 7 AM-5:30 PM
    410-822-1000,
    ext. 5645
Fax: 410-820-9489

MASSACHUSETTS

BOSTON

**Drug Information Services
Brigham and Women's
Hospital**
75 Francis St.
Boston, MA 02115
Mon.-Fri. 7 AM-3:30 PM
    617-732-7166
Fax: 617-566-2396

WORCESTER

**Drug Information Center
UMass Memorial
Healthcare Hospital**
55 Lake Ave. North
Worcester, MA 01655
Mon.-Fri. 8:30 AM-5 PM
    508-856-3456
    508-856-2775
    (24 hour)
Fax: 508-856-1850

MICHIGAN

ANN ARBOR

**Drug Information and
Pharmacy Services
University of Michigan
Health System**
1500 East Medical
Center Dr.
UHB2 D301 Box 0008
Ann Arbor, MI 48109-0008
Mon.-Fri. 8 AM-5 PM
    734-936-8200
Fax: 734-936-7027
www.pharm.med.edu/
public

DETROIT

**Drug Information Center
Department of Pharmacy
Services, Detroit Receiving
Hospital and University
Health Center**
4201 St. Antoine Blvd.
Detroit, MI 48201
Mon.-Fri. 9 AM-5 PM
    313-745-4556
Fax: 313-993-2522
www.dmcpharmacy.org

LANSING

**Drug Information Services
Sparrow Hospital**
1215 East Michigan Ave.
Lansing, MI 48912
7 days/week, 24 hours
    517-364-2444
Fax: 517-364-2088

PONTIAC

**Drug Information Center
St. Joseph Mercy Hospital**
44405 Woodward Ave.
Pontiac, MI 48341
Mon.-Fri. 8 AM-4:30 PM
    248-858-3055
Fax: 248-858-3010

ROYAL OAK

**Drug Information Services
William Beaumont Hospital**
3601 West 13 Mile Rd.
Royal Oak, MI 48073-6769
Mon.-Fri. 8 AM-4:30 PM
    248-551-4077
Fax: 248-551-3301

SOUTHFIELD

**Drug Information Service
Providence Hospital**
16001 West 9 Mile Rd.
Southfield, MI 48075
Mon.-Fri. 8 AM-4 PM
    248-849-3125
Fax: 248-849-5364

MISSISSIPPI

JACKSON

**Drug Information Center
University of Mississippi
Medical Center**
2500 N. State St.
Jackson, MS 39216
Mon.-Fri. 8 AM-4:30 PM
    601-984-2060
Fax: 601-984-2064

MISSOURI

KANSAS CITY
University of Missouri-Kansas City Drug Information Center
2411 Holmes St., MG-200
Kansas City, MO
64108-2792
Mon.-Fri. 8 AM-5 PM
816-235-5490
Fax: 816-235-5491
www.umkc.edu/druginfo

SPRINGFIELD
Drug Information Center St. Johns Regional Health Center
1235 E. Cherokee St.
Springfield, MO 65804
Mon.-Fri. 7:30 AM-4:30 PM
417-885-3488
Fax: 417-888-7788
E-mail:
tbarks@sprg.smhs.com

ST. JOSEPH
Drug Information Service Heartland Hospital West
801 Faraon St.
St. Joseph, MO 64501
Mon.-Fri. 9 AM-5:30 PM
816-271-7582
Fax: 816-271-7590

MONTANA

MISSOULA
Drug Information Service University of Montana School of Pharmacy and Allied Health Sciences
Missoula, MT 59812-1522
Mon.-Fri. 8 AM-5 PM
406-243-5254
Fax: 406-243-5256
www.umt.edu/druginfo
E-mail:
druginfo@selway.umt.edu

NEBRASKA

OMAHA
Drug Informatics Service School of Pharmacy Creighton University
2500 California Plaza
Omaha, NE 68178
Mon.-Fri. 8:30 AM-5:00 PM
402-280-5101
Fax: 402-280-5149
www.druginfo.creighton.edu

NEW JERSEY

NEWARK
New Jersey Poison Information and Education System
65 Bergen St.
Newark, NJ 07107
7 days/week, 24 hours
973-972-9280
800-222-1222
(poison control)
Fax: 973-643-2679
www.njpies.org
E-mail: bruck@njpies.org

NEW BRUNSWICK
Drug Information Service Robert Wood Johnson University Hospital
Pharmacy Department
1 Robert Wood Johnson Pl.
New Brunswick, NJ 08901
Mon.-Fri. 8:30 AM-4:30 PM
732-937-8842
Fax: 732-937-8584

NEW MEXICO

ALBUQUERQUE
New Mexico Poison & Drug Information Center University of New Mexico Health Sciences Center
Albuquerque, NM 87131
7 days/week, 24 hours
505-272-2222
800-222-1222
(NM only)
Fax: 505-272-5892
http://hsc.unm.edu/
pharmacy/poison

NEW YORK

BROOKLYN
International Drug Information Center Long Island University Arnold & Marie Schwartz College of Pharmacy & Health Sciences
1 University Plaza
RM-HS509
75 Dekalb Ave.
Brooklyn, NY 11201
Mon.-Fri. 9 AM-5 PM
718-488-1064
Fax: 718-780-4056
www.liu.edu

Drug Information Center Brookdale University Hospital and Medical Center
1 Brookdale Plaza
Brooklyn, NY 11212
Mon.-Fri. 8 AM-4 PM
718-240-5993
Fax: 718-240-6606

COOPERSTOWN
Drug Information Center Bassett Healthcare
1 Atwell Rd.
Cooperstown, NY 13326
7 days/week, 24 hours
607-547-3686
Fax: 607-547-3629

NEW HYDE PARK
Drug Information Center St. Johns University at Long Island Jewish Medical Center
270-05 76th Ave.
New Hyde Park, NY 11040
Mon.-Fri. 8 AM-3 PM
718-470-DRUG (3784)
Fax: 718-470-1742

NEW YORK CITY
Drug Information Center Memorial Sloan-Kettering Cancer Center
1275 York Ave.
RM S-712
New York, NY 10021
Mon.-Fri. 9 AM-5 PM
212-639-7552
Fax: 212-639-2171

Drug Information Center Mount Sinai Medical Center
1 Gustave Levy Pl.
New York, NY 10029
Mon.-Fri. 9 AM-5 PM
212-241-6619
Fax: 212-348-7927

Drug Information Service New York Presbyterian Hospital
Room K04
525 E. 68th St.
New York, NY 10021
Mon.-Fri. 9 AM-5 PM
212-746-0741
Fax: 212-746-4434

ROCHESTER
Finger Lakes Poison and Drug Information Center University of Rochester
601 Elmwood Ave.
Rochester, NY 14642
7 days/week, 24 hours
585-275-3718

ROCKVILLE CENTER
Drug Information Center Mercy Medical Center
1000 North Village Ave.
Rockville Center, NY 11570
Mon.-Fri. 8 AM-4 PM
516-705-1053
Fax: 516-705-1071

NORTH CAROLINA

BUIES CREEK
Drug Information Center School of Pharmacy Campbell University
P.O. Box 1090
Buies Creek, NC 27506
Mon.-Fri. 8:30 AM-4:30 PM
910-893-1200 x2701
800-760-9697 x2701
800-327-5467
(NC only)
Fax: 910-893-1476
E-mail: dic@mailcenter.
campbell.edu

CHAPEL HILL
University of North Carolina Hospitals Drug Information Center
101 Manning Dr.
Chapel Hill, NC 27514
Mon.-Fri. 8 AM-4:30 PM
919-966-2373
Fax: 919-966-8480
E-mail:
jphilli2@unch.unc.edu

DURHAM
Drug Information Center Duke University Health Systems
DUMC Box 3089
Durham, NC 27710
Mon.-Fri. 8 AM-5 PM
919-684-5125
Fax: 919-681-3895

GREENVILLE
Eastern Carolina Drug Information Center Pitt County Memorial Hospital Dept. of Pharmacy Service
P.O. Box 6028
2100 Stantonsburg Rd.
Greenville, NC 27835
Mon.-Fri. 8 AM-5 PM
252-816-4257
Fax: 252-816-7425
E-mail:
rbshafer@pcmh.com

WINSTON-SALEM
Drug Information Service Center Wake-Forest University Baptist Medical Center
Medical Center Blvd.
Winston-Salem, NC 27157
Mon.-Fri. 8 AM-5 PM
336-716-2037
(for healthcare professionals only)
Fax: 336-716-2186

OHIO

ADA

**Drug Information Center
Raabe College of Pharmacy
Ohio Northern University**
Ada, OH 45810
Mon.-Fri. 9 AM-5 PM
419-772-2307
Fax: 419-772-2289
www.onu.edu/pharmacy/
druginfo

CINCINNATI

**Drug Information Center
Children's Hospital
Medical Center**
3333 Burnet Ave. ML9004
Cincinnati, OH 45229
Mon.-Fri. 9 AM-5 PM
513-636-5054
513-636-5111
(24 hour)
Fax: 513-636-5069

CLEVELAND

**Drug Information Service
Cleveland Clinic Foundation**
9500 Euclid Ave.
Cleveland, OH 44195
Mon.-Fri. 8:30 AM-4:30 PM
216-444-6456
**(for healthcare
professionals only)**
Fax: 216-444-6157

COLUMBUS

**Drug Information Center
Ohio State University
Hospital Dept. of Pharmacy**
Doan Hall 368
410 W. 10th Ave.
Columbus, OH 43210-1228
Mon.-Fri. 8 AM-4 PM
614-293-8679
Fax: 614-293-3264
E-mail: visconti-1@medctr.
osu.edu

**Drug Information Center
Riverside Methodist
Hospital**
3535 Olentangy River Road
Columbus, OH 43214
Mon.-Fri. 8:30 AM-4 PM
614-566-5425
Fax: 614-566-5850

TOLEDO

**Drug Information Services
St. Vincent Mercy Medical
Center**
2213 Cherry St.
Toledo, Ohio 43608-2691
Mon.-Fri. 8 AM-4 PM
419-251-4227
Fax: 419-251-3662
www.rx.medctr.ohio-
state.edu

OKLAHOMA

OKLAHOMA CITY

**Drug Information Service
Integris Health**
3300 Northwest Expressway
Oklahoma City, OK 73112
Mon.-Fri. 8 AM-4:30 PM
405-949-3660
Fax: 405-951-8274

**Drug Information Center
OU Medical Center
Presbyterian Tower**
700 NE 13th St.
Oklahoma City, OK 73104
Mon.-Fri. 8 AM-4:30 PM
405-271-6226
Fax: 405-271-6281

TULSA

**Drug Information Center
Saint Francis Hospital**
6161 S. Yale Ave.
Tulsa, OK 74136
Mon.-Fri. 8 AM-4 PM
918-494-6339
**(for healthcare
professionals only)**
Fax: 918-494-1893

PENNSYLVANIA

PHILADELPHIA

**Drug Information Center
Temple University Hospital
Dept. of Pharmacy**
3401 N. Broad St.
Philadelphia, PA 19140
Mon.-Fri. 8 AM-4:30 PM
215-707-4644
Fax: 215-707-3463

**Drug Information Service
Tenet Health System
Hahnemann University
Hospital Department of
Pharmacy**
MS 451
Broad and Vine Streets
Philadelphia, PA 19102
Mon.-Fri. 8 AM-4 PM
215-762-DRUG (3784)
**(for healthcare
professionals only)**
Fax: 215-762-7993

**Drug Information Service
Dept. of Pharmacy
Thomas Jefferson
University Hospital**
111 S. 11th St.
Philadelphia, PA 19107-5098
Mon.-Fri. 8 AM-5 PM
215-955-8877
Fax: 215-923-3316

**University of Pennsylvania
Health System Drug
Information Service
Hospital of the University
of Pennsylvania
Department of Pharmacy**
3400 Spruce St.
Philadelphia, PA 19104
Mon.-Fri. 8:30 AM-4 PM
215-662-2903
Fax: 215-662-4319

PITTSBURGH

**The Christopher and Nicole
Browett Pharmaceutical
Information Center
Mylan School of Pharmacy
Duquesne University**
431 Mellon Hall
Pittsburgh, PA 15282
Mon.-Fri. 8 AM-4 PM
412-396-4600
Fax: 412-396-4488

**Drug Information Center
University of Pittsburgh**
137 Victoria Hall
200 Lothrop St.
Pittsburgh, PA 15261
Mon.-Fri. 8:30 AM-4:30 PM
412-624-3784
**(for healthcare
professionals only)**
Fax: 412-624-6350
E-mail: druginfo@msx.
upmc.edu

UPLAND

**Drug Information Center
Crozer-Chester Medical
Center Dept. of Pharmacy**
1 Medical Center Blvd.
Upland, PA 19013
Mon.-Fri. 8 AM-4:30 PM
610-447-2851
610-447-2862
(after hours)
**(both numbers are
for healthcare
professionals only)**
Fax: 610-447-2820

WILLIAMSPORT

**Drug Information
Pharmacy Dept.
Susquehanna Health
System**
Rural Avenue Campus
Williamsport, PA 17701
7 days/week, 5 AM-Midnight
570-321-3083
Fax: 570-321-3230

PUERTO RICO

PONCE

**Centro Informacion
Medicamentos
Escuela de Medicina de
Ponce**
P.O. Box 7004
Ponce, PR 00732-7004
Mon.-Fri. 8 AM-4:30 PM
787-259-7085
(Spanish and English)
787-840-2575
(switchboard)
Fax: 787-842-0461

SAN JUAN

**Centro de Informacion de
Medicamentos-CIM
Escuela de Farmacia-RCM**
P.O. Box 365067
San Juan, PR 00936-5067
Mon.-Fri. 8 AM-4:30 PM
787-758-2525,
ext. 1516
Fax: 787-763-0196
E-mail: cimrcm@rcm.upr.edu

SOUTH CAROLINA

CHARLESTON

**Drug Information Service
Medical University of
South Carolina**
150 Ashley Ave.
Rutledge Tower
Annex, Room 604
P.O. Box 250584
Charleston, SC 29425-0810
Mon.-Fri. 9 AM-5:30 PM
843-792-3896
800-922-5250
Fax: 843-792-5532

COLUMBIA

**Drug Information Service
University of South Carolina
College of Pharmacy
University of South Carolina**
Columbia, SC 29208
Mon.-Fri. 8 AM-Midnight
803-777-7804
Fax: 803-777-6127
www.pharm.sc.edu

SPARTANBURG

**Drug Information Center
Spartanburg Regional
Medical Center**
101 E. Wood St.
Spartanburg, SC 29303
Mon.-Fri. 8 AM-5 PM
864-560-6910
Fax: 864-560-7323

TENNESSEE

KNOXVILLE

Drug Information Center
University of Tennessee
Medical Center at Knoxville
1924 Alcoa Highway
Knoxville, TN 37920-6999
Mon.-Fri. 8 AM-4:30 PM
    865-544-9124
Fax: 865-525-0326
    865-544-8242

MEMPHIS

South East Regional Drug
Information Center
VA Medical Center
1030 Jefferson Ave.
Memphis, TN 38104
Mon.-Fri. 6:30 AM-3 PM
    901-523-8990,
    ext. 6720
Fax: 901-577-7306

Drug Information Center
University of Tennessee
875 Monroe Ave.
Suite 116
Memphis, TN 38163
Mon.-Fri. 7 AM-7 PM
    901-448-5555
Fax: 901-448-5419
E-mail: utdic@utmem.edu

TEXAS

AMARILLO

Drug Information Center
Texas Tech University
School of Pharmacy
1300 Coulter Rd.
Amarillo, TX 79106
Mon.-Fri. 8 AM-5 PM
    806-356-4008
    (for healthcare
    professionals only)
Fax: 806-356-4017

GALVESTON

Drug Information Center
University of Texas
Medical Branch
301 University Blvd. - G01
Galveston, TX 77555-0701
Mon.-Fri. 8 AM-5 PM
    409-772-2734
Fax: 409-747-5222

HOUSTON

Drug Information Center
Ben Taub General Hospital
Texas Southern
University/HCHD
1504 Taub Loop
Houston, TX 77030
Mon.-Fri. 8 AM-5 PM
    713-873-3710
Fax: 713-873-3711

LACKLAND A.F.B.

Drug Information Center
Dept. of Pharmacy
Wilford Hall Medical Center
2200 Berquist Dr.
Suite 1
Lackland A.F.B., TX 78236
7 days/week, 24 hours
    210-292-5414
Fax: 210-292-3722

LUBBOCK

Drug Information and
Consultation Service
Covenant Medical Center
3615 19th St.
Lubbock, TX 79410
Mon.-Fri. 8 AM-5 PM
    806-725-0408
Fax: 806-725-0305

SAN ANTONIO

Drug Information Service
University of Texas
Health Science Center
at San Antonio
Department of
Pharmacology
7703 Floyd Curl Drive
San Antonio, TX 78229-3900
Mon.-Fri. 8 AM-4 PM
    210-567-4280
Fax: 210-567-4305

TEMPLE

Drug Information Center
Scott and White
Memorial Hospital
2401 S. 31st St.
Temple, TX 76508
Mon.-Fri. 8 AM-6 PM
    254-724-4636
Fax: 254-724-1731

UTAH

SALT LAKE CITY

Drug Information Service
University of Utah Hospital
Dept. of Pharmacy
Services
Room A-050
50 N. Medical Dr.
Salt Lake City, UT 84132
Mon.-Fri. 8:30 AM-4:30 PM
    801-581-2073
Fax: 801-585-6688
E-mail:
drug.info@hsc.utah.edu

VIRGINIA

HAMPTON

Drug Information Service
Hampton University School
of Pharmacy
Kittrell Hall Room 208
Hampton, VA 23668
Mon.-Fri. 8 AM-5 PM
    757-728-6687
    757-728-6693
    (drug info hotline)
Fax: 757-727-5840
E-mail: druginfo@hamp-
tonu.edu

WEST VIRGINIA

MORGANTOWN

West Virginia Drug
Information Center
WV University-
Robert C. Byrd
Health Sciences Center
1124 HSN, P.O. Box 9550
Morgantown, WV 26506
Mon.-Fri. 8:30 AM-5 PM
    304-293-6640
    800-352-2501 (WV)
Fax: 304-293-7672

WYOMING

LARAMIE

Drug Information Center
University of Wyoming
P.O. Box 3375
Laramie, WY 82071
Mon.-Fri. 8 AM-5 PM
    307-766-6988
E-mail: rxinfo@uwyo.edu

POISON CONTROL CENTERS

There's now a single nationwide emergency phone number that automatically links callers with their regional poison control center. This toll-free number—**800-222-1222**—is being used by every state with the exception of a few local poison-control centers and the ASPCA/National Animal Poison Control Center. The ASPCA/NAPCC information appears at the end of this listing.

Most of the centers listed below are certified by the American Association of Poison Control Centers. **Certified centers are marked by an asterisk (*)** after the name. In order to be certified, a center must meet the following criteria: it must serve a large geographic area; it must be open 24 hours a day and provide direct-dial or toll-free access; it must be supervised by a medical director; and it must have registered pharmacists or nurses available to answer questions from the public.

Within each state, centers are listed alphabetically by city. Telephone numbers designated "TTY" are teletype lines for the hearing-impaired. "TDD" numbers reach a telecommunication device for the deaf.

ALABAMA

BIRMINGHAM

Regional Poison Control Center, The Children's Hospital of Alabama (*)

1600 7th Ave. South
Birmingham, AL 35233-1711
Business: 205-939-9201
Emergency: 800-222-1222
              800-292-6678
              (AL)
Fax: 205-939-9245
www.chsys.org

TUSCALOOSA

Alabama Poison Center (*)

2503 Phoenix Dr.
Tuscaloosa, AL 35405
Business: 205-345-0600
Emergency: 800-222-1222
              800-292-6678
              (AL)
Fax: 205-343-7410
www.alapoisoncenter.org

ALASKA

JUNEAU

Alaska Poison Control System

Section of Community Health and EMS
410 Willoughby, Room 109
Box 110616
Juneau, AK 99811-0616
Business: 907-465-5319
              907-465-3027
Emergency: 800-222-1222
Fax: 907-465-4101
www.chems.alaska.gov/
ems_poison_control.htm

(PORTLAND, OR)

**Oregon Poison Center (*)
Oregon Health Sciences University**

3181 SW Sam Jackson Park Rd., CB550
Portland, OR 97239
Business: 503-494-8600
Emergency: 800-222-1222
www.ohsu.edu/poison

ARIZONA

PHOENIX

**Samaritan Regional Poison Center (*)
Good Samaritan Regional Medical Center**

Ancillary 1
1111 East McDowell Rd.
Phoenix, AZ 85006
Business: 602-495-6360
Emergency: 800-222-1222
              602-253-3334
Fax: 602-256-7579

TUCSON

**Arizona Poison and Drug Information Center (*)
Arizona Health Sciences Center**

1501 N. Campbell Ave.
Room 1156
Tucson, AZ 85724
Business: 520-626-7899
Emergency: 800-222-1222
              800-362-0101
              (AZ)
Fax: 520-626-2720

ARKANSAS

LITTLE ROCK

Arkansas Poison and Drug Information Center College of Pharmacy - UAMS

4301 West Markham St.
Mail Slot 522
Little Rock, AR 72205-7122
Business: 501-686-5540
Emergency: 800-222-1222
TDD/TTY: 800-641-3805
Fax: 501-296-1451

CALIFORNIA

FRESNO/MADERA

**California Poison Control System-Fresno/Madera (*)
Valley Children's Hospital**

9300 Valley Children's Pl.
MB 15
Madera, CA 93638-8762
Business: 559-622-2300
Emergency: 800-222-1222
              800-876-4766
              (CA)
TDD/TTY: 800-972-3323
Fax: 559-622-2322
www.calpoison.org

SACRAMENTO

California Poison Control System-Sacramento (*)

UCDMC-HSF Room 1024
2315 Stockton Blvd.
Sacramento, CA 95817
Business: 916-227-1400
Emergency: 800-222-1222
              800-876-4766
              (CA)
TDD/TTY: 800-972-3323
Fax: 916-227-1414
www.calpoison.org

SAN DIEGO

**California Poison Control System-San Diego (*)
UCSD Medical Center**

200 West Arbor Dr.
San Diego, CA 92103-8925
Business: 858-715-6300
Emergency: 800-222-1222
              800-876-4766
              (CA)
Fax: 858-715-6323
TDD/TTY: 800-972-3323
www.calpoison.org

SAN FRANCISCO

**California Poison Control System-San Francisco (*)
School of Pharmacy University of California San Francisco**

Box 1262
San Francisco, CA 94143-1262
Business: 415-502-8600
Emergency: 800-222-1222
              800-876-4766
              (CA)
Voice mail: 800-582-3387
Fax: 415-502-8620
www.calpoison.org

COLORADO

DENVER

Rocky Mountain Poison and Drug Center (*)

1001 Yosemite St.
Suite 200
Denver, CO 80230-6800
Business: 303-739-1100
Emergency: 800-222-1222
TTY: 303-739-1127
              (CO)
Fax: 303-739-1119
www.RMPDC.org

CONNECTICUT

FARMINGTON

**Connecticut Regional
Poison Control Center (*)
University of Connecticut
Health Center**

263 Farmington Ave.
Farmington, CT 06030-5365
Business: 860-679-4540
Emergency: 800-222-1222
TDD/TTY: 866-218-5372
Fax: 860-679-1623
http://poisoncontrol.uchc.
edu

DELAWARE

(PHILADELPHIA, PA)

**The Poison Control
Center (*)
Children's Hospital of
Philadelphia**

34th St. & Civic Center Blvd.
Philadelphia, PA 19104-3309
Business: 215-590-2003
Emergency: 800-222-1222
TDD/TTY: 215-590-8789
Fax: 215-590-4419

DISTRICT OF COLUMBIA

WASHINGTON, DC

**National Capital
Poison Center (*)**

3201 New Mexico Ave., NW
Suite 310
Washington, DC 20016
Business: 202-362-3867
Emergency: 800-222-1222
TDD/TTY: 202-362-8563
or
800-222-1222
Fax: 202-362-8377
www.poison.org

FLORIDA

JACKSONVILLE

**Florida Poison Information
Center-Jacksonville (*)
SHANDS Jacksonville
Medical Center**

655 West 8th St.
Jacksonville, FL 32209
Business: 904-244-4465
Emergency: 800-222-1222
TDD/TTY: 800-282-3171
(FL)
800-222-1222
Fax: 904-244-4063
http://ora.umc.ufl.edu/pcc/
pic_jax/htm/index.html

MIAMI

**Florida Poison Information
Center-Miami (*)
University of Miami
Department of Pediatrics
Jackson Memorial
Medical Center**

P.O. Box 110626 (R-131)
Miami, FL 33101
Business: 305-585-5250
Emergency: 800-222-1222
Fax: 305-545-9762
www.pediatrics.med.miami.
edu/FPIC/index.html

TAMPA

**Florida Poison Information
Center-Tampa (*)
Tampa General Hospital**

P.O. Box 1289
Tampa, FL 33601
Business: 813-844-4444
Emergency: 800-222-1222
Fax: 813-844-4443

GEORGIA

ATLANTA

**Georgia Poison Center (*)
Hughes Spalding
Children's Hospital, Grady
Health System**

80 Jesse Hill Jr. Dr.
P.O. Box 26066
Atlanta, GA 30303-3030
Business: 404-616-9237
Emergency: 800-222-1222
TDD: 404-616-9287
Fax: 404-616-6657
www.georgiapoisoncenter.
org

HAWAII

HONOLULU

Hawaii Poison Center (*)
1319 Punahou St.
Honolulu, HI 96826
Business: 808-941-4411
Emergency: 800-222-1222
Fax: 808-535-7922

IDAHO

(DENVER, CO)

**Rocky Mountain Poison
& Drug Center (*)**
1001 Yosemite St.
Suite 200
Denver, CO 80230-6800
Business: 303-739-1100
Emergency: 800-222-1222
TTY: 303-739-1127
(ID)
Fax: 303-739-1119
www.RMPDC.org

ILLINOIS

CHICAGO

Illinois Poison Center (*)

222 South Riverside Plaza
Suite 1900
Chicago, IL 60606
Business: 312-906-6136
Emergency: 800-222-1222
TDD/TTY: 312-906-6185
Fax: 312-803-5400
www.mchc.org/ipc

INDIANA

INDIANAPOLIS

**Indiana Poison Center (*)
Methodist Hospital
Clarian Health Partners**

I-65 at 21st St.
P.O. Box 1367
Indianapolis, IN 46206-1367
Business: 317-962-2335
Emergency: 800-222-1222
TTY: 317-962-2336
Fax: 317-962-2337
www.clarian.org/clinical/
poisoncontrol

IOWA

SIOUX CITY

**Iowa Statewide Poison
Control Center
St. Luke's Regional
Medical Center**

2720 Stone Park Blvd.
Sioux City, IA 51104
Business: 712-279-3710
Emergency: 800-222-1222
Fax: 712-234-8775
www.iowapoison.org

KANSAS

KANSAS CITY

**Mid-America Poison
Control Center,
University of Kansas
Medical Center**

3901 Rainbow Blvd.
Room B-400
Kansas City, KS 66160-7231
Business 913-588-6638
Emergency: 800-222-1222
800-332-6633
(KS)
TDD: 913-588-6639
Fax: 913-588-2350

KENTUCKY

LOUISVILLE

**Kentucky Regional
Poison Center (*)**

Medical Towers South
Suite 572
234 East Gray St.
Louisville, KY 40202
Business: 502-629-7264
Emergency: 800-222-1222
502-589-8222
Fax: 502-629-7277
www.krpc.com

LOUISIANA

MONROE

**Louisiana Drug and Poison
Information Center (*)
University of Louisiana at
Monroe School of
Pharmacy**

Sugar Hall
Monroe, LA 71209-6430
Business: 318-342-3648
Emergency: 800-222-1222
Fax: 318-342-1744
www.lapcc.org

MAINE

PORTLAND

**Northern New England
Poison Center (*)**

Maine Medical Center
22 Bramhall St.
Portland, ME 04102
Business: 207-842-7220
Emergency: 800-222-1222
TDD/TTY: 877-299-4447
Fax: 207-874-6354

MARYLAND

BALTIMORE

**Maryland Poison Center (*)
University of Maryland at
Baltimore School of
Pharmacy**

20 North Pine St., PH 772
Baltimore, MD 21201
Business: 410-706-7604
Emergency: 800-222-1222
TDD: 410-706-1858
Fax: 410-706-7184
www.pharmacy.umaryland.
edu/~mpc/

(MONTGOMERY AND PRINCE GEORGE'S COUNTIES)
National Capital Poison Center
3201 New Mexico Ave., NW
Suite 310
Washington DC 20016
Business: 202-362-3867
Emergency: 800-222-1222
TTY: 202-362-8563
Fax: 202-362-8377
www.poison.org

MASSACHUSETTS

BOSTON
Regional Center for Poison Control and Prevention (*)
300 Longwood Ave.
Boston, MA 02115
Business: 617-232-2120
Emergency: 800-222-1222
TDD/TTY: 888-244-5313
Fax: 617-738-0032
www.maripoisoncenter.com

MICHIGAN

DETROIT
Regional Poison Control Center (*) Children's Hospital of Michigan
4160 John R. Harper
Professional Office Bldg.
Suite 616
Detroit, MI 48201
Business: 313-745-5335
Emergency: 800-222-1222
TDD/TTY: 800-356-3232
Fax: 313-745-5493

GRAND RAPIDS
DeVos Children's Hospital Regional Poison Center (*)
1840 Wealthy, SE
Grand Rapids, MI 49506
Emergency: 800-222-1222
TTY: 800-356-3232
Fax: 616-774-7204

MINNESOTA

MINNEAPOLIS
Hennepin Regional Poison Center (*) Hennepin County Medical Center
701 Park Ave.
Minneapolis, MN 55415
Business: 612-347-6000
Emergency: 800-222-1222
TTY: 612-904-4691
Fax: 612-904-4289
www.mnpoison.org

MISSISSIPPI

JACKSON
Mississippi Regional Poison Control Center, University of Mississippi Medical Center
2500 North State St.
Jackson, MS 39216
Business: 601-984-1675
Emergency: 800-222-1222
Fax: 601-984-1676

MISSOURI

ST. LOUIS
Missouri Regional Poison Center (*) Cardinal Glennon Children's Hospital
7980 Clayton Rd.
Suite 200
St. Louis, MO 63117
Business: 314-772-5200
Emergency: 800-222-1222
TTY: 314-577-5336
Fax: 314-577-5355

MONTANA

(DENVER, CO)
Rocky Mountain Poison and Drug Center (*)
1001 Yosemite St.
Suite 200
Denver, CO 80230-6800
Business: 303-739-1118
Emergency: 800-222-1222
Fax: 303-739-1119
www.RMPDC.org

NEBRASKA

OMAHA
The Poison Center (*) Children's Hospital
8200 Dodge St.
Omaha, NE 68114
Business: 402-955-6976
Emergency: 800-222-1222
Fax: 402-955-6987
www.poison-center.com

NEVADA

(DENVER, CO)
Rocky Mountain Poison and Drug Center (*)
1001 Yosemite St.
Suite 200
Denver, CO 80230-6800
Business: 303-739-1100
Emergency: 800-222-1222
Fax: 303-739-1119
www.RMPDC.org

(PORTLAND, OR)
Oregon Poison Center (*) Oregon Health Sciences University
3181 SW Sam Jackson Park Rd.,
CB550
Portland, OR 97239
Business: 503-494-8600
Emergency: 800-222-1222
Fax: 503-494-4980
www.ohsu.edu/poison

NEW HAMPSHIRE

LEBANON
New Hampshire Poison Information Center, Dartmouth-Hitchcock Medical Center
1 Medical Center Dr.
Lebanon, NH 03756
Business: 603-650-8000
Emergency: 800-222-1222
Fax: 603-650-8986
www.hitchcock.org

NEW JERSEY

NEWARK
New Jersey Poison Information and Education System (*)
65 Bergan St.
Newark, NJ 07101
Business: 973-972-9280
Emergency: 800-222-1222
TDD/TTY: 973-926-8008
Fax: 973-643-2679
www.njpies.org

NEW MEXICO

ALBUQUERQUE
New Mexico Poison and Drug Information Center (*) University of New Mexico
Health Science Center
Library, Room 130
Albuquerque, NM 87131-1076
Business: 505-272-4261
Emergency: 800-222-1222
Fax: 505-272-5892

NEW YORK

BUFFALO
Western New York Regional Poison Control Center (*) Children's Hospital of Buffalo
219 Bryant St.
Buffalo, NY 14222
Business: 716-878-7654
Emergency: 800-222-1222
Fax: 716-878-1150
www.chob.edu

MINEOLA
Long Island Regional Poison and Drug Information Center (*) Winthrop University Hospital
259 First St.
Mineola, NY 11501
Business: 516-663-2650
Emergency: 800-222-1222
TDD: 516-747-3323
              (Nassau)
              516-924-8811
              (Suffolk)
Fax: 516-739-2070
www.lirpdic.org

NEW YORK CITY
New York City Poison Control Center (*) NYC Dept. of Health
455 First Ave., Room 123
New York, NY 10016
Business: 212-447-8152
Emergency: 800-222-1222
(English)   212-340-4494
              212-POISONS
              (212-764-7667)

Emergency: 212-VENENOS
(Spanish)   (212-836-3667)
TDD: 212-689-9014
Fax: 212-447-8223

ROCHESTER
Finger Lakes Regional Poison and Drug Information Center (*) University of Rochester Medical Center
601 Elmwood Ave.
Box 321
Rochester, NY 14642
Business: 585-273-4155
Emergency: 800-222-1222
TTY: 585-273-3854
Fax: 585-244-1677
www.urmc.rochester.edu/
urmc/telemed/flrpc/about.
htm

SYRACUSE
**Central New York
Poison Center (*)
SUNY Upstate Medical
University**
750 East Adams St.
Syracuse, NY 13210
Business: 315-464-7078
Emergency: 800-222-1222
Fax: 315-464-7077
www.cnypoison.org

NORTH CAROLINA

CHARLOTTE
**Carolinas Poison Center (*)
Carolinas Medical Center**
5000 Airport Center Pkwy.
Suite B
Charlotte, NC 28208
Business: 704-395-3795
Emergency: 800-222-1222
Fax: 704-395-4100
www.carolinas.org/
services/poison

NORTH DAKOTA

FARGO
**North Dakota Poison
Information Center,
Meritcare Medical Center**
720 4th St. North
Fargo, ND 58122
Business: 701-234-5575
Emergency: 800-222-1222
Fax: 701-234-5090

OHIO

CINCINNATI
**Cincinnati Drug and
Poison Information
Center (*) Regional Poison
Control System**
3333 Burnet Ave.
Vernon Place, 3rd Floor
Cincinnati, OH 45229
Business: 513-636-5063
Emergency: 800-222-1222
TDD/TTY: 800-253-7955
Fax: 513-636-5069
www.cincinnatichildrens.
org/dpic

CLEVELAND
**Greater Cleveland
Poison Control Center**
11100 Euclid Ave.
Cleveland, OH 44106-6010
Business: 216-844-2749
Emergency: 216-231-4455
              800-222-1222
Fax: 216-844-3242

COLUMBUS
**Central Ohio
Poison Center (*)**
700 Children's Dr.
Room L032
Columbus, OH 43205-2696
Business: 614-722-2635
Emergency: 614-228-1323
              800-222-1222
              937-222-2227
              (Dayton area)
TTY: 614-228-2272
Fax: 614-228-2672

OKLAHOMA

OKLAHOMA CITY
**Oklahoma Poison Control
Center, University of
Oklahoma**
940 Northeast 13th St.
Room 3512
Oklahoma City, OK 73104
Business: 405-271-5062
Emergency: 800-222-1222
TDD/TTY: 405-271-1122
Fax: 405-271-1816

OREGON

PORTLAND
**Oregon Poison Center (*)
Oregon Health Sciences
University**
3181 S.W. Sam Jackson
Park Rd., CB550
Portland, OR 97239
Business: 503-494-8600
Emergency: 800-222-1222
www.ohsu.edu/poison

PENNSYLVANIA

HERSHEY
**Central Pennsylvania
Poison Center (*)
Pennsylvania State
University, Milton S.
Hershey Medical Center**
500 University Dr.
MC H043, P.O. Box 850
Hershey, PA 17033-0850
Business: 717-531-7057
Emergency: 800-222-1222
TTY: 717-531-8335
Fax: 717-531-6932
www.hmc.edu/ems/cppc/
cppc.htm

PHILADELPHIA
**The Poison Control
Center (*)**
3535 Market St.
Suite 985
Philadelphia, PA 19104-3309
Business: 215-590-2003
Emergency: 800-222-1222
TDD/TTY: 215-590-8789
Fax: 215-590-4419

PITTSBURGH
**Pittsburgh Poison
Center (*) Children's
Hospital of Pittsburgh**
3705 Fifth Ave.
Pittsburgh, PA 15213
Business: 412-390-3300
Emergency: 800-222-1222
Fax: 412-390-3311

PUERTO RICO

SANTURCE
**San Jorge Children's
Hospital Poison Center**
258 San Jorge St.
Santurce, PR 00912
Business: 787-727-1000,
              ext. 4437
Emergency: 800-222-1222
Fax: 787-726-5660
www.poisoncenter.net

RHODE ISLAND

(BOSTON, MA)
**Regional Center for Poison
Control and Prevention (*)**
300 Longwood Ave.
Boston, MA 02115
Business: 617-232-2120
Emergency: 800-222-1222
TDD/TTY: 888-244-5313
Fax: 617-738-0032
www.maripoisoncenter.com

SOUTH CAROLINA

COLUMBIA
**Palmetto Poison Center (*)
College of Pharmacy
University of South
Carolina**
Columbia, SC 29208
Business: 803-777-7909
Emergency: 800-222-1222
Fax: 803-777-6127
www.pharm.sc.edu/pps.htm

SOUTH DAKOTA

(MINNEAPOLIS, MN)
**Hennepin Regional Poison
Center (*) Hennepin County
Medical Center**
701 Park Ave.
Minneapolis, MN 55415
Business: 612-347-6000
Emergency: 800-222-1222
TTY: 612-904-4691
Fax: 612-904-4289
www.mnpoison.org

SIOUX FALLS
**Provides education only—
Does not manage expo-
sure cases.**
**Sioux Valley Poison
Control Center (*)**
1100 South Euclid Ave.
Box 5039
Sioux Falls, SD 57117-5039
Business: 605-333-6638
Fax: 605-333-1477

TENNESSEE

MEMPHIS
**Southern Poison Center (*)
University of Tennessee**
875 Monroe Ave.
Suite 104
Memphis, TN 38163
Business: 901-448-6800
Emergency: 800-222-1222
              800-288-9999
              (TN)
Fax: 901-448-5419

NASHVILLE
**Middle Tennessee
Poison Center (*)**
1161 21st Ave. South
501 Oxford House
Nashville, TN 37232-4632
Business: 615-936-0760
Emergency: 800-222-1222
TDD: 615-936-2047
Fax: 615-936-0756
www.poisonlifeline.org

TEXAS

AMARILLO
**Texas Panhandle
Poison Center (*)
Northwest Texas Hospital**
1501 S. Coulter Dr.
Amarillo, TX 79106
Business: 806-354-1630
Emergency: 800-222-1222
TDD/TTY: 800-764-7661
             (TX)
Fax: 806-354-1667
www.panhandlepoison.org

DALLAS
**North Texas Poison
Center (*) Texas Poison
Center Network, Parkland
Health and Hospital
System**
5201 Harry Hines Blvd.
Dallas, TX 75235
Business: 214-589-0911
Emergency: 800-222-1222
TDD/TTY: 800-764-7661
             (TX)
Fax: 214-590-5008

EL PASO
**West Texas Regional
Poison Center (*)
Thomason Hospital**
4815 Alameda Ave.
El Paso, TX 79905
Business   915-534-3800
Emergency: 800-222-1222
TDD/TTY: 800-764-7661
             (TX)
Fax: 915-534-3809
www.poisoncenter.org

GALVESTON
**Southeast Texas
Poison Center (*)
The University of Texas
Medical Branch**
3112 Trauma Bldg.
301 University Ave.
Galveston, TX 77555-1175
Business: 409-766-4403
Emergency: 800-222-1222
TDD/TTY: 800-764-7661
             (TX)
Fax: 409-772-3917
www.utmb.edu/setpc

SAN ANTONIO
**South Texas
Poison Center (*)
The University of Texas
Health Science Center–San
Antonio**
7703 Floyd Curl Dr., MC 7849
San Antonio, TX 78229-3900
Business: 210-567-5762
Emergency: 800-222-1222
TDD/TTY: 800-764-7661
             (TX)
Fax: 210-567-5718

TEMPLE
**Central Texas Poison
Center (*) Scott & White
Memorial Hospital**
2401 South 31st St.
Temple, TX 76508
Business: 254-724-7401
Emergency: 800-222-1222
             800-764-7661
             (TX)
Fax: 254-724-7408

UTAH

SALT LAKE CITY
**Utah Poison Control
Center (*)**
410 Chipeta Way
Suite 230
Salt Lake City, UT 84108
Business: 801-581-7504
Emergency: 800-222-1222
Fax: 801-581-4199

VERMONT

(PORTLAND, ME)
**Northern New England
Poison Center (*)**
Maine Medical Center
22 Bramhall St.
Portland, ME 04102
Business: 207-842-7220
Emergency: 800-222-1222
TDD/TTY: 877-299-4447
Fax: 207-874-6354

VIRGINIA

CHARLOTTESVILLE
**Blue Ridge Poison
Center (*) University of
Virginia Health System**
PO Box 800774
Charlottesville, VA
22908-0774
Business: 434-924-0347
Emergency: 800-222-1222
Fax: 434-971-8657

RICHMOND
**Virginia Poison Center (*)
Virginia Commonwealth
University**
P.O. Box 980522
Richmond, VA 23298-0522
Business: 804-828-4780
Emergency: 800-222-1222
TDD/TTY: 800-828-1120
Fax: 804-828-5291

WASHINGTON

SEATTLE
**Washington Poison
Center (*)**
155 NE 100th St.
Suite 400
Seattle, WA 98125-8012
Business: 206-517-2351
Emergency: 800-222-1222
TDD: 800-572-0638
             (WA)
             206-517-2394
Fax: 206-526-8490

WEST VIRGINIA

CHARLESTON
**West Virginia
Poison Center (*)**
3110 MacCorkle Ave. SE
Charleston, WV 25304
Business: 304-347-1212
Emergency: 800-222-1222
Fax: 304-388-9560

WISCONSIN

MILWAUKEE
**Children's Hospital
of Wisconsin Statewide
Poison Center**
9000 W. Wisconsin Ave.
P.O. Box 1997,
Mail Station 677A
Milwaukee, WI 53201-1997
Business: 414-266-2000
Emergency: 800-222-1222
TDD/TTY: 414-266-2542
Fax: 414-266-2820

WYOMING

(OMAHA, NE)
**The Poison Center (*)
Children's Hospital**
8301 Dodge St.
Omaha, NE 68114
Business: 402-955-6976
Emergency: 800-222-1222
Fax: 402-955-6987
www.poison-center.com

ASPCA/NATIONAL ANIMAL POISON CONTROL CENTER
1717 South Philo Rd.
Suite 36
Urbana, IL 61802
Business: 217-337-5030
Emergency: 888-426-4435
             900-680-0000
Fax: 217-337-0599
www.napcc.aspca.org

POPULAR HERBS

Reliable information on herbal remedies is still hard to come by, yet Americans spend more than $4 billion each year on herbal products. Even more surprising are the findings from a recent *Prevention* magazine survey: Nearly 23 million consumers use herbal remedies *instead* of taking prescription medicine, and about 20 million take botanicals along with either OTC or prescription drugs.

To prepare you for those times when patients ask about the latest herbal "discovery"—as they surely will—we've compiled a quick reference of the most commonly used herbs. The information is based on the findings of the German Regulatory Authority's "Commission E"—currently the most authoritative source of information on botanical medicines. For a more thorough discussion of more than 700 herbs, consult the second edition of the *PDR® for Herbal Medicines™*.

Aloe (Aloe vera). The gel from the Aloe plant is an ancient remedy used externally for its antibacterial, antiviral, anti-inflammatory, and pain-relieving effects. It is used topically in skin moisturizers and to treat burns, wounds, psoriasis, and frostbite. While the internal use of Aloe is suggested as a treatment for several conditions including constipation, there is no evidence of its efficacy. In fact, internal use is not recommended because of the risk of serious adverse effects.

Warning: Aloe should not be used by pregnant or breastfeeding women, or by people with severe intestinal disorders. Aloe should not be taken with certain drugs associated with potassium loss—such as diuretics, cortico-steroids, and antiarrhythmics and other heart medications—or with the herb Licorice.

Arnica (Arnica montana). The Arnica plant is used externally for pain and inflammation due to injury, and as an anti-infectious agent. Arnica should be discontinued immediately in the event of an allergic reaction to external application. The herb should not be used on open skin wounds.

Warning: Although Europeans take Arnica internally to treat respiratory infections, internal use is not recommended due to the risk of serious cardiac adverse effects.

Astragalus (Astragalus species). Astragalus, or Huang-Qi, is used to improve immune function and strengthen the cardiovascular system. Compounds in Astragalus may also have beneficial antiviral, antioxidant, memory-enhancing, and liver-protecting effects, although the nature of those effects on specific diseases has not been established.

Warning: The use of Astragalus must be carefully monitored by a physician due to its potentially dangerous adverse effects, particularly in people with immune disorders or those taking blood-thinning medications.

Barberry (Berberis vulgaris). Both the fruit and root bark of the Barberry plant are used in folk medicine. The berry is a source of vitamin C, which stimulates the immune system, improves iron absorption, and protects against scurvy. The fruit's acid content has a mild diuretic effect that is thought to aid in urinary tract infections. Barberry root bark may reduce blood pressure, relieve constipation, and have some antibiotic effects.

Warning: Pregnant and nursing women should not use Barberry.

Bilberry (Vaccinium myrtillus). The astringent effects of Bilberry fruit are used to treat inflammation of the mouth and throat, and both the fruit and leaves are used for diarrhea. Reports citing Bilberry as a treatment for diabetic retinopathy need further confirmation.

Warning: The herb should not be used with blood-thinning drugs, including aspirin.

Black Cohosh (Cimicifuga racemosa). The hormone-modulating effects of Black Cohosh make it useful for women with menopausal symptoms and premenstrual syndrome.

Warning: Due to a risk of spontaneous abortion, Black Cohosh should not be used during pregnancy. The herb should not be taken with drugs that lower blood pressure.

Butcher's Broom (Ruscus aculeatus). This herb, native to the Mediterranean regions of Europe, Africa, and western Asia, is used medicinally as a diuretic, anti-inflammatory, and for its beneficial effects on circulation. Butcher's Broom is used to relieve the discomforts of hemorrhoids, such as itching and burning, and the leg heaviness, pain, cramping, and swelling of chronic venous insufficiency.

Cat's Claw (Uncaria tomentosa). The root of the South American Cat's Claw contains compounds that have immune-stimulating, anti-inflammatory, and anticancer effects. Although human studies have yet to be conducted, Cat's Claw is often used to treat cancer; arthritis and rheumatic disorders; and AIDS and other viral diseases.

Warning: Cat's Claw should not be used by pregnant or breastfeeding women, or by people with autoimmune disorders, multiple sclerosis, tuberculosis, transplant recipients, and children under 2 years of age.

Cayenne (Capsicum annuum). Externally, Cayenne is used to relieve the pain of muscle tension and spasm, diabetic neuropathy, and rheumatism. Cayenne is sometimes taken internally to relieve gastrointestinal disorders, although human studies have yet to confirm such uses.

Warning: Topical Cayenne preparations should not be used for more than two consecutive days, with a two-week break between applications. It should never be used on broken skin or near the eyes. When used internally, Cayenne preparations should not be taken with aspirin, antifungal drugs, ACE inhibitors, or theophylline.

Chamomile (Matricaria recutita). Chamomile tea—which has anti-inflammatory, antispasmodic, and muscle-relaxing effects—is used to treat gastrointestinal disorders such as indigestion and gas.

Warning: Chamomile should not be used by pregnant women.

Comfrey (Symphytum officinale). This herb is applied topically as an anti-inflammatory; it is used for bruises and sprains and to promote bone healing.

Warning: Because of possible toxic adverse effects, Comfrey should not be taken internally. The herb is contraindicated in pregnant and breastfeeding women.

Dandelion (Taraxacum officinale). Dandelion, commonly used as an addition to the salad bowl, is recommended as an effective remedy for digestive and liver complaints, urinary tract infection, and as an appetite stimulant.

Warning: Although the herb is sometimes used for gallbladder complaints, this should only be done under a doctor's supervision. People with bile duct obstruction or stomach ulcer should not use Dandelion.

Dong Quai (Angelica sinensis). Dong Quai root is used in China as a women's health tonic. It is particularly used as a remedy for fibrocystic breast disease, premenstrual syndrome, painful periods, and menopausal symptoms. Dong Quai is also used in cardiovascular disease to treat high blood pressure and improve poor circulation.

Warning: Dong Quai should not be used by pregnant or breastfeeding women. The herb can also cause photosensitivity.

Echinacea (Echinacea purpurea). This species of Echinacea is a well-established immune-system stimulator; it is used to treat flu, coughs and colds, bronchitis, urinary tract infections, wounds and burns, and inflammation of the mouth and pharynx.

Warning: It should not be used in patients who have autoimmune disorders such as multiple sclerosis, collagen disease, AIDS, or tuberculosis. The herb is also contraindicated in patients who have diabetes and in pregnant or breastfeeding women. Echinacea should not be used with the following: amiodarone, methotrexate, ketoconazole, anticancer agents, anti-organ rejection drugs, steroids, or immunosuppressants.

Evening Primrose (Oenothera biennis). The anti-inflammatory compounds in Evening Primrose oil have been extensively studied, but no definitive indication has been accepted. Some herbalists consider the oil useful for treating breast pain, premenstrual syndrome, and menopausal symptoms. Capsules containing at least 500 milligrams of the oil are approved in Germany as a remedy for eczema.

Warning: People with seizure disorder or schizophrenia should not take Evening Primrose oil.

Feverfew (Tanacetum parthenium). Feverfew is used to treat migraine headaches, allergies, and arthritic and rheumatic diseases.

Warning: Feverfew should not be used during pregnancy or breastfeeding. It is also contraindicated in people with bleeding disorders, and in those who are taking anticoagulants, including aspirin.

Flax (Linum usitatissimum). Ground Flax (also known as Linseed) is used internally to relieve constipation. It is also used externally as a compress to relieve skin inflammation.

Warning: Flax should not be used internally in the cases of bowel or esophageal obstruction; or in the presence of gastrointestinal or esophageal inflammation.

Fo-Ti (Polygonum multiflorum). The Asian herb Fo-Ti is used for constipation, atherosclerosis, high cholesterol, and as an immune enhancer.

Warning: Because of its laxative action, the herb may cause diarrhea. Taking the unprocessed root may cause skin rash; and overdosage may cause numbness in the extremities.

Garlic (Allium sativum). Garlic is used as a treatment for hardening of the arteries, high blood pressure, and to reduce cholesterol levels. It may also have antibacterial and antiviral effects.

Warning: Garlic can cause allergic skin and respiratory reactions. It should not be used by people with bleeding disorders, or by those taking blood thinners (including aspirin) or NSAID therapy. Nursing women should also not use Garlic.

Ginger (Zingiber officinale). Ginger root is a treatment for motion sickness and loss of appetite. It is also indicated for nausea and vomiting associated with chemotherapy, and to help control nausea and vomiting in postoperative patients.

Warning: Ginger should not be used for morning sickness associated with pregnancy, or by nursing mothers.

People who have gallstones or bleeding disorders should not take Ginger. The herb is also contraindicated in those taking blood thinners (including aspirin) or NSAID therapy.

Ginkgo (Gingko biloba). Ginkgo has proven useful for dementia, Alzheimer's disease, peripheral arterial occlusive disease, vertigo, and tinnitus of vascular origin.

Warning: Ginkgo should not be used by people who have bleeding disorders, or who are taking blood thinners (including aspirin) or NSAID therapy.

Ginseng (Panax ginseng). The Ginseng root is used for fatigue and to improve concentration and stamina. Ginseng may also have antiviral, antioxidant, and anticancer effects.

Warning: Caution with Ginseng is urged in people with cardiovascular disease or diabetes. People who are taking diabetes drugs, diuretics, blood thinners (including aspirin), MAO inhibitors, digoxin, or NSAIDs should not take Ginseng. It should not be used during pregnancy or breastfeeding, or by those with bleeding disorders. Taking large amounts can result in Ginseng abuse syndrome, which is characterized by high blood pressure, insomnia, water retention, and muscle tension.

Goldenseal (Hydrastis canadensis). Goldenseal contains the compound berberine, which is used for gastritis, gastric ulcer, gallbladder disease, and acute diarrhea. It can be useful as an adjunct therapy in cancer treatment, and is also used to treat chronic eye infection.

Warning: Goldenseal should not be used by pregnant or breastfeeding women, or by people who have bleeding disorders; it should also not be combined with blood thinners (including aspirin) or NSAIDs. Use of Goldenseal for extended periods can result in digestive disorders, constipation, excitement, hallucination or delirium, and decreased vitamin B absorption. **Overdosage can result in convulsion, difficulty breathing, and paralysis.**

Gotu Kola (Centella asiatica). Gotu Kola is used internally for chronic venous insufficiency and venous hypertension. In animal and lab studies, Gotu Kola was also effective for ulcers and varicose veins. The herb is used externally to treat wounds; if a rash develops, discontinue topical use.

Great Burnet (Sanguisorba officinalis). Great Burnet may be used both externally and internally for its astringent, decongestant, and diuretic properties. Internal uses include menopausal symptoms, intestinal bladder problems, and venous disorders. It is also prepared for external use as a plaster for wounds and ulcers.

Green Tea (Camellia sinensis). Green Tea, which is rich in catechins and flavonoids, is used to help prevent cancer. The antibacterial effects of Green Tea mouthwash are useful in the prevention of dental cavities. Keep in mind that Green Tea contains caffeine and should be used sparingly by pregnant and breastfeeding women, and by those who are caffeine-sensitive.

Hawthorn (Crataegus laevigata). Hawthorn contains several compounds that are considered beneficial to the heart. It is used for cardiac insufficiency, angina, congestive heart failure, and irregular heartbeat.

Warning: Hawthorn should not be used in children under 12, or in the first trimester of pregnancy. People taking Hawthorn must be carefully monitored by a physician, especially in cases where it is combined with cardiac glycosides, beta-blockers, or calcium channel blockers. Hawthorn should not be taken with cisapride. Overuse can lead to low blood pressure, irregular heartbeat, and excessive sleepiness.

Horse Chestnut (Aesculus hippocastanum). Both the seed and leaf of Horse Chestnut are used medicinally. The seed is indicated for the symptoms of chronic venous insufficiency, including pain, cramping, swelling, sensations of heaviness, and night cramping. Horse Chestnut leaf is used for venous disorders such as varicose veins, hemorrhoids, and phlebitis.

Warning: People taking blood thinners (including aspirin) should not use Horse Chestnut.

Kava-kava (Piper methysticum). The active compounds in Kava are lactones, which have antispasmodic, muscle-relaxing, and anticonvulsive effects; Kava can also thin the blood. The herb is used for nervousness, insomnia, tension, stress, and agitation.

Warning: Kava can be addictive. Liver damage and/or failure has been linked to the herb. People who are depressed should not take Kava. The herb is also contraindicated in pregnant or nursing women and in those with liver disorders. Overuse of Kava can result in skin rash or weight loss. Kava use for more than 3 months should be supervised by a physician. The herb should not be combined with alcohol, anti-anxiety or mood-altering drugs (including barbiturates), levodopa, sleeping pills, or drugs that affect the liver.

Licorice (Glycyrrhiza glabra). The sweet root of the Licorice plant has a long history of use in traditional medicine. It contains various compounds with anti-inflammatory and other soothing effects that make it helpful as a treatment for ulcers and digestive disorders such as gastritis. It also acts as an expectorant for cough and bronchitis.

Warning: Licorice should not be taken with digoxin, diuretics, or medications that lower blood pressure. Licorice should also not be used in people with hepatitis and other liver disorders, kidney disease, diabetes, arrhythmias, high blood pressure, muscle cramping, low potassium levels, and pregnancy

Ma-Huang (Ephedra sinica). Ma-Huang contains compounds that alleviate bronchial constriction and is used in folk remedies as a treatment for coughs and bronchitis.

Warning: The adverse effects of Ma-Huang outweigh any possible benefits. The herb should not be taken by pregnant or breastfeeding women, or by people with the following: anxiety, high blood pressure, glaucoma, brain tumors, prostate disorders, adrenal tumors, cardiac arrhythmia, or thyroid disease. Ma-Huang should not be combined with caffeine, decongestants, stimulants, heart or glaucoma medication, MAO inhibitors, anesthetics, or labor-inducing drugs. **Overdosage can result in death.**

Milk Thistle *(Silybum marianum).* The compounds in Milk Thistle seed have protective and regenerative effects on the liver. It is used as a treatment for liver and gallbladder disorders such as jaundice, toxic liver damage, cirrhosis of the liver, and gallbladder pain.

Warning: The herb should not be used with antipsychotic drugs, yohimbine, or male hormones.

Pumpkin Seed *(Cucurbita pepo).* Pumpkin Seed has anti-inflammatory and antioxidant properties. It is used to treat irritable bladder and symptoms of benign prostatic hyperplasia (eg, obstructed urinary flow). It does not, however, appear to relieve an enlarged prostate.

Pygeum *(Pygeum africanum).* Pygeum bark contains compounds that inhibit the inflammation and swelling associated with benign prostatic hyperplasia.

Warning: The herb should not be used by pregnant or breastfeeding women. People with stomach disorders should check with their physician before using Pygeum.

Saw Palmetto *(Serenoa repens).* The anti-inflammatory and testosterone-moderating effects of Saw Palmetto make it useful for treating benign prostatic hyperplalsia; the herb is used for treating irritable bladder as well.

Warning: Saw Palmetto should not be used by pregnant or breastfeeding women. The herb should be avoided by those who have hormone-driven cancers or a family history of such cancers. People with stomach disorders and those who are taking hormones or hormone-like drugs should check with their physician before taking it.

St. John's Wort *(Hypericum perforatum).* St. John's Wort is one of the better studied herbs. Various compounds in St. John's Wort have antidepressant, anti-inflammatory, and antibacterial effects. It is used internally for depression and anxiety, and externally for wounds, burns, skin inflammation, and blunt injuries.

Warning: St. John's Wort can cause photosensitivity if taken for too long or at high doses. It can also cause gastrointestinal discomfort and headache. Combining St. John's Wort with other antidepressant medications such as MAO inhibitors, selective serotonin reuptake inhibitors (including fluoxetine, paroxetine, sertraline, fluvoxamine, or citalopram), or nefazodone could cause "serotonin syndrome"—a condition characterized by sweating, tremor, confusion, and agitation. The herb should also not be combined with the following: antibiotics that have photosensitizing effects, cyclosporine, indinavir, chemotherapy drugs, combination oral contraceptives, reserpine, barbiturates, theophylline, or digoxin.

Stinging Nettle *(Urtica dioica).* Both the flowers and root of the Stinging Nettle plant contain beneficial compounds used in various conditions. The flower is used internally and externally for rheumatism; it is used internally for urinary tract infections and kidney and bladder stones. The root is used for irritable bladder and to help relieve symptoms of benign prostatic hyperplasia (eg, obstructed urinary flow), although it does not reduce prostate enlargement.

Warning: Stinging Nettle should not be used by people who suffer from fluid retention due to impaired cardiac or kidney function.

Uva-Ursi *(Arctostaphylos uva-ursi).* Uva-ursi is used in the treatment of urinary tract infections because of its astringent and antibacterial effects.

Warning: The herb should not be used by pregnant or breastfeeding women; it should also not be used in children under 12 years of age, as it could cause liver damage. Uva-ursi should not be combined with diuretics, NSAIDs, or with substances (food or medication) that promote acidity in the urine.

Valerian *(Valeriana officinalis).* Valerian root contains sedative compounds that are useful in nervousness and insomnia. It is recommended for many other unproven uses such as headache, anxiety disorders, premenstrual syndrome, and menopausal symptoms.

Warning: Patients should avoid operating motor vehicles for several hours after taking Valerian. The herb should not be used by pregnant or breastfeeding women. Valerian extract or bath oils should not be used by people suffering from skin disorders, fever, infectious disease, heart disease, or muscle tension. Valerian should not be taken with, alcohol, barbituates, or benzodiazepenes.

Vitex *(Vitex agnus-castus).* Vitex (also known as Chaste Tree) is used as a treatment for premenstrual syndrome and menopausal symptoms.

Warning: Because of its hormonal effects, Vitex should not be used by pregnant or breastfeeding women. Occasionally, rash can occur. The herb should not be used with drugs that affect dopamine levels.

Wild Yam *(Dioscorea villosa).* Popular reports have led to the belief that Wild Yam is a "natural" source of the hormone progesterone. While Wild Yam is used as a constituent of artificial progesterone pharmaceutically, the body cannot complete the conversion process by itself. The herb can also be useful in treating high cholesterol.

Warning: Because of possible hormonal effects, pregnant and nursing women should not use Wild Yam. The herb should not be taken with estrogen-containing drugs or indomethacin.

Yohimbe *(Pausinystalia yohimbe).* Yohimbe is prepared pharmaceutically under the brand name Yocon and is used to treat erectile dysfunction. Compounds in Yohimbe stimulate norepinephrine, which improves blood flow to the penis. The risks, however, of unregulated ingestion of the herb are thought to outweigh the benefits. Therefore, it is recommended that Yohimbe be taken only under strict medical supervision.

Warning: Yohimbe should not be used by women, especially pregnant or breastfeeding women. It is also contraindicated in patients with liver or kidney disease, posttraumatic stress disorder, high blood pressure, panic disorder, or Parkinson's disease. The herb should not be taken with naltrexone, blood pressure medication, alcohol, or morphine. Patients should check with their doctor before taking Yohimbe with any OTC product.

HERB/DRUG INTERACTIONS

Shown below is a selection of common herbal remedies known to interact with conventional medications. Following the name of each herb is a list of the specific pharmaceutical categories with which it results.

This table is not all-inclusive. For further information on any herb of interest, please consult *PDR® for Herbal Medicines™*, a compendium of information on more than 700 medicinal herbs.

Adonis
(Adonis vernalis)
Calcium Increases action of Adonis
Digoxin Increases action of Adonis
Glucocorticoids Increases action of Adonis
Laxatives Increases action of Adonis
Quinidine Increases action of Adonis
Saluretics Increases action of Adonis

Aloe
(Aloe vera)
Antiarrhythmics Aloe-induced hypokalemia may affect cardiac rhythm
Cardiac Glycosides Increases effect of cardiac glycosides
Corticosteroids Increased potassium loss
Licorice Increased potassium loss
Thiazide Diuretics Increased potassium loss

Alpine Cranberry
(Vaccinium vitis-idaea)
Medication and Food that Increase Uric Acid Levels Decreases effect of Alpine Cranberry

Arnica
(Arnica montana)
Anticoagulant drugs, unspecified Coumarin component in Arnica may increase anticoagulant effect
Warfarin Sodium Additive anticoagulant effect

Astragalus
(Astragalus species)
Anticoagulant drugs, unspecified Astragalus may potentiate anticoagulant effects
Immunosuppressants Decreased effectiveness of immunosuppressive effect due to immunostimulant effect of Astragalus

Belladonna
(Atropa belladonna)
Amantadine Hydrochloride Increases anti-cholinergic effect of herb
Quinidine Increases anticholinergic effect of herb
Tricyclic Antidepressants Increases anti-cholinergic effect of herb

Bilberry
(Vaccinium myrtillus)
Salicylates Increases prothrombin time; caution should be observed when used concurrently
Warfarin Sodium Increases prothrombin time; caution should be observed when used concurrently

Bladderwrack
(Fucus vesiculosus)
Hypoglycemic Drugs Herb may have an additive hypoglycemic effect when with other hypoglycemic drugs

Brewer's Yeast
(Saccharomyces cerevisiae)
MAO Inhibitors Increase in blood pressure

Buckthorn
(Rhamnus catharticus)
Antiarrhythmics Increased effect due to potassium loss with chronic use of herb
Cardiac Glycosides Increased effect due to potassium loss with chronic use of herb
Corticosteroids Increases hypokalemic effects
Digoxin Herb may cause hypokalemia, which may increase digoxin toxicity
Licorice Root Increases hypokalemic effects
Thiazide Diuretics Increases hypokalemic effects

Bugleweed
(Lycopus virginicus)
Diagnostic Procedures Using Radioactive
Herb interferes with these isotopes
Thyroid Preparations Effect not specified

Cascara Sagrada
(Rhamnus purshiana)
Antiarrhythmics Potentiates arrhythmias with prolonged use of Cascara
Cardiac Glycosides Increased effect due to potassium loss with chronic use of herb

Corticosteroids Increases hypokalemic effect
Digoxin Herb may cause hypokalemia, which may increase digoxin toxicity
Indomethacin Decreases therapeutic effect of Cascara
Thiazide Diuretics Increases hypokalemic effect

Castor Oil Plant
(Ricinus communis)
Cardioactive Steroids Increased effect due to potassium loss with chronic use of herb

Cayenne
(Capsicum annuum)
Aspirin Decreased bioavailability of aspirin

Chaste Tree
(Vitex agnus-castus)
Dopamine Antagonists Decreased dopaminergic effect of herb

Chinese Rhubarb
(Rheum palmatum)
Cardiac Glycosides Increased effect due to potassium loss with chronic use of herb
Digoxin Herb may cause hypokalemia, which may increase digoxin toxicity

Coffee
(Coffea arabica)
Drugs, unspecified Herb can hinder (or decrease) resorption of other drugs

Digitalis
(Digitalis purpurea)
Methylxanthines Increases risk of cardiac arrhythmias
Phosphodiesterase Inhibitors Increases risk of cardiac arrhythmias
Quinidine Increases risk of cardiac arrhythmias
Sympathomimetic Agents Increases risk of cardiac arrhythmias

Echinacea Angustifolia
(Echinacea angustifolia)
Corticosteroids Echinacea may potentially interfere with the anti-cancer chemotherapeutic effect of corticosteroids
Immunosuppressants The immune-stimulating effect of Echinacea may interfere with drugs that have immunosuppressant effects

Evening Primrose
(Oenothera biennis)
Anticonvulsants Evening Primrose oil may lower seizure threshold and decrease effectiveness of anticonvulsant medications

Fenugreek
(Trigonella foenum-graecum)
Hypoglycemic Drugs Herb may have an additive hypoglycemic effect when taken with other hypoglycemic drugs

Feverfew
(Tanacetum parthenium)
Aspirin Increased antithrombotic effect
Warfarin Sodium Increased antithrombotic effect

Flax
(Linum usitatissimum)
Drugs, unspecified Absorption of other drugs may be delayed when taken simultaneously

Frangula
(Rhamnus frangula)
Cardiac Glycosides Increased effect due to potassium loss with chronic use of herb
Digoxin Herb may cause hypokalemia, which may increase digoxin toxicity

German Chamomile
(Matricaria recutita)
Alcohol May increase sedative effect
Benzodiazepines May increase sedative effect
Warfarin Sodium Hydroxycoumarin component in Chamomile may elevate prothrombin times

Ginkgo
(Ginkgo biloba)
Antithrombolytic Drugs Increases effect of antithrombolytic drugs

Ginseng
(Panax ginseng)
Hypoglycemic Drugs Increases hypoglycemic effect

Loop Diuretics Increases diuretic resistance
MAO Inhibitors Combination increases chance for headache, tremors, mania

Goat's Rue
(Galega officinalis)
Hypoglycemic Drugs Herb may have an additive hypoglycemic effect when taken with other hypoglycemic drugs

Green Tea
(Camellia sinensis)
Alkaline Drugs Decreased absorption of alkaline drugs due to tannin component in tea

Guarana
(Paullinia cupana)
Cardiac Glycosides Increased effect due to potassium loss with chronic use of herb
Digoxin Herb may cause hypokalemia, which may increase digoxin toxicity

Henbane
(Hyoscyamus niger)
Amantadine Hydrochloride Increased anticholinergic action
Antihistamines Increased anticholinergic action
Phenothiazines Increased anticholinergic action
Procainamide Increased anticholinergic action
Quinidine Increased anticholinergic action
Tricyclic Antidepressants Increased anticholinergic action

Horse Chestnut
(Aesculus hippocastanum)
Anticoagulant drugs, unspecified Horse Chestnut has a coumarin component and may interact with warfarin, salicylates, and other drugs with anticoagulant properties

Indian Squill
(Urginea indica)
Methylxanthines Can increase the risk of cardiac arrhythmias when given simultaneously with this herb
Phosphodiesterase Inhibitors Can increase the risk of cardiac arrhythmias when given simultaneously with this herb
Quinidine Can increase the risk of cardiac arrhythmias when given simultaneously with this herb
Sympathomimetic Agents Can increase the risk of cardiac arrhythmias when given simultaneously with this herb

Jimson Weed
(Datura stramonium)
Anticholinergics Co-administration of Jimson Weed with other anticholinergic drugs may increase the frequency and/or severity of anticholinergic side effects such as dry mouth, constipation, drowsiness, and others

Kombe Seed
(Strophanthus hispidus)
Calcium Salts Increases effects and side effects of herb
Diuretics Increases effects and side effects of herb
Glucocorticoids Increases effects and side effects of herb
Laxatives Increases effects and side effects of herb
Quinidine Increases effects and side effects of herb

Licorice
(Glycyrrhiza glabra)
Antiarrhythmics Licorice-induced hypokalemia increases risk of arrhythmias
Digitalis Glycoside Preparations Licorice-induced hypokalemia increases risk of digitalis toxicity
Glucocorticoids Licorice potentiates effect of glucocorticoids
Loop Diuretics Additive effect of hypokalemia
Thiazide Diuretics Additive effect of hypokalemia

Lily-of-the-Valley
(Convallaria majalis)
Calcium Increases the effect of Lily-of-the-Valley
Digoxin Increases the effect of Lily-of-the-Valley
Glucocorticoids Increases the effect of Lily-of-the-Valley
Laxatives Increases the effect of Lily-of-the-Valley
Quinidine Increases the effect of Lily-of-the-Valley
Saluretics Increases the effect of Lily-of-the-Valley

Ma-Huang
(Ephedra sinica)
Cardiac Glycosides Disturbance of heart rhythm
Central Nervous System Stimulants Ma-Huang has an additive effect on the CNS when combined with CNS stimulants
Guanethidine Increased sympathomimetic effects
Halothane Disturbance of heart rhythm

MAO Inhibitors Increases sympathomimetic effects of ephedrine

Oxytocin Development of high blood pressure

Milk Thistle
(Silybum marianum)

Haloperidol Silymarin in combination with haloperidol causes a decrease in lipid peroxidation

Phenothiazines Silymarin in combination with phenothiazines causes a decrease in lipid peroxidation

Phentolamine Mesylate Silymarin antagonizes the effect of phentolamine

Yohimbine Hydrochloride Silymarin antagonizes the effect of yohimbine

Niauli
(Melaleucea viridiflora)

Drugs, unspecified Co-administration may result in decreased effect of drugs that undergo liver metabolism

Oak
(Quercus robur)

Alkaline Drugs Absorption of alkaline drugs may be reduced or inhibited

Alkaloids Absorption of alkaloids may be reduced or inhibited

Oleander
(Nerium oleander)

Calcium Salts Increased efficacy and side effects when given simultaneously with herb

Glucocorticoids Increased efficacy and side effects when given simultaneously with herb

Laxatives Increased efficacy and side effects when given simultaneously with herb

Quinidine Increased efficacy and side effects when given simultaneously with herb

Saluretics Increased efficacy and side effects when given simultaneously with herb

Papaya
(Carica papaya)

Warfarin Sodium Increased INR levels

Psyllium
(Plantago ovata)

Drugs, unspecified Absorption of other drugs may be decreased if taken simultaneously with herb

Insulin Effect unspecified; insulin dose should be decreased

Psyllium Seed
(Plantago afra)

Drugs, unspecified Absorption of other drugs may be decreased if taken simultaneously with herb

Quinine
(Cinchona pubescens)

Drugs that Cause Thrombocytopenia Herb increases risk of thrombocytopenia

Rauwolfia
(Rauwolfia serpentina)

Alcohol Increases impairment of motor skills

Barbiturates Synergistic effect

Digitalis Glycoside Preparations Severe bradycardia when used in combination with digitalis glycosides

Levodopa Decreased effect; increases in extrapyramidal symptoms

Neuroleptics Synergistic effect

Sympathomimetic Agents Increases blood pressure

Saw Palmetto
(Serenoa repens)

Alpha Adrenergic Blockers Saw Palmetto has an additive alpha adrenergic blocking effect when given in combination with alpha blockers

Androgens Saw Palmetto antagonizes the effect of androgens

Scopolia
(Scopolia carniolica)

Amantadine Hydrochloride Increased effect when given simultaneously with herb

Quinidine Increased effect when given simultaneously with herb

Tricyclic Antidepressants Increased effect when given simultaneously with herb

Scotch Broom
(Cytisus scoparius)

MAO Inhibitors Increased risk of hypertensive crisis

Senna
(Cassia senna)

Antiarrhythmics Senna-induced hypokalemia may increase risk of arrhythmia

Digitalis Glycoside Preparations Senna-induced hypokalemia may increase toxicity of digitalis preparations

Estrogen Senna decreases estrogen levels when taken with estrogen supplements

Indomethacin Decreased therapeutic effect of Senna

Nifedipine Inhibits activity of Senna via calcium channel blockade

Squill
(Urginea maritima)

Calcium Increases effectiveness and side effects of herb

Digoxin Squill potentiates the positive inotropic and negative chronopic effects of digoxin

Glucocorticoids Increases effectiveness and side effects of herb

Laxatives Increases effectiveness and side effects of herb

Methylxanthines Increases risk of cardiac arrhythmias

Phosphodiesterase Inhibitors Increases risk of cardiac arrhythmias

Quinidine Increases risk of cardiac arrhythmias; increases effectiveness and side effects of herb

Saluretics Increases effectiveness and side effects of herb

Sympathomimetic Agents Increases risk of cardiac arrhythmias

St. John's Wort
(Hypericum perforatum)

Cyclosporine The herb induces the cytochrome P450 enzyme system and will lower cyclosporine serum levels

Digoxin Co-administration of the herb with digoxin has resulted in a significant decrease in the digoxin area under the curve

Indinavir Sulfate The herb induces the cytochrome P450 enzyme system and will lower indinavir serum levels

Oral Contraceptives Breakthrough bleeding has been reported with concomitant use of the herb with oral contraceptives

Photosensitizing Agents An additive photosensitizing effect is expected when the herb is used with photosensitizing drugs such as tetracyclines, sulfonamides, and thiazides

Reserpine Hypericum antagonizes the effect of reserpine

Selective Serotonin Reuptake Inhibitors Concomitant use with the herb will result in an additive serotonin effect and possible toxicity

Sympathomimetic Agents St. John's Wort may have MAO inhibitor properties and caution should be used with sympathomimetic agents

Theophylline The herb induces the cytochrome P450 enzyme system and will lower theophylline serum levels

Strophanthus
(Strophanthus kombe)
Calcium Salts Simultaneous administration with herb enhance both effects and side effects
Glucocorticoids Simultaneous administration with herb enhance both effects and side effects
Laxatives Simultaneous administration with herb enhance both effects and side effects
Quinidine Simultaneous administration with herb enhance both effects and side effects
Saluretics Simultaneous administration with herb enhance both effects and side effects

Uva-Ursi
(Arctostaphylos uva-ursi)
Loop Diuretics The sodium-sparing effect of Uva-Ursi may antagonize the diuretic effect of the loop diuretics
Medication and Food that Increase Uric Acid Levels Decreases effect of herb
Nonsteroidal Anti-Inflammatory Drugs Uva-Ursi may potentiate the gastrointestinal irritation caused by NSAIDs
Thiazide Diuretics The sodium-sparing effect of Uva-Ursi may antagonize the diuretic effect of thiazide diuretics

Urinary Tract Acidifiers Drugs or foods that acidify the urine will decrease the antibacterial effect of Uva-Ursi

Uzara
(Xysmalobium undulatum)
Digoxin Herb contains cardiac glycosides and may have additive effect when taken with digoxin, possibly increasing digoxin toxicity

Valerian
(Valeriana officinalis)
Alcohol Additive depressive effects with Valerian
Hypnotics Additive effect when taken with Valerian

White Willow
(Salix species)
Alcohol Enhances toxicity of salicylates
Antiplatelet Drugs Additive effect with salicylates
Barbiturates Enhances toxicity of salicylates
Carbonic Anhydrase Inhibitors Potentiates action of salicylates
Nonsteroidal Anti-Inflammatory Drugs Use with caution; effect not specified
Salicylates Use with caution; effect not specified

Wild Yam
(Dioscorea villosa)
Estrogen Additive effect
Indomethacin Wild Yam may decrease the anti-inflammatory effect of indomethacin

Wormwood
(Artemisia absinthium)
Phenothiazines Wormwood preparations should not be administered with drugs known to lower the seizure threshold
Trazodone Hydrochloride Wormwood preparations should not be administered with drugs known to lower the seizure threshold
Tricyclic Antidepressants Wormwood preparations should not be administered with drugs known to lower the seizure threshold

Yohimbe Bark
(Pausinystalia yohimbe)
Antihypertensive agents, unspecified May need to adjust antihypertensive medications due to hypertensive effect of Yohimbe
Ethanol Increased anxiogenic effects
Morphine Sulfate Potentiates effects of morphine
Naltrexone Hydrochloride Potentiates Yohimbe side effects
OTC stimulants Potentiates hypertensive effect